Clinical Veterinary Medicine

Clinical Veterinary Medicine

Editor: Mel Roth

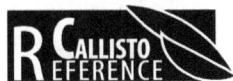

R CALLISTO REFERENCE

www.callistoreference.com

Callisto Reference,
118-35 Queens Blvd., Suite 400,
Forest Hills, NY 11375, USA

Visit us on the World Wide Web at:
www.callistoreference.com

ISBN: 978-1-63239-847-5 (Hardback)

Cataloging-in-publication Data

Clinical veterinary medicine / edited by Mel Roth.
   p. cm.
Includes bibliographical references and index.
ISBN 978-1-63239-847-5
   1. Veterinary medicine. 2. Animals--Diseases--Control. 3. Veterinary therapeutics. I. Roth, Mel.
SF745 .C55 2017
636.089--dc23

Table of Contents

Preface

The branch of medicine that deals with the causes, diagnosis and treatment of diseases and injuries of animals is called veterinary medicine. There has been rapid progress in this field and its applications are finding their way across multiple industries. It aims to cover a wide range of topics that are essential in understanding the field of clinical veterinary medicine. This book will also provide interesting topics for research which readers can take up. Different approaches, evaluations, methodologies and advanced studies in this field have been included in this book. For all those who are interested in veterinary sciences and medicine the case studies included in this book will serve as excellent guide to develop a comprehensive understanding.

This book is a result of research of several months to collate the most relevant data in the field.

When I was approached with the idea of this book and the proposal to edit it, I was overwhelmed. It gave me an opportunity to reach out to all those who share a common interest with me in this field. I had 3 main parameters for editing this text:

1. Accuracy – The data and information provided in this book should be up-to-date and valuable to the readers.

2. Structure – The data must be presented in a structured format for easy understanding and better grasping of the readers.

3. Universal Approach – This book not only targets students but also experts and innovators in the field, thus my aim was to present topics which are of use to all.

Thus, it took me a couple of months to finish the editing of this book.

I would like to make a special mention of my publisher who considered me worthy of this opportunity and also supported me throughout the editing process. I would also like to thank the editing team at the back-end who extended their help whenever required.

Editor

Deep 16S rRNA Pyrosequencing Reveals a Bacterial Community Associated with Banana *Fusarium* Wilt Disease Suppression Induced by Bio-Organic Fertilizer Application

Zongzhuan Shen[1], **Dongsheng Wang[3]**, **Yunze Ruan[2]**, **Chao Xue[1]**, **Jian Zhang[1]**, **Rong Li[1]**, **Qirong Shen[1]***

1 National Engineering Research Center for Organic-based Fertilizers, Key Laboratory of Plant Nutrition and Fertilization in Low-Middle Reaches of the Yangtze River, Ministry of Agriculture, Jiangsu Key Lab and Engineering Center for Solid Organic Waste Utilization, Jiangsu Collaborative Innovation Center for Solid Organic Waste Resource Utilization, Nanjing Agricultural University, Nanjing, China, **2** Hainan key Laboratory for Sustainable Utilization of Tropical Bio-resources, College of Agriculture, Hainan University, Haikou, China, **3** Nanjing Institute of Vegetable Science, Nanjing, China

Abstract

Our previous work demonstrated that application of a bio-organic fertilizer (BIO) to a banana mono-culture orchard with serious *Fusarium* wilt disease effectively decreased the number of soil *Fusarium* sp. and controlled the soil-borne disease. Because bacteria are an abundant and diverse group of soil organisms that responds to soil health, deep 16 S rRNA pyrosequencing was employed to characterize the composition of the bacterial community to investigate how it responded to BIO or the application of other common composts and to explore the potential correlation between bacterial community, BIO application and *Fusarium* wilt disease suppression. After basal quality control, 137,646 sequences and 9,388 operational taxonomic units (OTUs) were obtained from the 15 soil samples. *Proteobacteria*, *Acidobacteria*, *Bacteroidetes*, *Gemmatimonadetes* and *Actinobacteria* were the most frequent phyla and comprised up to 75.3% of the total sequences. Compared to the other soil samples, BIO-treated soil revealed higher abundances of *Gemmatimonadetes* and *Acidobacteria*, while *Bacteroidetes* were found in lower abundance. Meanwhile, on genus level, higher abundances compared to other treatments were observed for *Gemmatimonas* and *Gp4*. Correlation and redundancy analysis showed that the abundance of *Gemmatimonas* and *Sphingomonas* and the soil total nitrogen and ammonium nitrogen content were higher after BIO application, and they were all positively correlated with disease suppression. Cumulatively, the reduced *Fusarium* wilt disease incidence that was seen after BIO was applied for 1-year might be attributed to the general suppression based on a shift within the bacteria soil community, including specific enrichment of *Gemmatimonas* and *Sphingomonas*.

Editor: Gabriele Berg, Graz University of Technology (TU Graz), Austria

Funding: This work was supported by the National Natural Science Foundation of China (41101231 and 31372142), Natural Science Foundation of Hainan province (313045), the Priority Academic Program Development of Jiangsu Higher Education Institutions (PAPD), 111 project (B12009), the Agricultural Ministry of China (201103004), the Innovative Research Team Development Plan of the Ministry of Education of China (IRT1256), the China Postdoctoral Science Foundation (2011M501248 and 2012T50479), and the (KJ2011007) and The Central Financial Support to the Central and Western Nniversities to Specially Enhance the Comprehensive Strength (ZDZX2013023). The funders had no role in study design, data collection and analysis, decision to publish, or preparation of the manuscript.

Competing Interests: The authors have declared that no competing interests exist.

* E-mail: shenqirong@njau.edu.cn

⑨ These authors contributed equally to this work.

Introduction

Banana *Fusarium* wilt disease, which is caused by *Fusarium oxysporum* f. sp. *cubense* race 4 (FOC) and reported to be the most limiting factor in banana production worldwide, has spread quickly in *Cavendish*-production areas since 1996, and it affects approximately 90% of the banana industry in China [1–3]. Among the managements for controlling the disease, such as crop rotation, biocontrol, application of chemical fungicides and cropping of resistant banana cultivars [4–8], biocontrol is the most promising technique for disease prevention because of owning the advantages of environmental protection, safety, high economic benefits and longevity at the same time [9]. However, direct inoculation of functional microorganisms into the soil without a suitable organic substrate cannot be expected to be successful due to the absence of nutrients [10]. Many reports have demonstrated that biocontrol agents combined with organic materials to create novel bio-organic fertilizers (BIOs) can enhance the suppression of *Fusarium* wilt disease in the soil by ameliorating the structure of the microbial community [11–14].

The composition of the soil microbial community and induced changes caused by its amendment, provide useful information on soil health and quality [15]. Maintaining biodiversity of soil microbes is crucial to soil health because a decrease in soil microbial diversity is responsible for the development of soil-borne diseases [16]. Determining the responses of soil bacterial communities to different organic amendments is particularly important because the bacterial community is one of the main components that determine soil health and is believed to be one of the main drivers in disease suppression [17]. Despite the known key roles of bacteria in soil health and the significant change in soil bacterial composition and activity after BIO application, information regarding the variation of soil bacterial communities that are affected by different organic amendments is still lacking. More importantly, understanding soil microbial community structure shifts following implementation of various organic amendments is an important component when selecting fertilizer types to improve soil function and health.

As described in our previous work, *Fusarium* wilt disease was more effectively controlled by a 1-year application of BIO than by the other composts in a field experiment [12]. In that study, the effects of different types of composts on soil bacterial communities were mainly assessed using traditional PCR-DGGE fingerprinting and culture-dependent methods. Taking into account the large size of the bacterial community and the heterogeneity of the soils, only a tiny fraction of the bacterial diversity was unraveled by that study. Recently, pyrosequencing of 16 S rRNA gene fragments has been applied for in-depth analysis of soil bacterial communities [18,19]. This method could provide a large number of parallel reads to characterize the unseen majority of the soil microbial community and offer an opportunity to achieve a high throughput and deeper insight into the effects of different types of composts on soil bacterial communities [20], thus it is an improvement over previous fingerprinting techniques, such as PCR-DGGE or T-RFLP, which are not entirely specific and do not result in many sequences [15].

We used a deep 16 S rRNA pyrosequencing approach to further investigate how the soil bacteria community responded to the application of BIO or other common composts and to explore the potential correlation between bacterial community, BIO application and *Fusarium* wilt disease suppression. This study was the first to provide information on the banana soil bacterial community in a single soil type that was exposed to different organic amendments using deep 16 S rRNA pyrosequencing. Therefore, the aims of this study were to answer the following questions: (1) Does the soil bacteria community that is amended with BIO differ from that exposed to other common composts? (2) Does the *Fusarium* wilt disease incidence correlate with the bacterial community? (3) Does the disease suppression after BIO application correlate with the physicochemical properties of the soil?

Materials and Methods

Ethics statement

Our study was carried out on the farmers' land (18°23′ N, 108°44′ E) with property rights in China (1996-2035) and farmer Yusheng Li should be contacted for future permissions. No specific permits were required for the described field studies and the locations are not protected. The field studied did not involve endangered or protected species.

Field experiment

Five treatments were established as randomized, complete block designs with three replicates at the "Wan Zhong" banana orchard in Hainan, China and included a general operation control (GCK) and soil that was amended with four different types of organic amendments: bio-organic fertilizer (BIO), cattle manure compost (CM), Chinese medicine residue compost (CMR) and pig manure compost (PM). And each replicate was planted with 170 banana tissue culture plantlets (*Musa acuminate* AAA *Cavendish* cv. Brazil) with an area of 667 m^2. Worthy to notify, the bio-organic fertilizer

(BIO) contained a biocontrol agent *Bacillus* sp. and was prepared by a solid fermentation method according to Chen et al. [21]. The orchard has been continuously cropped banana for more than 10 years and was abandoned by farmers to growing banana for high *Fusarium* wilt disease incidence (50%). The detailed information regarding the field experiment setting and amendments were described in our previous report [12].

Soil sample collection and DNA extraction

The soil sample collection and DNA extraction methods were described in detail as supplementary information to our previous study [12]. Five individual, healthy banana trees that were at least 5 m apart in each treatment plot were randomly selected for sample collection, and the collected soil samples from each tree were mixed as a composite soil sample for each replicate plot. For each tree, composite soil from 4 random sites of the trunk base was collected using a 25-mm soil auger at a depth of 20 cm. All soil samples were transported to the laboratory and stored at −70°C for subsequent DNA extraction after sifting through a 2-mm sieve. Total soil DNA was extracted using PowerSoil DNA Isolation Kits (MoBio Laboratories Inc., Carlsbad, USA) according to the manufacturer's protocol. The concentration and quality (ratio of A260/A280) of the DNA were determined using a spectrophotometer (NanoDrop 2000, ThermoScientific, USA).

Polymerase chain reaction amplification and deep 16 S rRNA pyrosequencing

PCR reactions for each sample were performed in triplicate (including two negative control reactions) with 2 μM of each primer, 0.25 μM of dNTPs, 4 μL of 5 × FastPfu Buffer, 1 U of FastPfu DNA polymerase (2.5 U/μL, TransGen Biotech Co., Ltd., Beijing, China) and approximately 20 ng of soil DNA template at a final volume of 20 μL. The forward primer consisted of the 25-bp 454 adapter A, 2-bp linker A and 15-bp universal bacterial primer 27F [22], and the reverse primer consisted of the 25-bp 454 adapter B, 2-bp linker B, a 10-bp barcode and the 19-bp universal bacterial primer 533R [23]. Detailed information regarding the primer sequence is shown in Table S1. These primers target an approximately 500-bp region of the 16 S rRNA gene that contains variable regions 1 to 3 (V1–V3), which is well-suited for accurate phylogenetic placement of bacterial sequences [24].

Amplifications were performed using an Eppendorf Mastercycler thermocycler (Eppendorf North America, Hauppauge, NY) with the following temperature program: an initial denaturation step of 95°C for 4 min, followed by 25 cycles of denaturation at 95°C for 30 s, annealing at 55°C for 30 s, extension at 72°C for 30 s and a final elongation at 72°C for 5 min. PCR amplicon libraries were purified from a 1.2% agarose gel and quantified using the PicoGreen dsDNA reagent (Promega, USA). Equal amplicons from each sample were then pooled in equimolar concentrations into a single aliquot. After cleaning, precipitating, and re-suspending the amplicons in nuclease-free water, an emPCR was carried out to attach the single strands onto beads for further 454 pyrosequenicng. Pyrosequencing was performed on a Roche 454 GS-FLX Titanium System at Majorbio Biopharm Technology Co., Ltd (Shanghai, China).

Bioinformatic analysis

After pyrosequencing, raw sequences were analyzed using the Mothur software following the Schloss standard operating procedure [25]. Briefly, sequences with a minimum flow length of 450 flows were denoised using the Mothur-based reimplementation of the PyroNoise algorithm with the default parameters [26]. Sequences with more than 1 mismatch to the barcode, 2 mismatches to the primer, any ambiguous base call, homopolymers longer than 8 bases and reads shorter than 250 bp were eliminated, and the filtered sequences were then trimmed and assigned to soil samples based on unique 10-base barcodes. After removing the barcode and primer sequences, the unique sequences were aligned against the Silva bacteria database [27]. After screening, filtering, preclustering, and chimera removal, the retained sequences were used to build a distance matrix with a distance threshold of 0.2. Using the average neighbor algorithm with a cut-off of 97% similarity, bacterial sequences were clustered to operational taxonomic units (OTU), and the representative sequence for each OTU was picked and classified using a Ribosomal Database Project naive Bayesian rRNA classifier with a confidence threshold of 80% [28]. Lastly, the resulting matches for each set of sequence data were summarized at various levels of taxonomic hierarchal structure (e.g., phylum and genera). All raw sequences have been deposited in DDBJ SRA under the accession number DRA001282.

To correct for sampling effects, we used a randomly selected subset of 7,817 sequences per sample to further analyze the richness and diversity of the bacterial community. All analyses were based on the OTU clusters with a cut-off of 3% dissimilarity. The richness index of the Chao1 estimator (Chao1) [29] and the abundance-based Coverage estimator (ACE) [30] was calculated to estimate the number of observed OTUs that were present in the sampling assemblage. The diversity within each individual sample was estimated using the nonparametric Shannon diversity index [31]. Good's nonparametric Coverage estimator was used to estimate the percentage of the total species that were sequenced in each sample [32], and a rarefaction curve generated using the Mothur software was used to compare the relative levels of bacterial OTU diversity across all soil samples.

To compare bacterial community structures across all samples, a heat map based on the abundant phyla were performed in R (Version 3.0.2) with the gplots package [33,34], and principal coordinates analysis (PCoA) based on the OTU composition was performed using the Mothur software. To examine the relationship between the frequencies of abundant phyla, samples and environmental variables, redundancy analysis (RDA) was carried out using CANOCO for Windows [35].

Statistical analysis

The relationships between the selected taxonomy group (abundant phyla or genera) or bacterial community indices (Chao1, ACE and Shannon) and *Fusarium* wilt disease incidence (DI) were calculated using the SPSS 13.0 software program. For all parameters, data were compared using a one-way analysis of variance (ANOVA) at the end of each bioassay. Mean comparison was performed using Fisher's least significant difference test (LSD) and the Duncan multiple range test with a significance level of $p < 0.05$.

Results

After filtering the reads based on basal quality control, 137,646 sequences with an average length of 254 bases were obtained from 15 soil samples when using Mothur flowgrams strategy to analyze sequences. The number of high-quality sequences per sample varied from 7,817 to 11,234 (Table 1). Based on 97% species similarity, in total 9,388 OTUs were found, and 12,845 sequences (9.3% of the total sequences) were returned as unclassified.

Table 1. Good quality sequences that were used to further analysis after basic quality control for treatments: bio-organic fertilizer (BIO), cattle manure compost (CM), Chinese medicine residue compost (CMR), general operation control (GCK) and pig manure compost (PM).

Treatments	Good quality sequences
BIO1	9,382
BIO2	9,666
BIO3	7,817
CM1	9,937
CM2	8,521
CM3	8,459
CMR1	8,736
CMR2	9,280
CMR3	8,614
GCK1	8,192
GCK2	8,473
GCK3	11,234
PM1	8,695
PM2	11,185
PM3	9,455
Total	137,646

Bacterial community composition

As shown in Fig. 1, although the phyla compositions of the different soil samples were similar, some obvious variations in the relative abundances of phyla between different fertilizer treatments were still observed. The classified sequences for each sample were affiliated with 19 bacterial phyla, and the remaining sequences were unclassified. The most abundant phyla of *Proteobacteria*, *Acidobacteria* and *Bacteroidetes* were found in all treatments at a relative abundance of approximately 35%, 15% and 10%, respectively, and 9 phyla (*Actinobacteria*, *Gemmatimonadetes*, *Nitrospirae*, *Firmicutes*, *Chloroflexi*, *Verrucomicrobia*, *TM7*, *Armatimonadetes* and *Planctomycetes*) were found in all samples at a relative abundance of higher than 1%, but lower than 6%, with some obvious variations. The relative abundances of *Acidobacteria* and *Gemmatimonadetes* were highest, while those of *Bacteroidetes* were lowest, in the BIO-treated soil sample compared with the other treatments (CM, CMR, GCK and PM).

The most abundant classified genera (>1%) for each treatment are shown in Table 2, which shows 12, 16, 14, 12 and 15 most frequently classified genera for the BIO, CM, CMR, GCK and PM treatments, respectively. Among the most frequent genera, only 10, including *Gemmatimonas*, *Gp1*, *Gp4*, *Gp6*, *Burkholderia*, *Gp3*, *Nitrospira*, *Ohtaekwangia*, *TM7_genus_incertae_sedis* and *3_genus_incertae_sedis* were represented in all treatments. Moreover, in comparison to other treatments, significantly higher abundances of the genera *Gemmatimonas* and *Gp4* were observed in BIO-treated soil among the most 10 abundant genera.

Bacterial α-diversity

The bacterial richness and diversity of the different fertilizer treatments were calculated based on 7,817 randomly selected sequences (Table 3). The richness index, Chao1 and ACE showed that the CM-treated soil exhibited the lowest number of OTUs,

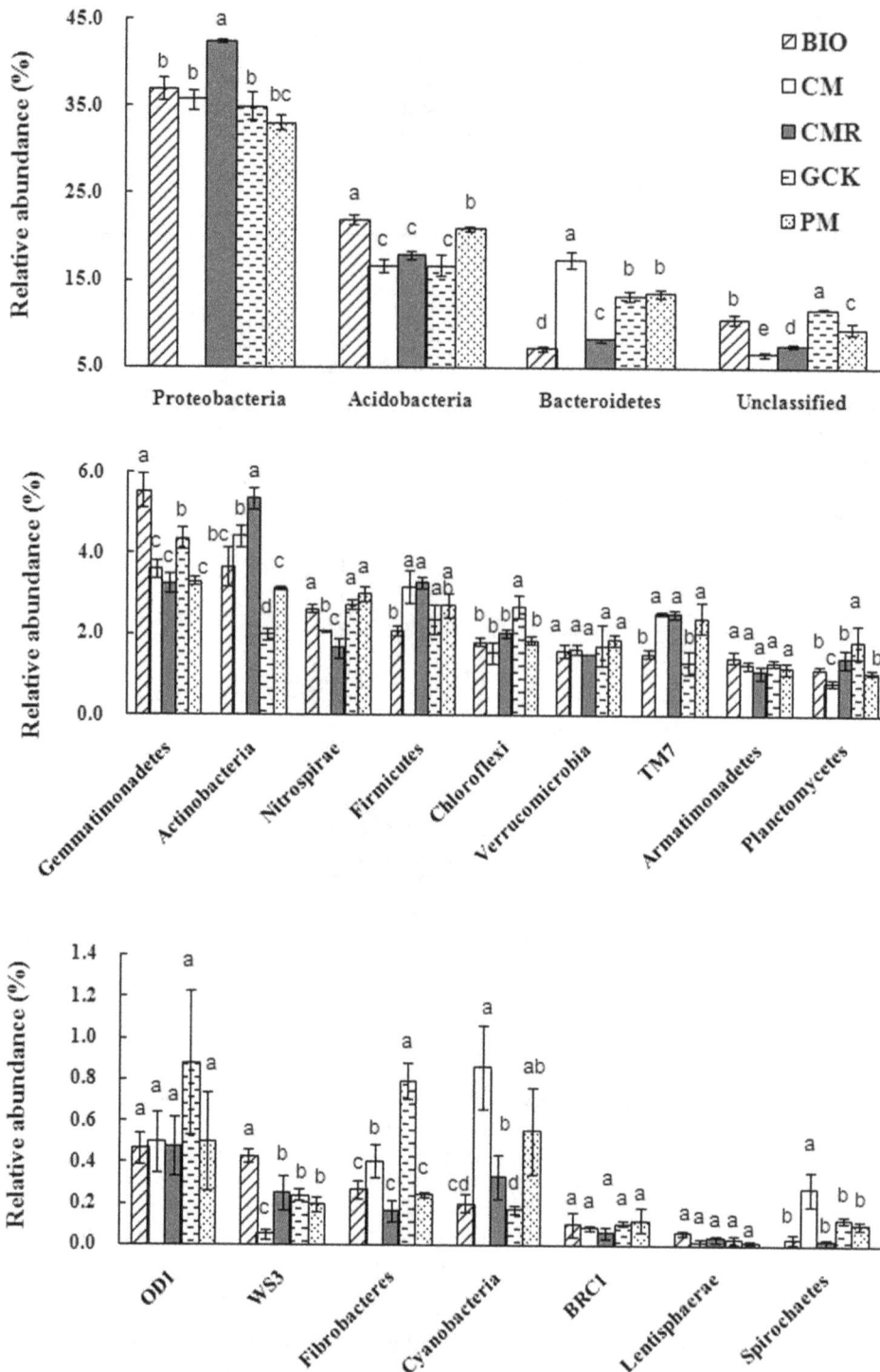

Figure 1. The relative abundance of the phyla for treatments with bio-organic fertilizer (BIO), cattle manure compost (CM), Chinese medicine residue compost (CMR), general operation control (GCK) and pig manure compost (PM). Bars represent the standard error of the three replicates and different letters above each phylum indicate significantly difference at 0.05 probability level according to the Duncan test.

while the BIO-treated soil showed the highest number with no significant difference between the CMR, PM and GCK treatments. The CM treatment had the lowest Shannon diversity index value (H'), while the highest values were of the GCK and PM treatments. CM treatment showed the highest Good's query

Coverage (ranging from 0.87 to 0.90 for all treatments), and no significant difference was observed for the other treatments.

Similar results were observed with 3% dissimilarity after comparing the rarefaction curves of the mean pooled sequences of 3 replicates of each treatment, with the GCK treatment showing the highest OTU number and CM treatment showing the lowest

Deep 16S rRNA Pyrosequencing Reveals a Bacterial Community Associated with Banana Fusarium Wilt...

5

Table 2. Frequency of the most abundant bacterial genera, indicated in % of all classified sequences, within each treatment of bio-organic fertilizer (BIO), cattle manure compost (CM), Chinese medicine residue compost (CMR), general operation control (GCK) and pig manure compost (PM).

%	BIO	CM	CMR	GCK	PM	Phylum
Gemmatimonas	5.56±0.42a	3.62±0.22c	3.27±0.25c	4.38±0.25b	3.33±0.10c	*Gemmatimonadetes*
Gp1	5.49±0.31c	6.54±0.17b	7.07±0.39a	2.43±0.07d	6.59±0.75b	*Acidobacteria*
Gp4	4.62±0.27a	2.15±0.08d	2.19±0.35d	3.55±0.46b	2.72±0.14c	*Acidobacteria*
Gp6	4.49±0.19a	1.49±0.07c	2.38±0.16b	5.31±1.07a	2.73±0.60b	*Acidobacteria*
Burkholderia	3.76±1.00d	8.68±0.77b	10.79±2.02a	1.46±0.43e	6.51±1.90c	*Proteobacteria*
Gp3	2.90±0.19a	2.84±0.45a	2.10±0.23b	2.35±0.68a	2.77±0.10a	*Acidobacteria*
Nitrospira	2.64±0.10b	2.07±0.01c	1.66±0.23d	2.73±0.12b	3.01±0.17a	*Nitrospirae*
Ohtaekwangia	1.70±0.19d	2.18±0.13c	1.32±0.06e	3.31±0.11a	2.83±0.16b	*Bacteroidetes*
TM7_genus_incertae_sedis	1.55±0.09b	2.54±0.04a	2.52±0.11a	1.33±0.30b	2.44±0.38a	*TM7*
3_genus_incertae_sedis	1.07±0.19a	1.13±0.12a	1.11±0.07a	1.17±0.42a	1.39±0.10a	*Verrucomicrobia*
Sphingomonas	1.71±0.49a	1.10±0.05b	1.47±0.05a			*Proteobacteria*
Gp5	1.17±0.12a			1.12±0.12a	1.12±0.17a	*Acidobacteria*
Bacillus		1.67±0.11a	1.78±0.06a		1.44±0.12b	*Firmicutes*
Niastella		2.96±0.23a			1.55±0.20b	*Bacteroidetes*
Gp2		1.48±0.19b	1.09±0.05c		1.68±0.05a	*Acidobacteria*
Beggiatoa				1.46±0.16		*Proteobacteria*
Gp13					1.49±0.06	*Acidobacteria*
Segetibacter		1.87±0.12				*Bacteroidetes*
Chitinophaga		1.36±0.04				*Bacteroidetes*
Frateuria			1.06±0.13			*Proteobacteria*

Only the genera frequency higher than 1% was listed in the table. Values are the means followed by standard error of the mean. Different letters indicate statistically significant differences at the 0.05 probability level according to Fisher's least significant difference test (LSD) and the Duncan test.

OTU number, However, the rarefaction curves did not reach saturation, which indicated that more sequencing efforts were needed (Fig. 2).

Bacterial community structure

The analysis of microbial communities using hierarchical cluster analysis showed that the bacterial communities from the same treatment were more similar to each other than those from different treatments, as observed for the 5 highly supported clusters that were made up of samples from different fertilizer-treated soils (Fig. 3). Bacterial community structure from soil samples that were amended with common composts (CM, CMR, and PM) clustered together while soil samples from BIO and GCK were clustered together based on weighted UniFrac algorithm (Fig. 3a). Bacterial community membership from soil samples that were amended with organic amendments (CM, CMR, PM and BIO) clustered together and were separated to general operation control (GCK) based on unweighted UniFrac algorithm (Fig. 3b). Moreover, BIO-treated soil grouped separately from common compost treatments (CM, CMR and PM), which were grouped together.

Heat map analysis of the abundant phyla within a hierarchical cluster based on Bray–Curtis distance indices showed different patterns of community structure among the different treatments

Table 3. Calculations of Chao1, ACE, Shannon and Good's Coverage indices for treatments with bio-organic fertilizer (BIO), cattle manure compost (CM), Chinese medicine residue compost (CMR), general operation control (GCK) and pig manure compost (PM) at a 97% similarity threshold.

Treatments	Chao1	ACE	Shannon	Coverage
BIO	3,751±220a	5,398±292a	6.60±0.04b	0.87±0.01b
CM	3,105±75b	4,085±91b	6.38±0.05c	0.90±0.01a
CMR	3,477±174a	4,904±216ab	6.46±0.03c	0.88±0.01b
GCK	3,588±173a	5,112±395a	6.76±0.05a	0.88±0.01b
PM	3,724±236a	5,573±108a	6.70±0.04a	0.88±0.01b

Values indicate the means followed by standard error of the mean. Different letters indicate statistically significant differences at the 0.05 probability level according to Fisher's least significant difference test (LSD) and the Duncan test.

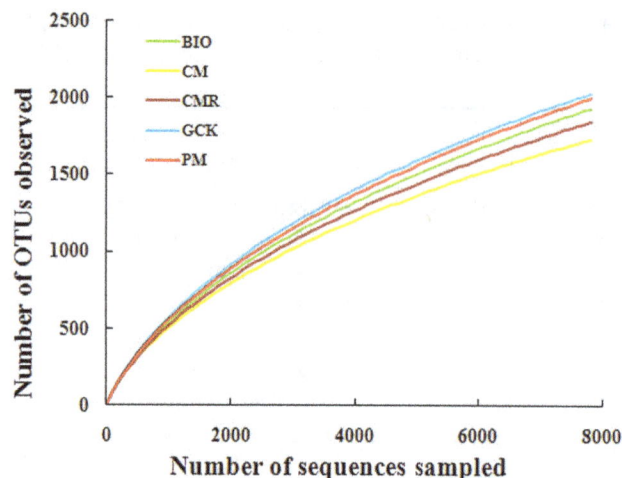

Figure 2. Rarefaction analysis at different 3% dissimilarity levels for treatments with bio-organic fertilizer (BIO), cattle manure compost (CM), Chinese medicine residue compost (CMR), general operation control (GCK) and pig manure compost (PM).

and similar patterns for the same treatment in triplicate (Fig. 4a). Moreover, BIO treatment showed a different pattern of community structure from those of other soil samples and enriched phyla of *Acidobacteria*, *Gemmatimonadetes*, *WS3* and *Lentisphaerae*, as shown in blue. Principal coordinates analysis (PCoA) based on the OTU composition also clearly showed variations among these different fertilizer treatments (Fig. 4b). The first two principal components could explain 83.1% of the variation of the individual samples of the total bacterial community. The bacterial community of the BIO-treated soil was well-separated from that of common compost-treated soils (CM, PM and CMR) along the first component (PCoA1) and was separated from the general control (GCK) along the second component (PCoA2).

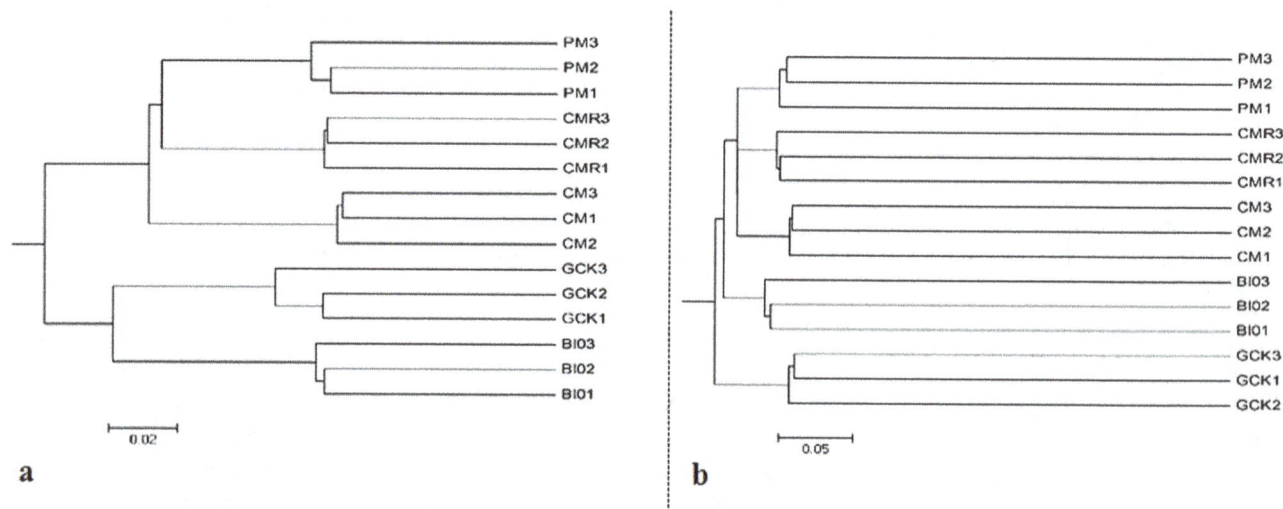

Relationship between disease incidence and the selected parameters

According to the disease incidence reported in our previous paper [12] and based on line regression analysis, a significant correlation between the abundance of the *Gemmatimonadetes*, *Bacteroidetes*, *Lentisphaerae* and *SR1* phyla and *Fusarium* wilt disease incidence was found (Table S2). Among these phyla, *Lentisphaerae* and *SR1* were not considered further due to their low abundance and random distribution. A clear negative correlation between *Gemmatimonadetes* (r = −0.579, p = 0.024) and the disease incidence and a clear positive correlation between *Bacteroidetes* (r = 0.600, p = 0.018) and the disease incidence were observed (Fig. 5a).

Line regression analysis between the 20 most-abundant classified genera and disease incidence showed that *Gemmatimonas*, *Ohtaekwangia* and *Sphingomonas* were significantly correlated to disease incidence (Table S3). A strong negative correlation between disease incidence and *Gemmatimonas* (r = −0.579, p = 0.024) and *Sphingomonas* (r = −0.689, p = 0.005) and a positive correlation with *Ohtaekwangia* (r = 0.764, p = 0.001) were observed (Fig. 5b). Unfortunately, some classified genera that were generally considered to contain plant growth-promoting rhizobacteria (PGPR) strains, which can suppress soil-borne fungi or promote plant growth, were only present in limited amounts, and their presence was not correlated with disease incidence (Table S4). Furthermore, in our research, no significant correlation was found between the whole bacteria community indices (richness and diversity) and disease incidence (Table S5).

The RDA that was performed on the phyla data and soil chemical properties showed that the first two RDA components could explain 88.6% of the total variation (Fig. 6). The first component (RDA1) separated the BIO and CMR treatments from the other fertilizer treatments and explained 61.1% of the variation, and the second component (RDA2), which separated the BIO from the CMR treatment, explained 27.5% of the variation. All soil chemical properties sufficiently explained the variation in phyla data (p = 0.002, Monte Carlo test). Ammonium nitrogen (NH_4-N) and electricity conductivity (EC) accounted for a large amount of the variation in the distribution of the BIO treatment from other treatments along the RDA1 and RDA2 axes.

a

b

Figure 3. Hierarchical cluster tree constructed based on the distance matrix that was calculated using the (a) weighted UniFrac algorithm and (b) unweighted UniFrac algorithm for treatments with bio-organic fertilizer (BIO), cattle manure compost (CM), Chinese medicine residue compost (CMR), general operation control (GCK) and pig manure compost (PM).

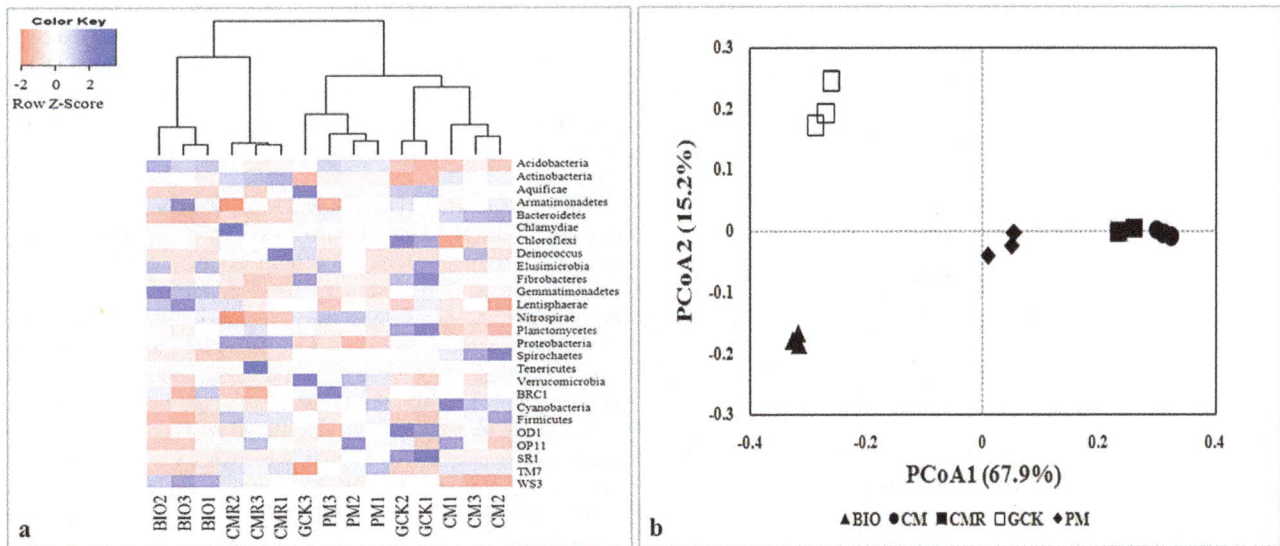

Figure 4. Heat map of the bacterial communities based on abundance of phyla (a) and Jackknifed principal coordination analysis (PCoA) plots with unweighted UniFrac distance metric (b) from treatments with bio-organic fertilizer (BIO), cattle manure compost (CM), Chinese medicine residue compost (CMR), general operation control (GCK) and pig manure compost (PM). Color from pink to blue indicates increasing abundance.

As shown by their close grouping and by the vectors, BIO-treated soil with the lowest disease incidence was positively related to the higher relative abundant phyla of *Gemmatimonadetes* and *Lentisphaerae*, the higher content of NH4-N and the EC, and it was negatively related to *Bacteroidetes*, a higher content of soil nitrate nitrogen (NO3-N) and higher total carbon to nitrogen ratio (C/N). Furthermore, the relative abundance of *Gemmatimonadetes* was positively correlated with soil pH, EC and NH4-N contents and negatively correlated with the soil total carbon (TOC) and C/N ratio. Moreover, the relative abundance of *Lentisphaerae* was

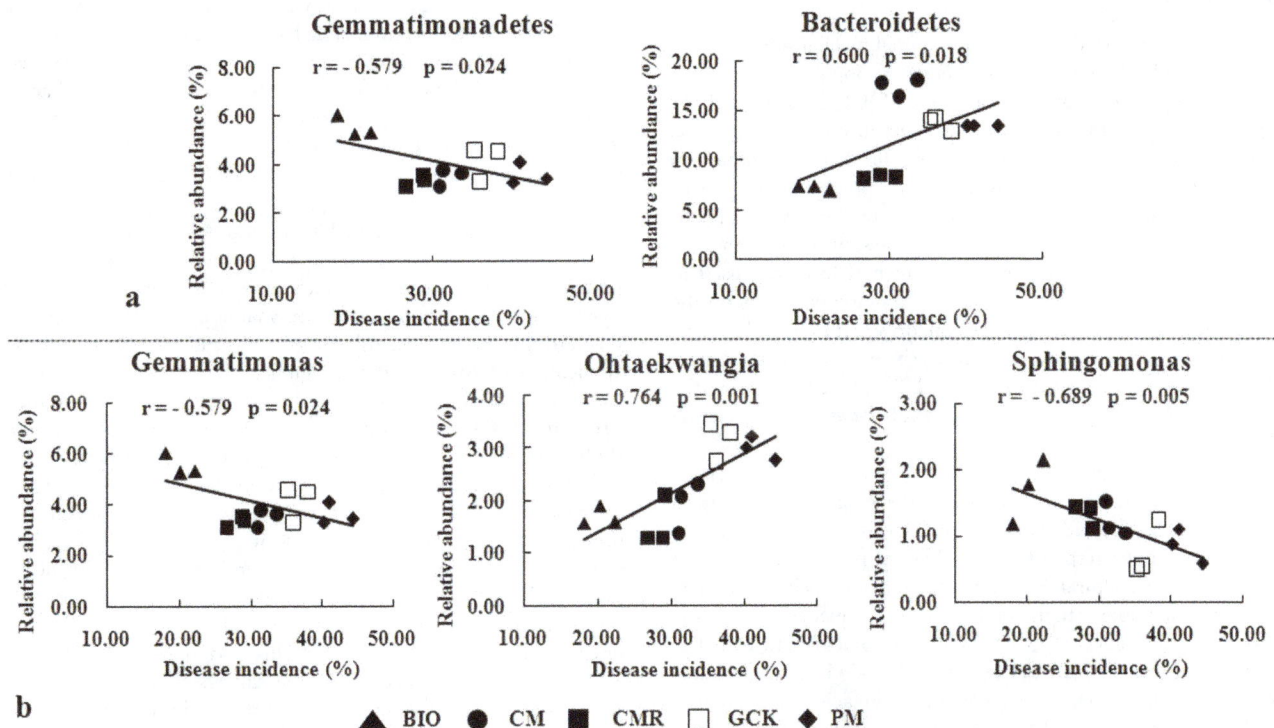

Figure 5. Correlation analysis between the relative abundance of two bacteria phyla (a), three of the most classified bacteria genera (b) and banana *Fusarium* wilt disease incidence for treatments with bio-organic fertilizer (BIO), cattle manure compost (CM), Chinese medicine residue compost (CMR), general operation control (GCK) and pig manure compost (PM).

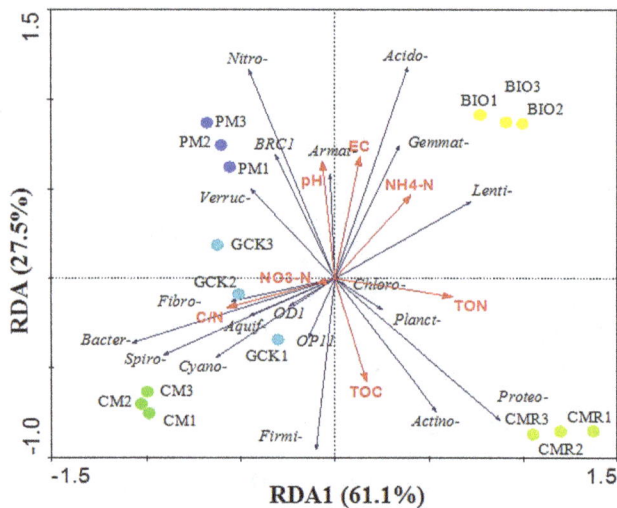

Figure 6. Redundancy analysis (RDA) of the abundant phyla and soil properties for soil samples from treatments with bio-organic fertilizer (BIO), cattle manure compost (CM), Chinese medicine residue compost (CMR), general operation control (GCK) and pig manure compost (PM).

positively correlated with the total nitrogen (TON) and NH4-N contents of the soil and negatively correlated with the soil C/N ratio. In contrast, the relative abundance of *Bacteroidetes* was positively correlated with the soil C/N ratio and negatively correlated with the soil TON and NH4-N contents (Fig. 6 and Table S6).

Discussion

In our previous study, the main potential mechanism by which the BIO application reduced the *Fusarium* population has been revealed by culture-depended and PCR-DGGE methods [12]. However, deeper research should be done to further explore the potential mechanism. To our knowledge, this detailed comparison of the soil bacteria community after the application of BIO or other common composts in a banana orchard with serious *Fusarium* wilt disease was the first to be assessed using deep 16 S rRNA pyrosequencing, although this method has been used to study the long-term effects of selected, common composts on the soil bacteria community composition or structure [15,36]. The obtained results supported the hypothesis that soil amended with different organic materials showed different responses by the bacterial community or suppression of *Fusarium* wilt disease [15,37–39].

Phyla analysis revealed that *Proteobacteria, Acidobacteria, Bacteroidetes, Gemmatimonadetes, Actinobacteria* and *Firmicutes* were the most common phyla, but with some variety in relative abundance. This finding roughly corresponded with those of previous articles that investigated agricultural or other type soils in which these phyla accounted for more than 74.0% of the sequences that were examined using deep 16 S rRNA pyrosequencing [18,19]. The relative abundance of *Acidobacteria* was relatively high in our study due to the experiment being conducted in acidic soil [40,41]. However, in our study, BIO and PM treatments with the higher pH showed the higher relative abundance of *Acidobacteria*. This finding was contrary to a previous study that showed that pH had a negative relation to *Acidobacteria* abundance [40,42]. The reason for this phenomenon is still unclear and may be due to the narrow

pH value range of the treated soil; however, a few articles have shown no obvious correlation between pH and abundance of *Acidobacteria* [15,36]. Analysis of the most abundant genera (>1%) also revealed significant differences between the bacterial communities of different treatments, a higher abundance of *Gemmatimonas* and *Gp4* in BIO-treated soil compared to other soil samples.

These changes could correspond to the decline of *Fusarium* wilt disease incidence. Thus, further correlation analysis was performed. Interestingly, the results showed that *Fusarium* wilt disease incidence might be related to the *Gemmatimonadetes* and *Bacteroidetes* phyla and/or *Gemmatimonas* genus, which belongs to *Gemmatimonadetes*, *Ohtaekwangia*, which belongs to *Bacteroidetes*, and *Sphingomonas*, which belongs to *Proteobacteria*. The high abundance of the *Bacteroidetes* phylum and the *Ohtaekwangia* genus that was observed in this study might positively correspond to *Fusarium* wilt disease incidence because this finding is in accordance with the report that the relative abundance of *Bacteroidetes* was similar between the initial and disease stages and followed by a significant decrease when suppressiveness was reached, as investigated using a 16 S rRNA-based microarray method [43], although, *Bacteroidetes* was also reported to possess the potential ability for biocontrol [44]. Moreover, we found the *Gemmatimonadetes* phylum and *Gemmatimonas* and *Sphingomonas* genera might respond to the suppression of *Fusarium* wilt disease via BIO application. *Gemmatimonas* and *Gemmatimonadetes* are a recently proposed genus and phylum, respectively, and they widely exist in multiple terrestrial and aquatic habitats. However, little is known about the ecological functions of this genus/phylum, except that Yin et al. [45] reported that the *Gemmatimonas* genus was found at a higher frequency in the rhizosphere of healthy plants using 454 pyrosequencing. *Sphingomonas*, which belongs to the *Sphingomonadaceae* order and *Proteobacteria* phylum, is widely distributed in natural habitats and is utilized for a wide range of biotechnological applications due to its remarkable biodegradative and biosynthetic capabilities [46]. Kyselková et al. [44] reported that bacteria affiliated with *Sphingomonadaceae* were more prevalent in tobacco-suppressive rhizosphere soil. Wachowska et al. [47] also reported that *Sphingomonas* could be used as biological agents to control winter wheat pathogens, such as *Fusarium*, under greenhouse conditions.

Analysis using rarefaction, Chao1 and ACE showed that the OTU numbers for BIO treatment were not significantly higher than for the other treatments. Furthermore, the diversity for BIO treatment that was estimated by the Shannon index and Coverage was also not the highest. All of the results indicated that a 1-year application of BIO could not significantly increase the bacteria community richness and diversity at the whole-community-structure level, which was in accordance with results of a previous study that used pyrosequencing to show that soil bacterial community richness and diversity were similar after a 5-year application of different organic amendments [15]. Although many previous articles indicated that the richness and/or diversity of the soil microbial community may respond to disease incidence [12,38], this phenomenon was not observed in this study because no obvious correlation between the indices and *Fusarium* wilt disease was observed (Table S5). This may be due to all 1-year treatments being performed on the same soil, which possessed similar bacteria community indices at the beginning.

In our study, the results of phylogenetic structure analyzed using the hierarchical cluster tree, heat map analysis based on the phyla frequency and PCoA analysis based on the OTU composition all showed that the bacterial community of BIO-treated soil differed from the common compost treatments (CM, CMR, and PM) and the control (GCK). All of the results confirmed that BIO application altered the bacterial community, which was roughly similar to the results of our previous investigation using PCR-DGGE that showed that BIO-treated soil grouped away from other soil samples [12]. Poulsen et al. [15] also reported similar results suggesting that soil amended with MSW-compost was separate from other amendments or the control, which indicated that the soil bacterial community responds differently to different compost amendments.

It has been reported that the chemical properties of soil can influence the suppressiveness of soil towards diseases [48]. In our RDA analysis, the BIO treatment with lowest *Fusarium* wilt disease incidence was highly correlated with the highest proportion of *Gemmatimonadetes* and lowest proportion of *Bacteroidetes*. Furthermore, the proportion of *Gemmatimonadetes* was positively correlated with soil pH, EC and NH4-N and negatively correlated with TOC and the C/N ratio. However, *Bacteroidetes* was positively correlated with the soil C/N ratio and negatively correlated with TON and NH4-N (Fig. 5, Table S6). Therefore, suppression of *Fusarium* wilt disease might be highly correlated with soil properties because *Fusarium* wilt disease incidence was positively correlated with the C/N ratio and negatively correlated to NH4-N and TON (Table S7), which was in agreement with reports from several previous studies. For example, Hamel et al. [49] reported a positive association between the TON content of the soil and the suppressiveness towards *Fusarium* spp. on asparagus. However, the form of N, either as NO3-N or NH4-N, is also important for disease suppression. Pérez-Piqueres et al. [50] reported that suppressive soil contained higher rates of NH4–N than conductive soil when studying the effect of compost amendment on soil suppressiveness toward *Rhizoctonia solani* disease, and Mallett and Maynard [51] reported that the incidence of *Armillaria* root disease significantly increased with decreasing NH4-N concentration on the organic surface horizon. In contrast, Oyarzun et al. [52] reported that the disease suppression ability of *Thielaviopsis basicola* was positively associated with a decreased C/N ratio.

In this study, after analyzing all of the data, the abundance of *Bacillus* was not enriched after BIO application. This finding combined with our previous results, the main mechanism reduced the *Fusarium* population for BIO application might be attributed to a general suppression that the BIO application altered the soil microbial composition and stimulated the population of soil bacteria, actinomycetes and some beneficial microorganisms [12], indicated that the genus might not necessarily reflect the individual species that has functional importance in suppressing endemic soil disease and all the results revealed by further deep 16S rRNA pyrosequencing confirmed that the main potential mechanism by which the BIO application reduced the *Fusarium* population was deduced to the fact that the specific bio-organic fertilizer containing functional microbes altered the soil microbial composition and stimulated the population of some beneficial microorganisms, thus resulting in a general suppression.

Conclusions

Deep 16 S rRNA pyrosequencing assessment of soil bacterial communities from different compost-treated soil in a monoculture banana orchard revealed significant differences among all treatments, including differences in community structure, composition, richness, diversity and bacterial phylogeny. Phyla of *Gemmatimonadetes* and *Acidobacteria* were significantly elevated in BIO treatment in comparison to other treatments. A decrease was also found for *Bacteroidetes* in BIO treatment. Moreover, genera of *Gemmatimonas* and *Gp4* were significantly elevated in BIO treatment

in comparison to other treatments. Additionally, the enrichment of *Gemmatimonas* and *Sphingomonas* and the TON and NH4-N soil content was positively correlated with disease suppression. Cumulatively, the reduction of the *Fusarium* wilt disease incidence after a 1-year application of BIO might be attributed to the fact that application of a BIO fertilizer containing *Bacillus* sp. induced general suppression in the soil by modulating the bacterial community and specific suppression by enriching *Gemmatimonas* and *Sphingomonas*.

Supporting Information

Table S1 Primer sequences used for preparation of samples for deep 16S rRNA pyrosequencing.

Table S2 Line regression coefficient of the most abundant phyla (>1%) and Fusarium wilt disease incidence. * in the table means correlation is significant at the 0.05 level, ** in the table means correlation is significant at the 0.01 level.

Table S3 Line regression coefficient of the most frequent classified genera (>1%) and Fusarium wilt disease incidence. * in the table means correlation is significant at the 0.05 level, ** in the table means correlation is significant at the 0.01 level.

Table S4   Line regression coefficient of selected bacteria genera and Fusarium wilt disease incidence. * in the table means correlation is significant at the 0.05 level, ** in the table means correlation is significant at the 0.01 level.

Table S5 Line regression coefficient of the bacteria community indices and Fusarium wilt disease incidence. * in the table means correlation is significant at the 0.05 level, ** in the table means correlation is significant at the 0.01 level.

Table S6 Line regression coefficient (r) between selected phyla in all samples and soil properties. * in the table means correlation is significant at the 0.05 level, ** in the table means correlation is significant at the 0.01 level.

Table S7 Line regression coefficient (r) between Fusarium wilt disease incidence in all samples and soil properties. * in the table means correlation is significant at the 0.05 level, ** in the table means correlation is significant at the 0.01 level.

Acknowledgments

We thank Majorbio Bio-pharm Biotech Company (Shanghai, China) for deep 16 S rRNA barcode pyrosequencing and Hainan Wanzhong Agriculture Company for huge help to us in banana planting.

Author Contributions

Conceived and designed the experiments: QS RL. Performed the experiments: ZS DW YR CX JZ. Analyzed the data: ZS DW YR. Contributed reagents/materials/analysis tools: CX JZ. Wrote the paper: ZS QS RL.

References

1. O'Donnell K, Kistler HC, Cigelnik E, Ploetz RC (1998) Multiple evolutionary origins of the fungus causing Panama disease of banana: concordant evidence from nuclear and mitochondrial gene genealogies. P Natl Acad Sci USA 95: 2044–2049.

2. Butler D (2013) Fungus threatens top banana. Nature 504: 195–196.

3. Chen YF, Chen W, Huang X, Hu X, Zhao JT, et al. (2013) Fusarium wilt-resistant lines of Brazil banana (*Musa* spp., AAA) obtained by EMS-induced mutation in a micro-cross-section cultural system. Plant Pathol 62: 112–119.

4. Getha K, Vikineswary S (2002) Antagonistic effects of *Streptomyces violaceusniger* strain G10 on *Fusarium oxysporum* f. sp. *cubense* race 4: Indirect evidence for the role of antibiosis in the antagonistic process. J Ind Microbiol Biot 28: 303–310.

5. Getha K, Vikineswary S, Wong W, Seki T, Ward A, et al. (2005) Evaluation of *Streptomyces* sp. strain g10 for suppression of *Fusarium* wilt and rhizosphere colonization in pot-grown banana plantlets. J Ind Microbiol Biot 32: 24–32.

6. Raguchander T, Jayashree K, Samiyappan R (1997) Management of Fusarium wilt of banana using antagonistic microorganisms. J Biol Control 11: 101–105.

7. Saravanan T, Muthusamy M, Marimuthu T (2003) Development of integrated approach to manage the fusarial wilt of banana. Crop Prot 22: 1117–1123.

8. Sivamani E, Gnanamanickam S (1988) Biological control of *Fusarium oxysporum* f. sp. *cubense* in banana by inoculation with *Pseudomonas fluorescens*. Plant Soil 107: 3–9.

9. Wang BB, Yuan J, Zhang J, Shen ZZ, Zhang MX, et al. (2012) Effects of novel bioorganic fertilizer produced by *Bacillus amyloliquefaciens* W19 on antagonism of *Fusarium* wilt of banana. Biol Fertil Soils 49: 435–446.

10. El-Hassan S, Gowen S (2006) Formulation and delivery of the bacterial antagonist *Bacillus subtilis* for management of lentil vascular wilt caused by *Fusarium oxysporum* f. sp. *lentis*. J Phytopathol 154: 148–155.

11. Kavino M, Harish S, Kumar N, Saravanakumar D, Samiyappan R (2010) Effect of chitinolytic PGPR on growth, yield and physiological attributes of banana (*Musa* spp.) under field conditions. Appl Soil Ecol 45: 71–77.

12. Shen ZZ, Zhong ST, Wang YG, Wang BB, Mei XL, et al. (2013) Induced soil microbial suppression of banana fusarium wilt disease using compost and biofertilizers to improve yield and quality. Eur J Soil Biol 57: 1–8.

13. Cotxarrera L, Trillas-Gay MI, Steinberg C, Alabouvette C (2002) Use of sewage sludge compost and *Trichoderma asperellum* isolates to suppress Fusarium wilt of tomato. Soil Biol Biochem 34: 467–476.

14. Zhao QY, Dong CX, Yang XM, Mei XL, Ran W, et al. (2011) Biocontrol of *Fusarium* wilt disease for *Cucumis melo* melon using bio-organic fertilizer. Appl Soil Ecol 47: 67–75.

15. Poulsen PHB, Al-Soud WA, Bergmark L, Magid J, Hansen LH, et al. (2013) Effects of fertilization with urban and agricultural organic wastes in a field trial-Prokaryotic diversity investigated by pyrosequencing. Soil Biol Biochem 57: 784–793.

16. Mazzola M (2004) Assessment and mangement of soil microbial community structre for disease suppression. Annu Rev Phytopathol 42: 35–59.

17. Garbeva P, Van VJ, Van EJ (2004) Microbial diversity in soil: selection of microbial populations by plant and soil type and implications for disease suppressiveness. Annu Rev Phytopathol 42: 243–270.

18. Acosta-Martinez V, Dowd S, Sun Y, Allen V (2008) Tag-encoded pyrosequencing analysis of bacterial diversity in a single soil type as affected by management and land use. Soil Biol Biochem 40: 2762–2770.

19. Roesch LF, Fulthorpe RR, Riva A, Casella G, Hadwin AK, et al. (2007) Pyrosequencing enumerates and contrasts soil microbial diversity. ISME J 1: 283–290.

20. Binladen J, Gilbert MTP, Bollback JP, Panitz F, Bendixen C, et al. (2007) The use of coded PCR primers enables high-throughput sequencing of multiple homolog amplification products by 454 parallel sequencing. PLoS One 2: e197.

21. Chen LH, Yang XM, Raza W, Luo J, Zhang FG, et al. (2011) Solid-state fermentation of agro-industrial wastes to produce bioorganic fertilizer for the biocontrol of *Fusarium* wilt of cucumber in continuously cropped soil. Bioresour Technol 102: 3900–3910.

22. Dethlefsen L, Huse S, Sogin ML, Relman DA (2008) The pervasive effects of an antibiotic on the human gut microbiota, as revealed by deep 16 S rRNA sequencing. PLoS Biol 6: e280.

23. Huse SM, Dethlefsen L, Huber JA, Welch DM, Relman DA, et al. (2008) Exploring microbial diversity and taxonomy using SSU rRNA hypervariable tag sequencing. PLoS Genet 4: e1000255.

24. Liu Z, Lozupone C, Hamady M, Bushman FD, Knight R (2007) Short pyrosequencing reads suffice for accurate microbial community analysis. Nucleic Acids Res 35: e120.

25. Schloss PD, Westcott SL, Ryabin T, Hall JR, Hartmann M, et al. (2009) Introducing mothur: open-source, platform-independent, community-supported software for describing and comparing microbial communities. Appl Environ Microb 75: 7537–7541.

26. Quince C, Lanzen A, Davenport RJ, Turnbaugh PJ (2011) Removing noise from pyrosequenced amplicons. BMC Bioinformatics 12: 38.

27. Pruesse E, Quast C, Knittel K, Fuchs BM, Ludwig W, et al. (2007) SILVA: a comprehensive online resource for quality checked and aligned ribosomal RNA sequence data compatible with ARB. Nucleic Acids Res 35: 7188–7196.

28. Wang Q, Garrity GM, Tiedje JM, Cole JR (2007) Naive Bayesian classifier for rapid assignment of rRNA sequences into the new bacterial taxonomy. Appl Environ Microb 73: 5261–5267.

29. Chao A (1984) Nonparametric estimation of the number of classes in a population. Scand J Stat 11: 265–270.

30. Eckburg PB, Bik EM, Bernstein CN, Purdom E, Dethlefsen L, et al. (2005) Diversity of the human intestinal microbial flora. Science 308: 1635–1638.

31. Washington H (1984) Diversity, biotic and similarity indices: a review with special relevance to aquatic ecosystems. Water Res 18: 653–694.

32. Bunge J, Fitzpatrick M (1993) Estimating the number of species: a review. J Am Stat Assoc 88: 364–373.

33. Warnes GR, Bolker B, Bonebakker L, Gentleman R, Huber W, et al. (2011) gplots: Various R programming tools for plotting data. R package version 2.

34. R Development Core Team (2012) R: A language and environment for statistical computing. Vienna, Austria, http://www.r-project.org.

35. Etten EV (2005) Multivariate analysis of ecological data using CANOCO. Austral Eco 30: 486–487.

36. Chaudhry V, Rehman A, Mishra A, Chauhan PS, Nautiyal CS (2012) Changes in bacterial community structure of agricultural land due to long-term organic and chemical amendments. Microbial Ecol 64: 450–460.

37. Bonanomi G, Antignani V, Pane C, Scala F (2007) Suppression of soilborne fungal diseases with organic amendments. J Plant Pathol 89: 311–324.

38. Qiu MH, Zhang RF, Xue C, Zhang SS, Li SQ, et al. (2012) Application of bio-organic fertilizer can control *Fusarium* wilt of cucumber plants by regulating microbial community of rhizosphere soil. Biol Fert Soils 48: 807–816.

39. Sun H, Deng S, Raun W (2004) Bacterial community structure and diversity in a century-old manure-treated agroecosystem. Appl Environ Microbiol 70: 5868–5874.

40. Lauber CL, Hamady M, Knight R, Fierer N (2009) Pyrosequencing-based assessment of soil pH as a predictor of soil bacterial community structure at the continental scale. Appl Environ Microb 75: 5111–5120.

41. Rousk J, Bååth E, Brookes PC, Lauber CL, Lozupone C, et al. (2010) Soil bacterial and fungal communities across a pH gradient in an arable soil. ISME J 4: 1340–1351.

42. Shen CC, Xiong JB, Zhang HY, Feng YZ, Lin XG, et al. (2012) Soil pH drives the spatial distribution of bacterial communities along elevation on Changbai Mountain. Soil Biol Biochem 57: 204–211.

43. Sanguin H, Sarniguet A, Gazengel K, Moënne-Loccoz Y, Grundmann G (2009) Rhizosphere bacterial communities associated with disease suppressiveness stages of take-all decline in wheat monoculture. New Phytol 184: 694–707.

44. Kyselková M, Kopecký J, Frapolli M, Défago G, Ságová-Marečková M, et al. (2009) Comparison of rhizobacterial community composition in soil suppressive or conducive to tobacco black root rot disease. ISME J 3: 1127–1138.

45. Yin C, Hulbert SH, Schroeder KL, Mavrodi O, Mavrodi D, et al. (2013) Role of bacterial communities in the natural suppression of *Rhizoctonia solani* bare patch of wheat (*Triticum aestivum* L.). Appl Environ Microb 79: 7428–7438.

46. Balkwill DL, Fredrickson JK, Romine MF (2006) Sphingomonas and related genera. In Dworkin M, Falkow S, Rosenberg E, Schleifer K, Stackebrandt E, editors. The Prokaryotes: Delta, Epsilon Subclass. Springer, New York. pp. 605–629.

47. Wachowska U, Irzykowski W, Jędryczka M, Stasiulewicz-Paluch AD, Głowacka K (2013) Biological control of winter wheat pathogens with the use of antagonistic *Sphingomonas* bacteria under greenhouse conditions. Biocontrol Sci Tech 23: 1110–1122.

48. Höper H, Alabouvette C (1996) Importance of physical and chemical soil properties in the suppressiveness of soils to plant diseases. Eur J Soil Biol 32: 41–58.

49. Hamel C, Vujanovic V, Jeannotte R, Nakano-Hylander A, St-Arnaud M (2005) Negative feedback on a perennial crop: Fusarium crown and root rot of asparagus is related to changes in soil microbial community structure. Plant Soil 268: 75–87.

50. Pérez-Piqueres A, Edel-Hermann V, Alabouvette C, Steinberg C (2006) Response of soil microbial communities to compost amendments. Soil Biol Biochem 38: 460–470.

51. Mallett K, Maynard D (1998) Armillaria root disease, stand characteristics, and soil properties in young lodgepole pine. Forest Eco Manag 105: 37–44.

52. Oyarzun P, Gerlagh M, Zadoks J (1998) Factors associated with soil receptivity to some fungal root rot pathogens of peas. Appl Soil Ecol 10: 151–169.

2

Livestock-Associated MRSA Carriage in Patients without Direct Contact with Livestock

Miranda M. L. van Rijen[1]*, Thijs Bosch[2], Erwin J. M. Verkade[1,3], Leo Schouls[2], Jan A. J. W. Kluytmans[1,4]* and on behalf of the CAM Study Group

1 Laboratory for Microbiology and Infection Control, Amphia Hospital, Breda, the Netherlands, 2 Center for Infectious Disease Control Netherlands, National Institute for Public Health and the Environment, Bilthoven, the Netherlands, 3 Laboratory for Medical Microbiology and Immunology, St. Elisabeth Hospital, Tilburg, the Netherlands, 4 Department of Medical Microbiology and Infection ControlJK, VUmc Medical University, Amsterdam, the Netherlands

Abstract

Background: Livestock-associated MRSA (MC398) has emerged and is related to an extensive reservoir in pigs and veal calves. Individuals with direct contact with these animals and their family members are known to have high MC398 carriage rates. Until now it was assumed that MC398 does not spread to individuals in the community without pig or veal calf exposure. To test this, we identified the proportion of MC398 in MRSA positive individuals without contact with pigs/veal calves or other known risk factors (MRSA of unknown origin; MUO).

Methods: In 17 participating hospitals, we determined during two years the occurrence of MC398 in individuals without direct contact with livestock and no other known risk factor (n = 271) and tested in a post analysis the hypothesis whether hospitals in pig-dense areas have higher proportions of MC398 of all MUO.

Results: Fifty-six individuals (20.7%) without animal contact carried MC398. In hospitals with high pig-densities in the adherence area, the proportion of MC398 of all MUO was higher than this proportion in hospitals without pigs in the surroundings.

Conclusions: One fifth of the individuals carrying MUO carried MC398. So, MC398 is found in individuals without contact to pigs or veal calves. The way of transmission from the animal reservoir to these individuals is unclear, probably by human-to-human transmission or by exposure to the surroundings of the stables. Further research is needed to investigate the way of transmission.

Editor: D. Ashley Robinson, University of Mississippi Medical Center, United States of America

Funding: This work was supported by The Netherlands Organisation for Health Research and Development [grant number 125020007]. ZonMw is a non-profit organisation working for the Ministry of Health, Welfare and Sport (VWS) and the Dutch Organisation for Scientific Research (NOW). ZonMw had no role in study design, data collection and analysis, decision to publish, or preparation of the manuscript. http://www.zonmw.nl/nl/

* Email: mvrijen@amphia.nl (MvR); jankluytmans@gmail.com (JK)

Introduction

Since 2003, the so-called livestock-associated MRSA (LA-MRSA) has emerged in animals and humans in areas with intensive animal farming in Europe, North America, and Asia [1]. Human carriage of LA-MRSA is strongly related to direct contact with pigs, veal calves and broilers [2,3]. The majority of these LA-MRSA strains belong to multilocus sequence type clonal complex 398 (CC398) [4]. After its emergence, the risk factor 'direct contact with living pigs, veal calves and broilers' was added to the Dutch national MRSA guideline and an active screening program in hospitals was implemented [5]. By the end of 2011, 39% of all newly identified MRSA strains in humans in the Netherlands belonged to this variant in the Netherlands [6].

Recent surveys showed that MRSA CC398 was 4 to 6-fold less transmissible than other MRSA strains in a hospital-setting [7–8]. At present, the human-to-human transmissibility of MRSA CC398 in a community setting is still unclear. Considering the extensive reservoir in animals and people who work with livestock, the occurrence of MRSA CC398 in people who are not directly involved in farming is strikingly low. So far, there are no indications that MRSA CC398 has spread extensively into the general population [9]. A cross-sectional survey in a livestock-dense region found that only 0.2% of adult individuals without livestock contact were positive for MRSA CC398 [10]. On the other hand, there are observations that proximity of farms is a potential risk factor, even in absence of direct contact between humans and animals [11–13]. In addition, in a recent exploratory study an association was found between consumption of poultry and MRSA carriage [14]. A spectrum of infections with MRSA CC398 have been documented, ranging from relatively minor or localized infections including abscesses [15–17] and various skin and soft tissue infections (SSTI) [18–20], urinary tract infections [16], wound infections [16], mastitis [4], and conjunctivitis [21], as

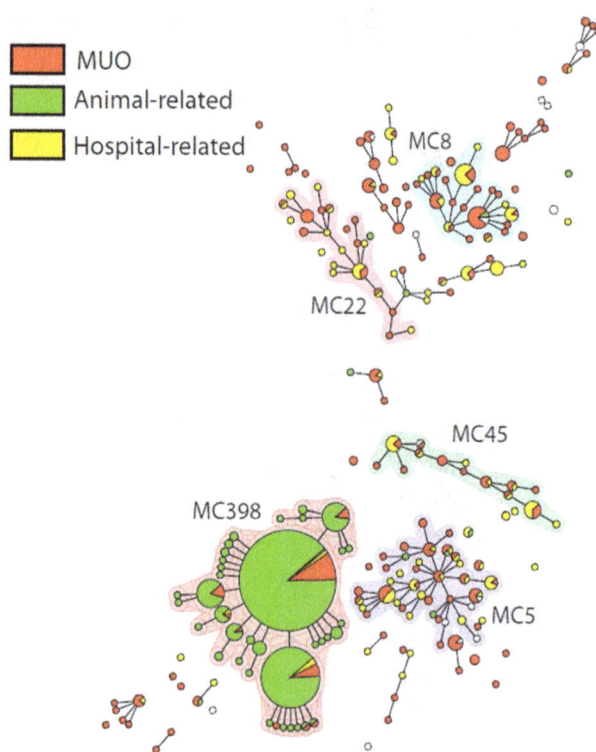

Figure 1. Genotypic relatedness of 1020 MRSA isolates represented as a minimum spanning tree based on MLVA types. Clustering of MLVA profiles was obtained using a categorical coefficient to create a minimum spanning tree in which the MLVA types are displayed as circles. The size of each circle indicates the number of isolates with this particular type. MLVA complexes (MC) are indicated in characters e.g. MC398 denotes MLVA complex 398.

well as more serious or invasive infections, including bacteremia [21–24], endocarditis [24,25], pneumonia (including necrotizing pneumonia, osteomyelitis, pyomyositis, and postoperative infections [26]. Despite the diverse array of infection types reported, it has been suggested that MRSA CC398 is less virulent than other human MRSA strains [27].

Apart from LA-MRSA and hospital-associated (HA)MRSA, MRSA rates also are rapidly increasing in community dwelling individuals without known healthcare- or livestock-associated risk factors. This third entity has been referred to as community-acquired (CA) MRSA [28] or MUO [29]. In this study, the proportion of CC398 in MUO isolates was determined. We hypothesized that people living in an area in which CC398 is common have more risk of MRSA CC398 carriage than persons living in an area in which CC398 is rare.

Methods

Ethics Statement

Ethical approval for the study was obtained by the medical ethics committee of the St. Elisabeth Hospital in Tilburg (NL 19489.008.07, protocol 0749, March 9th, 2009). Patient information was anonymized and de-identified prior to analysis.

MRSA source identification

To identify MRSA sources in the Netherlands, Infection Control Practitioners (ICP) from seventeen hospitals (three academic, seven teaching and seven general hospitals) throughout

the Netherlands were asked to complete a questionnaire on a website for all consecutive patients that were found to be MRSA positive (both infection and carriage) for the first time in the microbiological laboratory of the hospital from January 2009 until December 2010. Samples were taken during a visit to the outpatient's clinic or during a stay on a ward in the hospital. Patients who had already been found MRSA-positive in the past were not included. The questionnaire on the website contained data about patient type (in- or outpatient), demographics, positive body sites, molecular typing results and probable source of MRSA. The MRSA source was identified based on the patient's history combined with molecular typing results and then classified in risk groups described in the national infection prevention guidelines [5]. When neither of these risk groups was applicable, the MRSA was classified as 'MRSA of unknown origin (MUO)'.

Genotyping of MRSA isolates

All MRSA isolates were genotyped by multiple-locus variable number of tandem repeat analysis (MLVA) by the Dutch National Reference Center (RIVM, Bilthoven, the Netherlands) [30]. MLVA is known for its higher discriminatory power for LA-MRSA strains as compared to either multilocus sequence typing (MLST) or pulsed-field gel electrophoresis (PFGE) [30]. The MLVA profiles were clustered using a categorical clustering coefficient (unweighted-pair group method using arithmetic averages, UPGMA) and a minimum spanning tree was constructed to display the relationships between the various MLVA complexes (MC) and MRSA sources. For this study, we incorporated phiSa3 into the MLVA scheme. Furthermore, tetM was determined by use of DNA microarray (Identibac *S. aureus* Genotyping, Alere).

Data analysis

The percentage of MC398 in the group with individuals not reporting contact with pigs or veal calves was determined. We hypothesized that individuals without direct contact with pigs/veal calves living in a pig-dense area have more chance to become colonized with MC398 MUO than individuals living in areas without many pigs. Hospitals were divided into two categories: 1) Hospital with an adherence area with a high pig-density; 2) Hospital with an adherence area with a low pig-density. Municipality level data of the number of pigs were downloaded from the website of the Central Institute for Statistics (CBS) [31]. To test our hypothesis, the numbers of MC398 MUO positive individuals in these two categories were compared in a Chi-square test in a post analysis. To avoid bias by possible different screening policies of the 17 different hospitals, only MRSA infections were included in this analysis. In this way, unexpected findings in contract tracings were excluded.

Results

During 2009–2010, 1020 patients (368 inpatients and 652 outpatients) were found to be MRSA-positive in the seventeen participating hospitals. From 299 (29.3%) patients, MRSA-positive samples were obtained from body sites other than nose, throat, and perineum, mainly urine, sputum and wounds. Eight patients suffered from a bacteremia with MRSA (0.8%). In 39 patients (3.8%), MRSA was found in the perineum sample only, while other tested sites were found to be negative for MRSA.

MRSA source analysis is depicted in Table 1. MLVA typing of the strains showed that 649/1020 (63.6%) strains were MC398. Two-hundred and seventy one (26.6%) of all newly identified carriers were of unknown origin, and 56 (20.7%) of them were MC398. These 56 MC398 isolates were tetM positive and lacked

Legend

✚ Non-Academic Hospitals

✚ Academic Hospitals

Quartiles of Pig Density per Municipality

▢ Q1: 0.000 - 0.001

▢ Q2: 0.002 - 0.535

▢ Q3: 0.536 - 3.411

▢ Q4: 3.412 - 46.715

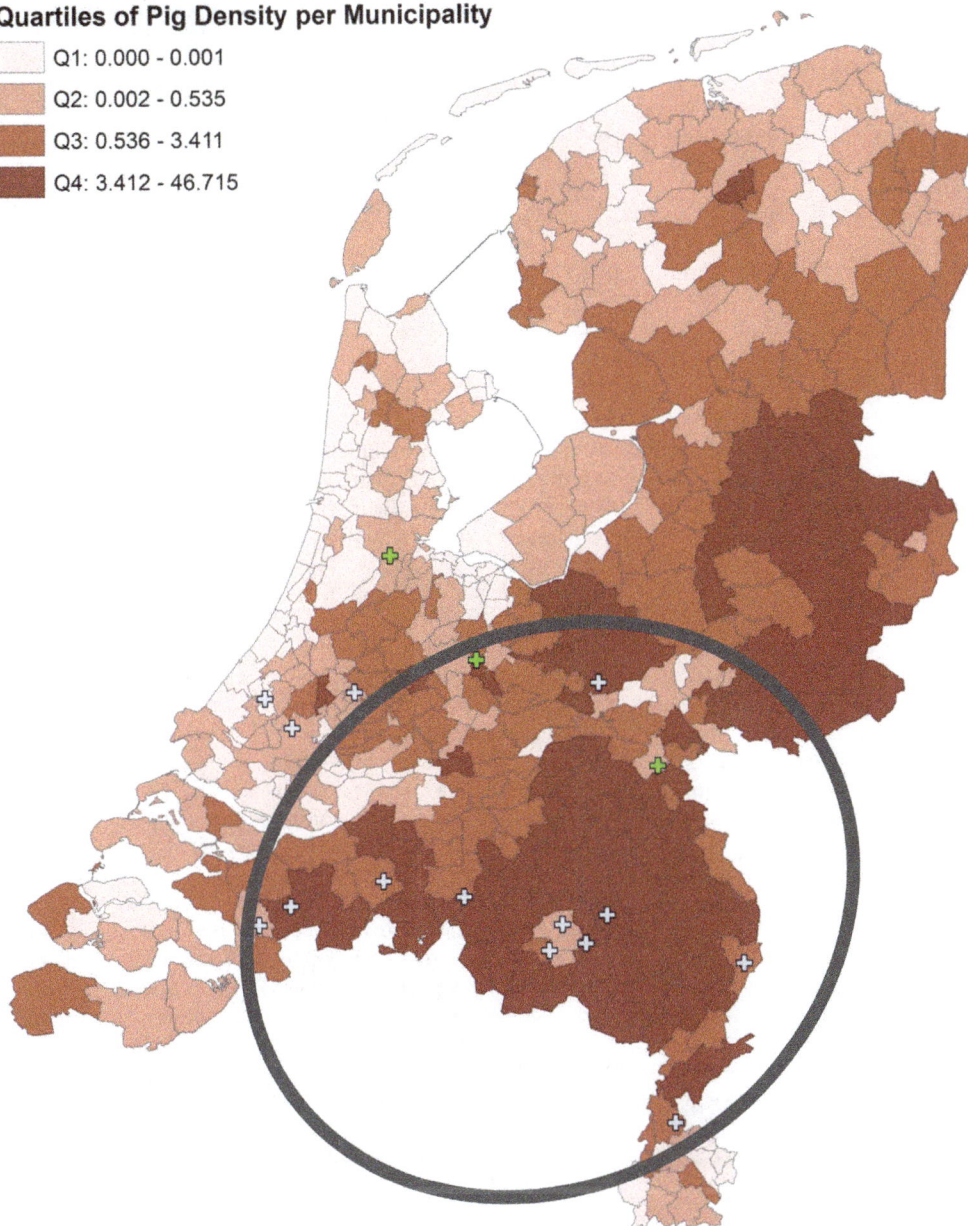

Figure 2. Pig-densities in the Netherlands. Hospitals with high pig-densities in the adherence areas are presented within the circle.

the prophage Sa3 (phiSa3). The mean risk to find a MC398 MUO in a participating hospital was estimated at 1 per 8 months (1 per 12 months for infections only). Thirty-five of the 56 (62.5%) individuals suffered from an infection. Figure 1 shows MUO, hospital- and animal-related MRSA and their MLVA complexes. MC398 MUO and MC398 of patients with animal contact cluster together. To test our hypothesis that individuals without animal contact have more chance to carry MC398 MRSA in pig-dense areas than in areas without many pigs, a Chi-square test was performed for hospitals with an adherence area with many pig farms compared to hospitals in an area without many pigs. Data of

all participating hospitals is shown in Table 2. Pig-densities in the Netherlands are shown in Figure 2. We found an indication that, in hospitals with high pig-densities in the adherence area, the proportion of MC398 infection of all MUO infection is higher than in hospitals without pigs in the surroundings (32/148 vs. 3/59; RR 4.25 95% CI 1.35–17.21, $P = 0.004$).

Discussion

The majority (n = 603, 59.1%) of newly identified MRSA-positive patients in 17 hospitals in 2009 and 2010 was related to

Table 1. MRSA sources in patients in 17 Dutch hospitals, 2009–2010.

Source	Total		MC398	
	N	% of total	n	% within source
Pigs/veal calves	603	59.1	587	97.3
Foreign hospital	75	7.4	3	4.0
Nosocomial transmission	44	4.3	3	6.8
Transmission in nursing home	5	0.5	0	0.0
Adoption children	18	1.8	0	0.0
Dialysis patients from foreign countries	2	0.2	0	0.0
Unknown origin (MUO)	271	26.6	56	20.7
No data	2	0.2		
Total	**1020**	**100**	**649**	**63.6**

exposure to livestock. A substantial proportion could not be classified to an established risk group (n = 271, 26.6%) and are therefore assumed to have acquired their MRSA in the community. One fifth (20.7%) of these MRSA strains belonged to MC398. The presence of the tetM resistance gene and the absence of the phiSa3 suggest that these isolates were animal-associated [22,32]. We found an indication that, in hospitals with high pig-density in the surroundings, the proportion of MC398 infection of all MUO infection was higher than in hospitals with a low pig-density in the surroundings. This indicates that LA-MRSA may be spreading through other sources than direct exposure to livestock. Until now it was assumed that LA-MRSA is able to spread to the pig/veal calf farmers and others who are in close contact with the animals, but is less able to spread from the farmer to household members who do not enter the stables, and is almost unable to spread to persons in the community without pig or veal calf exposure. Thus, it is assumed that constant pressure of LA-MRSA from animals with MRSA must be present to maintain the LA-MRSA colonization in humans. However, several recent studies have shown that persistent colonization with MC398 is possible [33–35]. Moreover, pig-, dairy cow-, and veal calf densities per municipality were also found to be independent risk factors for carriage of MRSA MC398 in two recently published case-control studies [11,14]. Although it cannot be excluded that human-to-human transmission occurs in areas with a high MRSA MC398 pressure, environmental contamination with MRSA MC398 may play a role as well. MRSA MC398 has been shown to be present in air and soil samples collected downwind of pig and swine barns [13]. Other transmission routes can play a role as well. For example, regular consumption of poultry was recently found to be associated with CA-MRSA transmission in an exploratory hospital-based case-control study [14]. De Boer et al. demonstrated that a substantial part of the meat products obtained from retail stores in the Netherlands were colonized with MRSA, including both MC398 and non-MC398 strain types [36]. However, meat consumption cannot explain the increased prevalence in people who live in pig-dense areas. We expect the risk, associated with meat consumption, to be the same for all areas over the country. Unless, locals consume more meat from their own area.

Limitations

We performed a post hoc analysis to study whether the proportion of MC398 MUO infection is higher in hospitals in pig-dense areas than in areas with a low pig-density. Our study was originally not designed for this purpose. Therefore, we have to be careful with the conclusions. An analysis in which pig-density was determined based on postal code of the individuals would have been more reliable. These data were not available because of privacy issues. Also, the stratification of hospitals in 'pig-dense' and 'pig-arm' areas is arbitrary. Based on the CBS data, we classified the hospitals that are known to be situated in the most urbanized parts of the country as 'pig-arm'. This resulted in four hospitals in pig-arm areas and 13 hospitals in pig-dense areas. So, more hospitals in pig-dense areas were included in the analysis. Furthermore, there may be detection bias due to differences in screening policies between hospitals. It is possible that physicians in some hospitals take more clinical samples than physicians in other hospitals. This may lead to an underestimation in the number of MUO findings. Also, classification bias may occur depending on the reliability of the history of risk factors. However, all participating hospitals screened the MRSA risk groups described in the national MRSA guideline [5]. After coincidental MRSA findings, patients were asked for these risk factors also.

In conclusion, this study shows that the majority of newly identified MRSA patients in these 17 hospitals were acquired by direct contact with pigs/veal calves. The second largest group is the group of unknown origin. One fifth of these MUO are MC398. We found a significant association between individuals living in pig-dense areas and the likelihood of MC398 MUO carriage. MC398 MUO infections were rarely detected, i.e. 1 per 12 months for every participating hospital, so, currently, this MC398 MUO seems not to cause many problems. Because of the absence of known risk factors and probable risk for transmission in the healthcare settings, it is worthwhile to monitor the number of MUO in general, and of MC398 separately, in the coming years.

Acknowledgments

CAM Study Group:
Amphia Hospital, Breda: Brigitte van Cleef, Yvonne Hendriks, Daniëlle op den Kamp, Jan Kluytmans, Marjolein Kluytmans – van den Bergh, Renée Ladestein, Rudolf Punselie, Miranda van Rijen, Erwin Verkade
Catharina Hospital, Eindhoven: Marieke Ernest, Mireille Wulf
Duke University, Durham, NC, USA: Beth Feingold
Elkerliek Hospital, Helmond: Mariëlla Brekelmans, Patricia Willemse, Mireille Wulf
Franciscus Hospital, Roosendaal: Nelleke ten Feld, Rob Wintermans
Hospital Gelderse Vallei, Ede: Bent Postma, Marja Terwee, Thuy-Nga
Groene Hart Hospital, Gouda: Truus de Ruiter, Eric van der Vorm, Antoinette Wijker

Table 2. Unknown risk factor (MUO) and proportion of MC398 within this group, shown per hospital.

Hospital	Hospital type	Newly identified MRSA (total)	Pig-density in adherence area	Unknown risk factor (MUO)		MC398 MUO	
				n_{total} ($n_{infection}$)	%	n_{total} ($n_{infection}$)	%
1	teaching	100	High	39 (32)	39.0	7 (5)	17.9
2	teaching	53	High	10 (7)	18.9	2 (2)	20.0
3	general	95	High	10 (7)	10.5	5 (5)	50.0
4	general	137	High	24 (18)	17.5	9 (6)	37.5
5	general	26	Low	17 (11)	65.4	2 (1)	11.8
6	general	19	High	4 (3)	21.1	0	0
7	teaching	54	High	6 (6)	11.1	1 (1)	16.7
8	general	30	High	19 (16)	63.3	1 (1)	5.3
9	teaching	18	Low	9 (9)	50.0	1 (0)	11.1
11	general	40	High	5 (5)	12.5	1 (1)	20.0
12	teaching	84	High	15 (9)	17.9	4 (0)	26.7
13	teaching	25	Low	18 (15)	72.0	1 (1)	5.6
14	academic	60	High	23 (16)	38.3	12 (9)	52.2
15	academic	48	High	23 (14)	47.9	6 (1)	26.1
16	academic	52	Low	30 (24)	57.7	1 (1)	3.3
17	general	26	High	9 (9)	34.6	2 (1)	22.2
18	teaching	151	High	10 (6)	6.6	1 (0)	10.0
Total		**1018[a]**		**271 (207)**	**26.6**	**56 (35)**	**20.7**

[a] in two individuals there were no data about the source.
Hospital 10 intended to participate, but completed no electronic forms.

Lievensberg Hospital, Bergen op Zoom: Henk Hamers, Rob Winter-mans

Maxima Medical Centre, Eindhoven/Veldhoven: Philo Das, Ellen Sanders, Kees Verduin

Orbis Medical Centre, Sittard: Dick van Dam, Jan Diederen

Regional Health Authority, Leiden: Peter ten Ham

Reinier de Graaf Hospital, Delft: Loes Nolles, Eric van der Vorm

St. Anna Hospital, Geldrop: Anouk Smeulders, Kees Verduin

St. Elisabeth Hospital, Tilburg: Anton Buiting, Helma Hörmann, Ellen Nieuwkoop

St. Franciscus Gasthuis, Rotterdam: Yvonne Muller

University Medical Centre St Radboud, Nijmegen: Diana Haverkate, Paul Verweij

University Medical Centre Utrecht, Utrecht: Marc Bonten, Marischka van der Jagt-Zwetsloot, Annet Troelstra

VieCuri Medical Centre, Venlo: Hanneke Berkhout, Liduine van den Hout

VU Medical Centre, Amsterdam: Annie Kaiser, Christina Vanden-broucke-Grauls

We want to thank Beth Feingold for creating figure 2.

Author Contributions

Conceived and designed the experiments: MvR JK. Performed the experiments: MvR TB LS EV. Analyzed the data: MvR TB LS JK. Contributed reagents/materials/analysis tools: MvR TB EV LS JK. Contributed to the writing of the manuscript: MvR TB LS EV JK. Making of figure 1: TB LS.

References

1. Smith TC, Pearson N (2011) The emergence of Staphylococcus aureus ST398. Vector Borne Zoonotic Dis 11: 327–9.

2. van Loo I, Huijsdens X, Tiemersma E, de Neeling A, van de Sande-Bruinsma N, et al. (2007) Emergence of methicillin-resistant Staphylococcus aureus of animal origin in humans. Emerg Infect Dis 13: 1834–9.

3. Mulders MN, Haenen AP, Greenen PL, Vesseur PC, Poldervaart ES, et al. (2010) Prevalence of livestock-associated MRSA in broiler flocks and risk factors for slaughterhouse personnel in The Netherlands. Epidemiol Infect 138: 743–55.

4. Huijsdens XW, van Dijke BJ, Spalburg E, van Santen-Verheuvel MG, Heck ME, et al. (2006) Community-acquired MRSA and pig-farming. Ann Clin Microbiol Antimicrob 5: 26.

5. Dutch Workingparty on Infection Prevention (2007) MRSA hospital. Available at http://www.wip.nl. Accessed 1 November 2012.

6. Infectieziekten Bulletin (2012) Surveillance of MRSA in the Netherlands in 2011 [in Dutch]. Available at http://www.rivm.nl/Onderwerpen/I/Infectieziekten_Bulletin. Accessed 4 November 2013.

7. Wassenberg MW, Bootsma MC, Troelstra A, Kluytmans JA, Bonten MJ (2011) Transmissibility of livestock-associated methicillin-resistant Staphylococcus aureus (ST398) in Dutch hospitals. Clin Microbiol Infect 17(2): 316–9. doi: 10. 1111/j. 1469-0691.2010.03260.x

8. Bootsma MC, Wassenberg MW, Trapman P, Bonten MJ (2011) The nosocomial transmission rate of animal-associated ST398 meticillin-resistant Staphylococcus aureus. J R Soc Interface 8(57): 578–84.

9. Cuny C, Nathaus R, Layer F, Strommenger B, Altmann D (2009) Nasal colonization of humans with methicillin-resistant Staplylococcus aureus (MRSA) CC398 with and without exposure to pigs. PLoS One 4(8):e6800. doi: 10. 1371/journal.pone.0006800.

10. van Cleef BA, Verkade EJ, Wulf MW, Buiting AG, Voss A, et al. (2010) Prevalence of livestock-associated MRSA in communities with high pig-densities in The Netherlands. PLoS One 5(2):e9385. doi: 10. 1371/journal.pone. 0009385.

11. Feingold BJ, Silbergeld EK, Curriero FC, van Cleef BA, Heck ME, et al. (2012) Livestock density as risk factor for livestock-associated methicillin-resistant Staphylococcus aureus, the Netherlands. Emerg Infect Dis 18: 1841–9.

12. van Cleef BA, Monnet DI, Voss A, Krziwanek K, Allerberger F, et al. (2011) Livestock-associated methicillin-resistant Staphylococcus aureus in humans, Europe. Emerg Infect Dis 17(3): 502–5.

13. Schulz J, Friese A, Klees S, Tenhagen BA, Fetsch A, et al. (2012) Longitudinal study of the contamination of air and of soil surfaces in the vicinity of pig barns by livestock-associated methicillin-resistant Staphylococcus aureus. Appl Environ Microbiol 78: 5666–71.

14. van Rijen MM, Kluytmans-van den Bergh MF, Verkade EJ, ten Ham PB, Feingold BJ, et al. (2013) Lifestyle-associated risk factors for community-acquired methicillin-resistant Staphylococcus aureus carriage in the Netherlands: an exploratory hospital-based case-control study. PLoS One 8(6): e65594.

15. Fanoy E, Helmhout LC, van der Vaart WL, Weijdema K, van Santen-Verheuvel MG, et al. (2009) An outbreak of non-typeable MRSA within a residential care facility. Euro Surveill 14.

16. van Belkum A, Melles DC, Peeters JK, van Leeuwen WB, van Duijkeren E, et al. (2008) Dutch Working Party on Surveillance and Research of MRSA-SOM. Methicillin-resistant and -susceptible Staphylococcus aureus sequence type 398 in pigs and humans. Emerg Infect Dis 14: 479–83.

17. Pan A, Battisti A, Zoncada A, Bernieri F, Boldini M, et al. (2009) Community-acquired methicillin-resistant Staphylococcus aureus ST398 infection, Italy. Emerg Infect Dis 15: 845–7.

18. Declercq P, Petre D, Gordts B, Voss A (2007) Complicated community-acquired soft tissue infection by MRSA from porcine origin. Infection 36: 590–2.

19. van Rijen MM, van Keulen PH, Kluytmans JA (2008) Increase in a Dutch hospital of methicillin-resistant Staphylococcus aureus related to animal farming. Clin Infect Dis 46: 261–3.

20. Krziwanek K, Metz-Gercek S, Mittermayer H (2009) Methicillin-resistant Staphylococcus aureus ST398 from human patients, upper Austria. Emerg Infect Dis 15: 766–9.

21. Grisold AJ, Zarfel G, Hoenigl M, Krziwanek K, Feierl G, et al. (2010) Occurrence and genotyping using automated repetitive-sequence-based PCR of methicillin-resistant Staphylococcus aureus ST398 in Southeast Austria. Diagn Microbiol Infect Dis 66: 217–21.

22. Valentin-Domelier AS, Girard M, Bertrand X, Violette J, François P, et al. (2011) Bloodstream Infection Study Group of the Réseau des Hygiénistes de Centre (RHC). Methicillin-susceptible ST398 Staphylococcus aureus responsible for bloodstream infections: an emerging human-adapted subclone? PLoS One 6: e28369.

23. Verkade E, Bergmans AM, Budding AE, van Belkum A, Savelkoul P, et al. (2012) Recent emergence of Staphylococcus aureus clonal complex 398 in human blood cultures. PLoS One 7: e41855.

24. Ekkelenkamp MB, Sekkat M, Carpaij N, Troelstra A, Bonten MJ (2006) Endocarditis due to meticillin-resistant Staphylococcus aureus originating from pigs [in Dutch]. Ned Tijdschr Geneeskd 150: 2442–7.

25. Tristan A, Rasigade JP, Ruizendaal E, Laurent F, Bes M, et al. (2012) Rise of CC398 lineage of Staphylococcus aureus among infective endocarditis isolates revealed by two consecutive population-based studies in France. PLoS One 7(12): e51172. doi: 10. 1371/journal.pone.0051172.

26. Witte W, Strommenger B, Stanek C, Cuny C (2007) Methicillin-resistant Staphylococcus aureus ST398 in humans and animals, Central Europe. Emerg Infect Dis 13: 255–8.

27. Grundmann H, Aanensen DM, van den Wijngaard CC, Spratt BG, Harmsen D, et al. (2010) Geographic distribution of Staphylococcus aureus causing invasive infections in Europe: a molecular-epidemiological analysis. PLoS Med 7(1):e1000215. Doi: 10. 1371/journal.pmed.1000215.

28. David MZ, Daum RS (2010) Community-associated methicillin-resistant Staphylococcus aureus: epidemiology and clinical consequences of an emerging epidemic. Clin Microbiol Rev 23: 616–87.

29. Lekkerkerk WS, van de Sande-Bruinsma N, van der Sande MA, Tjon-A-Tsien A, Groenheide A, et al. (2012) Emergence of MRSA of unknown origin in the Netherlands. Clin Microbiol Infect 18(7): 656–61.

30. Schouls LM, Spalburg EC, van Luit M, Huijsdens XW, Pluister GN, et al. (2009) Multiple-locus variable number tandem repeat analysis of Staphylococcus aureus: comparison with pulsed-field gel elctrophoresis and spa-typing. PLoS One 4(4): e5082 doi: 10. 1371/journal.pone.0005082.

31. CBS Central Bureau of Statistics: Statline (2009) Available: cbs.statline.nl. Accessed 2012 July.

32. Price LB, Stegger M, Hasman H, Aziz M, Larsen J, et al. (2013) Staphylococcus aureus CC398: host adaptation and emergence of methicillin resistance in livestock. MBio 31(1): e00305–11 doi: 10. 1128/mBio.00305-11.

33. Köck R, Loth B, Köksal M, Schulte-Wülwer J, Harlizius J, et al. (2012) Does nasal colonization with livestock-associated Methicillin-resistant Staphylococcus aureus (MRSA) in pig farmers persist after holidays from pig exposure? Appl Environ Microbiol 78(11): 4046–7.

34. Slingerland BC, Tavakol M, McCarthy AJ, Lindsay JA, Snijders SV, et al. (2012) Survival of Staphylococcus aureus ST398 in the human nose after artificial inoculation. PLoS One 7(11): e48896.

35. Verkade E, van Benthem B, Kluytmans-van den Bergh MF, van Cleef B, van Rijen M, et al. (2013) Dynamics and determinants of Staphylococcus aureus carriage in livestock veterinarians: a prospective cohort study. Clin Infect Dis 57: e11–7.

36. de Boer E, Zwartkruis-Nahuis JT, Wit B, Huijsdens XW, de Neeling AJ, et al. (2009) Prevalence of methicillin-resistant Staphylococcus aureus in meat. Int J Food Microbiol 134: 52–6.

3

Development to Term of Cloned Cattle Derived from Donor Cells Treated with Valproic Acid

Juliano Rodrigues Sangalli[1,2,3]*, **Marcos Roberto Chiaratti**[2,4], **Tiago Henrique Camara De Bem**[1,5],
Reno Roldi de Araújo[1,2], **Fabiana Fernandes Bressan**[1], **Rafael Vilar Sampaio**[1,2,3], **Felipe Perecin**[1],
Lawrence Charles Smith[6], **Willian Allan King**[3], **Flávio Vieira Meirelles**[1]

1 Departamento de Medicina Veterinária, Faculdade de Zootecnia e Engenharia de Alimentos, Universidade de São Paulo, Pirassununga, São Paulo, Brazil, **2** Departamento de Cirurgia, Faculdade de Medicina Veterinária e Zootecnia, Universidade de São Paulo, São Paulo, São Paulo, Brazil, **3** Department of Biomedical Science, Ontario Veterinary College, University of Guelph, Ontario, Canada, **4** Departamento de Genética e Evolução, Centro de Ciências Biológicas e da Saúde, Universidade Federal de São Carlos, São Carlos, Brazil, **5** Departamento de Genética, Faculdade de Medicina de Ribeirão Preto, Universidade de São Paulo, Ribeirão Preto, São Paulo, Brazil, **6** Centre de recherche em reproduction animale, Faculté de médecine vétérinaire, Université de Montréal, St. Hyacinthe, Québec, Canada

Abstract

Cloning of mammals by somatic cell nuclear transfer (SCNT) is still plagued by low efficiency. The epigenetic modifications established during cellular differentiation are a major factor determining this low efficiency as they act as epigenetic barriers restricting reprogramming of somatic nuclei. In this regard, most factors that promote chromatin decondensation, including histone deacetylase inhibitors (HDACis), have been found to increase nuclear reprogramming efficiency, making their use common to improve SCNT rates. Herein we used valproic acid (VPA) in SCNT to test whether the treatment of nuclear donor cells with this HDACi improves pre- and post-implantation development of cloned cattle. We found that the treatment of fibroblasts with VPA increased histone acetylation without affecting DNA methylation. Moreover, the treatment with VPA resulted in increased expression of *IGF2R* and *PPARGC1A*, but not of *POU5F1*. However, when treated cells were used as nuclear donors no difference of histone acetylation was found after oocyte reconstruction compared to the use of untreated cells. Moreover, shortly after artificial activation the histone acetylation levels were decreased in the embryos produced with VPA-treated cells. With respect to developmental rates, the use of treated cells as donors resulted in no difference during pre- and post-implantation development. In total, five clones developed to term; three produced with untreated cells and two with VPA-treated cells. Among the calves from treated group, one stillborn calf was delivered at day 270 of gestation whereas the other one was delivered at term but died shortly after birth. Among the calves from the control group, one died seven days after birth whereas the other two are still alive and healthy. Altogether, these results show that in spite of the alterations in fibroblasts resulting from the treatment with VPA, their use as donor cells in SCNT did not improve pre- and post-implantation development of cloned cattle.

Editor: Carlos Eduardo Ambrósio, Faculty of Animal Sciences and Food Engineering, University of São Paulo, Pirassununga, SP, Brazil, Brazil

Funding: JRS is supported by São Paulo Research Foundation (FAPESP), grant number 2013/06673-7, and previously by Coordination for the Improvement of Higher Level Personnel (CAPES/DFAIT). This work was granted by São Paulo Research Foundation (FAPESP; grant numbers 2011/51126-9, 2010/13384-3, 2010/19768-8). The funders had no role in study design, data collection and analysis, decision to publish, or preparation of the manuscript.

Competing Interests: The authors have declared that no competing interests exist.

* Email: jrsh5n1@yahoo.com.br

Introduction

In 1997, cloning of mammals by somatic cell nuclear transfer (SCNT) was shown feasible, becoming a promising technology because of its applications in medicine (e.g. derivation of patient-specific embryonic stem cells) and transgenesis [1]. However, SCNT is still plagued by low efficiency, as a multitude of successful steps are needed for a cloned animal to be born healthy [2]. These include oocyte-mediated reprogramming, pregnancy establishment, development of a functional placenta with adequate maternal–fetal interaction, finally successful delivery and adaptation to the extra uterine life [3]. Problems such as persistence of somatic cell methylation [4] and acetylation patterns in SCNT embryos [5], aberrant expression of imprinted genes [6], failure to produce a functional placenta and consequently poor fetal nutrition are frequently observed in animal clones [7]. These observations suggest that the nuclear reprogramming process is incomplete in most SCNT embryos representing an important target for strategies aiming to improve SCNT efficiency [8].

There are several epigenetic modifications that accompany cell differentiation, including DNA methylation, histone modifications (e.g. H3K9me2/3 methylation; deacetylation), incorporation of histone variants (e.g. macroH2A) and chromatin compaction. All these modifications act as epigenetic barriers restricting reprogramming of somatic nuclei [9]. Since histone deacetylation, followed by DNA compaction, is commonly associated with gene repression in differentiated cells, decondensation of chromatin is required to enable access of transcriptional regulators to genomic targets essential for successful reprogramming of somatic nuclei [10,11]. Corroborating this hypothesis, most factors that promote chromatin decondensation, including histone deacetylase inhibitors (HDACis), have been found to increase nuclear reprogramming efficiency, making their use common to improve SCNT rates [12,13].

The use of HDACis, including Valproic Acid (VPA) [14], Sodium Butyrate (NaBu) [15], Trichostatin A (TSA) [16] and Scriptaid [17] is associated with increased rates of successful nuclear reprogramming. An increase of up to five fold in the success rate of mouse cloning was reported when HDACi was used in SCNT [13]. For example, treatment of donor cells with TSA, markedly improved in vitro development of SCNT embryos in rabbits [18] and cattle [19]. In addition, the use of NaBu in cattle improved SCNT [15] whereas the use of VPA enhanced gene reactivation and reprogramming efficiency in pig SCNT [20] and mouse induced pluripotent stem cells (iPSCs) experiments [21]. VPA, a short-chain fatty acid, is widely used in humans as an anticonvulsant and mood stabilizer [22]. Recently, VPA was reported to be a powerful HDACi with low toxicity to the cells, both in vitro and in vivo [23]. VPA relieves HDAC-dependent transcriptional repression and causes hyperacetylation of histones in cultured cells and in vivo [24,25]. Since histone hyperacetylation promotes neutralization of positive charges of lysine residues, this reduces their DNA binding and may contribute directly to chromatin opening and indirectly to transcriptional upregulation [26]. For this reason, VPA has been used in cattle to investigate its effect on nuclear reprogramming. Treatment of cloned embryos with VPA greatly improved blastocyst formation rate, the number of cells in the inner cell mass (ICM) and trophectoderm (TE), and cell survival in cattle [27]. Recently, Selokar et al. demonstrated in cattle that the use of donor cells treated with VPA was beneficial for efficient reprogramming using handmade cloning procedures [28]. Nonetheless, the use VPA has been limited to experiments involving pre-implantation development as end-points, with no study having evaluated its effect on development of cattle clones to term.

Herein VPA was used in SCNT to test whether the treatment of nuclear donor cells with this HDACi affects pre- and post-implantation development of cattle clones. We hypothesized that the treatment of donor cells with VPA might relax the chromatin structure turning them more amenable cells for reprogramming. As a result, based on previous studies and the low- toxicity of VPA, an increase of the global levels of histone acetylation favoring nuclear reprogramming towards higher developmental rates was expected.

Materials and Methods

All chemicals and reagents used were purchased from Sigma-Aldrich Chemical Company (St. Louis, MO, USA) unless otherwise stated. In vitro experimental procedures were carried out in humidified incubators maintained at 38.5°C in air with 5% CO_2. Each experiment consisted of at least three replicates. The experiments were conducted in accordance with the International Guiding Principles for Biomedical Research Involving Animals (Society for the Study of Reproduction).

Ethics Statement

The present study was approved by the "Ethic Committee in the use of animals" of the School of Veterinary Medicine and Animal Science of University of São Paulo, protocol number 2546/2012, which complies with the ethical principles in animal research. We adopted the International Guiding Principles for Biomedical Research Involving Animals (Society for the Study of Reproduction) as well.

Treatment of nuclear donor cells with VPA

Nuclear donor cells were derived from a 14-year old Gir (*Bos indicus*) bull as described previously [29]. Fibroblasts at third passage were plated at a density of 7×10^4 cells per 35-mm Petri dish in Alpha Minimum Essential Medium (α-MEM; GIBCO BRL, Grand Island, NY, USA) supplemented with 10% (v/v) fetal calf serum (FCS) and 50 µg/ml gentamicin sulfate. After 48 h post plating, the medium was changed to α-MEM supplemented with 0.5% FCS and 50 µg/ml gentamicin sulfate, and the cells were cultured for another three days to arrest the cell cycle at the G1/G0 stages. The treatment with VPA was performed by adding 0, 1, 2 or 5 mM of VPA to the culture medium 24 h before the end of the culture. Based on the results from an MTT analysis (see below), only 0 mM (control) and 2 mM (treated) of VPA were used in the following experiments.

MTT cell proliferation assay

To evaluate fibroblast viability and proliferation after VPA treatment, we used the 3-(4,5-dimethylthiazol-2-yl)-2, 4-diphenyl-tetrazolium bromide assay [30] (MTT) as previously described [29], with a few modifications. Briefly, fibroblasts were seeded in 96-well plates at 7×10^3 cells per well and treated with 0, 1, 2 and 5 mM of VPA as described above. Thereafter, 100 µl of the MTT solution (0.5 mg/ml final concentration) were added into each well of the 96-well plates and cultured in a humidified incubator with 5% CO_2 at 38.5°C. After 3 h, the MTT solution was removed and 200 µl of acidic isopropanol (0.04 M HCl in absolute isopropanol) were added into each well to dissolve the formed formazan crystals. Each plate was read using a spectrophotometer Thermo Scientific Multiskan FC (Thermo Scientific, Wilmington, DE, USA) at 570 nm wavelength. Absorbance values are expressed as percentages in relation to a control group (without VPA).

Somatic cell nuclear transfer

Somatic cell nuclear transfer was performed as described by Sangalli et al. [29]. Briefly, cumulus-oocyte complexes (COCs) were aspirated from ovaries obtained from local abattoirs and selected based on morphological characteristics. COCs were then subjected to in vitro maturation (IVM) and the oocytes denuded of cumulus cells by gentle pipetting. The oocytes with visible first polar body (PB) were enucleated by removing the 1st PB and metaphase-II (MII) plate by gentle aspiration using a 15-µm (internal diameter) glass pipette (ES transferTip; Eppendorf, Hamburg, Germany). Enucleated oocytes were reconstructed by injection of a single fibroblast (previously untreated or treated with VPA) into the perivitelline space. The resulting couplet was fused in electrofusion solution (0.28 M mannitol, 0.1 mM $MgSO_4$, 0.5 mM HEPES and 0.05% BSA in ultra-pure water) by applying one pulse of alternating current (0.05 kV/cm for 5 s) and two pulses of continuous current (1.75 kV/cm for 45 µs). Successfully fused couplets were fixed immediately before activation (see below) or artificially activated 26 h post-IVM. Artificial activation was performed by treatment with 5 µM ionomycin for 5 min, washing in 3% BSA solution and treatment with 2 mM of 6-dimethyla-minopurine (6-DMAP) for 3 h [29]. Presumptive zygotes were cultured for an additional period of 2 h post-activation (h.p.a.) and fixed for immunocytochemistry analysis (5 h.p.a.) or cultured for 7 days in SOF supplemented with 2.5% v/v FCS, 0.5% bovine serum albumin (BSA), 0.2 mM sodium pyruvate and 50 µg/ml gentamicin sulfate. Cleavage and blastocyst rates were evaluated at 48 and 168 h.p.a., respectively. In all experiments, parallel parthenogenetic embryos were generated and used as controls.

Embryo transfer and pregnancy evaluation

Blastocysts at day 7 of development were individually transferred non-surgically into the uterus of previously synchronized recipient cows [31]. Recipients were evaluated for pregnancy by transrectal palpation/ultrasonography at 30, 60, 90 and 270 days after embryo transfer. Abortion rate was evaluated on a monthly basis.

Immunodetection of H3K9ac and 5-methylcytosine

Immunocytochemistry for histone 3 lysine 9 acetylation (H3K9ac) was performed using fused couplets (immediately before the activation) or presumptive zygotes (5 h.p.a.). Nuclear donor cells were also evaluated by immunocytochemistry for H3K9ac and global levels of DNA methylation (5-mC) as previously reported [32–34], with a few modifications. Briefly, samples were fixed for 12 min in 4% (w/v) paraformaldehyde diluted in phosphate buffer solution (PBS) with 0.1% (w/v) polyvinylpyrrolidone (PBS-PVP) and permeabilized for 20 min in PBS-PVP with 1% (v/v) Triton X-100, washed in PBS-PVP containing 0.1% (v/v) Tween 20 (TW-PBS) and incubated for 15 min in 4 N HCl. Afterwards, samples were extensively washed in TW-PBS and non-specific binding sites were blocked by incubation overnight at 4°C in a blocking buffer consisting of PBS-PVP containing 0.4% (w/v) BSA. Samples were incubated for 3 h at 37°C with primary antibodies diluted at 1:1000. DNA methylation staining (fibroblasts) was performed using the anti-mouse 5-mC (Santa Cruz Biotechnology, Santa Cruz, CA, USA) whereas the anti-rabbit H3K9ac (Millipore, Bedford, MA, USA) was used for histone acetylation staining (fibroblasts, fused couplets and presumptive zygotes). Next, samples were washed in TW-PBS and incubated for 1 h at room temperature with secondary antibodies diluted at 1:500. The goat anti-rabbit conjugated with fluorescein isothiocyanate-FITC (Vector Laboratories, Burlingame, CA, USA) was used for histone acetylation staining and the rabbit anti-mouse conjugated with rhodamine (Santa Cruz Biotechnology) for DNA methylation staining. After several washes in TW-PBS, fibroblasts, fused couplets and presumptive zygotes were mounted on glass slides with coverslips using Prolong Antifade reagent (Invitrogen). An epifluorescent microscope (Axioplan; Carl Zeiss, Zeppelingstrasse, Germany) was used for evaluation of both DNA methylation and histone acetylation. As negative control, PBS was used in place of primary antibody.

Images were captured using a digital camera (Zeiss MC 80 DX; Carl Zeiss) and the same settings for all samples subject to the same staining (e.g. methylation or acetylation) procedure. The acetylation status was analyzed using at least 15 images of individual couplets for each experimental group. With regards to donor cells, 5 images of a monolayer of fibroblasts were evaluated for each experimental group to evaluate both acetylation and methylation status. Individual nuclei were outlined (excluding overlapping and folded nuclei) using the Adobe Photoshop v. 7 (Adobe Systems, San Jose, CA, USA). About 30 nuclei were outlined in each fibroblast image. The background was subtracted from pixel intensity in all analysis and the averaged signal intensity was calculated using the ImageJ software (ImageJ, National Institute of Health, Bethesda, MD, USA). Here, intensity refers to the degree of brightness of colored pixels (in a gray scale: 0–255; 0 = black and 255 = white) where brighter intensity indicates greater immunocytochemistry reactivity.

Gene expression analysis

RNA was extracted from control and treated fibroblasts using TRIzol reagent (Invitrogen, Carlsbad, CA, USA) according to the manufacturer's recommendations, with a few modifications. In brief, a mix containing 100 µl of TRIzol reagent, 5 µg of linear acrylamide (Ambion Inc., Austin, TX, USA) and 5 µl of diethylene pyrocarbonate-treated H_2O was added to each sample. The extracted RNA was directly dissolved in 10 µl of DNase I solution (Invitrogen) plus 1 unit/µl RNase OUT for DNA degradation, as suggested by the manufacturer. Then, the RNA was immediately reverse transcribed into cDNA using the High-Capacity cDNA Reverse Transcription kit (Applied Biosystems) according to manufacturer's protocol and stored at −20°C until use.

The target genes of interest were *POU5F1*, *IGF2R* and *PPARGC1A* whereas *ACTB* was used as a reference gene. Primers used for real-time reverse transcription PCR (RT-PCR) were designed using the Primer Express software v.3.1 (Applied Biosystems) based upon sequences available in GenBank (Table 1). Relative quantification of gene-specific mRNA transcripts was performed in 20-µl reactions containing 0.2 µM of primers (*POU5F1*, *IGF2R*, *PPARGC1A* and *ACTB*) plus 1× Power SYBR Green PCR Master Mix (Applied Biosystems) and 2 µl of a 8-fold diluted cDNA. All gene-specific cDNAs amplified for a particular sample were run in triplicate in the same PCR plate. A non-template control was always run in parallel with samples using 2 µl of water instead of cDNA. The following cycling conditions were applied for amplification: initial denaturation at 95°C for 10 min followed by 40 cycles consisting of 95°C for 15 sec and 60°C for 1 min. The SYBR Green fluorescence was read at the end of each extension step (60°C). Pilot experiments using five different concentrations of cDNA (spanning a 60-fold range) were run to set up real time RT-PCR conditions. The specificity of PCR products was confirmed by analysis of melting curves. Target transcript amounts were determined using the following formula: $E_{(target)}^{-\Delta Ct(target)}/E_{(ref)}^{-\Delta Ct(ref)}$, in which E corresponds to the amplification efficiency and ΔCt to the difference of cycle threshold (Ct) between control and treated samples. Values of Ct were averaged from sample duplicates whereas E referred to the mean efficiency estimated for each primer set (which varied from 93.6% to 95.2%) using LinRegPCR program [35–37]. Gene expression data from seven biological replicates are presented.

Statistical analysis

All experiments were repeated at least three times. Statistical analysis was performed using the SAS System v. 9.3 (SAS/STAT, SAS Institute Inc., Cary, NC). Developmental rates were analyzed using chi-square test. Remaining data were tested for normality of residuals and homogeneity of variances, and analysed as follows. MTT and immunocytochemistry data were analysed by regression analysis and t-Student's test, respectively. Gene expression data were analyzed by one-way ANOVA followed by Tukey post-hoc test. Gene expression data are presented in natural log (Ln) scale because of the log normal distribution considered for analysis. Differences with probabilities (P)<0.05 were considered significant. In the text, values are presented as means ± the standard error of the mean (SEM).

Results

Valproic Acid increases proliferation/viability of donor cells

In order to ascertain whether VPA-treated cells were suitable as nuclear donors and monitor the changes caused by VPA treatment, bovine fibroblasts were evaluated by the MTT assay after the treatment with 0, 1, 2 and 5 mM VPA for 24 h. The rate of proliferation/viability of these cells fitted (P = 0.0001) a second grade polynomial regression (Figure 1). The cells treated with 1, 2

Table 1. Primer sequences used in real time RT-PCR.

Gene Symbol	Gene Name	Accession number	Primer Sequences (5'-3')	Product (bp)	Annealing Temp. (°C)
POU5F1	POU class 5 homeobox 1	NM_174580.2	F: CAGGCCCGAAAGAGAAAGC	78	60
			R: CGGGCACTGCAGGAACA		
IGF2R	Insulin-like growth factor 2 receptor	NM_174352.2	F: CAGGTCTTGCAACTGGTGTATGA	83	60
			R: ACGAAGCTGATGACGCTCTTG		
PPARGC1A	Peroxisome proliferator-activated receptor gamma, coactivator 1 alpha	NM_177945.3	F: ACCATGCAAACCATAATCACAGGAT	82	60
			R: CTCTTCGCTTTATTGCTCCATGAAT		
ACTB	Actin beta	NM_173979.3	F: CAGCAGATGTGGATCAGCAAGC	91	60
			R: AACGCAGCTAACAGTCCGCC		

and 5 mM VPA increased proliferation/viability by 134±5,32%, 135±5,53% and 127±4,97%, respectively, compared to untreated cells (100±5,60%). Thus it was concluded that since the treatment did not impair cell viability the cells treated with VPA were suitable as nuclear donors.

VPA treatment increases H3K9 acetylation without affecting DNA methylation of donor cells

In order to confirm the effect of VPA treatment on histone acetylation, global histone acetylation levels of fibroblasts treated with 2 mM VPA were evaluated by immunocytochemistry (Figure 2). Compared to control cells, the treatment with VPA increased H3K9ac by about 1.9 fold (P<0.0001). Moreover, since VPA has been shown to decrease DNA methylation in cultured cells [38], we evaluated the global DNA methylation levels, but no differences were found between control and treated cells (Figure 2).

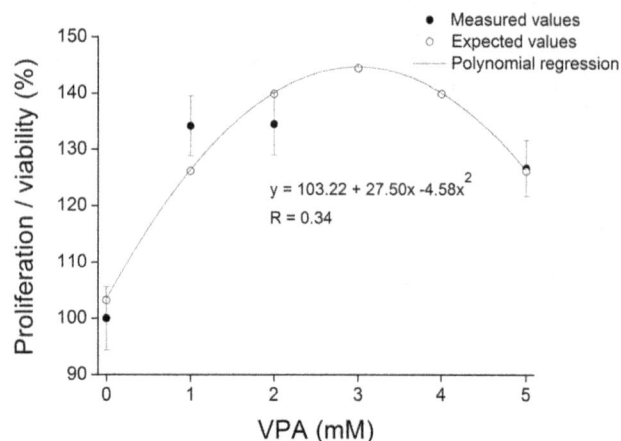

Figure 1. Valproic Acid increases proliferation/viability of donor cells. Proliferation/viability rates of donor cells treated with 0, 1, 2 and 5 mM VPA measured by the MTT assay. Values fitted a second grade polynomial regression (P=0.0001).

Expression of *IGF2R* and *PPARGC1A* is increased in donor cells treated with VPA

In order to further understand the effect of VPA on the cells, we evaluated expression of *POU5F1*, *IGF2R* and *PPARGC1A* by real-time RT-PCR (Figure 3). The genes evaluated are known for their role in regulating fetal growth (*IGF2R*) [39], promoting pluripotency (*POU5F1*) [40] and metabolism regulation (*PPARGC1A*) [41]. With respect to *IGF2R*, it was found that the treatment with VPA increased (P<0.0001) transcript abundance by about two fold compared to control cells (Figure 3a). No difference in expression of *POU5F1* was found (Figure 3b). Finally, expression of *PPARGC1A* was increased (P<0.0001) over five fold in the cells treated with VPA (Figure 3c). In summary, treatment of cells with VPA increased expression of *IGF2R* and *PPARGC1A*, but not of *POU5F1*.

The higher levels of histone acetylation in donor cells are not maintained after nuclear transfer

Fibroblasts with increased levels of histone acetylation after VPA treatment were used as SCNT donors cells. To confirm whether the higher acetylation levels were maintained after nuclear transfer, global histone acetylation levels were measured in fused couplets before and after artificial activation concerning their global histone acetylation levels (Figure 4). Although H3K9ac was marginally superior in the VPA group (28.0±4.44 versus 36.5±3.37, respectively for control and VPA), no significant difference was found between groups before activation (P=0.12). Unexpectedly, when H3K9ac was evaluated after artificial activation (5 h.p.a.), a significant decrease of about 1.3 fold was verified in the VPA group (P=0.03). Taken together, it appears that the higher levels of histone acetylation of donor cells treated with VPA are not maintained after nuclear transfer.

Higher levels of histone acetylation in donor cells has no effect on pre- and post-implantation development of clones

Since the cells treated with VPA showed higher levels of histone acetylation, they were used as donors in SCNT to evaluate the effect of donor cell acetylation levels on developmental rates (Table 2). A total of 254 cloned embryos were produced in four experimental replicates, 180 controls and 168 treated, but no

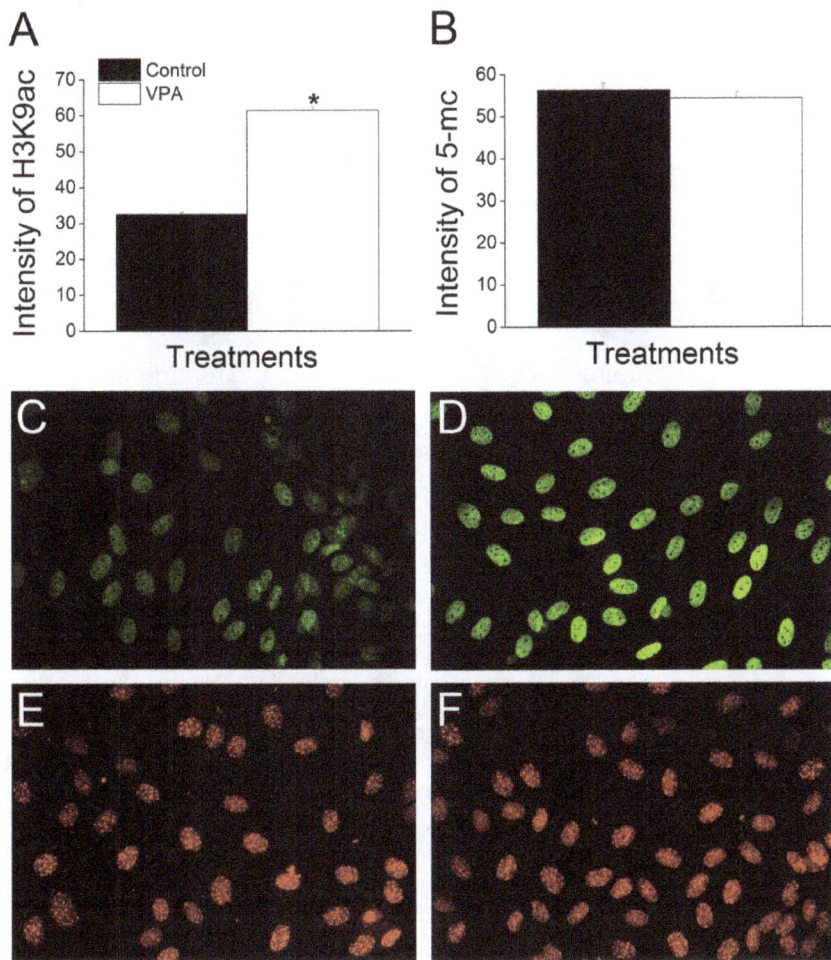

Figure 2. VPA treatment increases H3K9 acetylation without affecting DNA methylation of donor cells. (A) Relative average intensity of H3K9 acetylation (H3K9ac) of control and VPA-treated cells. (B) Relative average intensity of 5-methylcytosine (5-mC) of control and VPA-treated cells. (C–D) Immunofluorescence labeling for H3K9ac of control (C) and VPA-treated cells (D). (E–F) Immunofluorescence labeling for 5-mC of control (E) and VPA-treated cells (F). The (*) denotes a significant difference between experimental groups (P<0.0001). All images were taken in the same magnification (200×).

difference in overall rates of fusion, cleavage or blastocyst rates were found between groups. Although this finding indicates that the treatment of donor cells with VPA does not affect the development of SCNT embryos, blastocysts produced from both groups were transferred to recipients to evaluate whether the treatment affected post-implantation development (Table 3). Sixty-four blastocysts, 34 controls and 30 treated, were transferred individually into synchronized recipients. Although fewer full term gestations were obtained from VPA-treated donor cells, no significant difference was found between control and treated groups at any stage during pregnancy, further indicating that the treatment of donor cells with VPA does not affect developmental rates of cattle clones.

Analysis of the health status of cloned calves

Five calves were born after SCNT; two from the VPA group and three from the control group (Table 3). The recipient that delivered one of the calves from the VPA group showed signs of severe hydrallantois on day 270 of gestation (Figure 5A). We performed an emergency cesarean section, and delivered a stillborn calf, in spite of intensive care management and attempts of resuscitation. The calf was born with enlarged umbilical cord and ascites (Figure 5B). The other four calves that developed to term were delivered by cesarean section as well, but on day 289 of pregnancy. Among these, the remaining calf from the VPA group presented intestinal atony and died 12 h after birth due to gastrointestinal complications. One calf from the control group, showed poor viability after birth, received intensive care, including intranasal oxygen supplementation and colostrum via an esophageal tube, but died seven days after birth from septicemia secondary to omphalitis. The other two calves from the control group had no apparent abnormality, showed strong suckling reflex and drank colostrum with vigor. Both had clinical parameters monitored (e.g. glycemia, respiratory and heart rate, rectal temperature, blood gas) during the first 24 h. After this period, as they showed no clinical abnormalities they were discharged to a ventilated and clean stall. At the time of writing this manuscript, the surviving clones (both from the control group) were 13 months old, healthy and normal (Figure 5C) compared to their age-matched peers derived from natural reproduction at the time of preparation of this manuscript. It is noteworthy that between the two survivors calves, one is morphologically normal, adjusted all vital parameters and nursed the surrogate cow (Figure 5D) faster than the other calf. Surprisingly, the four calves (two from VPA

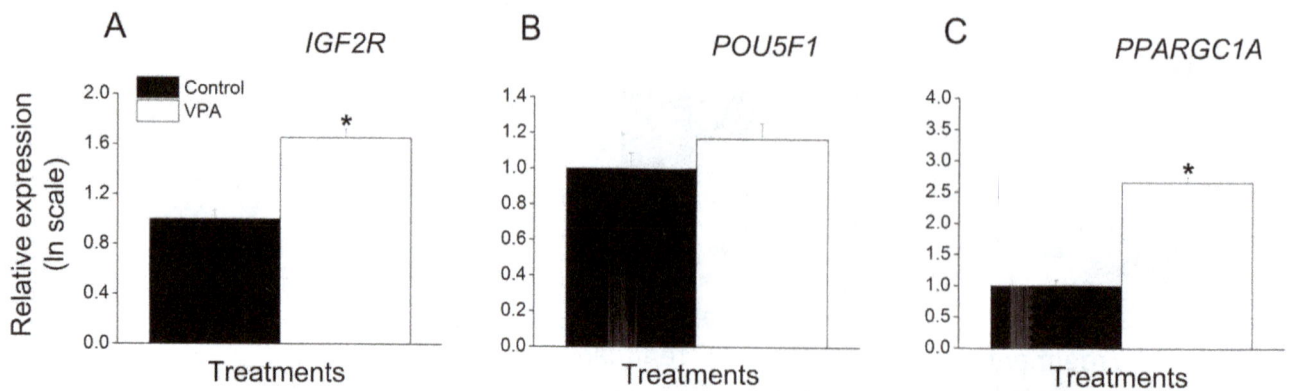

Figure 3. Expression of *IGF2R* and *PPARGC1A* is increased in donor cells treated with VPA. The amounts of *IGF2R* (A), *POU5F1* (B) and *PPARGC1A* (C) transcripts are expressed in relation to the control group. The asterisk (*) denotes difference between control and VPA-treated groups ($P < 0.0001$).

and two from control) had some degree of brachygnathism (Figure 5B and 5E). Furthermore, the surviving calf that had brachygnathism also had monorchidism (Figure 5F).

Discussion

Almost two decades have passed since the first mammal was cloned by using donor cells from an adult animal [1]. Yet, SCNT is still an inefficient procedure in which less than 10% of the embryos transferred to recipients results in the birth of viable offspring [2,42,43]. Among the factors affecting SCNT efficiency, chromatin compaction is thought to be a challenge for reprogramming donor cells as it acts as an epigenetic barrier to complete nuclear reprogramming [9,11]. HDAC inhibitors such as VPA are molecules that increase the global levels of histone

acetylation [25] and the treatment of donor cells with HDAC inhibitors have been reported to effectively increase in vitro cloning efficiency [15,19]. Thus, we hypothesized that the treatment of donor cells with VPA should increase the global levels of histone acetylation, leading to an "open chromatin" state. The use of these cells in SCNT might result in increased development rates of SCNT as their nuclei are expected to be more amenable to reprogramming [9,25]. To address this hypothesis, we investigated the effects of donor cells treatment with VPA on cellular proliferation/viability, epigenetic remodeling, gene expression, and pre- and post-implantational development of cattle clones derived from them. Our results showed that, albeit VPA treatment increased cellular proliferation/viability, expression of *PPARGC1A* and *IGF2R*, and the levels of H3K9ac in

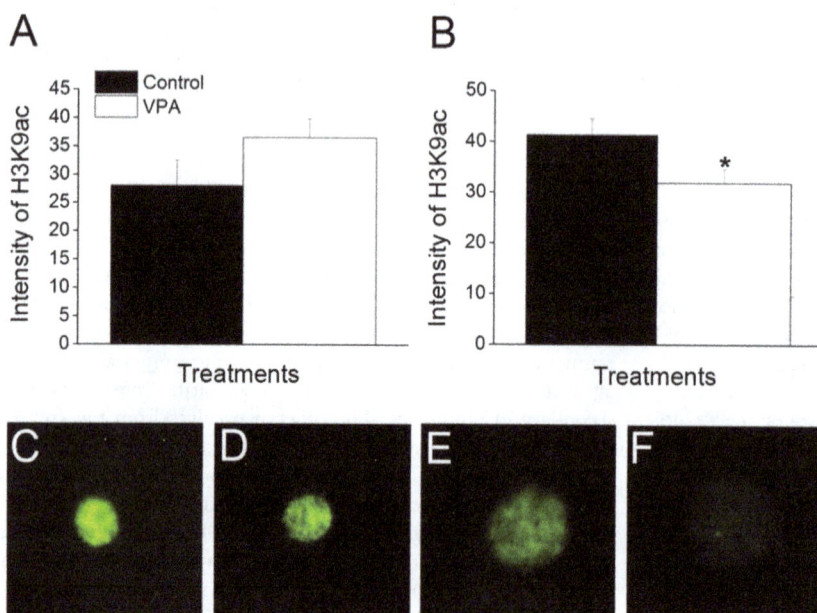

Figure 4. The higher levels of histone acetylation in donor cells are not maintained after nuclear transfer. (A) Relative average intensity of H3K9ac of fused couplets from control and VPA-treated groups. (B) Relative average intensity of H3K9ac of presumptive zygotes 5 h.p.a from control and VPA-treated groups. (C–D) Immunofluorescence labelling for H3K9ac of fused couplets from (C) control and (D) VPA-treated groups. (E–F) Immunofluorescence labelling for H3K9ac of presumptive zygotes 5 h.p.a. from (E) control and (F) VPA-treated groups. The asterisk (*) denotes difference between control and VPA-treated groups ($P = 0.03$). All images were taken in the same magnification (200×).

Table 2. Effect of treating nuclear-donor cells with Valproic Acid on pre-implantation developmental rates of cloned embryos.

Groups	Oocytes N	Fused embryos N (%)	Cleavage N (%)	Blastocysts N (%)
Control	180	139 (77.22)	112 (80.57)	44 (31.65)
VPA	168	115 (68.45)	90 (78.26)	38 (33.04)

Values within the same column did not differ statistically.
Fusion rate: number of embryos fused/number embryos reconstructed.
Cleavage rate: number of cleaved embryos/number of fused embryos.
Blastocyst rate: number of blastocysts/number of fused embryos.

donor cells, no effect on efficiency of SCNT was found when treated cells were used as nuclear donors.

The viability of the cells used as nucleus donors is a major point in SCNT as their nuclei drive development of SCNT embryos after oocyte reconstruction. Previous studies have shown that development of clones is negatively impacted when donor cells are treated with chromatin modifying agents (CMAs) that compromise cell cycle distribution, morphological characteristics and cellular proliferation [19,29,44,45]. Therefore, donor fibroblasts were treated for 24 h with increasing concentrations of VPA (1, 2 and 5 mM) and evaluated based on an MTT assay. Since all doses resulted in significantly higher proliferation/viability according to the MTT assay, 2 mM of VPA was used in the subsequent experiments as this concentration has been shown to increase the rates of induced pluripotent stem cells (iPSCs) [21] production and SCNT in mice [14]. It is noteworthy that based on the MTT assay, the treatment with VPA increased cell proliferation/viability while these cells were not expected to proliferate because of serum starvation to synchronize the cell cycle [46,47]. However, this increase might be caused as a side effect of VPA on cell metabolism as the MTT assay is based on activity of metabolic enzymes that reduces tetrazolium salts [30]. According to a recent paper, inhibition of HDAC doubled the activity of enzymes related to intermediate cell metabolism [48]. *PPARGC1A* is a transcriptional coactivator with a central role in mitochondrial biogenesis and metabolism regulation in the cell [41]. The finding that VPA treatment increased expression of *PPARGC1A* further supports its effect on cell metabolism as previously reported [49,50]. Based on these findings, 2 mM of VPA were found to be a suitable concentration to be used in the subsequent experiments.

In a second experiment we confirmed the effect of VPA on histone acetylation by evaluation of fibroblasts treated with 2 mM of VPA for 24 h in comparison to untreated cells. In addition, since VPA has been shown to cause DNA demethylation [38], the global levels of DNA methylation were evaluated, but no difference was found between control and treated cells. Since VPA causes demethylation by stimulating accessibility of a demethylase to DNA [38], we believe that a more prolonged treatment may be needed in order to obtain detectable levels of DNA demethylation. Next, since we hypothesized that the effects of VPA treatment would persist into embryo development, we attempted to confirm that the higher acetylation levels of donor cells were maintained after nuclear transfer. However, similar levels of histone acetylation were found between cloned embryos produced with control and treated cells. Moreover, a significant decrease in acetylation levels was found in SCNT couplets at 5 h.p.a. when fibroblasts treated with VPA were used as nuclear donors. This is in contrast with a report in the mouse, in which histone modifications caused by treatment of 8-cell embryos with VPA were maintained at least until the blastocyst stage [51]. On the other hand, oocytes are known to have special enzymatic activities, such as histone-modifying and DNA demethylating enzymes [11], that are responsible for reprogramming the sperm after fertilization [52]. Gao et al. showed that reprogramming by nuclear transfer uses the developmental program that is normally used after fertilization, termed by the authors as "erase-and-rebuild" process [53]. Furthermore, we speculate that the oocyte might have erased the epigenetic marks brought by the transferred nucleus, to reestablish a new developmental program. According to our data, this erasing process begins immediately after nuclear transfer, as no difference of acetylation was seen between control and treated groups immediately before artificial activation (approximately 1 to 2 h after couplet fusion). The ability of the oocyte to reverse the hyperacetylation caused by VPA, lowering the acetylation levels compared to a control group (5 h.p.a.), raises questions about the relevance of pretreating donor cells with CMAs. Enright et al. also found hypoacetylation in SCNT embryos produced by treatment of donor cells with TSA [19]. The authors suggested this was caused by a rebound effect from drug treatment, because the effect of HDACis is reversible [19]. In rabbits, similar results were found after treatment with NaBu and the authors argued that the aberrant epigenetic marks of clones cannot be corrected by the treatment with HDAC inhibitors [18]. In summary, although the treatment of donor cells with VPA caused histone hyperacetylation, this epigenetic state was reversed

Table 3. Effect of treating nuclear-donor cells with VPA on post-implantation developmental of clones.

Groups	Transferred embryos N	Pregnancies N (%)				Live born offspring
		Day 30	Day 60	Day 90	Day 270	Day 289
Control	34	7 (20.58)	3 (8.82)	3 (8.82)	3 (8.82)	3 (8.82)
VPA	30	6 (20.00)	2 (6.66)	2 (6.66)	2 (6.66)	1 (3.33)

Values within the same column did not differ statistically.
Pregnancy rate: number of pregnancies/number transferred embryos.

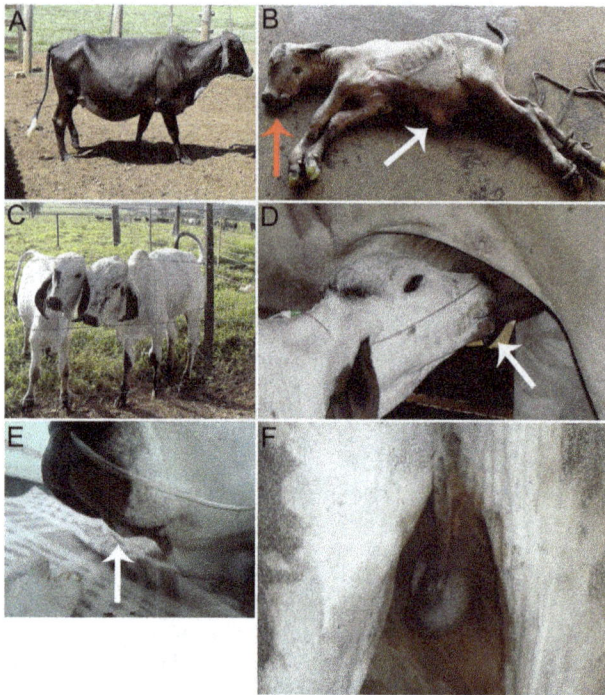

Figure 5. Analysis of health status of cloned calves. (A) Recipient female from the VPA-treated group showing signals of severe hydroallantois on day 270 of gestation. (B) Stillborn calf from VPA-treated group with enlarged umbilical cord and ascites (white arrow) and brachygnatism (red arrow). (C) Viable calves from the control group. (D) Calf from control group nursing, picture highlighting the correct morphology of the mandible (white arrow). (E) Mandible of cloned calf from control group with moderate brachygnatism (white arrow). (F) Picture highlighting the inguinal region of the calf from the control group evidencing monorchidism.

after oocyte reconstruction resulting in zygotes from treated group with lower levels of H3K9ac than the control group.

In a third experiment we investigated the effect of VPA treatment on gene expression in fibroblasts. It was reported that the treatment with VPA, even for a short period, had a significant effect on gene expression in cultured cells [25,54]. Since treatment of donor cells has been reported to improve SCNT rates [15,28], we hypothesized that this effect might be mediated, among other factors, by an effect of VPA on expression of key genes to SCNT. Since an appropriate expression of *POU5F1* [55] and *IGF2R* [56] during early embryogenesis is critical to the success of SCNT, we evaluated whether the expression of these genes is altered in fibroblasts treated with VPA. We found no effect of the treatment on the expression of *POU5F1*, but VPA did increase expression of *IGF2R* compared to untreated cells. *POU5F1* plays an essential role in controlling cellular pluripotency and therefore is a key factor in nuclear reprogramming in SCNT [40]. Treatment of myogenic cells with VPA was been shown to increase expression of *POU5F1* [57]. Thus, SCNT might benefit from an overexpression of *POU5F1* in donor cells as SCNT embryos frequently fail to express this gene [55]. However, as we found that VPA did not affect *POU5F1* expression, we believe that other epigenetic modifications than histone acetylation are involved in the control of *POU5F1* expression [58]. With respect to *IGF2R*, this gene plays an important role as a negative effector in fetal growth since it promotes *IGF2* arrest into lysosomes followed by degradation [59,60]. It has been hypothesized that dysregulation of imprinted

genes such as *IGF2R* are the cause of poor developmental rates observed in SCNT [56], and alterations of *IGF2R* expression has often been associated to common problems in cloned embryos [61]. For instance, in sheep, parthenogenetic embryos that express low levels of *IGF2* and high levels of *IGF2R* and *H19*, have retarded growth when compared to control embryos [62–64]. On the other hand, the reduced *IGF2R* expression in ovine embryos cultured in vitro is associated with Large Offspring Syndrome [39]. Baqir et al. observed that most imprinted genes have their expression increased following exposure of mouse embryonic stem cells to TSA [65]. Interestingly, they also found that expression of several imprinted genes remained high and in some cases, increased further, after drug removal or even after cell passageing, indicating a long lasting and retarded effect of the treatment on gene expression [65]. Herein we confirmed the effect of VPA on increased expression of an imprinted gene, providing further evidence that acetylation is involved in regulation of imprinting [65,66]. The higher expression levels of *IGF2R* induced by the treatment of donor cells with VPA might affect SCNT as the epigenetic modifications induced by VPA on *IGF2R* have a long lasting effect on development [65]. Hence, the treatment of donor cells with VPA resulted on increased expression of *IGF2R* without affecting expression of *POU5F1*.

Although the hyperacetylation caused by VPA on donor cells was reversed after nuclear transfer, we decided to evaluate development of cloned embryos to further characterize the effect of VPA on SCNT. It is possible that some of the modifications induced by VPA on donor cells (e.g. overexpression of *IGF2R*) remain after nuclear transfer, with a consequent effect on cloning efficiency. Several groups have reported increased rates of SCNT when donor cells were treated with HDAC inhibitors, including VPA [28], TSA (cattle) [19,32] and NaBu (cattle [15] and rabbits [18]). Yet, here we found no effect of donor cells treated with VPA on pre-implantation development of SCNT embryos. Although surprisingly this finding is in agreement with a previous reports in which NaBu was used to produce pig clones [45]. This report described that the treatment of donor cells with NaBu resulted in histone hyperacetylation, but the use of these cells in SCNT did not affect development of cloned embryos. These contradictory results provide evidence that the effect of CMAs may diverge depending on several factors including species and reprogramming system (e.g. SCNT or iPSCs). This notion is supported by a recent report with cloned mice which showed that several HDAC inhibitors such as TSA, scriptaid, suberoylanilide hydroxamic acid and oxamflatin reduced the rate of apoptosis in blastocysts and improved full term development, whereas VPA had no effect on SCNT efficiency [67]. The authors argued that VPA is an inhibitor of HDAC classes I and IIa, whereas the others are inhibitors of HDAC classes I and IIa/b, suggesting that inhibition of HDAC class IIb is a key step for successful reprogramming in the mouse [67]. In contrast, Costa-Borges et al. found that VPA improved in vitro development, blastocyst quality, and full term development of cloned mice, at comparable level to TSA [14]. Treatment with VPA also improved pre-implantation development of cattle [68] and pigs [69] when the cloned embryos were treated during in vitro culture. The treatment resulted in an increase of blastocyst rate and cell number in the inner cell mass (ICM) [68,69]. Selokar et al showed that the treatment of donor cells with VPA improved bovine SCNT blastocysts production, reduced the apoptosis and H3K9 methylation levels, similar to those of embryos derived from IVF [28]. While these results differ from our, it should be noted that Selokar et al used handmade cloning, which is characterized by significant differences in the technique from that used in the present study, which might explain the differences observed in pre-implantation development. In addition, VPA was recently found to regulate pluripotency in iPSCs, increasing the efficiency as measured by the number of colonies, and up-regulation of pluripotency genes [21]. In summary, the effect of CMAs such as VPA on SCNT is not clear [70], but here we found no effect of VPA on developmental rates of SCNT embryos.

Taking into account that VPA might have affected SCNT embryos later during development, the blastocysts derived from the previous experiment were transferred to recipients to evaluate post-implantation development. Cloning of cattle by SCNT is typically associated with a high incidence of pregnancy failure throughout gestation [7,71]. Our data are in accordance with previous reports, showing that the majority of established pregnancies (60–70%) were lost around the time of implantation [56,72]. In cloned cattle, the losses that occur between days 30 and 60 of pregnancy are frequently associated to morphological (placentomegaly and faulty vascularization) and functional (steroidogenesis) abnormalities in placentas [71]. With respect to VPA, no effect of its treatment was seen on post-implantation development as the rate of pregnancy failure between 60 and 270 days and rate of development to term did not appreciably differ between groups. This unexpected result supports the hypothesis that all the modifications induced by the treatment were either inconsequential for post blastocyst development or reversed after nuclear transfer. Moreover, whereas two out of three clones produced with untreated cells were healthy at birth, the two clones that derived from VPA-treated cells died after caesarian section. This highlights the importance of evaluating post-implantation development and survival rate when CMAs are employed in SCNT. This agrees with the report by Kang et al. with pigs who described that VPA improved in vitro development of cloned embryos but did not improve survival to adulthood [73]. Interestingly, herein four out of five calves produced by SCNT (two from untreated cells and two from treated cells) presented brachygnatism. This trait is widely accepted to be a congenital and heritable abnormality [74]. However, the bull whose donor cells

were derived did not present this phenotype. We speculate that the cell culture environment or an incomplete nuclear reprograming might have led to such abnormality. In a previous study, Johnson et al. also reported the occurrence of brachygnatism in foals derived by SCNT, trait that was not present in the horse used to donor cell derivation [74]. Strikingly, one of the viable calves, in addition to brachygnatism, had monorchidism whereas the other calf did not present noticeable abnormalities. After birth, the calf without abnormalities, stood up, drank colostrum and adjusted the physiological parameters faster than the other one with brachygnatism and monorchidism. This suggests that the process of nuclear reprogramming is stochastic, with calves derived from the same cell line presenting variable levels of "reprogramming" and health status. In summary, the treatment of donor cells with VPA did not affect developmental rates resulting in one stillborn and one calf that survived only 12 h after birth.

In conclusion, accumulated evidence suggests that CMAs are highly important to aid nuclear reprogramming with a consequent increase in SCNT efficiency in the mouse [75]. In cattle the use of CMAs remains largely controversial [70,76]. Altogether, our results show that in spite of the alterations caused in fibroblasts by the treatment with VPA, their use as donor cells in SCNT does not improve pre- and post-implantation development of cloned cattle. In the future, it will be interesting to dissect the roles that CMAs have in donor cells and cloned embryos, to gain mechanistic insights on their use.

Acknowledgments

The authors gratefully acknowledge the help provided by Dr. Paulo Fantinato Neto and Dr. Flávio José Minieri Marchese.

Author Contributions

Conceived and designed the experiments: JRS MRC FVM. Performed the experiments: JRS MRC THCDB RRA FFB RVS. Analyzed the data: JRS MRC FP LCS WAK FVM. Contributed reagents/materials/analysis tools: JRS FP FVM. Wrote the paper: JRS MRC LCS WAK FVM.

References

1. Wilmut I, Schnieke AE, McWhir J, Kind AJ, Campbell KH (1997) Viable offspring derived from fetal and adult mammalian cells. Nature 385: 810–813.
2. Wilmut I, Beaujean N, de Sousa PA, Dinnyes A, King TJ, et al. (2002) Somatic cell nuclear transfer. Nature 419: 583–586.
3. Meirelles F V, Birgel EH, Perecin F, Bertolini M, Traldi AS, et al. (2010) Delivery of cloned offspring: experience in Zebu cattle (Bos indicus). Reprod Fertil Dev 22: 88–97.
4. Santos F, Zakhartchenko V, Stojkovic M, Peters A, Jenuwein T, et al. (2003) Epigenetic marking correlates with developmental potential in cloned preimplantation embryos. Curr Biol 13: 1116–1121.
5. Wee G, Koo DB, Song BS, Kim JS, Kang MJ, et al. (2006) Inheritable histone H4 acetylation of somatic chromatins in cloned embryos. J Biol Chem 281: 6048–6057.
6. Suzuki J, Therrien J, Filion F, Lefebvre R, Goff AK, et al. (2011) Loss of methylation at H19 DMD is associated with biallelic expression and reduced development in cattle derived by somatic cell nuclear transfer. Biol Reprod 84: 947–956.
7. Arnold DR, Fortier AL, Lefebvre R, Miglino MA, Pfarrer C, et al. (2008) Placental insufficiencies in cloned animals - a workshop report. Placenta 29 Suppl A: S108–10.
8. Dean W, Santos F, Stojkovic M, Zakhartchenko V, Walter J, et al. (2001) Conservation of methylation reprogramming in mammalian development: Aberrant reprogramming in cloned embryos. Proc Natl Acad Sci U S A 24: 13734–13738.
9. Pasque V, Jullien J, Miyamoto K, Halley-Stott RP, Gurdon JB (2011) Epigenetic factors influencing resistance to nuclear reprogramming. Trends Genet 27: 516–525.
10. Gaspar-Maia A, Alajem A, Meshorer E, Ramalho-Santos M (2011) Open chromatin in pluripotency and reprogramming. Nat Rev Mol Cell Biol 12: 36–47.
11. Gurdon JB, Wilmut I (2011) Nuclear transfer to eggs and oocytes. Cold Spring Harb Perspect Biol 3 (6).
12. Zhao J, Hao Y, Ross JW, Spate LD, Walters EM, et al. (2010) Histone deacetylase inhibitors improve in vitro and in vivo developmental competence of somatic cell nuclear transfer porcine embryos. Cell Reprogram 12: 75–83.
13. Kishigami S, Mizutani E, Ohta H, Hikichi T, Thuan N Van, et al. (2006) Significant improvement of mouse cloning technique by treatment with trichostatin A after somatic nuclear transfer. Biochem Biophys Res Commun 340: 183–189.
14. Costa-borges N, Santaló J, Ibáñes E. (2010) Comparison between the effects of valproic acid and trichostatin A on in vitro development, blastocyst quality, and full-term development of mouse somatic cell nuclear transfer embryos. Cell Reprogram 12: 437–446.
15. Shi W, Hoeflich A, Flaswinkel H, Stojkovic M, Wolf E, et al. (2003) Induction of a senescent-like phenotype does not confer the ability of bovine immortal cells to support the development of nuclear transfer embryos. Biol Reprod 69: 301–309.
16. Lee MJ, Kim SW, Lee HG, Im GS, Yang BC, et al. (2011) Trichostatin A promotes the development of bovine somatic cell nuclear transfer embryos. J Reprod Dev 57: 34–42.
17. Zhao J, Ross JW, Hao Y, Spate LD, Walters EM, et al. (2009) Significant improvement in cloning efficiency of an inbred miniature pig by histone deacetylase inhibitor treatment after somatic cell nuclear transfer. Biol Reprod 81: 525–530.
18. Yang F, Hao R, Kessler B, Brem G, Wolf E, et al. (2007) Rabbit somatic cell cloning: effects of donor cell type, histone acetylation status and chimeric embryo complementation. Reproduction 133: 219–230.
19. Enright BP, Kubota C, Yang X, Tian XC (2003) Epigenetic characteristics and development of embryos cloned from donor cells treated by trichostatin A or 5-aza-2′-deoxycytidine. Biol Reprod 69: 896–901.
20. Miyoshi K, Mori H, Mizobe Y, Akasaka E, Osawa A, et al. (2010) Valproic acid enhances in vitro development and OCT-3/4 expression of miniature pig somatic cell nuclear transfer embryos. Cell Reprogram 12: 67–74.

21. Huangfu D, Maehr R, Guo W, Eijkelenboom A, Snitow M, et al. (2008) Induction of pluripotent stem cells by defined factors is greatly improved by small-molecule compounds. Nat Biotechnol 26: 795–797.

22. Phiel CJ, Zhang F, Huang EY, Guenther MG, Lazar M a, et al. (2001) Histone deacetylase is a direct target of valproic acid, a potent anticonvulsant, mood stabilizer, and teratogen. J Biol Chem 276: 36734–36741.

23. Göttlicher M, Minucci S, Zhu P, Krämer OH, Schimpf A, et al. (2001) Valproic acid defines a novel class of HDAC inhibitors inducing differentiation of transformed cells. EMBO J 20: 6969–6978.

24. Marchion DC, Bicaku E, Daud AI, Sullivan DM, Munster PN (2005) Valproic acid alters chromatin structure by regulation of chromatin modulation proteins. Cancer Res 65: 3815–3822.

25. Hezroni H, Sailaja BS, Meshorer E (2011) Pluripotency-related, valproic acid (VPA)-induced genome-wide histone H3 lysine 9 (H3K9) acetylation patterns in embryonic stem cells. J Biol Chem 286: 35977–35988.

26. Turner BM (2007) Defining an epigenetic code. Nat Cell Biol 9: 2–6.

27. Xu W, Wang Y, Li Y, Wang L, Xiong X, et al. (2012) Valproic acid improves the in vitro development competence of bovine somatic cell nuclear transfer embryos. Cell Reprogram 14: 138–145.

28. Selokar NL, St John L, Revay T, King WA, Singla SK, et al. (2013) Effect of histone deacetylase inhibitor valproic acid treatment on donor cell growth characteristics, cell cycle arrest, apoptosis, and handmade cloned bovine embryo production efficiency. Cell Reprogram 15: 531–542.

29. Sangalli JR, De Bem THC, Perecin F, Chiaratti MR, Oliveira LDJ, et al. (2012) Treatment of nuclear-donor cells or cloned zygotes with chromatin-modifying agents increases histone acetylation but does not improve full-term development of cloned cattle. Cell Reprogram 14: 235–247.

30. Mosmann T (1983) Rapid Colorimetric Assay for Cellular Growth and Survival: Application to Proliferation and Cytotoxicity Assays. J Immunol Methods 65: 55–63.

31. Nasser LF, Reis EL, Oliveira MA, Bó GA, Baruselli PS (2004) Comparison of four synchronization protocols for fixed-time bovine embryo transfer in Bos indicus x Bos taurus recipients. Theriogenology 62: 1577–1584.

32. Ding X, Wang Y, Zhang D, Guo Z, Zhang Y (2008) Increased pre-implantation development of cloned bovine embryos treated with 5-aza-2′-deoxycytidine and trichostatin A. Theriogenology 70: 622–630.

33. Giraldo AM, Lynn JW, Purpera MN, Godke RA (2007) DNA methylation and histone acetylation patterns in cultured bovine fibroblasts for nuclear transfer. Mol Reprod Dev 74: 1514–1524.

34. Martinez-Diaz MA, Che L, Albornoz M, Seneda MM, Collis D, et al. (2010) Pre- and postimplantation development of swine-cloned embryos derived from fibroblasts and bone marrow cells after inhibition of histone deacetylases. Cell Reprogram 12: 85–94.

35. Ramakers C, Ruijter JM, Deprez RHL, Moorman AF. (2003) Assumption-free analysis of quantitative real-time polymerase chain reaction (PCR) data. Neurosci Lett 339: 62–66.

36. Pfaffl MW, Horgan GW, Dempfle L (2002) Relative expression software tool (REST) for group-wise comparison and statistical analysis of relative expression results in real-time PCR. Nucleic Acids Res 30: e36.

37. Livak KJ, Schmittgen TD (2001) Analysis of relative gene expression data using real-time quantitative PCR and the 2(-Delta Delta C(T)) Method. Methods 25: 402–408.

38. Detich N, Bovenzi V, Szyf M (2003) Valproate induces replication-independent active DNA demethylation. J Biol Chem 278: 27586–27592.

39. Young LE, Fernandes K, McEvoy TG, Butterwith SC, Gutierrez CG, et al. (2001) Epigenetic change in IGF2R is associated with fetal overgrowth after sheep embryo culture. Nat Genet 27: 153–154.

40. Boiani M, Eckardt S, Schöler HR, McLaughlin KJ (2002) Oct4 distribution and level in mouse clones: consequences for pluripotency. Genes Dev 16: 1209–1219.

41. Austin S, St-Pierre J (2012) PGC1α and mitochondrial metabolism—emerging concepts and relevance in ageing and neurodegenerative disorders. J Cell Sci 125: 4963–4971.

42. Gurdon JB, Melton DA (2008) Nuclear reprogramming in cells. Science 322: 1811–1815.

43. Yang X, Smith SL, Tian XC, Lewin HA, Renard JP, et al. (2007) Nuclear reprogramming of cloned embryos and its implications for therapeutic cloning. Nat Genet 39: 295–302.

44. Enright BP, Sung LY, Chang CC, Yang X, Tian XC (2005) Methylation and acetylation characteristics of cloned bovine embryos from donor cells treated with 5-aza-2′-deoxycytidine. Biol Reprod 72: 944–948.

45. Das ZC, Gupta MK, Uhm SJ, Lee HT (2010) Increasing histone acetylation of cloned embryos, but not donor cells, by sodium butyrate improves their in vitro development in pigs. Cell Reprogram 12: 95–104.

46. Campbell KH (1999) Nuclear equivalence, nuclear transfer, and the cell cycle. Cloning 1: 3–15.

47. Miranda MDS, Bressan FF, Zecchin KG, Vercesi AE, Mesquita LG, et al. (2009) Serum-starved apoptotic fibroblasts reduce blastocyst production but enable development to term after SCNT in cattle. Cloning Stem Cells 11: 565–573.

48. Zhao S, Xu W, Jiang W, Yu W, Lin Y, et al. (2010) Regulation of cellular metabolism by protein lysine acetylation. Science 327: 1000–1004.

49. Chiang MC, Cheng YC, Lin KH, Yen CH (2013) PPARγ regulates the mitochondrial dysfunction in human neural stem cells with tumor necrosis factor alpha. Neuroscience 229: 118–129.

50. Aouali N, Palissot V, El-Khoury V, Moussay E, Janji B, et al. (2009) Peroxisome proliferator-activated receptor gamma agonists potentiate the cytotoxic effect of valproic acid in multiple myeloma cells. Br J Haematol 147: 662–671.

51. VerMilyea MD, O'Neill LP, Turner BM (2009) Transcription-independent heritability of induced histone modifications in the mouse preimplantation embryo. PLoS One 4: e6086.

52. Jullien J, Pasque V, Halley-Stott RP, Miyamoto K, Gurdon JB (2011) Mechanisms of nuclear reprogramming by eggs and oocytes: a deterministic process? Nat Rev Mol Cell Biol 12: 453–459.

53. Gao T, Zheng J, Xing F, Fang H, Sun F, et al. (2007) Nuclear reprogramming: the strategy used in normal development is also used in somatic cell nuclear transfer and parthenogenesis. Cell Res 17: 135–150.

54. Felisbino MB, Tamashiro WMSC, Mello MLS (2011) Chromatin remodeling, cell proliferation and cell death in valproic acid-treated HeLa cells. PLoS One 6: e29144.

55. Bortvin A, Eggan K, Skaletsky H, Akutsu H, Berry DL, et al. (2003) Incomplete reactivation of Oct4-related genes in mouse embryos cloned from somatic nuclei. Development 130: 1673–1680.

56. Smith LC, Suzuki J, Goff AK, Filion F, Therrien J, et al. (2012) Developmental and epigenetic anomalies in cloned cattle. Reprod Domest Anim 47 Suppl 4: 107–114.

57. Teng HF, Kuo YL, Loo MR, Li CL, Chu TW, et al. (2010) Valproic acid enhances Oct4 promoter activity in myogenic cells. J Cell Biochem 110: 995–1004.

58. Simonsson S, Gurdon J (2004) DNA demethylation is necessary for the epigenetic reprogramming of somatic cell nuclei. Nat Cell Biol 6: 984–990.

59. Ludwig T, Eggenschwiler J, Fisher P, D'Ercole a J, Davenport ML, et al. (1996) Mouse mutants lacking the type 2 IGF receptor (IGF2R) are rescued from perinatal lethality in Igf2 and Igf1r null backgrounds. Dev Biol 177: 517–535.

60. Lau MM, Stewart CE, Liu Z, Bhatt H, Rotwein P, et al. (1994) Loss of the imprinted IGF2/cation-independent mannose 6-phosphate receptor results in fetal overgrowth and perinatal lethality. Genes Dev 8: 2953–2963.

61. Perecin F, Méo SC, Yamazaki W, Ferreira CR, Merighe GKF, et al. (2009) Imprinted gene expression in in vivo- and in vitro-produced bovine embryos and chorio-allantoic membranes. Genet Mol Res 8: 76–85.

62. Feil R, Khosla S, Cappai P, Loi P (1998) Genomic imprinting in ruminants: allele-specific gene expression in parthenogenetic sheep. Mamm Genome 9: 831–834.

63. Hagemann LJ, Peterson AJ, Weilert LL, Lee RS, Tervit HR (1998) In vitro and early in vivo development of sheep gynogenones and putative androgenones. Mol Reprod Dev 50: 154–162.

64. Young LE, Schnieke AE, McCreath KJ, Wieckowski S, Konfortova G, et al. (2003) Conservation of IGF2-H19 and IGF2R imprinting in sheep: effects of somatic cell nuclear transfer. Mech Dev 120: 1433–1442.

65. Baqir S, Smith LC (2006) Inhibitors of histone deacetylases and DNA methyltransferases alter imprinted gene regulation in embryonic stem cells. Cloning Stem Cells 8: 200–213.

66. Hu JF, Pham J, Dey I, Li T, Vu TH, et al.(2000) Allele-Specific histone acetylation accompanies genomic imprinting of the insulin-like growth factor II receptor gene. 141: 4428–4435.

67. Ono T, Li C, Mizutani E, Terashita Y, Yamagata K, et al. (2010) Inhibition of class IIb histone deacetylase significantly improves cloning efficiency in mice. Biol Reprod 83: 929–937.

68. Xu W, Wang Y, Li Y, Wang L, Xiong X, et al. (2012) Valproic acid improves the in vitro development competence of bovine somatic cell nuclear transfer embryos. Cell Reprogram 14: 138–145.

69. Kim YJ, Ahn KS, Kim M, Shim H (2011) Comparison of potency between histone deacetylase inhibitors trichostatin A and valproic acid on enhancing in vitro development of porcine somatic cell nuclear transfer embryos. In Vitro Cell Dev Biol Anim 47: 283–289.

70. Akagi S, Geshi M, Nagai T (2013) Recent progress in bovine somatic cell nuclear transfer. Anim Sci J 84: 191–199.

71. Chavatte-Palmer P, Camous S, Jammes H, Le Cleac'h N, Guillomot M, et al. (2012) Review: Placental perturbations induce the developmental abnormalities often observed in bovine somatic cell nuclear transfer. Placenta 33 Suppl: S99–S104.

72. Hill JR, Burghardt RC, Jones K, Long CR, Looney CR, et al. (2000) Evidence for placental abnormality as the major cause of mortality in first-trimester somatic cell cloned bovine fetuses. Biol Reprod 63: 1787–1794.

73. Kang JD, Li S, Lu Y, Wang W, Liang S, et al. (2013) Valproic acid improved in vitro development of pig cloning embryos but did not improve survival of cloned pigs to adulthood. Theriogenology 79: 306–11.

74. Johnson AK, Clark-Price SC, Choi YH, Hartaman DL, Hinrichs K, (2010) Physical and clinicopathologic findings in foals derived by use of somatic cell nuclear transfer: 14 cases (2004–2008). J Am Med Vet Assoc 236: 983–990.

75. Ogura A, Inoue K, Wakayama T (2013) Recent advancements in cloning by somatic cell nuclear transfer. Philos Trans R Soc Lond B Biol Sci 368: 20110329.

76. Galli C, Duchi R, Colleoni S, Lagutina I, Lazzari G (2014) Ovum pick up, intracytoplasmic sperm injection and somatic cell nuclear transfer in cattle, buffalo and horses: from the research laboratory to clinical practice. Theriogenology 81: 138–151.

4

Efficacy of a Crosslinked Hyaluronic Acid-Based Hydrogel as a Tear Film Supplement: A Masked Controlled Study

David L. Williams[1]*, Brenda K. Mann[2,3]

1 Department of Veterinary Medicine, Cambridge University, Cambridge, United Kingdom, **2** SentrX Animal Care, Inc., Salt Lake City, Utah, United States of America,
3 Department of Bioengineering, University of Utah, Salt Lake City, Utah, United States of America

Abstract

Keratoconjunctivitis sicca (KCS), or dry eye, is a significant medical problem in both humans and dogs. Treating KCS often requires the daily application of more than one type of eye drop in order to both stimulate tear prodcution and provide a tear supplement to increase hydration and lubrication. A previous study demonstrated the potential for a crosslinked hyaluronic acid-based hydrogel (xCMHA-S) to reduce the clinical signs associated with KCS in dogs while using a reduced dosing regimen of only twice-daily administration. The present study extended those results by comparing the use of the xCMHA-S to a standard HA-containing tear supplement in a masked, randomized clinical study in dogs with a clinical diagnosis of KCS. The xCMHA-S was found to significantly improve ocular surface health (conjunctival hyperaemia, ocular irritation, and ocular discharge) to a greater degree than the alternative tear supplement ($P = 0.0003$). Further, owners reported the xCMHA-S treatment as being more highly effective than the alternative tear supplement ($P = 0.0024$). These results further demonstrate the efficacy of the xCMHA-S in reducing the clinical signs associated with KCS, thereby improving patient health and owner happiness.

Editor: Elisabeth Engel, 1Biomaterials for Regenerative Therapies Group, Institute for Bioengineering of Catalonia, Baldiri Reixac 15-21, Barcelona 08028, Spain, 2Technical University of Catalonia, Av. Diagonal 647, Barcelona 08028, Spain, 3CIBER-BBN, María de Luna 11, Zaragoza 50, Spain

Funding: The authors have no support or funding to report.

Competing Interests: B.K. Mann is employed by and owns stock in SentrX Animal Care where the hydrogel used in the study was developed. D.L. Williams has no competing interests.

* E-mail: dlw33@cam.ac.uk

Introduction

Dry eye or keratoconjunctivitis sicca (KCS), is a widespread problem in both the human and canine populations. The prevalence of KCS in humans may vary between 5 and 33%, in different reports and with different methods of ocular evaluation [1]. The prevalence in the canine species varies between 1 to 4% [2]. Topical cyclosporine has been developed as a widely efficacious lacrimogenic agent in dogs [3] and more recently in man, [4] but not all individuals in either affected population respond adequately to the drug by a higher rate of tear production. Also, the high price of the product puts it out of the financial reach of many dog owners. For these reasons an effective, less expensive tear replacement eyedrop is still required. Many of these are available as topical medications containing a wide number of lubricating agents, including polyacrylic acid, polyvinyl alcohol, and hyaluronic acid (HA) [2,5]. Since HA is a naturally occurring polysaccharide found as a lubricative agent in joint fluid, its use as a similar agent on the ocular surface is particularly appropriate [6,7]. For tear supplements containg HA, previous reports have shown that the viscoelasticity of the polysaccharide leads to an increase in tear stability and a consequent reduction in many of the symptoms of dry eye [8–10].

The viscoelasticity of HA-based products can vary significantly, depending on the molecular weight and concentration of the HA used, as well as the concentration of salts present due to interaction with the polyanionic HA [8,11,12]. Such variation in rheologic properties, such as viscoelasticity, can lead to differences in comfort and efficacy for a dry eye formulation [13]. Typical HA-based tear supplements have been a simple solution of high molecular weight, low concentration HA. However, by covalently crosslinking HA, such as the formulation documented herein, leads to a more viscoelastic material. This increase in viscoelasticity extends the contact time of the HA with the ocular surface and will thus allow for less frequent application, reducing the overall cost and burden on the patient, and in the case of dogs, the owner. The covalent HA crosslinking described here, acts in a different manner than the physical or ionic crosslinking occurring in solutions of simple high molecular weight HA.

The crosslinked modified HA, thiolated carboxymethyl HA (CMHA-S), used in the present study has previously been used in other formulations to treat skin and corneal wounds [14,15]. The hydrogel formulation used in this study was specifically developed as a tear supplement for the treatment of canine KCS. We have previously characterised the hydrogel rheologically to compare with non-crosslinked solutions of HA [16]. We also compared the ocular surface effects of this product to a previous study using a different tear replacement drop, evaluating tear production by use of the Schirmer tear test, conjunctival hyperaemia, ocular discharge and ocular irritation as determined by blink frequency and palpebral apperture narrowing [17]. Although the previous study demonstrated promising results, it was neither masked nor randomised, and the comparison of the products relied on two populations of KCS-affected dogs. Here we present the results of a study in which KCS-affected dogs were randomly assigned to treatment with either the CMHA-S product or a commercial tear replacement drop. Importantly, the medication was dispensed in such a manner that the investigator could not know which medication was being provided. Only after completion of the study and all assessments made following medication was the treatment regime for each dog unmasked, thus allowing a truly masked study. The statistical analyses of the data were also blinded in that statisticians were provided only "treatment one" and "treatment two" identification for each dog.

Materials and Methods

Crosslinked CMHA-S hydrogel

CMHA-S was synthesized and analyzed as previously described [15,16]. A CMHA-S solution was then filter-sterilized, crosslinked to form a hydrogel, and packaged aseptically into sterile 10-ml eye drop bottles as previously described [16].

Animals

The study was reviewed and accepted by the Ethics and Welfare Committee of the Department of Veterinary Medicine, University of Cambridge, Cambridge, UK and all animals were treated in accordance with the welfare guidelines in the Royal College of Veterinary Surgeons Guide to Professional Conduct.

Twenty dogs affected with KCS (as diagnosed clinically) and for whom treatment with topical cyclosporine (Optimmune, Schering-Plough UK) was either ineffective or not available for financial reasons were entered into the study with full informed owner consent. The gender, breed, and age of the dogs in the study is given in Table 1.

Clinical evaluation and treatment

All dogs underwent full clinical and ophthalmic examination using a direct and indirect ophthalmoscopy and slit lamp biomicroscopy. Tear production was measured using the Schirmer tear test and ocular surface health assessed with the clinical measurements of conjunctival hyperaemia, ocular discharge and ocular irritation, graded as absent (0), mild (1), moderate (2) or severe (3). Tear supplement, either the crosslinked modified HA product (xCMHA-S) or the HA-based iDrop® Vet Plus Eye Lubricant (ITRD; I-MED Animal Health), was dispensed without the investigator being made aware of the treatment given. Dogs were treated for three weeks before reassessment. Owners were requested to use the trial medication alone three times daily. On re-examination a full ophthalmic examination was undertaken with conjunctival hyperaemia, ocular discharge and ocular irritation assessed and graded as previously. Owners were asked for their own subjective assessment of whether the treatment given was effective in ameliorating their animal's ocular symptoms, rating this from not effective (0) to highly effective (3).

The number of dogs included in the study was determined by a power analysis [18]. Using a desired effect size (the difference in mean between the treatment groups) for the composite score of 2.5, a standard deviation of 1.9 (based on the previous prospective study [16]), a type I error of 0.05, and power of 0.8, a sample size needed for each treatment group was 10.

Table 1. Demographics and composite pre-treatment and post-treatment scores of ocular health for xCMHA-S and ITRD treatment of 10 dogs each.

Dog ID#	Breed	Age	Sex/neuter	Pre-score	Post-score
xCMHA-S Treatment					
601	Boxer	12	fn	6	1
606	WHWT	6	fn	14	5
608	JRT	11	fe	4	2
609	WHWT	12	fn	9	0
610	CKCS	9	fn	6	0
611	Shih Tzu	8	mn	4	0
614	ECS	12	fn	15	2
615	ACS	9	me	9	0
617	CKCS	10	fn	10	4
618	WHWT	12	fn	11	2
ITRD Treatment					
602	WHWT	7	fn	11	6
603	Lhasa Apso	8	me	6	3
604	CKCS	5	mn	9	4
605	CKCS	7	fn	9	3
607	X-bred	8	fn	8	3
612	X-bred	12	me	12	6
613	Labrador	10	fn	6	3
616	Lhasa Apso	8	fe	13	8
619	Cairn terrier	14	fe	14	6
620	ECS	9	mn	10	7

In Breed: WHWT = West Highland white terrier; JRT = Jack Russell terrier; CKCS = Cavalier King Charles spaniel; ECS = English cocker spaniel; ACS = American cocker spaniel; X-bred = mixed breed. In Gender: Fn = neutered female; Fe = unaltered female; Mn = neutered male; Me = unaltered male.

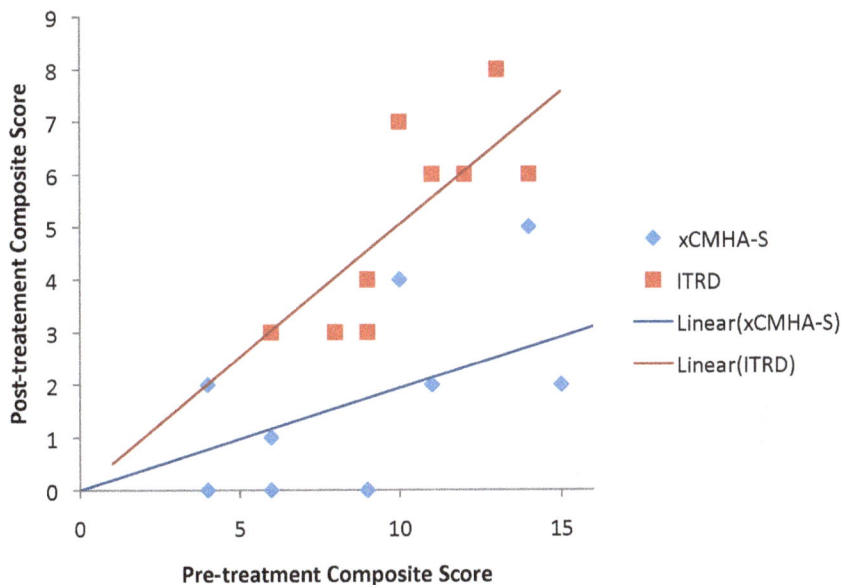

Figure 1. Composite score results. Post-treatment composite score plotted against pre-treatment composite score for xCMHA-S and ITRD treatments for all 20 dogs in the study. Note that for xCMHA-S, 2 dogs had a pre-treatment composite of 9 and post-treatment composite of 0; for ITRD, 2 dogs had a pre-treatment composite of 6 and post-treatment composite of 3. Lines indicate linear fits for each treatment.

Statistical analysis

The primary outcome was defined as the composite post-treatment score, as the sum of the six post-treatment scores for each dog (hyperaemia, irritation, and discharge for each eye). This score was compared with the composite pre-treatment score using an analysis of covariance (ANCOVA) with the post-treatment score as the dependent variable, treatment as the main effect and pre-treatment score as the covariate. The pre-treatment score was used as a covariate because dogs that started with low scores cannot improve to the same extent as can dogs starting with higher scores, and thus improvement depends to some degree on the pre-treatment scores. A two-tailed t-test was used to compare the average age of dogs in the two groups, as well as owner happiness after treatment for the two groups. As previously mentioned, statistical analyses were made with the statistician blinded to the treatment given.

Results

The treatment provided to each dog is shown in Table 1 together with composite pre-treatment and post-treatment scores. Dogs of a range of species were included with breeds predisposed to KCS such as West Highland White terriers, Lhasa Apsos, Shih Tzus, Cocker Spaniels and Cavalier King Charles spaniels predominating. The genders of the dogs were 7 female neutered animals, one entire bitch, one entire dog and one neutered dog in the xCHMA-S arm and 4 female neutered animals, two entire bitches, two entire dogs and one neutered dog in the ITRD arm of the study. The average age of dogs in the xCHMA-S arm (10.1±2.1 years) was not significantly different than in the ITRD arm (8.8±2.6 years) ($P = 0.23$).

Pre-treatment and post-treatment scores for STT, hyperaemia, irritation, and discharge for each dog are provided in Table 2, along with the owner happiness ratings at the end of the treatment period. Figure 1 shows the difference between pre-treatment and post-treatment composite scores for all dogs, demonstrating that xCHMA-S gives a substantially better resolution of KCS-associated ocular surface signs than does ITRD. The linear fits are forced through the origin, as no improvement is expected for cases with pre-scores of 0. For both treatments, the trends of the post-treatment scores are roughly proportional to the pre-treatment scores. There was no significant increase in STT following treatment with either xCMHA-S or ITRD (right eye: $P = 0.1773$ for both treatments; left eye: $P = 0.5086$ for xCMHA-S, 0.2695 for ITRD). Additionally, there was no significant difference between treatment groups for post-treatment STT, using pre-treatment STT as a covariate (right eye: $P = 0.9445$; left eye: $P = 0.6170$).

Table 3 provides the ANCOVA p-value for composite scores, showing that the coefficient for treatment, adjusted for pre-treatment scores, is highly significant ($P = 0.0003$). These results indicate that xCHMA-S treatment significantly improved composite ocular surface health compared to ITRD treatment. The adjustment for pre-score was also highly significant ($P = 0.0018$). The effects of age, sex, and neuter status were also tested, but were not found to be significant ($P = 0.4405$, 0.6298, and 0.3841, respectively). Additionally, a test of the slopes in Figure 1 indicated that they were highly significantly different ($P = 0.00006$). The post-scores for ITRD treatment were higher than the post-scores for xCMHA-S treatment, despite accounting for differences in pre-scores between the two treatments.

ANCOVA analysis was performed on each of the six assessment criteria as well, and the resulting P-values are also shown in Table 3. Conjunctival hyperaemia and degree of irritation show statistically significantly greater improvement with xCMHA-S treatment than ITRD treatment, although the degree of irritation result for the right eye is not significant with the Bonferroni adjustment for multiple testing. The amount of discharge was not significantly different, likely because it is a much more variable clinical sign than conjunctival hyperaemia or ocular irritation. In fact, several dogs had low discharge scores pre-treatment in both groups, leading to this non-significant difference. The eyes are shown separately since conflating the results in eyes in which

Table 2. STT values and scores of ocular health pre- and post-treatment, and owner happiness post-treatment with xCMHA-S or ITRD.

Dog ID#	STT pre (mm/min)	STT post (mm/min)	Hyperaemia pre	Hyperaemia post	Irritation pre	Irritation post	Discharge pre	Discharge post	Owner happiness
xCMHA-S Treatment									
601	3/11	5/12	3/0	1/0	2/0	0/0	1/0	0/0	3
606	0/1	0/2	3/3	1/0	2/2	1/1	3/1	1/1	3
608	5/5	6/4	2/2	1/0	0/0	1/0	0/0	0/0	2
609	6/4	6/5	2/2	0/0	2/1	0/0	1/1	0/0	3
610	7/5	6/6	2/1	0/0	2/1	0/0	0/0	0/0	3
611	8/9	10/8	1/1	0/0	0/0	0/0	1/1	0/0	2
614	0/0	0/0	3/3	0/1	2/2	0/0	3/2	1/0	3
615	3/3	2/2	2/2	0/0	1/1	0/0	2/1	0/0	3
617	4/3	5/4	2/2	0/0	2/2	1/1	1/1	1/1	3
618	0/1	1/1	2/2	0/0	2/2	0/0	2/1	1/1	3
Mean ± SD	3.60±2.95/4.20±3.52	4.10±3.25/4.40±3.60	2.20±0.63/1.80±0.92	0.30±0.48/0.10±0.32	1.50±0.85/1.10±0.88	0.30±0.48/0.20±0.42	1.40±1.07/0.80±0.63	0.40±0.52/0.30±0.48	2.80±0.42
ITRD Treatment									
602	1/1	3/1	3/3	1/1	1/1	1/1	1/2	1/1	1
603	3/4	5/4	1/1	0/1	2/1	1/1	1/0	0/0	2
604	5/3	6/2	1/2	1/1	2/2	1/1	1/1	0/0	1
605	4/4	3/5	2/2	1/1	2/1	0/1	1/1	0/0	2
607	4/4	4/5	1/1	0/0	1/1	0/1	2/2	1/1	2
612	0/0	0/0	3/3	1/1	1/1	1/1	2/2	1/1	3
613	0/16	0/18	3/0	1/0	3/0	1/0	0/0	1/0	3
616	2/1	1/3	3/3	2/2	1/2	1/1	2/2	1/1	1
619	2/2	3/2	3/3	1/1	2/2	1/1	2/2	1/1	2
620	4/3	5/2	2/2	1/1	2/2	2/1	1/1	1/1	1
Mean ± SD	2.50±1.78/3.80±4.52	3.00±2.11/4.20±5.12	2.20±0.92/2.00±1.05	0.90±0.57/0.90±0.57	1.70±0.67/1.30±0.67	0.90±0.57/0.90±0.32	1.30±0.67/1.30±0.82	0.70±0.48/0.60±0.52	1.80±0.79

STT = Schirmer tear test; values given are for right eye/left eye. Scores given for hyperaemia, irritation, and discharge are for right eye/left eye and indicate: absent (0), mild (1), moderate (2), or severe (3). Owner happiness scores were rated from not effective (0) to highly effective (3).

Table 3. Results of ANCOVAs for composite scores and individual assessments.

Assessment	P-value
Composite score	0.0003
Conjunctival hyperaemia (right)	0.0060
Conjunctival hyperaemia (left)	0.0003
Degree of irritation (right)	0.0261
Degree of irritation (left)	0.0002
Amount of discharge (right)	0.1094
Amount of discharge (left)	0.6093

The p-value provided compares the xCMHA-S treatment to the ITRD treatment, with post-treatment score as the dependent variable, treatment as the main effect, and pre-treatment score as the covariate.

clinical signs are likely to be correlated would give inappropriately elevated degrees of significance [19].

Owner happiness with the results of treatment was significantly higher with xCHMA-S treatment than with ITRD ($P = 0.0024$). For xCMHA-S treatment, the average score was 2.8 ± 0.4, with eight of the 10 owners rating the treatment as highly effective (score of 3). For ITRD treatment, the average score was 1.8 ± 0.8, with only two of the 10 owners rating the treatment as highly effective.

Discussion

Treatment for dry eye (KCS) can be taxing, whether in canine patients or humans. The advent of topical cyclosporine has substantially improved the lot of individuals in which this treatment is effective, but there are dogs in which the medication does not have the desired lacrimomimetic effects and for many owners the drug is too expensive, given as it must be used for the lifetime of the animal. Yet regular treatment with topical tear replacers can be difficult for owner and pet, and for human patients also.

In a previous study we reported the use of a crosslinked HA-based hydrogel as a tear supplement in a clinical study of 25 dogs with KCS [16]. Although the study demonstrated the potential for the xCMHA-S to reduce the clinical signs associated with KCS, the study was not masked or randomized. Thus, here we

conducted a masked, randomized study comparing the xCMHA-S hydrogel and a standard tear replacement eye drop containing HA.

The results show a statistically significantly better therapeutic efficacy, based on ocular surface health, with the xCMHA-S gel applied three times daily than with the standard tear replacement drop. ANCOVA analysis was necessary here, with the pre-treatment score as a covariate, since the pre-treatment score will affect the degree to which the score can improve. Because the pre-treatment score estimate is not equal to 1.0, it underlines the idea that the treatment cannot have the same effect if a component of the composite pre-treatment score is coded as 0 as it can if that component is coded 3.

Although ocular surface health was improved, there was no significant improvement in STT value with either treatment. This was expected since both types of drops are merely tear supplements and do not stimulate the production of tears [16]. Additionally, owners were happier with the outcome of using the xCMHA-S gel compared to the standard tear replacement drop. Since this clinical study involved canine patients, it was not possible to assess any potential disruption in vision due to the increased viscosity of the xCMHA-S gel compared to the ITRD drops. However, if the owners had observed any vision issues, it is likely that the owner happiness scores would have been lower.

These findings have important implications for the canine population where an effective ocular surface lubricant will be welcomed by owners and canine patients alike. This crosslinked CMHA-S hydrogel may have potential translational importance as well, as an effective tear replacement drop with a long ocular surface residence time and thus a low required dose frequency would be highly valuable for the sizeable population of humans with dry eye.

Acknowledgments

The authors would like to thank Barbara Thomson and Professor David Andrews of Thomson Data Analysis (Toronto, Canada) for their assistance with the statistical analysis.

Author Contributions

Conceived and designed the experiments: DLW BKM. Performed the experiments: DLW. Analyzed the data: DLW BKM. Contributed reagents/materials/analysis tools: DLW BKM. Wrote the paper: DLW BKM.

References

1. Smith JA (2007) The epidemiology of dry eye disease: Report of the epidemiology subcommittee of the International Dry Eye Work Shop (2007). Ocul Surf 5: 93–107.
2. Williams DL (2008) Immunopathogenesis of keratoconjunctivitis sicca in the dog. Vet Clin North Am Small Anim Pract 38: 251–268.
3. Kaswan RL, Salisbury MA, Ward DA (1989) Spontaneous canine keratoconjunctivitis sicca. A useful model for human keratoconjunctivitis sicca: treatment with cyclosporine eye drops. Arch Ophthalmol 107: 1210–1216.
4. Stonecipher K, Perry HD, Gross RH, Kerney DL (2005) The impact of topical cyclosporine A emulsion 0.05% on the outcomes of patients with keratoconjunctivitis sicca. Curr Med Res Opin. 21: 1057–1063.
5. Bron AJ, Mangat H, Quinlan M, Foley-Nolan A, Eustace P, et al. (1998) Polyacrylic acid gel in patients with dry eyes: a randomised comparison with polyvinyl alcohol. Eur J Ophthalmol 8: 81–89.
6. Barbucci R, Lamponi S, Borzacchiello A, Ambrosio L, Fini M, et al. (2002) Hyaluronic acid hydrogel in the treatment of osteoarthritis. Biomaterials 23: 4503–4513.
7. Rah MJ (2011) A review of hyaluronan and its ophthalmic applications. Optometry 82: 38–43.
8. Kobayashi Y, Okamoto A, Nishinari K (1994) Viscoelasticity of hyaluronic acid with different molecular weights. Biorheology 31: 235–244.
9. Hamano T, Horimoto K, Lee M, Komemushi S (1996) Sodium hyaluronate eyedrops enhance tear film stability. Jpn J Ophthalmol 40: 62–65.
10. Guillaumie F, Furrer P, Felt-Baeyens O, Fuhlendorff BL, Nymand S, et al. (2010) Comparative studies of various hyaluronic acids produced by microbial fermentation for potential topical ophthalmic applications. J Biomed Mater Res Part A 92A: 1421–1430.
11. Gibbs DA, Merrill EW, Smith KA, Balazs EA (1968) Rheology of hyaluronic acid. Biopolymers 6: 777–791.
12. Higashide T, Sugiyama K (2008) Use of viscoelastic substance in ophthalmic surgery – focus on sodium hyaluronate. Clin Ophthalmol 2: 21–30.
13. Nakamura S, Okada S, Umeda Y, Saito F (2004) Development of a rabbit model of tear film instability and evaluation of viscosity of artificial tear preparations. Cornea 23: 390–397.
14. Yang G, Prestwich GD, Mann BK (2011) Thiolated carboxymethyl hyaluronic acid-based biomaterials enhance wound healing in rats, dogs, and horses. ISRN Vet Sci Article ID 851593: 1-7. Available: http://www.hindawi.com/isrn/veterinary.science/2011/851593/. Accessed 20 February 2014.
15. Yang G, Espandar L, Mamalis N, Prestwich GD (2010) A crosslinked hyaluronan gel accelerate healing of corneal epithelial abrasion and alkali burn injuries in rabbits. Vet Ophthalmol 13: 144–150.

16. Williams DL, Mann BK (2013) A crosslinked HA-based hydrogel ameliorates dry eye symptoms in dogs. Int J Biomater Article ID 460437. Available: http://www.hindawi.com/journals/ijbm/2013/460437/. Accessed 20 February 2014.

17. Williams DL, Middleton S, Fattahian H, Moridpour R (2012) Comparison of hyaluronic acid-containing topical eye drops with carbomer-based topical ocular gel as a tear replacement in canine keratoconjunctivitis sicca; a prospective study in twenty-five dogs. Vet Res Forum 3: 229–232.

18. Festing MF, Altman DG (2002) Guidelines for the design and statistical analysis of experiments using laboratory animals. ILAR J 43: 244–258.

19. Newcombe RG, Duff GR (1987) Eyes or patients? Traps for the unwary in the statistical analysis of ophthalmological studies. Br J Ophthalmol 71: 645–646.

5

Long-Term Health Effects of Neutering Dogs: Comparison of Labrador Retrievers with Golden Retrievers

Benjamin L. Hart[1]*, Lynette A. Hart[2], Abigail P. Thigpen[2], Neil H. Willits[3]

1 Department of Anatomy, Physiology and Cell Biology, School of Veterinary Medicine, University of California Davis, Davis, California, United States of America,
2 Department of Population Health and Reproduction, School of Veterinary Medicine, University of California Davis, Davis, California, United States of America,
3 Department of Statistics, University of California Davis, Davis, California, United States of America

Abstract

Our recent study on the effects of neutering (including spaying) in Golden Retrievers in markedly increasing the incidence of two joint disorders and three cancers prompted this study and a comparison of Golden and Labrador Retrievers. Veterinary hospital records were examined over a 13-year period for the effects of neutering during specified age ranges: before 6 mo., and during 6–11 mo., year 1 or years 2 through 8. The joint disorders examined were hip dysplasia, cranial cruciate ligament tear and elbow dysplasia. The cancers examined were lymphosarcoma, hemangiosarcoma, mast cell tumor, and mammary cancer. The results for the Golden Retriever were similar to the previous study, but there were notable differences between breeds. In Labrador Retrievers, where about 5 percent of gonadally intact males and females had one or more joint disorders, neutering at <6 mo. doubled the incidence of one or more joint disorders in both sexes. In male and female Golden Retrievers, with the same 5 percent rate of joint disorders in intact dogs, neutering at <6 mo. increased the incidence of a joint disorder to 4–5 times that of intact dogs. The incidence of one or more cancers in female Labrador Retrievers increased slightly above the 3 percent level of intact females with neutering. In contrast, in female Golden Retrievers, with the same 3 percent rate of one or more cancers in intact females, neutering at all periods through 8 years of age increased the rate of at least one of the cancers by 3–4 times. In male Golden and Labrador Retrievers neutering had relatively minor effects in increasing the occurrence of cancers. Comparisons of cancers in the two breeds suggest that the occurrence of cancers in female Golden Retrievers is a reflection of particular vulnerability to gonadal hormone removal.

Editor: Roger A. Coulombe, Utah State University, United States of America

Funding: This work was supported by the Canine Health Foundation (#01488-A) and the Center for Companion Animal Health University of California, Davis (# 2009-54-F/M). The funders had no role in study design, data collection and analysis, decision to publish, or preparation of the manuscript.

Competing Interests: The authors have declared that no competing interests exist.

* Email: blhart@ucdavis.edu

Introduction

In the last three decades, the practice of spaying female dogs and castrating males (both referred to herein as neutering) has greatly increased. The current estimate is that in the U.S., 83 percent of all dogs are neutered [1] and, increasingly, neutering is being performed prior to 6 mo., as advocated by many veterinarians and animal activists. The impetus for this widespread practice is presumably pet population control, and the belief that mammary gland and prostate cancers are prevented and aggressive male behavior is markedly less likely than in those neutered later. This societal practice in the U.S. continues to contrast with the general attitudes in many European countries, where neutering is commonly avoided and not promoted by animal health authorities [2–4].

In the last decade or so, studies have pointed to some of the adverse effects of neutering in dogs on several long-term health parameters by looking at one disease syndrome in one breed or in pooling data from several breeds. With regard to cancers, a study on osteosarcoma (OSA) in several breeds found a 2-fold increase in neutered dogs relative to intact dogs [5], and in Rottweilers neutering prior to 1 year of age was associated with an increased occurrence of OSA to 3–4 times that of intact dogs [6].

A study of cardiac hemangiosarcoma (HSA) in spayed females found that the incidence of this cancer was 4 times greater than that of intact females [7] and another on splenic HSA in spayed females found rates 2 times greater than of intact females [8]. A study on lymphosarcoma (lymphoma, LSA) found that neutered females had a higher incidence of the disease than intact females [9]. Cutaneous mast cell tumors (MCT) were studied in several dog breeds revealing an increase in incidence in neutered females to 4 times that of intact females [10]. Another cancer of concern is prostate cancer that, in contrast to humans, is potentiated by the removal of testosterone. One extensive study found that this cancer occurred in neutered males 4 times as frequently as in intact males [11].

The most frequently mentioned advantage of early neutering of female dogs is protection against mammary cancer (MC) [12]. However, a recent meta-analysis of published studies on neutering females and MC found that the evidence linking neutering to a reduced risk of MC is weak [13].

Three very recent studies are particularly relevant in the discussion of neutering and cancers. One was a comprehensive study, from this center, on neutering in 759 Golden Retrievers where males were compared with females and effects of neutering were evaluated in early-neutered (<1 year), late-neutered (>1 year) and intact dogs [14]. Almost 10 percent of early-neutered males were diagnosed with LSA, 3 times more than intact males. There were no cases of MCT in intact females, but in late-neutered females the rate was nearly 6 percent. The incidence of HSA in late-neutered females was also higher than that of intact females. The occurrence of MC was very low and was only seen in a couple of late-neutered females.

A study utilizing the Veterinary Medical Database of over 40,000 dogs found that neutered males and females were more likely to die of cancer than intact dogs, especially of OSA, LSA and MCT [15]. This study included no information on age of neutering. The most recent publication in this area is a study of Vizslas utilizing owner-reported disease occurrence in an online survey, in which the incidence of cancers was reported higher in neutered dogs than in intact dogs [16]. The main cancers related to neutering were LSA, HSA and MCT. The occurrence of MC was very low in females left intact.

With regard to joint disorders, one study of effects of neutering in larger breeds documents a 3-fold increase in excessive tibial plateau angle – a known risk factor for development of cranial cruciate ligament tears or rupture (CCL) [17]. Across several breeds, a study of CCL found that neutered males and females were 2 to 3 times more likely than intact dogs to have this disorder [18]. Neither study examined early versus late neutering with regard to this disorder. The study from this center of neutering in Golden Retrievers (mentioned above with regard to cancers [14]) included examination of joint disorders. Of the early-neutered males, 10 percent were diagnosed with hip dysplasia (HD), double the occurrence of that in intact males. There were no cases of CCL diagnosed in intact males or females, but in early-neutered males and females the occurrences were 5 percent and 8 percent, respectively.

One factor that merits attention with regard to the effects of neutering on joint disorders relates to documented effects of neutering in increasing body weight [19], as reflected in body condition score (BCS). Additional weight on the joints is considered to play a role in the onset of joint disorders [19,20]. While neutering is expected to increase BCS, the issue of concern here is whether neutered dogs with a joint disorder have consistently higher BCSs at the time of diagnosis than do neutered dogs without the joint disorder in the same age range. In the previous analyses on Goldens [14] there was no consistent and major difference in BCS between early neutered dogs with and without a joint disorder. For dogs diagnosed with a joint disorder, some increase in BCS would be expected as a function of less activity due to discomfort from painful joints. Therefore, a modestly higher BCS was predicted for neutered dogs with a joint disorder than in the neutered counterparts without a joint disorder.

The above study on Golden Retrievers [14] raised a major question about breed differences in the effects of neutering, which are relevant for breeders and caregivers of puppies when deciding if, and when, to neuter. A more basic issue concerns insights into the possible pathogenic factors triggering the occurrence of the cancers under consideration. The present study, using the same veterinary hospital database, explored the effects of neutering on joint disorders and cancers in the popular Labrador Retriever to compare with the Golden Retriever, with an addition of several years to the database. The age periods of neutering were refined as

<6 mo., 6–11 mo., 12–23 mo. (1 year), and 2 through 8 years to provide more detailed information on the effects of gonadal hormone removal. The Golden is known for being particularly vulnerable to cancers [21], so we expected some major differences from the Labrador where cancer-related deaths are less frequent than in Goldens [21].

In addition to reporting on the incidence of the individual joint disorders and cancers, a new slant on analyses in the present study combined the incidence of all three joint disorders that have shown evidence of being increased by neutering (HD, CCL, and elbow dysplasia, ED) for one data-point representing the incidence of dogs diagnosed with at least one of the joint disorders, after controlling for multiple diagnoses. This analysis was based on the perspective that for dog owners or breeders, avoidance of any of the debilitating joint disorders would be of prime interest. This analysis was also deemed logical for pathophysiological reasons because a disruption of the growth plate closure by gonadal hormone removal in the joint developmental stage would be expected to apply to all the joint disorders. The study also combined the incidence of dogs diagnosed with at least one of the cancers (LSA, HSA, MCT) for one data point, after controlling for multiple diagnoses, because for dog owners avoidance of any of the cancers would be important. This analysis seemed logical, as there may be a common factor involved in increasing these three particular cancers in neutered dogs because these cancers are repeatedly reported as being increased by neutering in several studies.

Methods

Ethics Statement

No animal care and use committee approval was required because, in conformity with campus policy, the only data used were from retrospective veterinary hospital records. Upon approval, faculty from the University of California, Davis (UCD), School of Veterinary Medicine, are allowed use of the record system for research purposes by the Veterinary Medical Teaching Hospital (VMTH). The co-authors of this study were given permission by the VMTH to use their veterinary hospital records for this study.

Data Collection

The dataset used in this study was obtained from the computerized hospital record system (Veterinary Medical and Administrative Computer System) of the Veterinary Medical Teaching Hospital (VMTH) at UCD. The subjects included were gonadally intact and neutered female and male Labrador Retrievers and Golden Retrievers, from 1 through 8 years of age and admitted to the hospital between January 1, 2000 and December 31, 2012, for 13 years of data. If a disease of interest occurred before 12 months of age or before January 1, 2000, that case was removed for that specific disease analysis, but included in other disease analyses.

Data on patients at 9 years of age or older were not considered. This was deemed an appropriate cut-off point in order to exclude disease information on advanced-aged dogs where the effects of aging would confound interpreting the disease effects related to neutering. Additional inclusion criteria were requirements for information on date of birth, age at neutering (if neutered) and age of diagnosis (or onset of clinical signs) of the joint disorder or cancer. The age at neutering was classified as <6 mo., 6–11 mo., 1 year (12 - <24 mo.), and 2–8 years (2 - <9 years). For all neutered dogs, the neuter status at the time of each visit was reviewed to ensure that neutering occurred prior to onset of the first clinical signs or diagnosis of any disease of interest. If a disease of interest occurred before neutering, the diseased dog was recorded as intact for that specific disease analysis. For the same dog where a different disease occurred after neutering, the dog was recorded as neutered for that disease analysis. Detailed reviews of patient records were performed for evidence of disease occurrence meeting specific diagnostic criteria (see below). Using this screening, only diseases with at least 15 cases in the database were included in the study.

For both breeds, many cases with neutering did not include detailed data on age at neutering. With a very large database for the Labrador, there was a sufficient number of dogs with these data to restrict the analyses to cases for which the age at time of neutering was available from the record system. For the Golden with fewer cases, where additional neutering date information was necessary, telephone calls to the referring veterinarians were made to obtain the neutering dates for case patients born after 2000. Because of the number of neutered dogs where age at neutering was not available from either the record or by phone call, there were proportionately more intact cases in the final data set than would be expected in the population at large.

Golden Retriever cases with complete data for analyses totaled 1,015, with 543 males (315 neutered and 228 intact) and 472 females (306 neutered and 166 intact). Labrador Retriever cases with complete data for analyses totaled 1,500 cases with 808 males (272 neutered and 536 intact) and 692 females (347 neutered and 345 intact). The number of cases analyzed for each disease varied somewhat among diseases because a case could be excluded for one disease analysis, if the diagnosis was made prior to 1 year of age, was unconfirmed, or was outside of study range, but would be included for other diseases if no diagnosis was made or where the diagnoses were confirmed after 1 year of age and within the study range.

Table 1 defines the categories of diagnoses based on information in the record of each case. A patient was considered as having a disease of interest if the diagnosis was made at the VMTH or by a referring veterinarian and later confirmed at the VMTH. Patients diagnosed with HD, ED and/or CCL presented with clinical signs such as difficulty moving, standing up, lameness, and/or joint pain; diagnoses were confirmed with radiographic evidence, orthopedic physical examination and/or surgical confirmation. Diagnoses of the various cancers (LSA, HSA, MCT, MC) were accompanied by clinical signs such as enlarged lymph nodes, lumps on the skin or presence of masses, and confirmed by imaging, appropriate blood cell analyses, chemical panels, histopathology and/or cytology. Pyometra was confirmed by ultrasonic evidence and/or post-surgically after removal of the uterus. When a diagnosis was listed in the record as "suspected" based on clinical signs, but the diagnostic tests were inconclusive, the case was excluded from the analysis for that specific disease, but included for other diseases.

The analyses used in Figures 1 and 2 portray single data-points representing the incidence of dogs diagnosed with at least one joint disorder or at least one cancer, after controlling for multiple diagnoses. The data for incidence of individual joint disorders and cancers are presented in Tables 2 through 5.

Given that body weights are difficult to compare among dogs because of the confounding factor of variations in body height, BCSs were used. The BCS system used by the VMTH is the standard 1–9 range where a score of 5 is the goal [22]. Typically, the clinician assigns the BCS at the time of a patient's visit to the hospital. For this study the BCSs at the time of diagnosis (or clinical signs) of neutered dogs with joint disorders were compared with BCSs of neutered dogs without the disorder at an age that fell within the range representing 80 percent of the ages of dogs with the disorder at the time of diagnosis. The BCSs were compared between neutered dogs with and without joint disorders for the disorders that were significantly increased in incidence over that of intact dogs and for just the neuter periods where there were such differences. For the few joint disorders associated with neutering at one year or beyond, the BCSs were not included for comparison to maintain uniformity across comparisons. The data are represented as medians to reduce the impact of outliers.

Statistical Analyses

While the study set out to estimate incidence rates of each disease related to age at neutering, patients were diagnosed at different ages and with differing durations of the disease as well as varying years at risk from the effects of gonadal hormone removal. Cox proportional hazard models (CPH) [23,24] were used to test for group differences with respect to the hazard of a disease while adjusting for the time of neutering and the animal's age at diagnosis. All analyses were run using the SAS software package, version 9.3. Post hoc comparisons among the subgroups were based on least squares means of the hazard within each subgroup. In the Results section the p-values were based on these proportional hazard models. For all statistical tests the two-tailed statistical level of significance was set at $p < 0.05$.

Data Availability

In compliance with journal policy the final dataset used for statistical analyses, with the client information removed for confidentiality, is publically available at figshare.com: http://dx.doi.org/10.6084/m9.figshare.1038819.

Results

With regard to joint disorders and cancers, the incidence rates at various neuter ages were much more pronounced in the Golden Retrievers than in the Labrador Retrievers. Therefore, results will be presented first for the Golden, and then the Labrador, with the two breeds contrasted. For joint disorders, BCSs are reported for those that differed significantly from the intact dogs, only for the neuter periods where the differences occurred. The mean age of diagnosis of joint disorders and cancers for each sex and breed is given to the nearest 0.5 years.

Golden Retriever Males: Joint Disorders

Figure 1-A presents the incidence of dogs having at least one of the joint disorders. The incidence of at least one joint disorder occurring in intact males was 5 percent. At neuter age <6 mo., at least one of the joint disorders occurred in 27 percent of the males, or five times the incidence of intact males ($p < 0.0001$). At neuter age 6–11 mo., this incidence was 14 percent or almost three times that of intact males ($p < 0.005$). In the 2–8 year neutering period there was a moderate rise in this measure to double that of intact males ($p = 0.02$).

As shown in Figure 1-A and in Table 2, the main joint disorder related to neutering in males was HD, which was significantly higher than that of intact males for the <6 mo. and 6–11 mo. neuter periods ($p < 0.001$; $p < 0.05$, respectively). The mean age of diagnosis of HD in males was 4 years. The other important joint disorder was CCL, which was never diagnosed in intact males, and was significantly higher than intact males in the <6 mo. and 6–11 mo. neuter periods ($p < 0.001$; $p = 0.004$, respectively). The mean age of diagnosis of this joint disorder in males was 5 years. In this breed the occurrence of ED was relatively minor compared with the other joint disorders and not significantly above that of

Table 1. Categories used in determining diagnosis for joint disorders and cancers of interest in Golden Retrievers and Labrador Retrievers (1–8 years old) admitted to the Veterinary Medical Hospital, University of California, Davis, from 2000–2012.

Classification	Definition
No disease	No evidence of a joint disorder or cancer of interest in the medical records
VMTH	Diagnosed at the VMTH
Referring Veterinarian/VMTH	Diagnosed by referring veterinarian and confirmed at the VMTH through treatment or further testing
Referring Veterinarian	Diagnosed by referring veterinarian but no confirming diagnostic tests done at the VMTH. Unconfirmed cases were excluded from analysis for the specific joint disorder or cancer
Invalid (suspected)	Diagnosis was suspected based on clinical signs, but diagnostic tests were inconclusive or not done. Unconfirmed cases were excluded from analysis for the suspected joint disorder or cancer
Invalid (confirmed)	Diagnosed prior to January 2000 or before 1 year of age. Invalid cases were excluded from analysis for the specific joint disorder or cancer.

intact males for any neuter period. When it did occur, mean age of diagnosis of ED was 2.5 years.

The median BCS of neutered males with HD was 6.0, and the median BCS of neutered males without HD was 5.5. In intact males with and without HD the median BCS was 5. For neutered males with CCL, the median BCS was 5.5 and for neutered males without CCL, 6.0. In intact males without CCL the median BCS was 5.0.

Golden Retriever Males: Cancers

Figure 2-A presents the incidence in dogs having at least one of the cancers followed. The level in the intact males was 11 percent. At neuter ages <6 mo. and 6–11 mo. the occurrence of one or more cancers was 15–17 percent, but not significantly different than intact males. However, as Table 3 reveals, the main cancer elevated by neutering in males, LSA, reached 11.5 percent at the 6–11 mo. period, significantly higher than the 4 percent level of intact males ($p = 0.007$). The mean age of diagnosis of LSA in males was 5.5 years.

Golden Retriever Females: Joint Disorders

Figure 1-A portrays the incidence of dogs having at least one of the joint disorders at different neuter periods. The incidence of at least one joint disorder occurring in intact females was 5 percent, virtually the same as males. At neuter age <6 mo. at least one of the joint disorders occurred in 20 percent of dogs, four times that of the intact females ($p<0.001$). At the 6–11 mo. neuter age, 13 percent had at least one joint disorder, which was over twice that of intact females, but did not reach significance.

As shown in Table 2, the main joint disorders related to neutering females at the <6 mo. period were HD and CCL, occurring at 10–11 percent. The occurrence of HD did not reach significance compared with intact females (4 percent), but CCL, which was not seen in any of the intact females, was significantly higher at the <6 mo., 6–11 mo. and 2–8 year neuter periods ($p< 0.001$ to $p = 0.03$). The mean age of diagnosis of CCL in females was 5.5 years. As with males, the occurrence of ED in neutered females was not significant over that of intact females. The mean age of diagnosis of ED in females, when it did occur, was 1.5 years.

The median BCS of neutered females with CCL was 6.0 and the median BCS of the neutered females without CCL was 5.5. In intact females without CCL the median BCS was 5.0.

Golden Retriever Females: Cancers

Figure 2-A presents the incidence of females having at least one of the cancers where the incidence of cancers in intact females was just 3 percent. The increase in cancers over all the neuter periods ranged from 8 to 14 percent. Combining all of the neuter periods beyond 6 mo. (to have a larger data set for analyses), the elevated incidence level across all these neuter periods was significantly higher than that of intact females ($p = 0.049$). The results reveal that neutering through 8 years of age increases the risk of acquiring at least one of the cancers to a level 3–4 times that of leaving the female dog intact.

Examination of Table 3 shows that the main cancer resulting from neutering females at <6 mo. and 6–11 mo. was LSA where at 6–11 mo. the increased risk over that of intact females reached significance ($p = 0.014$). The mean age of diagnosis of LSA in females was 5.5 years. The main cancer that was increased at the 2–8 year period of neutering was MCT ($p = 0.013$). The occurrence of HSA, although increased by neutering beyond 1 year, did not reach significance over intact females. The mean age of diagnosis of both MCT and HSA in females was 6.5 years.

The occurrence of MC was not seen in any of the intact females. This cancer was seen only in dogs neutered in the 2–8 year period where the incidence was 3.5 percent. The occurrence of pyometra in intact females was 1.8 percent, which was diagnosed at the mean age of 6 years.

Labrador Retriever Males: Joint Disorders

Figure 1-B illustrates the incidence of males having at least one of the joint disorders. The only neuter period where this measure was significantly increased above the 5 percent level of intact males, was at <6 mo., where this measure was 12.5 percent ($p = 0.014$). Examining the joint disorders individually (Table 4), HD was not increased by neutering at any time. However, at the <6 mo. neuter period, both CCL and ED were significantly increased over that of intact males ($p = 0.02$; 0.02). For ED, there was a moderate increased risk with the 2–8 year neuter period to about 2 percent compared with the low 0.57 percent incidence in intact males ($p = 0.006$). The mean age of diagnosis of ED in males was 3 years, considerably less than that for CCL, which was 4.5 years.

The median BCS of neutered males with CCL was 6.0 and the median BCS of the neutered males without CCL was 5.0. In intact males with CCL the median BCS was 6.0 and for intact males without CCL the median BCS was 5. The median BCS of neutered males with ED was 6.5 and the median BCS of the neutered males without ED was 5.0. In intact males with and without ED the BCS was 5.0.

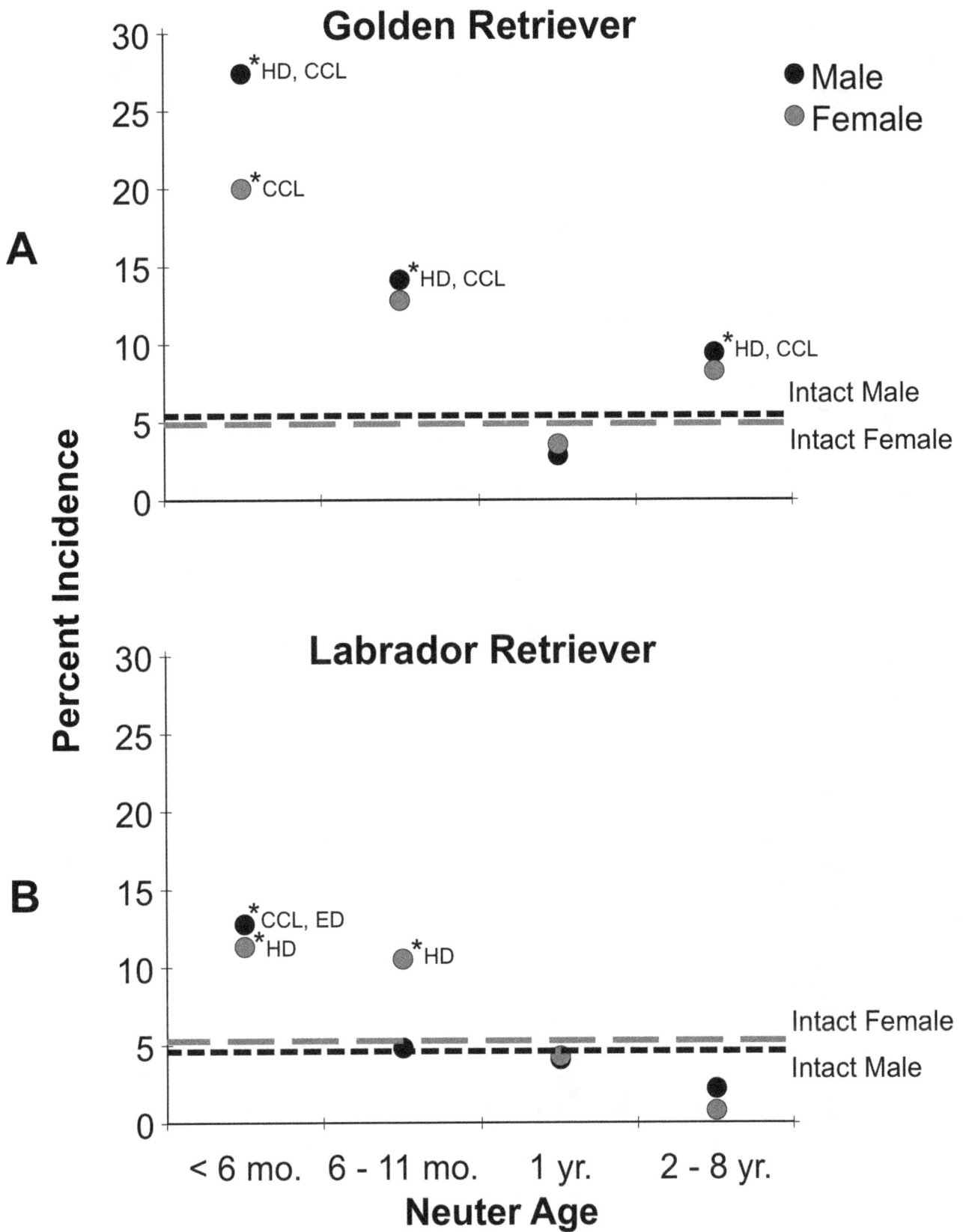

Figure 1. Incidence of the occurrence of at least one joint disorder in male and female Golden Retrievers (top) and Labrador Retrievers (bottom), as a function of age at neutering. The occurrences in intact males and females for the same measure are shown by the horizontal lines. The asterisks indicate significance from the intact level, and the abbreviations reveal the joint disorders contributing to the dots when significant.

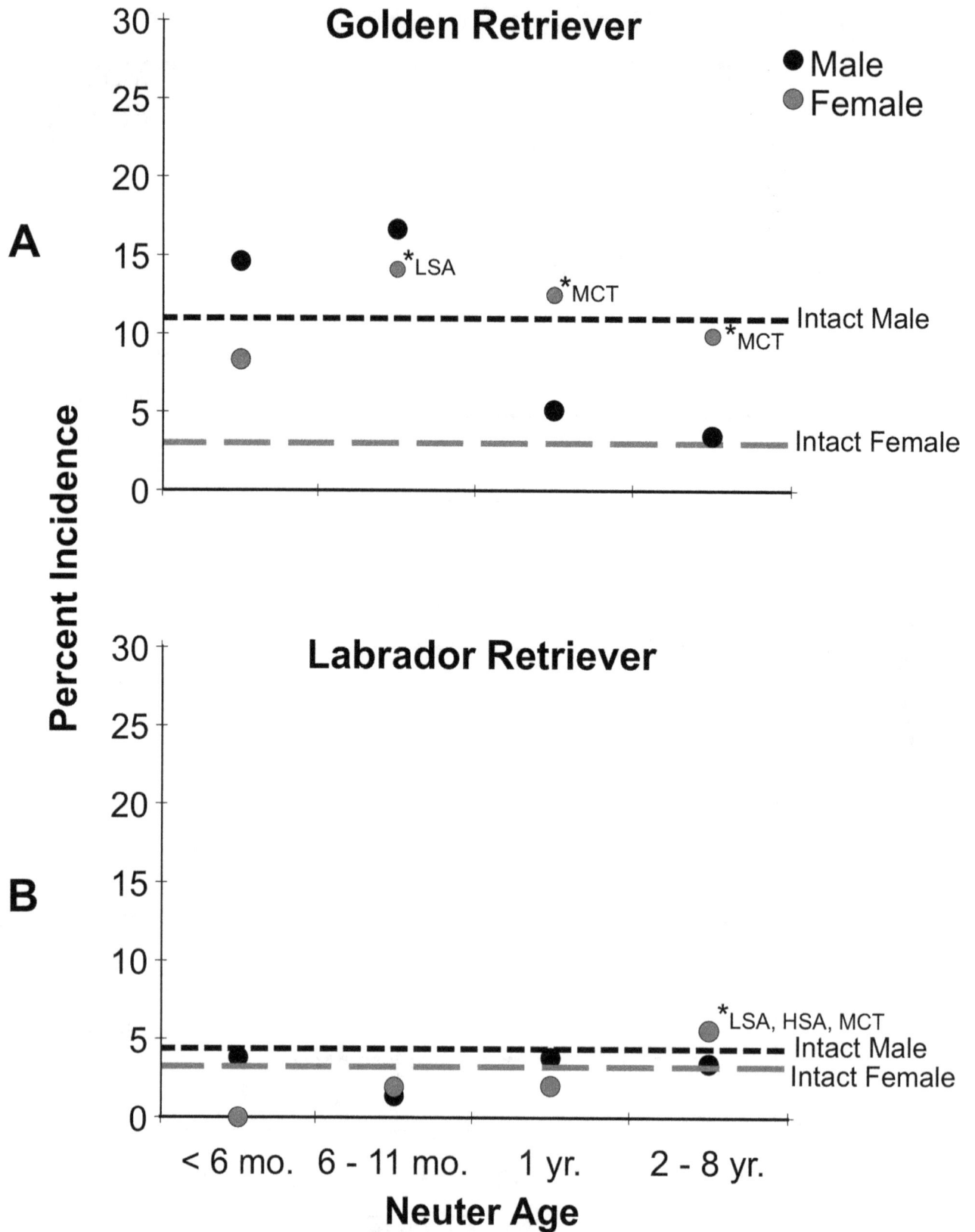

Figure 2. Incidence of the occurrence of at least one cancer in male and female Golden Retrievers (top) and Labrador Retrievers (bottom), as a function of age at neutering. The occurrences in intact males and females for the same measures are shown by the horizontal lines. The asterisks indicate significance from the intact level, and the abbreviations reveal the cancers contributing to the dots when significant.

Table 2. Golden Retriever males and females, joint disorders.

	HD	CCL	ED
Male <6 months	**11/75 (14.67)**	**8/89 (8.99)**	5/84 (5.95)
Male 6–11 months	**9/113 (7.96)**	**4/123 (3.25)**	4/116 (3.45)
Male 1 year	1/38 (2.63)	0/41 (0)	0/38 (0)
Male 2–8 years	**4/55 (7.27)**	**2/59 (3.39)**	0/59 (0)
Male Intact	9/221 (4.07)	0/226 (0)	5/222 (2.25)
Female <6 months	9/92 (9.78)	**11/101 (10.89)**	0/97 (0)
Female 6–11 months	4/79 (5.06)	**4/81 (4.94)**	3/81 (3.7)
Female 1 year	0/30 (0)	0/32 (0)	1/30 (3.33)
Female 2–8 years	4/86 (4.65)	**3/89 (3.37)**	0/88 (0)
Female Intact	6/163 (3.68)	0/165 (0)	2/164 (1.22)

For ages 1 through 8 years, for each neuter period, the joint disorders are: hip dysplasia (HD), cranial cruciate ligament tear or rupture (CCL), and elbow dysplasia (ED). Shown are number of cases over number in the pool, with percentages given in parentheses. When bolded the incidence is significantly above that of intact dogs.

Labrador Retriever Males: Cancers

The underlying rate of intact males having at least one of the cancers was 4.6 percent. Neutering at any age period had virtually no effect on this measure of cancer occurrence above the level of intact males (Figure 2-B and Table 5).

Labrador Retriever Females: Joint Disorders

As portrayed in Figure 1-B, at neuter periods <6 mo. and 6–11 mo. the risk of dogs having at least one of the joint disorders increased to about double the 5 percent level of intact females ($p = 0.044$; 0.043). In contrast to male Labradors, the females seemed to be vulnerable to the effects of early neutering on HD but not on ED. The neutering effects on HD were evident through 1 year, where the incidence was 4–5 percent compared to 1.5 percent in intact females (Table 4) ($p = 0.02$–0.046). The mean age of diagnosis of HD was 3.5 years, and for ED, 2.5 years. As in male Labradors, CCL in females was increased by early neutering, but in this sex, not significantly so. The mean age of diagnosis of CCL in females was 5.5 years.

The median BCS of neutered females with HD was 5.5, and the median BCS of neutered females without HD was 5.5. In intact females with HD the median BCS was 7 and for those without HD the median BCS was 5.0.

Labrador Retriever Females: Cancers

As seen in Figure 2-B, the underlying rate of intact females having at least one cancer of those tracked was 3.2 percent, close to that of males. In contrast to female Goldens, the only increase in the incidence of dogs having at least one cancer, was with the 2–8 year neuter period where the incidence was modestly increased to 5.6 percent ($p = 0.03$), a reflection of the increased occurrence of LSA and MCT (Table 5). The mean age of diagnosis of these two cancers in females was 5.5 and 6.5 years, respectively.

With regard to MC, only 1.4 percent of the intact females were diagnosed with MC. With the 2–8 year neuter period MC was diagnosed in 2 percent of females. Pyometra was diagnosed in just less than 4 percent of intact females. The mean age of diagnosis of pyometra was 5.5 years.

Discussion

Both the Golden Retriever and Labrador Retriever are very popular breeds that have found wide acceptance as family pets and

Table 3. Golden Retriever males and females, cancers.

	LSA	MCT	HSA
Male <6 months	6/89 (6.74)	3/90 (3.33)	5/90 (5.56)
Male 6–11 months	**14/122 (11.48)**	4/124 (3.23)	2/122 (1.64)
Male 1 year	0/41 (0)	1/40 (2.5)	1/39 (2.56)
Male 2–8 years	0/58 (0)	2/60 (3.33)	0/59 (0)
Male Intact	9/226 (3.98)	8/225 (3.56)	8/220 (3.64)
Female <6 months	4/98 (4.08)	**3/102 (2.94)**	1/102 (0.98)
Female 6–11 months	**9/82 (10.98)**	1/81 (1.23)	1/79 (1.27)
Female 1 year	2/32 (6.25)	**1/32 (3.13)**	1/32 (3.13)
Female 2–8 years	1/84 (1.19)	**5/88 (5.68)**	2/84 (2.38)
Female Intact	3/166 (1.81)	0/165 (0)	2/165 (1.21)

For ages 1 through 8 years, for each neuter period, the cancers are: lymphosarcoma (LSA), mast cell tumor (MCT), and hemangiosarcoma (HSA). Shown are number of cases over number in the pool, with percentages given in parentheses. When bolded the incidence is significantly above that of intact dogs.

Table 4. Labrador Retriever males and females, joint disorders.

	HD	CCL	ED
Male <6 months	0/48 (0)	**4/53 (7.55)**	**2/48 (4.17)**
Male 6–11 months	1/68 (1.47)	2/72 (2.78)	0/67 (0)
Male 1 year	1/50 (2.00)	1/52 (1.92)	0/49 (0)
Male 2–8 years	0/92 (0)	0/93 (0)	**2/93 (2.15)**
Male Intact	9/528 (1.7)	12/531 (2.26)	3/525 (0.57)
Female <6 months	**3/56 (5.36)**	3/59 (5.08)	1/57 (1.75)
Female 6–11 months	**5/99 (5.05)**	5/101 (4.95)	0/103 (0)
Female 1 year	**2/47 (4.26)**	0/50 (0)	0/50 (0)
Female 2–8 years	0/131 (0)	1/128 (0.78)	0/132 (0)
Female Intact	6/345 (1.74)	8/343 (2.33)	4/343 (1.17)

For ages 1 through 8 years, for each neuter period, the joint disorders are: hip dysplasia (HD), cranial cruciate ligament tear or rupture (CCL), and elbow dysplasia (ED). Shown are number of cases over number in the pool, with percentages given in parentheses. When bolded the incidence is significantly above that of intact dogs.

as service dogs for those with disabilities. The two breeds are similar in body size, conformation and in behavioral characteristics [25], and they share a similar developmental background as upland game retrievers. Using the same database and methodology, the two breeds were contrasted with regard to the effects of neutering on three joint disorders (HD, CCL, ED) and three cancers (LSA, HSA, MCT). In addition to reporting the occurrence of the three joint disorders and the three cancers, an analysis of cases with at least one of the joint disorders, or at least one of the cancers, was plotted graphically (Figures 1 and 2). The findings on the Golden Retriever closely resemble the picture presented in the earlier study drawn from this same database with a somewhat smaller data set [14].

The present study reveals that the breeds respond very differently to the effects of neutering on joint disorders and certain devastating cancers. With regard to the occurrence of one or more joint disorders, in Golden Retrievers, neutering at <6 mo. resulted in an incidence of 27 percent in males and 20 percent in females, 4–5 times the 5 percent level for intact males and females. In male and female Labrador Retrievers, with the same underlying occurrence of joint disorders in intact dogs, neutering at <6 mo. resulted in an incidence of 11–12 percent for one or more joint

disorders, roughly double that of intact males and females. Thus, for both breeds, neutering at the standard <6 mo. period markedly and significantly increased the occurrence of joint disorders, although the increase was worse in the Golden than the Labrador. A difference in the specific joints affected was that in male Goldens HD and CCL were mostly increased, but in male Labradors CCL and ED were increased. The effects of neutering in the first year of a dog's life, especially in larger breeds, undoubtedly reflects the vulnerability of joints to delayed closure of long-bone growth plates from gonadal hormone removal [26,27]. Differences in the two breeds studied here could be due to differences in sensitivities of the growth plates to gonadal hormone removal.

The BCSs in neutered dogs with the different joint disorders were compared with neutered dogs without the joint disorders. Although dogs with the disorders were expected to have a modestly higher BCS as a function of reduced activity from painful joints, the issue of concern was if those with a joint disorder had a consistently and markedly higher BCS than comparable neutered dogs without a joint disorder. The BCS comparisons revealed variable differences, in the range of 0.5 to 1.0 (except for ED in male Labradors where the difference was 1.5). The general picture

Table 5. Labrador Retriever males and females, cancers.

	LSA	MCT	HSA
Male <6 months	0/52 (0)	2/53 (3.77)	0/53 (0)
Male 6–11 months	0/72 (0)	0/73 (0)	1/73 (1.37)
Male 1 year	1/52 (1.92)	0/51 (0)	1/51 (1.96)
Male 2–8 years	0/93 (0)	2/89 (2.25)	1/93 (1.08)
Male Intact	4/530 (0.75)	12/533 (2.25)	7/531 (1.32)
Female <6 months	0/59 (0)	0/60 (0)	0/60 (0)
Female 6–11 months	0/104 (0)	2/103 (1.94)	0/104 (0)
Female 1 year	0/49 (0)	1/50 (2)	0/50 (0)
Female 2–8 years	2/131 (1.53)	5/126 (3.97)	0/133 (0)
Female Intact	4/342 (1.17)	6/344 (1.74)	1/345 (0.29)

For ages 1 through 8 years, for each neuter period, the cancers are: lymphosarcoma (LSA), mast cell tumor (MCT), and hemangiosarcoma (HSA). Shown are number of cases over number in the pool, with percentages given in parentheses. When bolded the incidence is significantly above that of intact dogs.

of BCSs of neutered dogs with joint disorders being usually, but not always, a bit higher than the BCSs of neutered dogs without joint disorders, is consistent with the perspective that the increase in joint disorders in neutered dogs is primarily due to the effect of gonadal hormonal removal on bone growth plates and not to greater weight on the joints.

Data on the effects of neutering on the occurrence of cancers in the two breeds also reveal important breed differences. In both breeds the occurrence of one more cancers in intact dogs ranged from 3 to 5 percent, except for Golden Retriever males where the level in intact dogs was 11 percent. In Golden Retriever females neutering females at any neuter period beyond 6 months elevated the risk of one or more cancers to 3 to 4 times the level of intact females (Figure 2). In male Golden Retrievers neutering appeared to have little effect in the occurrence of one or more of the three cancers. An exception was LSA that was increased significantly at the <6 mo. period. In both male and female Labrador Retrievers, neutering at any period appeared to have little effect in increasing cancers.

The striking effect of neutering in female Golden Retrievers compared to male and female Labradors, and male Golden Retrievers, suggests that for this gender and breed the presence of gonadal hormones has a protective effect against cancers over most years of the dog's life. This may reflect a particular sensitivity of receptor sites of some potentially metastatic cancer cells to gonadal hormone removal and/or prolonged levels of the gonadotropin hormone, follicle stimulating hormone [28]. Gonadotropin receptors have been identified in some extragonadal tissues. For example, in the dog these receptor sites have been found in the skin [29] and urinary tract [30]. Treatment of one or more of these cancers by a receptor-site blocking agent may be worth exploring. The relatively high occurrence of one or more of

these cancers in intact male Goldens, coupled with the relative absence of an effect of neutering, except with regard to LSA, points to a relatively high underlying rate of cancer occurrence in this gender and breed that is not affected by gonadal hormone removal.

The findings presented here are clinically relevant in two realms. For dog owners of the popular Golden Retrievers and Labrador Retrievers, the study points to the importance of acquiring information needed to decide if, and when, to neuter. Aside from avoiding increased risks of joint disorders and cancers, there is an indication that age-related cognitive decline could be accelerated by neutering [31]. This is particularly relevant for service dogs where active cognition is important for the expected tasks.

The findings of this study also have important implications for investigators looking for canine models for research on various forms of cancer [32,33]. For some cancers of interest, not only may breeds vary in predisposition but also the possibility of interactions between gender, gonadal hormone influences, and timing of gonadal hormone alteration should be taken into account in selecting the model and in investigating causal factors to be explored.

Acknowledgments

Special thanks are extended to Marty Bryant, Cristina Bustamante, Valerie Caceres, Madeline Courville, Siobhan Aamoth and Roger Pender.

Author Contributions

Conceived and designed the experiments: BLH LAH. Performed the experiments: APT BLH LAH. Analyzed the data: NHW APT BLH LAH. Wrote the paper: BLH LAH APT. Edited manuscript: NHW.

References

1. Trevejo R, Yang M, Lund EM (2011) Epidemiology of surgical castration of dogs and cats in the United States. J Am Vet Med Assoc 238: 898–904.
2. Sallander M, Hedhammar A, Rundgren M, Lindberg JE (2001) Demographic data of population of insured Swedish dogs measured in a questionnaire study. Acta Vet Scand 42: 71–80.
3. Kubinyi E, Turcsan B, Miklosi A (2009) Dog and owner demographic characteristics and dog personality trait associations. Behav Processes 81: 392–401.
4. Diesel G, Brodbelt D, Laurence C (2010) Survey of veterinary practice policies and opinions on neutering dogs. Vet Rec 166: 455–458.
5. Ru G, Terracini B, Glickman LT (1998) Host related risk factors for canine osteosarcoma. Vet J 156:31–39.
6. Cooley DM, Beranek BC, Schlittler DL, Glickman MW, Glickman LT, et al. (2002) Endogenous gonadal hormone exposure and bone sarcoma risk. Cancer Epidemiol Biomarkers Prevent 11: 1434–1440.
7. Ware WA, Hopper DL (1999) Cardiac tumors in dogs: 1982–1995. J Vet Intern Med 13: 95–103.
8. Prymak C, McKee LJ, Goldschmidt MH, Glickman LT (1988) Epidemiologic, clinical, pathologic, and prognostic characteristics of splenic hemangiosarcoma and splenic hematoma in dogs: 217 cases (1985). J Am Vet Med Assoc 193: 706–712.
9. Villamil JA, Henry CJ, Hahn AW, Bryan JN, Tyler JW, et al. (2009) Hormonal and sex impact on the epidemiology of canine lymphoma. J Cancer Epidemiol 2009: 1–7. doi:10.1155/2009/591753
10. White CR, Hohenhaus AE, Kelsey J, Procter-Grey E (2011) Cutaneous MCTs: Associations with spay/neuter status, breed, body size, and phylogenetic cluster. J Am Anim Hosp Assoc 47: 210–216.
11. Teske E, Naan EC, van Dijk E, Van Garderen E, Schalken JA (2002) Canine prostate carcinoma: epidemiological evidence of an increased risk in castrated dogs. Mol Cell Endocrinol 197: 251–255.
12. Root Kustritz MV (2007) Determining the optimal age for gonadectomy of dogs and cats. J Am Vet Med Assoc 231: 1665–1675.
13. Beauvais W, Cardwell JM, Brodbelt DC (2012) The effect of neutering on the risk of mammary tumours in dogs – a systematic review. J Small Anim Pract 53: 314–322.
14. Torres de la Riva G, Hart BL, Farver TB, Oberbauer AM, McV Messam LL, et al. (2013) Neutering Dogs: Effects on Joint Disorders and Cancers in Golden Retrievers. PLOS ONE 2013; 8(2): e55937. doi:10.1371/journal.pone.0055937

15. Hoffman JM, Creevy KE, Promislow DEL (2013) Reproductive capability is associated with lifespan and cause of death in companion dogs. PLOS ONE 2013; 8(4): e6 1082. doi: 10.1371/journal.pone.0061082
16. Zink MC, Farhoody P, Elser SE, Ruffini LD, Gibbons TA, et al. (2014) Evaluation of the risk and age of onset of cancer and behavioral disorders in gonadectomized Vizslas. J Am Vet Med Assoc 244: 309–319.
17. Duerr FM, Duncan CG, Savicky RS, Park RD, Egger EL, et al. (2007) Risk factors for excessive tibial plateau angle in large-breed dogs with cranial cruciate disease. J Am Vet Med Assoc 231: 1688–1691.
18. Witsberger TH, Villamil JA, Schultz LG, Hahn AW, Cook JL (2008) Prevalence of, and risk factors for, hip dysplasia and cranial cruciate ligament deficiency in dogs. J Am Vet Med Assoc 232: 1818–1824.
19. Dobson JM (2013) Breed-predispositions to cancer in pedigree dogs. Vet Sci 2013: 1–23.
20. Kasström H (1975) Nutrition, weight gain and development of hip dysplasia. An experimental investigation in growing dogs with special reference to the effect of feeding intensity. Acta Radiologica 344: 135–179, Supplementum.
21. Duval JM, Budsberg SC, Flo GL, Sammarco Jl (1999) Breed, sex, and body weight as risk factors for rupture of the cranial cruciate ligament in young dogs. J Am Vet Med Assoc 215: 811–814.
22. Baldwin K, Bartges J, Buffington T, Freeman LM, Grabow M, et al. (2010) AAHA nutritional assessment guidelines for dogs and cats. J Am Anim Hosp Assoc 46: 285–296.
23. Cox DR (1972) Regression models and life tables (with discussion). Journal of the Royal Statistical Society, series B, 34: 187–220.
24. Rothman KJ, Greenland S (1998) Modern Epidemiology. Philadelphia: Lippincott Williams & Wilkins.
25. Hart BL, Hart LA (1988) The Perfect Puppy. How to Choose Your Dog by Its Behavior. New York: W.H. Freeman and Co.
26. Salmeri KR, Bloomberg MS, Scruggs SL, Shille V (1991) Gonadectomy in immature dogs: Effects on skeletal, physical, and behavioral development. J Am Vet Med Assoc 198: 1193–1203.
27. Grumbach M (2000) Estrogen, bone growth and sex: a sea of change in conventional wisdom. J Ped Endocrinol Metab 13: 1439–1455.
28. Concannon PW (1993). Biology of gonadotrophin secretion in adult and prepubertal female dogs. J Reprod Fert Supp 47: 3–27.
29. Reichler IM, Welle M, Eckrich C, Sattler U, Barth A, et al. (2008) Spaying-induced coat changes: the role of gonadotropins, GnRH and GnRH treatment on the hair cycle of female dogs. Vet Dermatol 19: 77–87.

30. Fields MJ, Shemesh M (2004) Extragonadal luteinizing hormone receptors in the reproductive tract of domestic animals. Biol Reprod 71: 1412–1418.

31. Hart BL (2001) Effects of gonadectomy on subsequent development of age-related cognitive impairment in dogs. J Am Vet Med Assoc 219: 51–56.

32. Vail DM, MacEwen EG (2002) Spontaneously occurring tumors of companion animals as models for human cancer. Cancer Invest 18: 781–792.

33. Khanna C, Lindblad-Toh K, Vail D, London C, Bergman P, et al. (2006) The dog as a cancer model. Nat Biotechnol 24: 1065–1066.

6

Sox9 Duplications Are a Relevant Cause of Sry-Negative XX Sex Reversal Dogs

Elena Rossi[1], Orietta Radi[1], Lisa De Lorenzi[2], Annalisa Vetro[3], Debora Groppetti[4], Enrico Bigliardi[5], Gaia Cecilia Luvoni[6], Ada Rota[7], Giovanna Camerino[1], Orsetta Zuffardi[1], Pietro Parma[2]*

1 Department of Molecular Medicine, Pavia University, Pavia, Italy, 2 Department of Agricultural and Environmental Sciences, Milan University, Milan, Italy, 3 Biotechnology Research Laboratories, Fondazione IRCCS Policlinico San Matteo, Pavia, Italy, 4 Department of Veterinary Science and Public Health, Milan University, Milan, Italy, 5 Department of Veterinary Science, Parma University, Parma, Italy, 6 Department of Health, Animal Science and Food Safety, Milan University, Milan, Italy, 7 Department of Veterinary Science, Torino University, Torino, Italy

Abstract

Sexual development in mammals is based on a complicated and delicate network of genes and hormones that have to collaborate in a precise manner. The dark side of this pathway is represented by pathological conditions, wherein sexual development does not occur properly either in the XX and the XY background. Among them a conundrum is represented by the XX individuals with at least a partial testis differentiation even in absence of SRY. This particular condition is present in various mammals including the dog. Seven dogs characterized by XX karyotype, absence of SRY gene, and testicular tissue development were analysed by Array-CGH. In two cases the array-CGH analysis detected an interstitial heterozygous duplication of chromosome 9. The duplication contained the *SOX9* coding region. In this work we provide for the first time a causative mutation for the XXSR condition in the dog. Moreover this report supports the idea that the dog represents a good animal model for the study of XXSR condition caused by abnormalities in the SOX9 locus.

Editor: Bin He, Baylor College of Medicine, United States of America

Funding: These authors have no support or funding to report.

Competing Interests: The authors have declared that no competing interests exist.

* Email: pietro.parma@unimi.it

Introduction

Gonadal differentiation in mammals is initiated, controlled, and regulated by the coordinated action of several genes and hormones.

During the last two decades many genes involved in this process have been identified [1], and in recent times, epigenetic factors have also come into play [2].

The scepter of power remains firmly in the hands of *SRY*, the sex determination key gene [3] located on the Y chromosome that is necessary and sufficient to induce the primordial undifferentiated gonad to develop into a testis [4]. In the absence of *SRY*, that is in the XX embryos a different set of genes is activated, and the undifferentiated gonad becomes an ovary [5]. *SRY* role takes place in a short period of timeand ceases after the activation of *SOX9*. This gene is a main actor in testis differentiation and in several other embryogenetic fields [6]. Normally this process follows well-defined tracks: the XY embryos develop the testis and a male phenotype, while the XX embryos develop ovaries and a female phenotype. However, this complex process can result in the appearance of developmental errors on account of the discordance between the chromosomal, gonadic, and phenotypic sex.

One of the most interesting issues is represented by the XX sex-reversal cases. In humans most of them do have the SRY gene that is transposed to the tip of Xp due a recurrent Non Allelic Homologous Recombination between of PRKX and PRKY in a particular Y haplotypic background [7]. However, in both humans and other mammals SRY-negative XX males have been observed displaying testicular tissue, with or without ovarian tissue. It has been observed, at least in pig, that in these cases *SOX9* gene is surprisingly activated in the absence of *SRY* [8]. Subjects with XX sex reversal have been observed in different species: human, pig, goat, llama, dog, and horse [9–14]. In the dog this pathology appears with a relatively high frequency compared to the other species and has been described in various breeds [15]. XX sex-reversal in dogs can show a very different structure of gonads, ranging from bilateral testis to one ovo-testis and one ovary. With regard to the causes of occurrence of this anomaly in different species, to date, only three genetic causes have been identified: *FOXL2* in goat [16] and *SOX9* [17] and RSPO1 [18] in humans. *SOX9* alterations in XXSR cases include duplications, triplications, and reciprocal translocations [17,19–21]. Surprisingly, despite the many cases investigated in XXSR dogs, till date no causative mutations have been reported, but only a linkage for a genomic region has been detected in a single specific pedigree [22].

In this article, we report the molecular analysis of seven XX sex-reversal dogs and we clearly show, for the first time in literature, that two of them carry *SOX9* gene duplication.

Materials and Methods

Case Description

Seven dogs from different breeds have been considered in this study: Four of these have already been described, while three are still unreported. Case C2, C9, C10, and C44 [23–25] have been

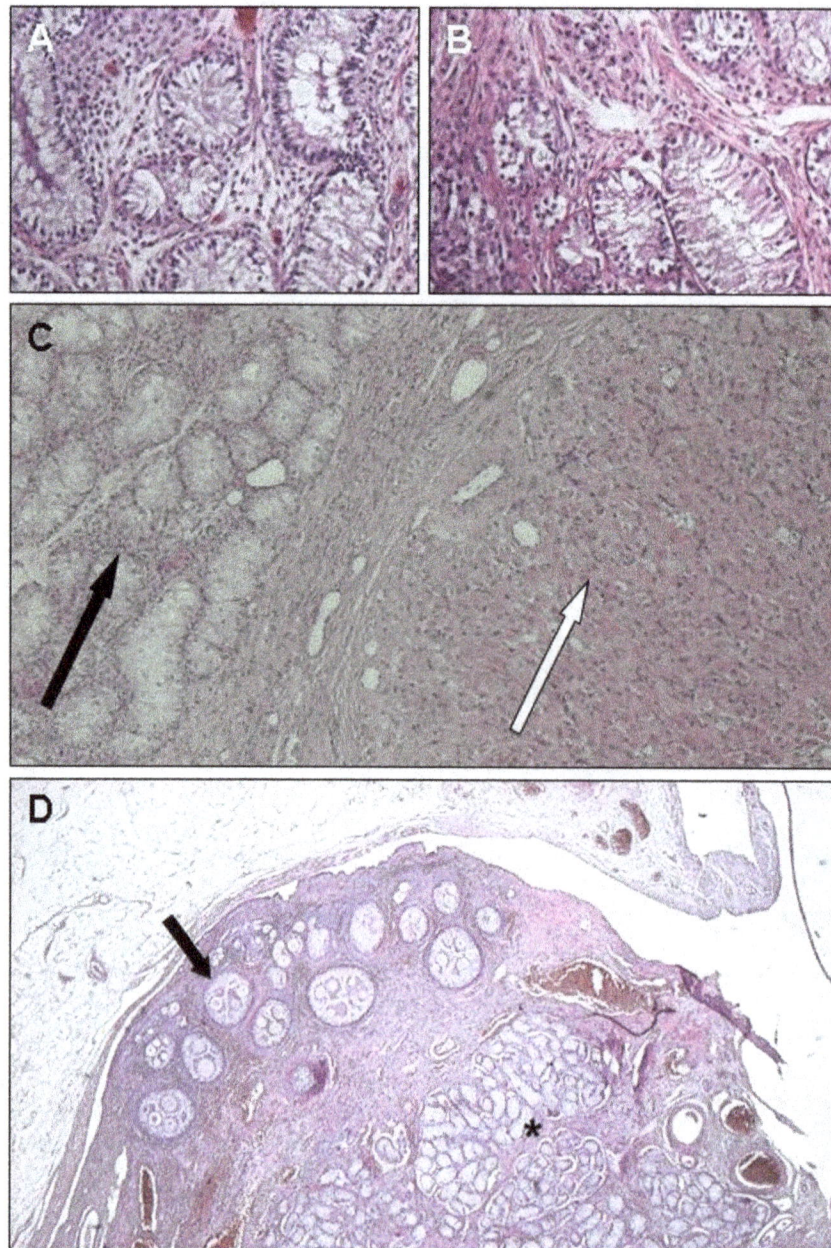

Figure 1. Histological examination of the new cases reported. Case C61: Histologic section of the right (A) and left (B) gonad showing seminiferous tubules with diffuse atrophy of the seminal line. Case C64: Right Ovotestis (C): The gonads were surrounded by ovarian bursa and shown some follicular structures and corpora lutea (white arrow). In the medulla hypoplastic seminiferous tubules were present (black arrow). Case C65 (D): Dog ovotestis. In the gonad, follicular structures including oocytes (arrow) coexist with testicular tubuli lined by Setoli cells (asterisc) (Courtesy of Valeria Grieco, University of Milan).

previously characterized to show a presence of testicular tissue with a XX karyotype in the absence of the *SRY* gene. The other three cases, C61, C64, and C65, have been characterized in this study.

Histological Examination

All clinical activities and surgical experiments on the dogs were carried out at the Veterinary Hospital of the University of Milan by veterinary surgeons. During the research no animals were sacrificed. The anesthetic and surgical protocol fulfilled the Federation of European Laboratory Animal Science Association's

recommendations and European Union legislation (Council Directive 86/609/EEC). Blood (1.5 ml) and gonad samples were collected for a routine medical procedure and stored for further analysis. Consistent with Italian regulation (D.L. 116/1992), the owners signed a voluntary consent, for their animals before undergoing surgery. This consent includes the possibility that the removed tissue may be used in scientific researches without economic interest.

After surgical excision of the gonads, they were fixed in 10% neutral buffered formalin for at least three days. For histological examination, several slices of gonads were processed histotechno-

Table 1. List of CNVs identified with array-CGH in the seven cases with the indication of their code, type, location and size (CanFam2 assembly).

Case code	CFA	DEL /DUP	CNV code	Log ratio	Size Kb	Last unaffected bp	First affected bp	Last affected bp	First unaffected bp	Already Described (Y/N)	Genes
C2	9	DEL	1	-0.7	459	20,436,097	20,465,561	20,924,123	20,924,097	Y	
	9	DUP	2	0.5	541		21,021,894	21,562,129	21,574,304	Y	
C9	9	DEL	1	-0.8	459	20,439,097	20,465,561	20,924,123		Y	
	9	DUP	2	0.5	541		21,021,894	21,562,129	21,574,304	Y	
C10	9	DUP	3	0.5	577	10,414,955	11,016,965	11,593,933	12,062,144	N	SOX9
	9	DUP	4	0.3	414	19,864,938	20,022,338	20,436,297	20,447,061	Y	
	9	DEL	1	-0.75	458	20,447,061	20,465,561	20,924,123		Y	
	9	DUP	2	0.5	541		21,021,894	21,574,304	21,589,624	Y	
C44	9	DUP	3	0.57	577	10,414,955	11,016,965	11,593,933	12,062,144	N	SOX9
	9	DEL	5	-0.9	1300	19,766,692	19,819,256	21,119,179	21,292,889	Y	
C61	9	DEL	6	-0.8	809	20,097,414	20,115,306	20,924,123		Y	
	9	DUP	2	0.5	541		21,021,894	21,562,129	21,574,304	Y	
C64	9	DEL	6	-0.8	809	20,097,414	20,115,306	20,924,123		Y	
	9	DUP	2	0.5	541		21,021,894	21,562,129	21,574,304	Y	
C65	9	DEL	6	-0.8	809	20,097,414	20,115,306	20,924,123		Y	
	9	DUP	2	0.5	541		21,021,894	21,562,129	21,574,304	Y	

CNVs were checked for occurrence in the Database of Genomic Copy Number Variants in the dog genome (http://dogs.genouest.org/LUPA.dir/CNV.html) and in several papers [29–33].

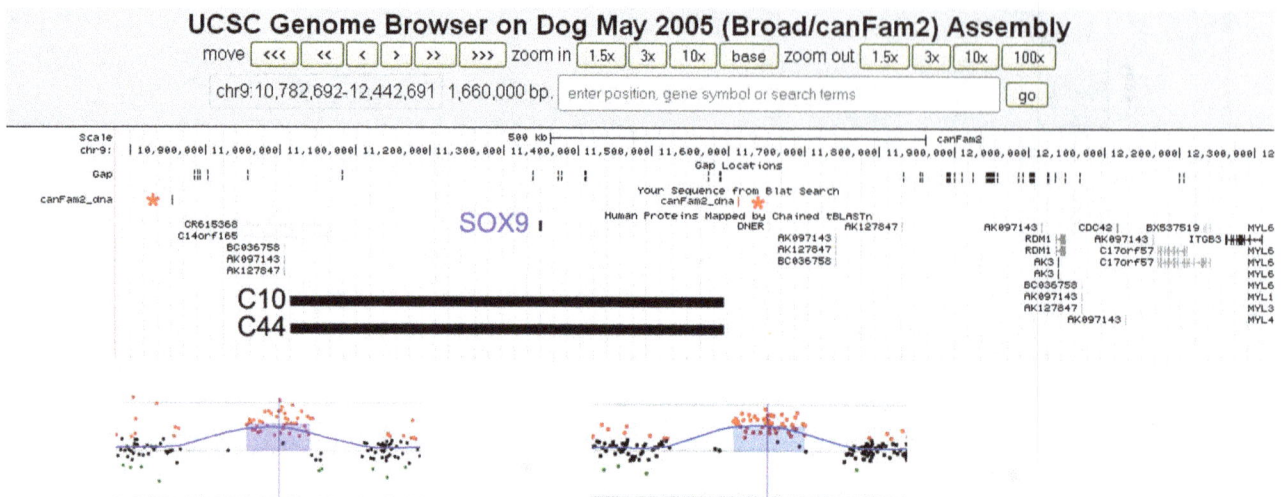

Figure 2. Graphical representation of the SOX9 locus duplications discovered. The figure shows a 1,6 Mb region of CFA 9 in the UCSC Genome Browser (canFam2 assembly) and magnified views of the two SOX9 duplications detected, by array-CGH, in cases C10 (left) and C44 (right), respectively. The shaded areas indicate a gain in DNA copy number (duplication, average log2 ratios: +0, 5) detected by red dots. Asterisks indicate the 168 bp repeats.

logically according to standard laboratory procedures, cut at 5 μm, and stained with hematoxylin and eosin [26].

Cell Cultures and Genetic Analyses

Peripheral blood lymphocyte cultures were performed following the standard procedures [27]. *SRY* gene analysis was performed as reported [23]. Briefly, the entire SRY coding region (GenBank AF107021) was amplified by polymerase chain reaction (PCR) using the following primers: (5'-3'): SRY-Dog-F: ctttccaacttccctccgta and SRY-Dog-R: ggacgtttcgttagccagag. The PCR product was 813 bp long. PCR was performed using AmpliTaq Gold DNA Polymerase (Applied Biosystems) according to the manufacturer's instructions.

Array-CGH Analyses

Array-CGH was performed using a custom Agilent Canine Genome CGH Microarray 180 K (Agilent Technologies, Santa Clara, California, USA) and processed as reported [28]. Briefly, 500 ng of purified DNA of a subject and a control, were double-digested with RsaI and AluI for two hours at 37°C. After 20 minutes at 65°C, each digested sample was labeled by the Agilent random primers; labeling was performed for two hours using Cy5-dUTP for the subject DNA and Cy3-dUTP for the control DNA. The labeled products were columns purified and prepared according to the Agilent protocol. After probe denaturation and pre-annealing with 5 μl of Cot-1 DNA, hybridization was performed at 65°C, with rotation for 40 hours. After two washing steps, the arrays were analyzed with the Agilent scanner and the Feature Extraction software (v10.7.3.1). A graphical overview was obtained using the CGH analytics software (v7.0.4.0). The DNA extracted from a normal female (boxer breed) was used as the control in all cases. All experimental data were submitted to GEO repository with the following Series accession number: GSE57137.

Quantitative real Time PCR

Sox9 duplications detected by array CGH were confirmed by Real-Time-qPCR with SYBR Green detection (Brilliant II SYBR Green QPCR master mix, Agilent Technologies), using one non-

polymorphic marker located within the duplicated region. The primers were designed by using the Primer3 Software online (http://frodo.wi.mit.edu/primer3/), with the following criteria: Amplicon size 80–200 bp, GC content of 20–80%, and melting temperature (Tm) of 59–61°C. The primer sequences are available on request. Real-time detection was performed using the Stratagene Mx3000P. The Real-Time-qPCRs were performed in triplicate for each reaction.

The comparative CT method ($\Delta\Delta$CT method) was used to discriminate between two and three allele copies of the DNA target sequence (Sox9) in the two dogs (resulted duplicated by a-CGH) relative to five normal control dogs DNA samples. The data have been normalized against two different reference sequences (Abs17, Bglr2).

Results

All the three new cases, C61, C64, and C65, showed a normal 78,XX karyotype in all the observed metaphases, and PCR analyses confirmed the absence of the *SRY* gene (not shown). Moreover, the histological analyses revealed the presence of testicular tissue in all the three cases, indicating that the male pathway was active during the fetal period in the absence of *SRY*. The testes of Case 61 are composed of testicular parenchyma with absence of the germline. In Cases 64 and 65 the right and left gonads are ovotestes (Figure 1a, b, c, d).

The results of array-CGH in the seven cases analyzed are listed in Table 1.

In cases C10 and C44, the array-CGH analysis detected an interstitial heterozygous duplication of chromosome 9, of 577 Kb (from 11,016,965 to 11,593,933; all data are referred to CanFam2 genome assembly) (Figure 2). The duplication contained the *SOX9* gene. This was confirmed by *reverse transcriptase* (RT)-PCR (Figure 3) and it was never described as *copy number variation*s (CNVs) in different dog breeds [29–33]. The duplicated region was flanked by small, 168 bp, directly oriented repeats of >97,6% sequence identity, suggesting that non-allelic homologous recombination (NAHR) might have mediated these duplications. Furthermore, array-CGH identified several CNVs (data not

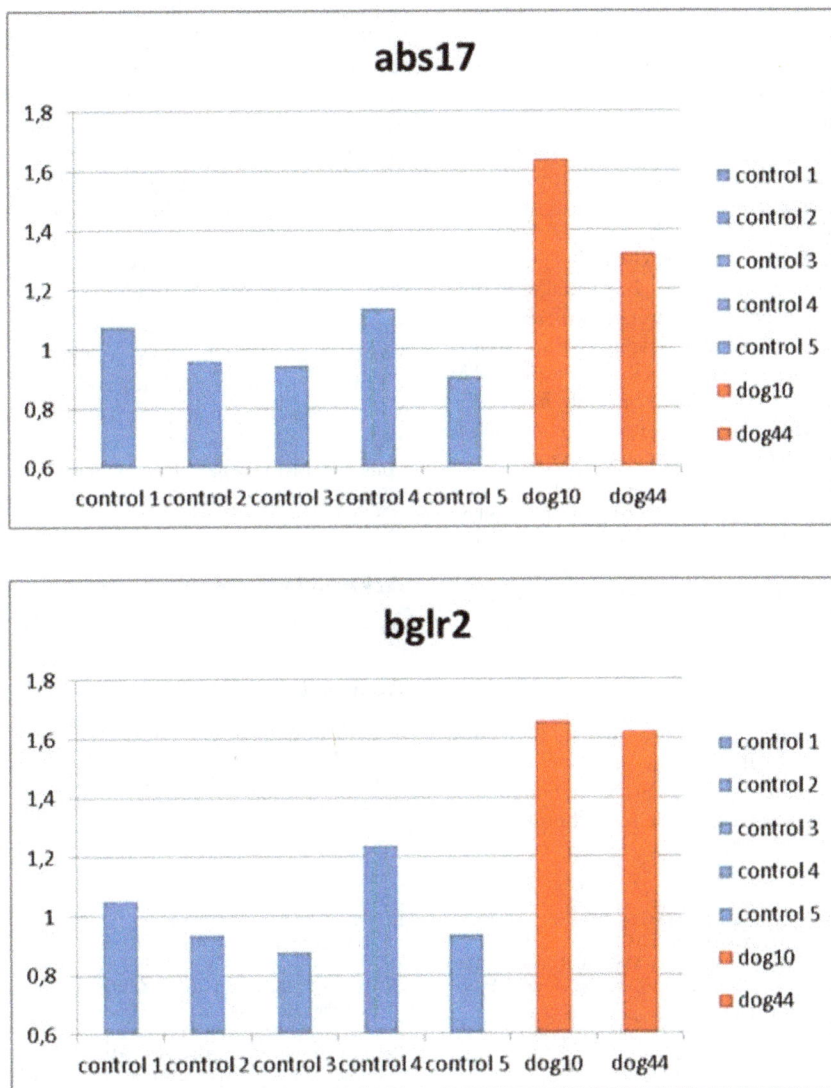

Figure 3. Q-RT PCR results. Histograms represent the copy numbers ratio of a non-polymorphic probe within Sox9 gene in the two duplicated dogs (dog10 and dog44, red bars) relative to five normal control dogs (blue bars). The data have been normalized against two different reference sequences (Abs17, Bglr2).

shown) in our cases; all of them were described as polymorphic in previous dog aCGH reports [29–33]. The complex CNV region on CFA9:19,761,852–21,600,512 has been observed, and reported with slightly different boundaries depending on the array platform used, in multiple studies [29–33]. Several CNV patterns have been described: gains or losses across the whole region, gains or losses of only a part of the region or alternate gains and losses within a single individual. The desert region between 20,115,306 and 21,119,179 is orthologous (61.9% of bases, 84.0% of span; http://genome.ucsc.edu/index.html) to the human region chr17:68,723,331–69,717,418 (genome assembly Hg19), located 500–600 Kb upstream of SOX9, which is suggested to be the human regulatory region critical for gonadal SOX9 expression [20]. It is particularly interesting because, taking into account that the Dog Genome Assembly is a working progress and contains many assembly errors (Rossi E. personal communication), the actual distance between SOX9 and this region within the dog genome could be the same of the human one. A more stable and defined dog assembly will demonstrate the actual distance between

the two regions and will help to clarify the related effects. As shown in Table 1, in our cases the CNV from CFA9:19,761,852–21,600,512 has different patterns: complex in cases 2, 9, 10, 61, 64, 65 and simple as a deletion in case 44.

Discussion

Genes in the SOX family play a critical role in the sex determination process. *SRY* is the master gene of this process [34] while *SOX9* represents the genetic factor that, activated by *SRY*, starts and regulates testis development. Although *SRY* is mammal-specific (with very few exceptions) *SOX9* plays an important role in bird also [35]. *SOX3* and *SOX8* genes are also involved in the sex determination process [36–37]. Chromosomal duplications as well as triplications involving the *SOX9* locus on HSA17q24.3, have been reported to be the causative mutations of the XX sex-reversal condition [38], however, all these duplications/triplications, except one, do not involve the *SOX9* coding region (CDS), but all are located 5′ to this gene. Indeed only the first reported *SOX9* duplication includes the SOX9 CDS [39]. This duplication, characterized by *Variable-Number Tandem Repeat* (VNTR) analyses, is at least 11.7 Mb long and is starts at 9.4 Mb 5′ and ends at 2.2 Mb 3′ of SOX9 CDS.

The mechanism underlying the XXSR condition in the presence of SOX9 duplications is still not clear, although it is clear that a *Sox9* over expression is required to induce the testis development in a XX background.

Therefore all different Sox9 locus duplications must be organized to allow this possibility. The Sox9 transgenic mouse effectively develops the XXSR phenotype. Incidentally, in this case, the gene is under the regulation of a strong promoter, which is able to activate the Sox9 expression in the right place at the right time, also in the absence of *Sry* [40]. *SOX9* is initially expressed in both the developing gonads (XY and XX), but only in the XY gonads its expression increases greatly. This upward regulation is due to *SRY* activation, and later on, to an auto-loop reinforced by additional positive feed-forward signals (Fgf9). In the XX developing gonad the auto-loop is not able by itself to up-regulate *Sox9* expression; moreover, female-specific genes repress additional feed-forward signals.

The analyses of human duplications in XXSR suggest a model of action. In these subjects two CDS SOX9 doses are present (as in normal subject), but the upstream region in one allele is duplicated, and this condition probably induces Sox9 over-expression.

The perturbation of sex determination process may be caused either by gain of function (GOF) or Loss of function (LOF) mechanisms. In the first case male gene (i.e. SOX9 in human and probably in pig) are involved whereas in the second ones female genes are involved (i.e. RSPO1 in human and FOXL2 in goat). In addition, the mechanisms of LOF are often associated with more severe phenotypes that include other abnormalities. For this reason we believe that SOX9 GOF remains the most reasonable candidate mechanism to explain the remaining unexplained XXSR cases in the involved species.

The dog represents a good animal model for the study of this disease because it shows relative high frequencies of XXSR cases and more precisely it can be a valuable model for the study of XXSR cases caused by SOX9 locus duplication.

In addition, the dog could represent an alternative animal model to the mouse considering that it seems to be different from other mammals at least for: a) SRY expression [41]; b) role of TESCO genomic region [42] and gene-dosage sensibility [43].

Unfortunately the genome assembly around the *SOX9* gene in the dog (CanFam3) seems to possess many assembly problems and consequently comparative analyses between this locus and the homolog locus in other species is quite difficult (Rossi E. personal communication).

Acknowledgments

We are grateful to the owners of the analyzed subjects for their willingness.

Author Contributions

Conceived and designed the experiments: OR GC OZ PP ER. Performed the experiments: ER OR LDL. Analyzed the data: ER OR PP AV. Contributed reagents/materials/analysis tools: DG EB GCL AR. Wrote the paper: ER OR GC OZ PP.

References

1. Quinn A, Koopman P (2012) The molecular genetics of sex determination and sex reversal in mammals. Semin Reprod Med 30: 351–363.
2. Kuroki S, Matoba S, Akiyoshi M, Matsumura Y, Miyachi H, et al. (2013) Epigenetic regulation of mouse sex determination by the histone demethylase Jmjd1a. Science 341: 1106–1109.
3. Kashimada K, Koopman P (2010) Sry: the master switch in mammalian sex determination. Development 137: 3921–3930.
4. Sekido R, Lovell-Badge R (2013) Genetic control of testis development. Sex Dev 7: 21–32.
5. Chassot AA, Gregoire EP, Magliano M, Lavery R, Chaboissier MC (2008) Genetics of ovarian differentiation: Rspo1, a major player. Sex Dev 2: 219–227.
6. Sekido R, Lovell-Badge R (2008) Sex determination involves synergistic action of SRY and SF1 on a specific Sox9 enhancer. Nature 453: 930–934.
7. Jobling MA, Williams GA, Schiebel GA, Pandya GA, McElreavey GA, et al. (1998) A selective difference between human Y-chromosomal DNA haplotypes. Curr Biol 8: 1391–1394.
8. Pailhoux E, Parma P, Sundström J, Vigier B, Servel N, et al. (2001) Time course of female-to-male sex reversal in 38,XX fetal and postnatal pigs. Dev Dyn 222: 328–340.
9. Wachtel SS (1994) XX sex reversal in the human. In: Wachtel SS, editor. Molecular genetics of sex determination. San Diego: Academic. p. 267.
10. Pailhoux E, Popescu PC, Parma P, Boscher J, Legault C, et al. (1994) Genetic analysis of 38XX males with genital ambiguities and true hermaphrodites in pigs. Anim Genet 25: 299–305.
11. Pailhoux E, Cribiu EP, Chaffaux S, Darre R, Fellous M, et al. (1994) Molecular analysis of 60,XX pseudohermaphrodite polled goats for the presence of SRY and ZFY genes. J Reprod Fertil 100: 491–496.
12. Wilker CE, Meyers-Wallen VN, Schlafer DH, Dykes NL, Kovacs A, et al. (1994) XX sex reversal in a llama. J Am Vet Med Assoc 204: 112–115.
13. Selden JR, Moorhead PS, Koo GC, Wachtel SS, Haskins ME, et al. (1984) Inherited XX sex reversal in the cocker spaniel dog. Hum Genet 67: 62–69.
14. Bannasch D, Rinaldo C, Millon L, Latson K, Spangler T, et al. (2007) SRY negative 64,XX intersex phenotype in an American saddlebred horse. Vet J 173: 437–439.
15. Meyers-Wallen VN (2009) Review and update: genomic and molecular advances in sex determination and differentiation in small animals. Reprod Domest Anim 44: 40–46.
16. Pailhoux E, Vigier B, Chaffaux S, Servel N, Taourit S, et al. (2001) A 11.7-kb deletion triggers intersexuality and polledness in goats. Nat Genet 29: 453–458.
17. Cox JJ, Willatt L, Homfray T, Woods CG (2011) A SOX9 duplication and familial 46,XX developmental testicular disorder. (Letter) New Eng J Med 364: 91–363.
18. Parma P, Radi O, Vidal V, Chaboissier MC, Dellambra E, et al. (2006) R-spondin1 is essential in sex determination, skin differentiation and malignancy. Nat Genet 38: 1304–1309.
19. Vetro A, Ciccone R, Giorda R, Patricelli MG, Della Mina E, et al. (2011) XX males SRY negative: a confirmed cause of infertility. J Med Genet 48: 710–712.
20. Benko S, Gordon CT, Mallet D, Sreenivasan R, Thauvin-Robinet C, et al. (2011) Disruption of a long distance regulatory region upstream of SOX9 in isolated disorders of sex development. J Med Genet 48: 825–830.
21. Xiao B, Ji X, Xing Y, Chen YW, Tao J (2013) A rare case of 46, XX SRY-negative male with a ~74-kb duplication in a region upstream of SOX9. Eur J Med Genet 56: 695–698.
22. Pujar S, Kothapalli KS, Göring HH, Meyers-Wallen VN (2007) Linkage to CFA29 detected in a genome-wide linkage screen of a canine pedigree segregating Sry-negative XX sex reversal. J Hered 98: 438–444.
23. De Lorenzi L, Groppetti D, Arrighi S, Pujar S, Nicoloso L, et al. (2008) Mutations in the RSPO1 coding region are not the main cause of canine SRY-negative XX sex reversal in several breeds. Sex Dev 2: 84–95.
24. Groppetti D, Genualdo V, Bosi G, Pecile A, Iannuzzi A, et al. (2012) XX SRY-negative true hermaphrodism in two dogs: clinical, morphological, genetic and cytogenetic studies. Sex Dev 6: 135–142.
25. Rota A, Cucuzza AS, Iussich S, De Lorenzi L, Parma P (2010) The case of an Sry-negative XX male Pug with an inguinal gonad. Reprod Domest Anim 45: 743–745.
26. Bigliardi E, Parma P, Peressotti P, De Lorenzi L, Wohlsein P, et al. Clinical, genetic, and pathological features of male pseudohermaphroditism in dog. Reprod Biol Endocrinol 9: 12.
27. De Grouchy J, Roubin M, Passage E (1964) Microtechnique pour l'étude des chromosomes humains a partir d'une culture de leucocytes sanguins. Ann Génét 7: 45–46.
28. De Lorenzi L, Kopecna O, Gimelli S, Cernohorska H, Zannotti M, et al. (2010) Reciprocal translocation t(4;7)(q14;q28) in cattle: molecular characterization. Cytogenet Genome Res 129: 298–304.
29. Chen WK, Swartz JD, Rush LJ, Alvarez CE (2009) Mapping DNA structural variation in dogs. Genome Res 19: 500–509.
30. Nicholas TJ, Cheng Z, Ventura M, Mealey K, Eichler EE, et al. (2009) The genomic architecture of segmental duplications and associated copy number variants in dogs. Genome Res 39: 491–499.

31. Nicholas TJ, Baker C, Eichler EE, Akey JM (2011) A high-resolution integrated map of copy number polymorphisms within and between breeds of the modern domesticated dog. BMC Genomics 12: 414.

32. Quilez J, Short AD, Martínez V, Kennedy LJ, Ollier W, et al. (2011) A selective sweep of >8 Mb on chromosome 26 in the Boxer genome. BMC Genomics 12: 339.

33. Berglund J, Nevalainen EM, Molin AM, Perloski M, André C, et al. (2012) Novel origins of copy number variation in the dog genome. Genome Biol 13: R73.

34. Sinclair AH, Berta P, Palmer MS, Hawkins R, Griffiths BL, et al. (1990) A gene from the human sex-determining region encodes a protein with homology to a conserved DNA-binding motif. Nature 346: 240–245.

35. Morais da Silva S, Hacker A, Harley V, Goodfellow P, Swain A, et al. (1996) Sox9 expression during gonadal development implies a conserved role for the gene in testis differentiation in mammals and birds. Nature Genet 14: 62–68.

36. Sutton E, Hughes J, White S, Sekido R, Tan J, et al. (2011) Identification of SOX3 as an XX male sex reversal gene in mice and humans. J Clin Invest 121: 328–341.

37. Chaboissier MC, Kobayashi A, Vidal VI, Lützkendorf S, van de Kant HJ, et al. (2004) Functional analysis of Sox8 and Sox9 during sex determination in the mouse. Development 131: 1891–1901.

38. Fonseca AC, Bonaldi A, Bertola DR, Kim CA, Otto PA, et al. (2013) The clinical impact of chromosomal rearrangements with breakpoints upstream of the SOX9 gene: two novel de novo balanced translocations associated with acampomelic campomelic dysplasia. BMC Med Genet 14: 50.

39. Huang B, Wang S, Ning Y, Lamb AN, Bartley J (1999) Autosomal XX sex reversal caused by duplication of SOX9. Am J Med Genet 87: 349–353.

40. Vidal VPI, Chaboissier M-C, de Rooij DG, Schedl A (2001) Sox9 induces testis development in XX transgenic mice. Nature Genet 28: 216–217.

41. Montazer-Torbati F, Kocer A, Auguste A, Renault L, Charpigny G, et al. (2010) A study of goat SRY protein expression suggests putative new roles for this gene in the developing testis of a species with long-lasting SRY expression. Dev Dyn 239: 3324–3335.

42. Georg I, Bagheri-Fam S, Knower KC, Wieacker P, Scherer G, et al. (2010) Mutations of the SRY-responsive enhancer of SOX9 are uncommon in XY gonadal dysgenesis. Sex Dev 4: 321–325.

43. Chen YS, Racca JD, Phillips NB, Weiss MA (2013) Inherited human sex reversal due to impaired nucleocytoplasmic trafficking of SRY defines a male transcriptional threshold. Proc Natl Acad Sci U S A 110: E3567–3576.

7

Lactic Acid and Thermal Treatments Trigger the Hydrolysis of *Myo*-Inositol Hexakisphosphate and Modify the Abundance of Lower *Myo*-Inositol Phosphates in Barley (*Hordeum vulgare* L.)

Barbara U. Metzler-Zebeli[1,2], Kathrin Deckardt[1], Margit Schollenberger[3], Markus Rodehutscord[3], Qendrim Zebeli[1]*

1 Institute of Animal Nutrition and Functional Plant Compounds, Department for Farm Animals and Veterinary Public Health, Vetmeduni Vienna, Vienna, Austria, **2** University Clinic for Swine, Department for Farm Animals and Veterinary Public Health, Vetmeduni Vienna, Vienna, Austria, **3** Institute of Animal Nutrition, University of Hohenheim, Stuttgart, Germany

Abstract

Barley is an important source of dietary minerals, but it also contains *myo*-inositol hexakisphosphate ($InsP_6$) that lowers their absorption. This study evaluated the effects of increasing concentrations (0.5, 1, and 5%, vol/vol) of lactic acid (LA), without or with an additional thermal treatment at 55°C (LA-H), on $InsP_6$ hydrolysis, formation of lower phosphorylated myo-inositol phosphates, and changes in chemical composition of barley grain. Increasing LA concentrations and thermal treatment linearly reduced ($P<0.001$) $InsP_6$-phosphate ($InsP_6$-P) by 0.5 to 1 g compared to the native barley. In particular, treating barley with 5% LA-H was the most efficient treatment to reduce the concentrations of $InsP_6$-P, and stimulate the formation of lower phosphorylated myo-inositol phosphates such as *myo*-inositol tetraphosphate ($InsP_4$) and *myo*-inositol pentaphosphates ($InsP_5$). Also, LA and thermal treatment changed the abundance of $InsP_4$ and $InsP_5$ isomers with $Ins(1,2,5,6)P_4$ and $Ins(1,2,3,4,5)P_5$ as the dominating isomers with 5% LA, 1% LA-H and 5% LA-H treatment of barley, resembling to profiles found when microbial 6-phytase is applied. Treating barley with LA at room temperature (22°C) increased the concentration of resistant starch and dietary fiber but lowered those of total starch and crude ash. Interestingly, total phosphorus (P) was only reduced ($P<0.05$) in barley treated with LA-H but not after processing of barley with LA at room temperature. In conclusion, LA and LA-H treatment may be effective processing techniques to reduce $InsP_6$ in cereals used in animal feeding with the highest degradation of $InsP_6$ at 5% LA-H. Further in vivo studies are warranted to determine the actual intestinal P availability and to assess the impact of changes in nutrient composition of LA treated barley on animal performance.

Editor: Wagner L. Araujo, Universidade Federal de Vicosa, Brazil

Funding: The authors have no support or funding to report.

Competing Interests: The authors have declared that no competing interests exist.

* Email: Qendrim.Zebeli@vetmeduni.ac.at

Introduction

Barley is an important cereal crop used for livestock feeding and human consumption. It contains relatively large amounts of starch, protein, dietary fiber, and minerals which make this cereal a highly valuable ingredient of the diet [1]. It represents an important source of phosphorus (P), with total P content exceeding 4 g per kg dry matter (DM). However, the availability of P for non-ruminants in barley, like in other cereals and legumes, is low because the major part of P is stored in form of *myo*-inositol hexakisphosphate ($InsP_6$) [2], and its salts, also called phytate, serving as a P source for germination [3]. *Myo*-inositol hexakisphosphate is considered an antinutritional factor due to its low digestibility in monogastric animals but also due to its ability to build mineral complexes which inhibit the absorption of cations (e.g., Ca^{2+}, Fe^{2+} and Zn^{2+})

and protein in the gastrointestinal tract [4,5]. Endogenous cereal phytases that catalyse the hydrolysis of $InsP_6$ to inorganic P and lower *myo*-inositol phosphates (InsP), most importantly *myo*-inositol pentaphosphates ($InsP_5$), *myo*-inositol tetraphosphates ($InsP_4$), and *myo*-inositol triphosphates ($InsP_3$) [6], during germination can be activated by luminal conditions (i.e., pH) in the gastrointestinal tract, rendering a certain amount of P available for the host [7]. Compared with other cereals such as rye and wheat, barley grain possesses lower endogenous phytase activity [2], emphasizing the necessity to treat barley grain to improve intestinal P availability.

Up to now intestinal availability of plant P is mostly enhanced by supplementation of microbial phytases in diets for monogastric livestock species [8], thereby relying on optimal gastrointestinal conditions for maximum phytase activity. Because gastrointestinal pH and digesta passage rate may not always support phytase activity, the degradation of InsP$_6$ prior to feeding to animals is of particular interest as lower InsP can be almost completely used by monogastric animals [9]. Traditional processing methods of cereals for human consumption like soaking, malting, germination, and dough fermentation activate endogenous phytase activity thereby promoting the hydrolysis of InsP$_6$ [2,5,10–12]. Similar processing techniques may apply in livestock animal nutrition. However, because these processing methods reduce availability and concentration of other nutrients and thus lower the nutritional value, processing of feed (e.g., soaking and fermentation) prior to feeding is mostly restricted to liquid feeding systems for pigs by far [13–15]. Lowering pH in the grain stimulates endogenous phytase activity [7]. Therefore, treatment of cereal grains with lactic acid (LA), which is naturally produced during soaking and fermentation in cereal grains, may favor InsP$_6$ hydrolysis [5]. Lower concentrations (0.2–0.9%) of LA previously showed to reduce InsP$_6$ in barley [16] and may be a suitable processing method to treat barley grain. Also, hydrothermal treatment can reduce InsP$_6$ in grains and could therefore lead to a further reduction in InsP$_6$ concentration when combined with LA treatment [16–18]. Because LA treatment can have additional benefits on health and performance in livestock animals [19–24], treatment of barley with LA may be of interest in animal feeding. We hypothesized that soaking barley in increasing concentrations of LA in combination with heat may exert an additive effect on InsP$_6$ hydrolyzing properties. The main aim of this study was to evaluate the hydrolyzing capacity of increasing concentrations (0.5, 1 and 5%) of LA alone or in conjunction with heat on InsP$_6$ degradation in barley grain and the appearance of intermediate InsP such as InsP$_3$, InsP$_4$, and InsP$_5$, and their respective isomers. We were also interested in the effects of chemical and thermal processing on changes in the overall chemical composition of barley, which might have consequences for the feeding value of barley grain for livestock animals.

Materials and Methods

Barley Grain and Lactic Acid

Winter 2-row *Eufora* barley (*Hordeum vulgare* L.) grown during the 2011 season in Eastern Austria was used in this experiment [25]. *Eufora* barley represents a common barley variety used in animal feed and human nutrition in Austria and was provided by the Department of Crop Sciences, Division of Plant Breeding, University of Natural Resources and Life Sciences Vienna, Vienna (research group: H. Grausgruber). After harvesting, grains were carefully cleaned and freed of extraneous matter. Food-grade DL-lactic acid solution (85%, wt/wt) used in this study was purchased from Alfa Aesar GmbH & Co KG (Karlsruhe, Germany). LA solutions (0.5, 1 and 5% LA) were prepared using deionized water (vol/vol). The pH of LA solutions was 2.4, 2.2, and 1.8 for 0.5%, 1% and 5% LA, respectively, prior to treatment.

Soaking and Thermal Treatment of Grains

The procedure of LA and thermal treatments was the same as described in our previous study [25]. Triplicate barley subsamples were randomly taken and soaked in increasing concentrations of LA, without or with heat treatment (LA-H; only 1% and 5% LA), resulting in an orthogonally designed experiment (i.e., 0.5% LA, 1% LA, 5% LA, 1% LA-H, and 5% LA-H). Based on our previous study [25], where the impact of heat treatment on changes in nutrient composition of barley was small for 0.5% LA, only effects of heat treatment with 1 and 5% LA were investigated in this study. For treatment, a barley subsample (50 g) was soaked in the respective LA solution (1:1.6 wt/wt) at room temperature (22°C)

or heated at 55°C in an oven for 48 hours. Attention was paid that every grain was sufficiently soaked in the treatment solution. After the 48-hours incubation, treated barley samples were spread on Petri dishes and air-dried at 22°C for 24 hours before being ground prior to chemical analysis. Samples of LA-H treatment were cooled to 22°C prior to air-drying. Triplicate subsamples of the untreated *Eufora* barley were used as control (native barley). Only the barley grains were used for subsequent analyses. Drip losses, and thus potential nutrient losses, of the wet barley samples onto the Petri dish were not recovered after air-drying.

Sample Preparation

Native and dry treated barley samples were ground to pass a 0.5 mm sieve (Type 738, Fritsch, Rudolstadt, Germany). Barley subsamples used for InsP analyses were ground to pass a 0.2 mm sieve, and attention was paid that the ground mass of barley was fine and uniform for analysis. Milled samples were packed in sealed plastic bags and stored at 4°C until further analyses.

Analyses of Inositol Phosphates

For the analysis of InsP$_3$ to InsP$_6$ isomers, the ground material was extracted twice with a solution containing 0.2 M EDTA and 0.1 M sodium fluoride (pH 10) using a rotary shaker. Sample to extractant ratio was 1 g to 15 mL, and the total time of extraction was 1 h. After centrifugation the combined supernatants were ultracentrifuged using a Microcon filter (cut-off 30 kDa) devise (Millipore, Bedford, MA, USA) at $14,000 \times g$ for 30 minutes. Throughout the whole extraction procedure the samples were kept below 5°C. Filtrates were analyzed by high-performance ion chromatography (HPIC) and InsP were detected using a UV detector at 290 nm after postcolumn derivatization using an ICS-3000 system (Dionex, Idstein, Germany) equipped with a Carbo Pac PA 200 column and corresponding guard column. Gradient elution was done with increasing amounts of hydrochloric acid (0.05 M to 0.5 M within 33 minutes). Fe(NO$_3$)$_3$ solution (0.1% Fe(NO$_3$)$_3$ × 9 H$_2$O in HClO$_4$ was used as reagent for derivatization according to Philippy and Bland [26].

InsP$_6$ dipotassium salt was obtained from Sigma (Deisenhofen, Germany), InsP$_5$ isomers from Sirius Fine Chemicals (Bremen, Germany), InsP$_3$ and InsP$_4$ isomers, as far as available, were from Santa Cruz Biotechnology (Heidelberg, Germany). These standards were used for peak identification. InsP$_6$ was used for calibration. Quantification of lower inositol phosphates was done according to Skoglund et al. [27]. Calibration curves were linear from quantification limit to approximately 10 to 30 μmol/g depending on the InsP isomer.

Quantification limits for InsP-isomers (S/N>10) were 1 μmol/g DM for InsP$_3$ and InsP$_4$ and 0.5 μmol/g DM for InsP$_5$, whereas the detection limits (S/N>5) were 0.5 μmol/g DM for InsP$_3$ to InsP$_4$ and 0.25 μmol/g DM for InsP$_5$. The InsP concentrations were determined as μmol InsP/g DM, and subsequently converted to g P pertaining to each InsP category (i.e., InsP$_3$-P, InsP$_4$-P, InsP$_5$-P, and InsP$_6$-P) based on their molecular weight and the respective content of P in the InsP molecule. Samples were analyzed in duplicate. The abundance of the different InsP$_3$, InsP$_4$ and InsP$_5$ isomers was in untreated barley samples as well as in LA and LA-H treated barley was used to evaluate the nature of the InsP$_6$ degradation caused by LA and heat treatment.

Nutrient Analyses

Dry matter, crude ash (CA), crude protein (CP), starch (total, non-resistant (NRS) and resistant starch (RS)), neutral detergent fiber (NDF), and acid detergent fiber (ADF) of the native and treated barleys were determined. Samples were analyzed for DM by oven-drying at 103°C for 4 h [27]. Crude ash was determined by combustion of samples over night at 580°C [28]. Crude protein was analyzed by the Kjeldahl method [28]. The concentrations of NDF and ADF were determined according to official methods [28,29] using Fiber Therm FT 12 (Gerhardt GmbH & Co. KG, Königswinter, Germany) including heat-stable α-amylase digestion for NDF determination, and were expressed exclusive of residual ash ($aNDF_{OM}$ and ADF_{OM}, respectively). The difference between $aNDF_{OM}$ and ADF_{OM} was considered as the hemicelluloses (HC) fraction. For P determination, samples were analyzed using ICP-OES (Vista Pro, Varian, Darmstadt, Germany) after acid digestion using a combination of sulphuric and nitric acid as described previously [30]. Samples were also analyzed for resistant starch (RS) and non-resistant starch (NRS) using a commercial enzymatic RS assay kit (Megazyme International Ireland Ltd., Bray, Ireland) following manufacturer's protocol, as previously described [25]. Total starch was calculated from RS and NRS fractions. Three subsamples per treatment were analyzed in duplicate.

Statistical Analysis

Data were subjected to two-way ANOVA using the PROC MIXED of SAS (SAS 9.2, SAS Institute Inc., Cary, NC, USA) with polynomial contrasts between control barley and barley treated with 0.5%, 1% and 5% LA as well as orthogonal contrasts between 1% and 5% LA treatments and 1% and 5% LA-H treatments. Linear patterns were analyzed using contrast statement of SAS accounting for unequal spacing among Control and treatments with 0.5, 1, and 5% LA or Control and treatments 1% LA-H and 5% LA-H. Interactions between LA concentration × heat were assessed where applicable. Duplicates per subsample were averaged and used as the experimental unit in the statistical analysis. Processing method served as fixed effect and sample nested within treatment as random effect. Degrees of freedom were approximated by Kenward-Roger method. Differences at $P<0.05$ level were declared significant.

Results

Impact of Lactic Acid and Heat Treatment on the Hydrolysis of Inositol Hexakisphosphate

The concentration of total P was not different between native and LA treated barley. Additional heat treatment reduced total P concentration by 0.3 g in LA-H treated barley compared to the native barley (Table 1). However, total P concentration did not differ between LA and LA-H treated barley. *Myo*-inositol hexakisphosphate concentration decreased in response to LA treatment and, in particular, when barley was treated with LA and oven-heated at 55°C (Figure 1). Gradual increase in LA concentration from 0 to 5% resulted in a linear decrease in $InsP_6$-P concentration from 2.55 g $InsP_6$-P/kg DM for control barley to 2.24, 2.04, and 1.75 g $InsP_6$-P/kg DM for 0.5, 1, and 5% LA, respectively. The additional heat treatment further lowered the $InsP_6$-P concentration to 1.55 and 1.49 g/kg DM for 1 and 5% LA-H, respectively. $InsP_3$ was present in all treatments in amounts of 0.05–0.11 g $InsP_3$-P/kg DM. $InsP_4$ and $InsP_5$ isomers were only quantifiable for 5% LA as well as 1 and 5% LA-H, ranging from 0.10–0.14 g $InsP_4$-P/kg and 0.16–0.22 g $InsP_5$-P/kg DM.

Proportions of $InsP_6$-P and total InsP-P relative to total P in barley are shown in Figure 2. The $InsP_6$-P proportion decreased ($P<0.01$) in barley when treated with LA (from 62.1 in control to 54.7, 50.8, 45.3% for 0.5%, 1% and 5% LA, respectively), and the extent of reduction was greater ($P<0.001$) when the LA-H treatment was applied (41.4 and 40.5% for 1 and 5% LA-H treatments, respectively; Figure 2), compared to the control. Also,

when comparing LA-H with LA treated barley, LA-H treatment reduced the proportion of $InsP_6$-P compared to LA treatment ($P=0.012$). The $InsP_3$-P was only a very small proportion of total InsP-P in the control barley and barley treated with 0.5% and 1% LA; therefore, total InsP-P mainly comprised $InsP_6$-P for these treatments. Due to the increase in $InsP_4$-P and $InsP_5$-P with 5% LA and 1 and 5% LA-H, the proportion of total InsP-P was similar for LA and LA-H treated barley but lower ($P<0.01$) when compared to the control barley (Figure 2).

The $Ins(1,5,6)P_3$ was quantifiable for the control barley and all treatments. In the control group as well as in the treatment with 0.5% LA a peak deriving from one or more of the coeluting isomers $Ins(1,2,6)P_3$, $Ins(1,4,5)P_3$ and $Ins(2,4,5)P_3$ was not detectable, whereas a peak from coeluting isomers was detectable but not quantifiable in barley treated with 5% LA and 1 and 5% LA-H (Figure 3). The $Ins(1,2,5,6)P_4$ was the predominant $InsP_4$ isomer in barley treated with 5% LA and 1 and 5% LA-H (Figure 3). The $InsP_4$ isomer was found in barley treated with 0.5 and 1% LA in amounts below the quantification limit but was not detected in control barley. Furthermore, $Ins(1,2,3,4)P4$ was found in 5% LA and 1 and 5% LA-H treated barley but not in the other treatments. In 5% LA and 1 and 5% LA-H treated barley, $Ins(1,2,3,4,5)P_5$ was the primary $InsP_5$ isomer. $Ins(1,2,3,4,6)P_5$ was detected in the control group and in LA-H treatments, $Ins(1,2,4,5,6)P_5$ were above the detection limit but not quantifiable for all treatments (Figure 4).

Impact of Chemical and Heat Treatment on Barley's Chemical Composition

After soaking barley for 48 h, pH values of barley treated with LA or LA-H raised by 0.3 to 1.2 units (pH 2.5, 2.7, 2.1, 2.7 and 2.1 for 0.5% LA, 1% LA, 5% LA, 1% LA-H and 5% LA-H pre-incubation; and pH 3.7, 3.2, 2.4, 3.9 and 3.0 for 0.5% LA, 1% LA, 5% LA, 1% LA-H and 5% LA-H after 48 h of incubation, respectively).

The greatest change in the chemical composition was observed for the starch content when comparing treated barley samples with the native barley grain (Table 1, Figure 5). In general, LA and in particular LA-H treatment decreased ($P<0.05$) total starch content of barley. Resistant starch, both as g/kg DM and as proportion of total starch, was higher ($P<0.001$) in LA treated barley than in control barley (Figure 5) and peak increase was attained by 5% LA (RS relative to total starch: 0.9 in control vs. 5% in 5% LA). However, when the barley samples that were treated with 5% LA underwent thermal treatment, RS content was comparable to the native barley grain (Figure 5).

The CP content of barley did not change when barley was treated with LA, but additional heat treatment lowered the concentration of CP by 0.4% units compared to the control barley (Table 1). Moreover, LA and LA-H treatment modified the fiber fractions of barley. The contents of $aNDF_{OM}$ and ADF_{OM} increased by 1.7 and 0.8% in response to LA treatment, respectively, whereas the content of HC remained similar for LA treated and control barley. The heat treatment increased $aNDF_{OM}$ and ADF_{OM} concentrations in barley when 1% LA treatment was used compared to the control, whereas heat decreased the $aNDF_{OM}$ concentration by approximately 2% when barley was soaked in 5% LA (Table 1). This finding suggests an interaction ($P<0.01$) between LA and heat treatment for these variables. As a consequence, HC content was reduced by approximately 2.5% with the 5% LA-H treatment compared to the control barley. Barley treated with LA and LA-H also contained less crude ash than the native control barley.

Table 1. Nutrient composition of native barley (CON) or barley steeped in various concentrations of lactic acid at room temperature at 22°C (LA) or oven-heated at 55°C (LA-H).

Item[2]	CON	LA			LA-H		SEM[1]	P-value[3]		
		0.5%	1%	5%	1%	5%		1	2	3
Dry matter (%)	90.7	93.0	92.2	93.1	91.8	92.2	0.09	<0.001	<0.001	<0.001
Starch (% DM)	59.5	55.2	52.5	54.7	55.3	54.5	0.57	<0.001	<0.001	0.038
Crude protein (% DM)	13.4	13.1	13.6	13.1	13.0	12.9	0.07	0.352	0.004	<0.001
NDF (% DM)	14.5	15.0	16.9	16.8	16.1	12.2	0.30	<0.010	0.490	<0.010
ADF (% DM)	5.34	5.97	6.36	6.20	6.36	5.30	0.220	0.010	0.130	0.110
HC (% DM)	9.15	9.04	10.5	10.6	9.77	6.94	0.360	0.090	0.150	<0.010
Ash (% DM)	2.39	1.98	1.97	1.97	1.90	1.83	0.028	<0.001	<0.001	0.002
P (g/kg DM)	4.11	4.07	3.99	3.85	3.79	3.71	0.084	0.220	<0.010	0.100

[1]SEM = standard error of the mean (n = 3).
[2]DM = dry matter, NDF = neutral detergent fiber, ADF = acid detergent fiber, HC = hemicelluloses (NDF – ADF), P = total phosphorus.
[3]Contrasts, 1 = Control vs. LA, 2 = Control vs. LA-H, 3 = LA (1 and 5%) vs. LA-H (1 and 5%+oven-heating).

Discussion

There is an increasing interest in enhancing utilization of minerals from cereal grains used in animal nutrition. This strategy alleviates the dependency on inclusion of large amounts of inorganic P in animal diets with great economical and ecological importance [8,31]. Because of the low availability of P in cereals for monogastric livestock species, a range of feed processing techniques has been applied to reduce their $InsP_6$ concentration. Yet, in the feeding of monogastric livestock species such as swine and poultry, processing techniques used to increase P availability of feeds are often restricted to microbial phytase supplementation [8,32]. Our data indicated that treatment of barley grain with LA and LA-H was able to decrease the $InsP_6$ concentration and thus potentially increase P availability in barley. Most previous studies investigating the effect of LA on phytate degradation focused only on $InsP_6$ disappearance [16,18]. Here, we could show characteristic changes in the accumulation of lower InsP, such as $InsP_3$ to $InsP_5$, related to the LA concentration and heat treatment. These lower InsP may interfere less in intestinal mineral availability than $InsP_6$; however, $InsP_3$ to $InsP_5$ still bind P and can have an inhibitory effect on mineral absorption [33]. Because soaking of cereals in water is current practice in liquid feeding systems for livestock, we abstained from comparing the effects of LA treatment with soaking barley in water in the present study. Also, the present processing of barley grain aimed at being applied in dry feeding systems; therefore, the comparison between the native barley and the LA-treated barley was more relevant for the present study than the comparison between soaking in water and LA.

Overall, the concentration of total P and $InsP_6$ in native barley were in accordance with data from previous studies [34–37] showing comparable $InsP_6$ disappearances when barley was treated with LA and and LA-H [16,18,38]. Accordingly, the $InsP_6$ reducing effect of LA was more pronounced at higher concentrations and potentiated by the heat treatment [16,18,38]. The most effective treatments in the present study, i.e. 5% LA, 1% LA-H and 5% LA-H, converted 17 to 22% of $InsP_6$-P into inorganic P or lower InsP-P in barley grain and the disappearance of $InsP_6$-P was about 10% greater with heat treatment than at room temperature.

Plant phytases and $InsP_6$ are mostly localized in the aleurone layer of cereal grains [39–41]. The two phytases isolated from barley are activated in wet conditions when a slightly acidic pH of 5 and 6 is reached, respectively [39]. Soaking of cereal grains stimulates endogenous LA production causing lower pH with progressing incubation time [16,36,40,42]. Treating barley grains with LA solutions might therefore mimic the endogenous LA production, shortening the time until the critical pH value is reached for phytase activation. However, in this experiment pH values of LA treated barley were much more acidic than the actual pH values for optimum endogenous phytase activity. Possible explanations for $InsP_6$ removal during treatment with LA without or with heat may therefore be that endogenous phytases of barley may have been shortly activated during the soaking process and a certain phytase activity during the drying process cannot be excluded, thereby contributing to the inorganic P release with LA and LA-H treatment. Yet, a reduction in phytase activity was previously found in barley grains soaked in 0.8% LA when compared to barley soaked in water after 48 and 96 h of incubation [16]. Endogenous phytase activity was not determined in the present study. However, it can be assumed that other processes, such as leaching of nutrients and acidic ester hydrolysis, than an enhancement of phytase activity likely contributed to the $InsP_6$ degradation in the present study. Soaking processes are

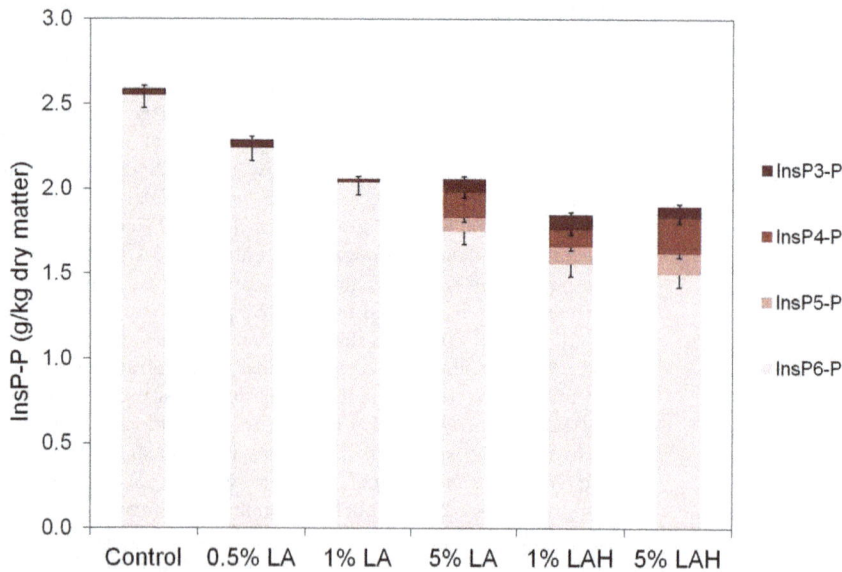

Figure 1. The concentrations of P pertaining to *myo*-inositol tri- to hexakisphosphate (InsP$_3$-P, InsP$_4$-P, InsP$_5$-P, and InsP$_6$-P) and to the sum of them (total InsP-P) in untreated barley (control) or barley soaked in increasing concentrations of lactic acid at room temperature in 22°C (LA) or oven-heated at 55°C (LA-H). Data are shown as least square means ± standard error of the mean (n = 3). For InsP$_3$-P: all contrasts $P > 0.10$; for InsP$_4$-P: control vs. LA $P = 0.50$, control vs. LA-H $P = 0.030$, LA vs. LA-H $P = 0.097$; for InsP$_5$-P: control vs. LA $P = 0.10$, control vs. LA-H $P < 0.001$, LA vs. LA-H $P = 0.006$; for InsP$_6$-P: control vs. LA $P < 0.001$, control vs. LA-H $P < 0.001$, LA vs. LA-H $P < 0.001$; for the sum of InsP-P: control vs. LA $P < 0.001$, control vs. LA-H $P < 0.001$, LA vs. LA-H $P = 0.055$.

generally associated with leaching of nutrients including minerals [3,31,43]. Leaching of minerals into the soaking medium may have been indicated by the lower crude ash concentration in treated barley samples and the higher pH of the soaking medium after the 48-hour incubation compared with initial pH values. Heat treatment can potentiate the soaking effect as the heat causes structural changes in the grain leading to a more rapid hydration (i.e. swelling) of the grain [31,40,44]. As we could only observe a reduction in total P of barley when treated with 1 and 5% LA-H, loss of P and with this of InsP$_6$ by leaching may have been mostly restricted to these treatments. Haraldsson and coworkers [16] estimated that a loss of 5% of InsP$_6$ during soaking and heat treatment (48°C) of barley with 0.8% LA could be explained by leaching processes in their study.

Another explanation for the reduction in InsP$_6$ in response to LA and LA-H treatment of barley could be related to the low pH in the soaking medium. Phosphate groups are esterified to the inositol ring of InsP, and can be removed by acidic ester hydrolysis [16,31,45]. Our data suggest an acceleration of acid hydrolysis of InsP$_6$ in response to additional heat treatment, which is indicated by the lower InsP$_6$ concentration and the accumulation of InsP$_4$ and InsP$_5$ for LA-H treated barley. Because only small amounts of InsP$_5$ to InsP$_3$ were detected, it is likely that this treatment might have triggered a complete degradation of lower InsP as soon as the first phosphate group was released from InsP$_6$ [44]. The accumulation pattern of lower InsP isomers may help to differentiate whether InsP$_6$ hydrolysis was more related to endogenous phytase activity or pH and heat. In this experiment, the occurrence of Ins(1,2,3,4,5)P$_5$, Ins(1,2,3,4)P$_4$, Ins(1,2,5,6)P$_4$ and Ins(1,2,6)P$_3$ with 5% LA and 1 and 5% LA-H may indicate the action of cereal phytases because these phytases, like barley phytases P1 and P2, are suggested to be 6-phytases [E.C.3.1.3.26] [35,46,47]. However, an ultimate distinction between endogenous 6-phytase action and pH and heat effects cannot be made using the present experimental design.

In line with previous studies evaluating soaking procedures [43], the LA and LA-H treatment of barley resulted in small losses of other nutrients. Observed changes in nutrient composition may reduce the feed value of LA and LA-H treated barley, with the decrease in total starch as the most critical loss for the feed value as it affects the energy concentration of barley. Despite its indigestibility for the host animal, the greater RS concentration of LA treated barley may increase the functional and thus health-promoting potential of barley for livestock animals, such as pigs [48] and ruminants [19–22,49]. Aside from leaching of nutrients, e.g. minerals, starch, and water-soluble protein into the soaking medium and potentiation of this effect by heat treatment [43], it is thinkable that the low pH in the soaking medium modified the molecule structure of some nutrients; for instance leading to the higher RS content of barley with increasing LA concentration [25]. Interestingly, the combination of the highest LA concentration and heat likely abolished the effect on RS formation, which confirms previous findings [25].

The leaching of certain nutrients into the soaking medium likely caused an increase in concentrations of other nutrients in barley such as fiber fractions. Here, aNDF$_{OM}$ and ADF$_{OM}$ contents increased for all LA and 1% LA-H treated barley samples thereby maintaining a similar HC content among treatments. Yet, low pH combined with heat treatment seemed to catalyze degradation of fibrous components in barley grain as indicated by the lower aNDF$_{OM}$, ADF$_{OM}$ and HC contents for 5% LA-H treatment compared to all LA and 1% LA-H treatments. Fibrous components can be mostly found in the three aleurone layers of the barley grain and mainly consist of cellulose, arabinoxylan and mixed-linked β-glucan [50]. According to previous studies, the arabinoxylan fraction may be more susceptible to low pH and heat than the cellulose and β-glucan fractions [16,51,52]. The β-glucan fraction in barley may even be stabilized by LA and heat treatment [16].

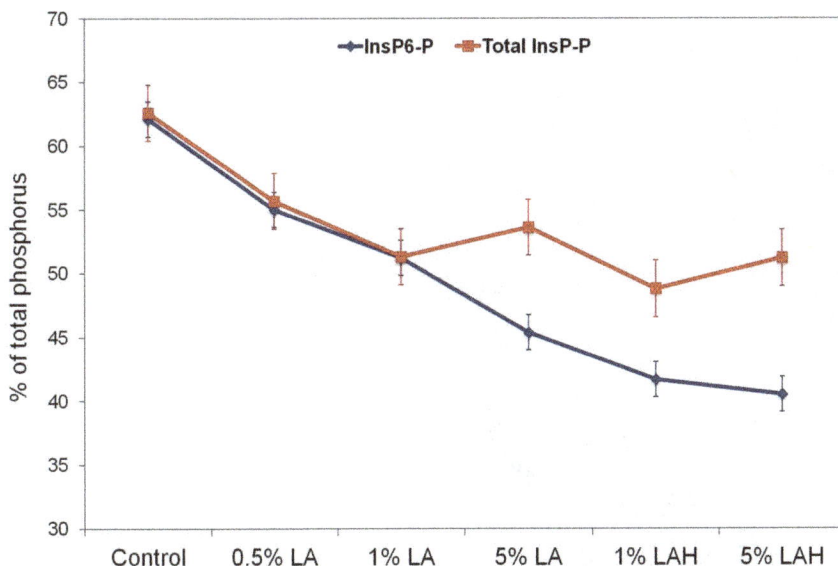

Figure 2. Changes in *myo*-inositol hexakisphosphate (InsP₆-P) and the sum of InsP₃-P to InsP₆-P (total InsP-P) relative to total phosphorus of untreated barley (control) or barley soaked in increasing concentrations of lactic acid at room temperature in 22°C (LA) or oven-heated at 55°C (LA-H). Data are shown as least square means ± standard error of the mean (n = 3). LA and LA-H effects on InsP₆-P: Control vs. LA $P<0.01$, Control vs. LA-H $P<0.001$, LA vs. LA-H $P = 0.012$; LA and LA-H effects on total InsP-P: Control vs. LA $P<0.01$, Control vs. LA-H $P< 0.001$, LA vs. LA-H $P = 0.14$.

Finally, the total InsP₆ degradation by LA and LA-H treatment may remain below the degradation extent reported by dietary supplementation of microbial phytase [34]. Yet, the conditions for the pre-treatment of barley grain may be more easily controlled and stabilized than luminal conditions in the gastrointestinal tract which are necessary to guarantee sufficient InsP₆ degradation.

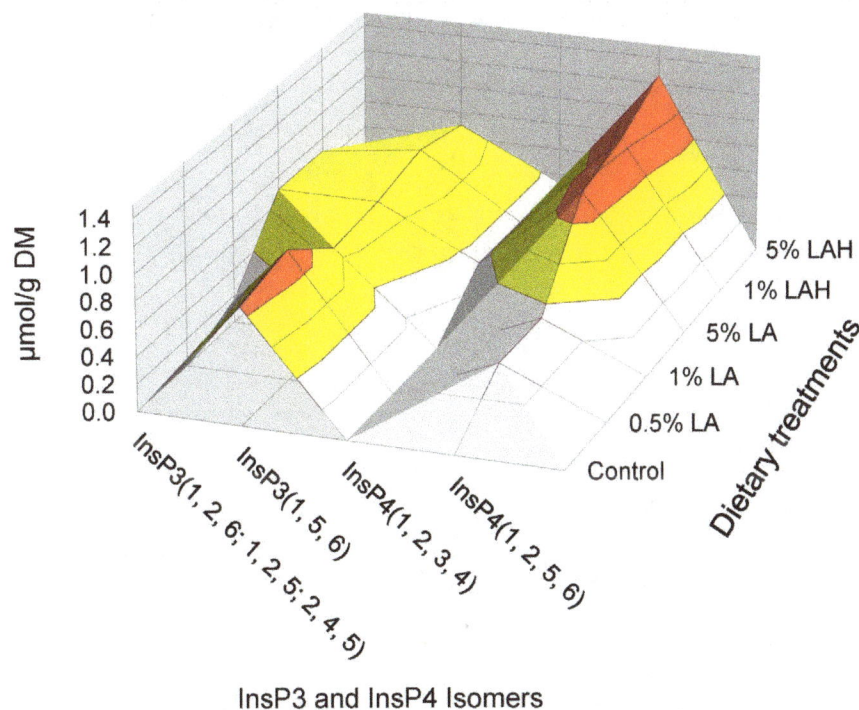

Figure 3. Concentrations of various isomers of *myo*-inositol triphosphate (InsP₃) and tetraphosphate (InsP₄) in untreated barley grain (control) or barley grain soaked in increasing concentrations of lactic acid at room temperature in 22°C (LA) or oven-heated at 55°C (LA-H). Data are shown as least square means (n = 3). Isomers exceeding a concentration of 1 μmol/g dry matter were quantified (area labeled in red color); isomers having concentrations between 0.5 to 1 μmol/g dry matter (detection limit and measurement threshold, respectively) were detected but could not be quantified (area labeled in yellow color); are below detection limit of these isomers is shown in white color (< 0.5 μmol/g dry matter).

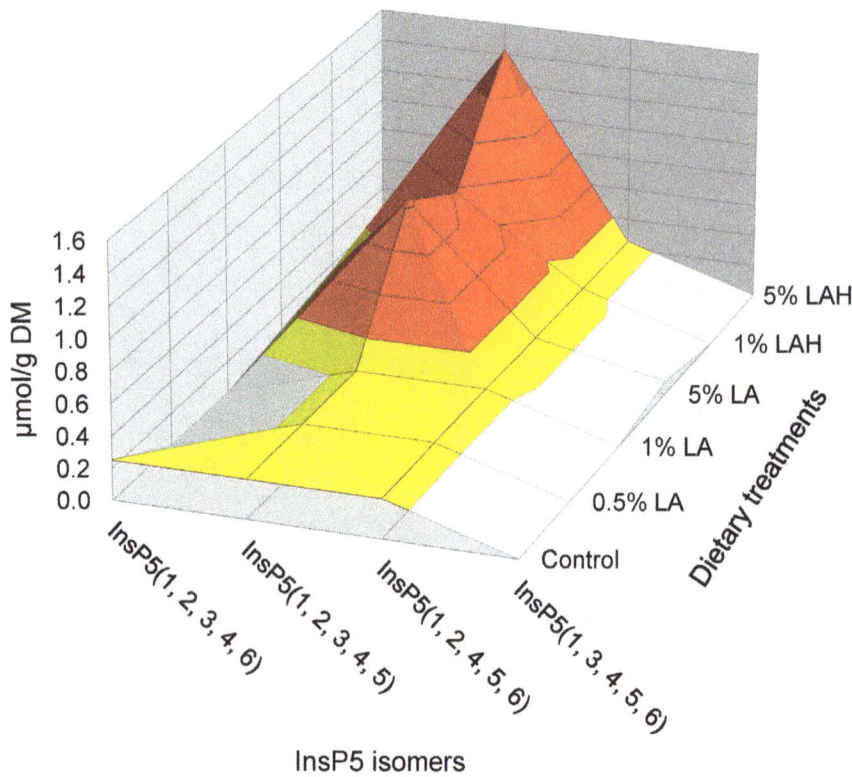

Figure 4. Concentrations of various isomers of *myo*-inositol pentaphosphate (InsP₅) in untreated barley (control) or barley soaked in increasing concentrations of lactic acid at room temperature in 22°C (LA) or oven-heated at 55°C (LAH). Data are shown as least square means (n = 3). Isomers exceeding a concentration of 0.5 μmol/g dry matter were quantified (area labeled in red color); isomers having a concentration between 0.25 to 0.5 μmol/g dry matter (detection limit and measurement threshold, respectively) were detected but could not be quantified (area labeled in yellow); area below detection limit of these isomers is shown in white color (<0.25 μmol/g dry matter).

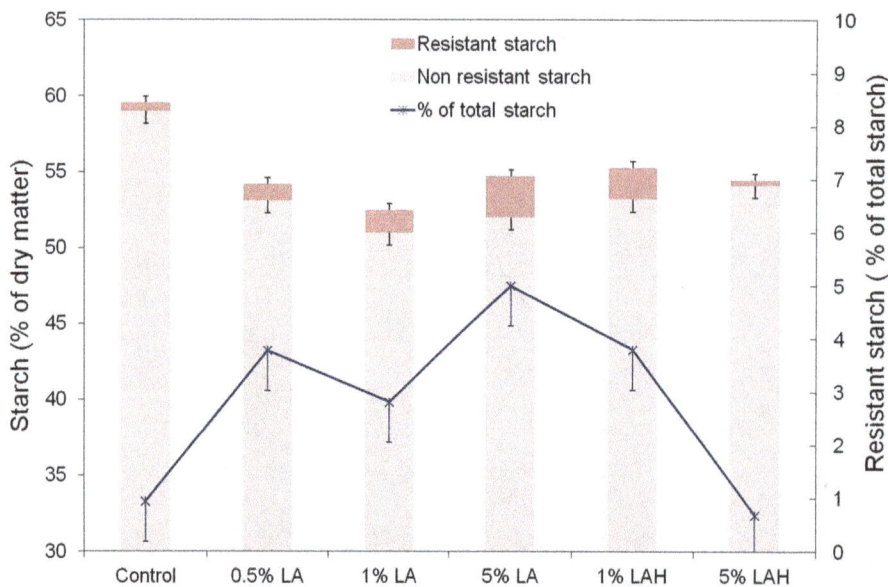

Figure 5. Changes in concentrations of resistant starch (RS) and non-resistant starch (NRS) of untreated barley (Control) or barley soaked in increasing concentrations of lactic acid at room temperature in 22°C (LA) or oven-heated at 55°C (LA-H). Data are shown as least square means ± standard error of the mean (n = 3). LA and LA-H effects on RS: Control vs. LA $P = 0.006$, Control vs. LA-H $P = 0.202$, LA vs. LA-H $P = 0.049$; LA and LA-H effects on RS relative to total starch: Control vs. LA $P = 0.006$, Control vs. LA-H $P = 0.186$, LA vs. LA-H $P = 0.051$; LA and LA-H effects on NRS: Control vs. LA $P<0.001$, Control vs. LA-H $P<0.001$, LA vs. LA-H $P = 0.033$.

Optimum microbial or cereal phytase activity depends on gastrointestinal pH and passage rate and may be biased in case luminal conditions are suboptimal in vivo. For instance, in pigs after weaning gastric pH may not reach the necessary acidic pH for microbial phytase activation [53]. Even in cattle nutrition, the inclusion of phytases has been suggested to optimize the utilization of dietary P [54] which indicates that, despite the highly complex rumen microbiota and long ruminal retention times of about 30–48 hours of ingested feed [55], $InsP_6$ hydrolyzing capacity may be limited, in particular when short forage particle size is fed [54]. Additional advantages of LA treatment of barley are improved storage stability by decreasing molding of the grain post-harvest and, when eaten, support of gastric barrier function in monogastric livestock animals [56]. In dairy cows, treating the barley fraction of the diet with 0.5 and 1% LA proved beneficial for rumen fermentation and immune-metabolic health status of the animals [19–22].

In conclusion, treating barley grain with LA or LA-H may be effective processing techniques to reduce the $InsP_6$ concentration of cereals used in animal feeding. The greatest $InsP_6$ hydrolysis was observed with the highest investigated LA concentration of 5% and heat treatment. Lower InsP profiles obtained with 5% LA, 1% LA-H and 5% LA-H treatments are similar to profiles found when microbial 6-phytase is applied. Changes in nutrient composition of barley grain due to LA and LA-H treatment, i.e. lower starch and ash concentrations and accumulation of fiber fractions, may impact the feed value of barley, but might increase its health-enhancing properties, in particular, due to greater concentrations of RS and dietary fiber. To determine the actual intestinal P availability and to assess the effects of changes in nutrient composition and functional abilities of LA and LA-H treated barley, further in vivo studies are needed.

Acknowledgments

The assistance of A. Dockner, S. Leiner and M. Wild (Institute of Animal Nutrition and Functional Plant Compounds, University of Veterinary Medicine Vienna, Austria) for the feed chemical analyses is gratefully acknowledged.

Author Contributions

Conceived and designed the experiments: QZ. Performed the experiments: KD MS. Analyzed the data: BM. Contributed reagents/materials/analysis tools: MS MR QZ. Contributed to the writing of the manuscript: BM QZ MS MR.

References

1. Baik BK, Ullreich E (2008) Barley for food: Characteristics, improvement, and renewed interest. J Cereal Sci 48: 233–242.

2. Egli I, Davidsson L, Juillerat MA, Barclay D, Hurrell RF (2002) The influence of soaking and germination on the phytase activity and phytic acid content of grains and seeds potentially useful for complementary feeding. J Food Sci 67: 3484–3488.

3. Stewart A, Nield H, Lott JNA (1988) An investigation of the mineral content of barley grains and seedlings. Plant Physiol 86: 93–97.

4. Sandberg AS (1991) The effect of food processing on phytate hydrolysis and availability of iron and zinc. Adv Exp Med Biol 289: 499–508.

5. Leenhardt F, Levrat-Verny MA, Chanliaud E, Rémésy C (2005) Moderate decrease of pH by sourdough fermentation is sufficient to reduce phytate content of whole wheat flour through endogenous phytase activity. J Agric Food Chem 53: 98–102.

6. Ariza A, Moroz OV, Blagova EV, Turkenburg JP, Waterman J, et al. (2013) Degradation of phytate by the 6-phytase from hafnia alvei : A combined structural and solution study. PLoS ONE 8: e65062.

7. Pable A, Gujar P, Khire JM (2014) Selection of phytase producing yeast strains for improved mineral mobilization and dephytinization of chickpea flour. J Food Biochem 38: 18–27.

8. Kiarie E, Romero LF, Nyachoti CM (2013) The role of added feed enzymes in promoting gut health in swine and poultry. Nutr Res Rev 26: 71–88.

9. Blaabjerg K, Jørgensen H, Tauson AH, Poulsen HD (2011) The presence of inositol phosphates in gastric pig digesta is affected by time after feeding a nonfermented or fermented liquid wheat- and barley-based diet. J Anim Sci 89: 3153–3162.

10. Proulx AK, Reddy MB (2007) Fermentation and lactic acid addition enhance iron bioavailability of maize. J Agric Food Chem 55: 2749–2754.

11. Afify AE-MMR, El-Beltagi HS, Abd El-Salam SM, Omran AA (2011) Bioavailability of iron, zinc, phytate and phytase activity during soaking and germination of white sorghum varieties. PLoS ONE 6: e25512.

12. Sanz-Penella JM, Frontela C, Ros G, Martinez C, Monedero V, et al. (2012) Application of bifidobacterial phytases in infant cereals: Effect on phytate contents and mineral dialyzability. J Agric Food Chem 60: 11787–11792.

13. Canibe N, Jensen BB (2003) Fermented and nonfermented liquid feed to growing pigs: effect on aspects of gastrointestinal ecology and growth performance. J Anim Sci 81: 2019–2031.

14. Canibe NH, Miettinen H, Jensen BB (2008) Effect of adding Lactobacillus plantarum or a formic acid containing-product to fermented liquid feed on gastrointestinal ecology and growth performance of piglets. Livest Sci 114: 251–262.

15. Plumed-Ferrer C, von Wright A (2009) Fermented pig liquid feed: nutritional, safety and regulatory aspects. J Appl Microbiol 106: 351–368.

16. Haraldsson A-K, Rimsten L, Alminger ML, Andersson R, Andlid T, et al. (2004) Phytate content is reduced and β-glucanase activity suppressed in malted barley steeped with lactic acid at high temperature. J Sci Food Agric 84: 653–662.

17. Tabekhia MM, Luh BS (1980) Effect of germination, cooking, and canning on phosphorus and phytate retention in dry beans. J Food Sci 45: 406–408.

18. Fredlund K, Asp N-G, Larsson M, Marklinder I, Sandberg AS (1997) Phytate reduction in whole grains of wheat, rye, barley and oats after hydrothermal treatment. J Cereal Sci 25: 83–91.

19. Iqbal S, Zebeli Q, Mazzolari A, Bertoni G, Dunn SM, et al. (2009) Feeding barley grain steeped in lactic acid modulates rumen fermentation patterns and increases milk fat content in dairy cows. J Dairy Sci 92: 6023–6032.

20. Iqbal S, Zebeli Q, Mazzolari A, Dunn SM, Ametaj BN (2010) Feeding rolled barley grain steeped in lactic acid modulated energy status and innate immunity in dairy cows. J Dairy Sci 93: 5147–5156.

21. Iqbal S, Terrill SJ, Zebeli Q, Mazzolari A, Dunn SM et al. (2012) Treating barley grain with lactic acid and heat prevented sub-acute ruminal acidosis and increased milk fat content in dairy cows. Anim Feed Sci Technol 172: 141–149.

22. Iqbal S, Zebeli Q, Mazzolari A, Dunn SM, Ametaj BN (2012) Barley grain-based diet treated with lactic acid and heat modulated plasma metabolites and acute phase response in dairy cows. J Anim Sci 90: 3143–3152.

23. Tanaka T, Imai Y, Kumagae N, Sato S (2010) The effect of feeding lactic acid to Salmonella typhimurium experimentally infected swine. J Vet Med Sci 72: 827–831.

24. Willamil J, Creus E, Pérez JF, Mateu E, Martín-Orúe SM (2011) Effect of a microencapsulated feed additive of lactic and formic acid on the prevalence of Salmonella in pigs arriving at the abattoir. Arch Anim Nutr 65: 431–444.

25. Deckardt K, Khiaosa-ard R, Grausgruber H, Zebeli Q (2014) Evaluation of various chemical and thermal feed processing methods for their potential to enhance resistant starch content in barley grain. Starch/Stärke 66: 558–565.

26. Philippy BQ, Bland JM (1988) Gradient ion chromatography of inositol phosphates. Anal Biochem 175: 162–166.

27. Skoglund E, Carlsson NG, Sandberg AS (1997) Determination of isomers of inositol mono- to hexaphosphates in selected foods and intestinal contents using high-performance ion chromatography. J Agric Food Chem 45: 431–436.

28. VDLUFA (Verband Deutscher Landwirtschaftlicher Untersuchungs- und Forschungsanstalten), in: Handbuch der Landwirtschaftlichen Versuchs- und Untersuchungsmethodik, Bd. III Die chemische Untersuchung von Futtermitteln, 4. Erg.-Lfg., VDLUFA-Verlag, Darmstadt, Germany, 1997.

29. Van Soest PJ, Robertson JB, Lewis BA (1991) Methods for dietary fiber, neutral detergent fiber, and nonstarch polysaccharides in relation to animal nutrition. J Dairy Sci 74: 3583–3597.

30. Shastak Y, Witzig M, Hartung K, Rodehutscord M (2012) Comparison of retention and prececal digestibility measurements in evaluating mineral phosphorus sources in broilers. Poultry Sci 91: 2201–2209.

31. Bohn L, Meyer AS, Rasmussen SK (2008) Phytate: impact on environment and human nutrition. A challenge for molecular breeding. J Zhejiang Univ Sci B 9: 165–191.

32. Rutherfurd SM, Chung TK, Moughan PJ (2014) Effect of microbial phytase on phytate P degradation and apparent digestibility of total P and Ca throughout the gastrointestinal tract of the growing pig. J Anim Sci 92: 189–197.

33. Sandberg AS, Brune M, Carlsson NG, Hallberg L, Skoglund E, et al. (1999) Inositol phosphates with different numbers of phosphate groups influence iron absorption in humans. Am J Clin Nutr 70: 240–246.

34. Shen Y, Yin YL, Chavez ER, Fan MZ (2005) Methodological aspects of measuring phytase activity and phytate phosphorus content in selected cereal grains and digesta and feces of pigs. J Agric Food Chem 53: 853–859.

35. Pontoppidan K, Pettersson D, Sandberg AS (2007) The type of thermal feed treatment influences the inositol phosphate composition. Anim Feed Sci Technol 132: 137–147.

36. Blaabjerg K, Nørgaard JV, Poulsen HD (2012) Effect of microbial phytase on phosphorus digestibility in non-heat-treated and heat-treated wheat-barley pig diets. J Anim Sci 90: 206–208.

37. Esmaeilipour O, van Krimpen MM, Jongbloed AW, De Jonge LH, Bikker P (2012) Effects of temperature, pH, incubation time, and pepsin concentration on the in vitro stability of 2 intrinsic phytase of wheat, barley, and rye. Anim Feed Sci Technol 175: 168–174.

38. Bergman EL, Fredlund K, Reinikainen P, Sandberg AS (1999) Hydrothermal processing of barley (cv. Blenheim): optimisation of phytate degradation and increase of free myo-inositol. J Cereal Sci 29: 261–272.

39. Greiner R, Jany KD, Alminger ML (2000) Identification and properties of myo-inositol hexakisphosphate phosphohydrolases (Phytases) from barley (Hordeum vulgare). J Cereal Sci 31: 127–139.

40. Raboy V (2003) Myo-Inositol-1,2,3,4,5,6-hexakisphosphate. Phytochemistry 64: 1033–1043.

41. Dionisio G, Holm PB, Brinch-Pedersen H (2007) Wheat (Triticum aestivum L.) and barley (Hordeum vulgare L.) multiple inositol polyphosphate phosphatases (MINPPs) are phytases expressed during grain filling and germination. Plant Biotech J 5: 325–338.

42. Beal JD, Niven SJ, Brooks PH, Gill BP (2005) Variation in short chain fatty acid and ethanol concentration resulting from the natural fermentation of wheat and barley for inclusion in liquid diets for pigs. J Sci Food Agric 85: 433–440.

43. Hurrell RF (2004) Phytic acid degradation as a means of improving iron absorption. Int J Vitam Nutr Res. 74: 445–452.

44. Blaabjerg K, Jørgensen H, Tauson AH, Poulsen HD (2010) Heat-treatment, phytase and fermented liquid feeding affect the presence of inositol phosphates in ileal digesta and phosphorus digestibility in pigs fed a wheat and barley diet. Animal 4: 876–85.

45. March JG, Simonet BM, Grases F, Salvador A (1998) Indirect determination of phytic acid in urine. Analytica Chimia Acta 1–3: 63–68.

46. Sandberg AS (2001) In vitro and in vivo degradation of phytate. In: Food phytases, Eds. R Reddy and SK Sathe. CRC Press, Boca Raton, FL, USA; 139–156.

47. Greiner R, Farouk AE, Carlsson NG, Konietzny U (2007) myo-inositol phosphate isomers generated by the action of a phytase from a Malaysian waste-water bacterium. Protein J 26: 577–584.

48. Regmi PR, Metzler-Zebeli BU, Gänzle MG, Van Kempen TAG, Zijlstra RT (2011) Starch with high amylose content and low in vitro digestibility increases intestinal nutrient flow and microbial fermentation and selectively promotes bifidobacteria in pigs. J Nutr 141: 1273–1280.

49. Deckardt K, Khol-Parisini A, Zebeli Q (2013) Peculiarities of enhancing resistant starch in ruminants using chemical methods: opportunities and challenges. Nutrients 5: 1970–1988.

50. Selvendran RR, Stevens BJH, DuPont MS, (1987) Dietary fiber: chemistry, analysis and properties. Adv Food Res 31: 117–209.

51. Agger J, Johansen KS, Meyer AS (2011) pH catalyzed pretreatment of corn bran for enhanced enzymatic arabinoxylan degradation. N Biotechnol 28: 125–135.

52. Holopainen-Mantila U, Marjamaa K, Merali Z, Käsper A, de Bot P, et al. (2013) Impact of hydrothermal pre-treatment to chemical composition, enzymatic digestibility and spatial distribution of cell wall polymers. Bioresour Technol. 138: 156–62.

53. de Lange CFM, Pluske J, Gong J, Nyachoti CM (2010) Strategic use of feed ingredients and feed additives to stimulate gut health and development in young pigs. Livest Sci 134: 124–134.

54. Jarrett JP, Wilson JW, Ray PP, Knowlton KF (2014) The effects of forage particle length and exogenous phytase inclusion on phosphorus digestion and absorption in lactating cows. J Dairy Sci. 97: 411–418.

55. Zebeli Q, Tafaj M, Weber I, Dijkstra J, Steingass H, et al. (2007) Effects of varying dietary forage particle size in two concentrate levels on chewing activity, ruminal mat characteristics, and passage in dairy cows. J Dairy Sci. 90: 1929–1942.

56. Heo JM, Opapeju FO, Pluske JR, Kim JC, Hampson DJ, et al. (2013) Gastrointestinal health and function in weaned pigs: a review of feeding strategies to control post-weaning diarrhoea without using in-feed antimicrobial compounds. J Anim Physiol Anim Nutr (Berl) 97: 207–237.

8

Transcriptional Profiling of Disease-Induced Host Responses in Bovine Tuberculosis and the Identification of Potential Diagnostic Biomarkers

Elihu Aranday-Cortes[1], Philip J. Hogarth[1], Daryan A. Kaveh[1], Adam O. Whelan[1], Bernardo Villarreal-Ramos[1], Ajit Lalvani[2], H. Martin Vordermeier[1]*

1 TB Research Group, Animal Health & Veterinary Laboratories Agency Weybridge, New Haw, Addlestone, Surrey, United Kingdom, 2 Tuberculosis Immunology Group, National Heart and Lung Institute, Imperial College London, London, United Kingdom

Abstract

Bovine tuberculosis (bTb) remains a major and economically important disease of livestock. Improved ante-mortem diagnostic tools would help to underpin novel control strategies. The definition of biomarkers correlating with disease progression could have impact on the rational design of novel diagnostic approaches for bTb. We have used a murine bTb model to identify promising candidates in the host transcriptome post-infection. RNA from *in vitro*-stimulated splenocytes and lung cells from BALB/c mice infected aerogenically with *Mycobacterium bovis* were probed with high-density microarrays to identify possible biomarkers of disease. In antigen-stimulated splenocytes we found statistically significant differential regulation of 1109 genes early (3 days) after infection and 1134 at a later time-point post-infection (14 days). 618 of these genes were modulated at both time points. In lung cells, 282 genes were significantly modulated post-infection. Amongst the most strongly up-regulated genes were: granzyme A, granzyme B, cxcl9, interleukin-22, and ccr6. The expression of 14 out of the most up-regulated genes identified in the murine studies was evaluated using *in vitro* with antigen-stimulated PBMC from uninfected and naturally infected cattle. We show that the expression of cxcl9, cxcl10, granzyme A and interleukin-22 was significantly increased in PBMC from infected cattle compared to naïve animals following PPD stimulation *in vitro*. Thus, murine transcriptome analysis can be used to predict immunological responses in cattle allowing the prioritisation of CXCLI9, CXCL10, Granzyme A and IL-22 as potential additional readout systems for the ante-mortem diagnosis of bovine tuberculosis.

Editor: Pere-Joan Cardona, Fundació Institut d'Investigació en Ciències de la Salut Germans Trias i Pujol. Universitat Autònoma de Barcelona. CIBERES, Spain

Funding: This work was funded by the Department for Environment, Food and Rural Affairs, United Kingdom. The funders had no role in study design, data collection and analysis, decision to publish, or preparation of the manuscript.

Competing Interests: The authors have declared that no competing interests exist.

* E-mail: martin.vordermeier@ahvla.gsi.gov.uk

Introduction

Bovine tuberculosis (bTb), mainly caused by mainly by *Mycobacterium bovis*, remains an economically important disease of livestock such as cattle [1] and is also a disease of zoonotic importance. Host biomarkers for bTb are needed urgently in several areas to underpin disease control strategies. For example, correlates of disease and/or pathology could improve the sensitivity of immunological ante-mortem diagnosis which is at present mainly based on tuberculin skin testing and ancillary blood tests. Furthermore, predictors of protection and correlates of protective immunity after vaccination would greatly facilitate vaccine development.

Although IFN-γ production has been a useful tool for the blood-based detection of *M. bovis* infection in cattle and other species [2,3,4] as well as for the detection of *M. tuberculosis* infected humans, additional biomarkers could improve the accuracy of *in vitro* blood tests [5]. For example, it has been shown recently that simultaneous measurement of antigen-stimulated IL-1β and TNF-α production enhances IFN-γ test sensitivity to diagnose bTb in cattle [6]. Previously, we have shown in a mouse model of *M. bovis* infection that studying cellular immune responses in BCG vaccinated compared to control animals can guide the study of

corresponding responses found in cattle [7]. Therefore, in the present study we applied a systematic approach to discover potential diagnostic biomarkers based on the definition of biomarkers in a cost-effective murine bTb model followed by validation of promising markers in cattle.

The paucity of reagents for cattle for the study of immunologically relevant markers by antibody-based assays such as the luminex multiplex system applied to human tuberculosis (e.g. [8]), makes host transcriptome analysis in cattle an attractive alternative. Therefore, in this study we report our application of microarray technology in combination with murine *M. bovis* infection experiments to select the most strongly up-regulated genes expressed from the whole transcriptomes of lung and spleen cells to predict biomarkers of disease in *M. bovis* infected cattle.

Results

Gene expression profiling of early disease in spleen and lung from mice infected with *M. bovis*

In order to identify potential biomarkers of tuberculosis infection, two groups of 5 BALB/C mice each were infected with *M. bovis*. After 3 and 14 days post-infection (p.i.) mice were euthanized and their splenocytes stimulated *in vitro* for 3 days with a protein pool of seven defined mycobacterial antigens, termed M7. Lung cells were collected and stimulated only at the 14 day p.i. time point. Following stimulation the fold change of gene expression was established using Whole Mouse Genome Oligo Microarrays. First, we compared the global transcriptional response in the spleen of mice infected with *M. bovis* against uninfected mice, and genes were considered significant when their corrected p-values were below 0.05 with more than a 2-fold change of expression. In antigen-stimulated splenocytes we found significant modulation of 1109 genes early after infection (day 3 p.i., Table S1) and 1134 at later time-point post-infection (day 14 p.i.) (Table S1). Unsupervised hierarchical cluster was performed using a centered linkage with a Person centered measure showing that 618 of these genes were modulated at both time points (Figure 1). Amongst the genes most strongly up-regulated at both time points p.i. was granzyme A (gzmA) with 21-fold and 26-fold changes in expression in infected animals compared to naïve controls after 3 days and 14 days p.i. respectively (Table 1). Amongst the genes significantly modulated only at 14 days p..i. were histocompatibility 28 (H28), and ubiquitin D, suggesting that they are associated with early disease progression (data not shown).

In antigen-stimulated lung cells we found 282 genes that were significantly modulated after 14 days post-infection (see Table S2 for list of genes and Figure 2 for heat-map of this signature of 282 genes). As expected [9], ifn-γ was strongly up-regulated (82-fold) in the lungs of infected animals after 14 days p.i. compared with naïve mice. Following the same trend were il-22 and cxcl9 with 74-fold and 22-fold change in their expression, respectively (Tables 1 and S2). Other genes that were differentially expressed in lungs after *M. bovis* infection were granzyme B, lymphocyte activation gene-3, il-17E receptor, and ccr6 (Tables 1 and S2).

Pathway Analysis

Pathway Analysis using IPA was performed on the 282 genes that were significantly modulated in antigen-stimulated lung cells after 14 days post-infection. The two most significantly associated canonical pathways were related to T Helper Cell Differentiation ($-\log[\text{p-value}] = 9.47\text{E}00$ and ratio $= 1.53\text{E}-01$) and B Cell Development ($-\log[\text{p-value}] = 7.88\text{E}00$ and ratio $= 1.53\text{E}-01$) (Figure 3A). The five networks most significantly associated with these genes were inflammatory response (60 genes, p-value $= 2.83\text{E}-15$), Cell-To-Cell Signalling and Interaction (63 genes, ρ-value $= 2.95\text{E}-15$), Cellular Growth and Proliferation

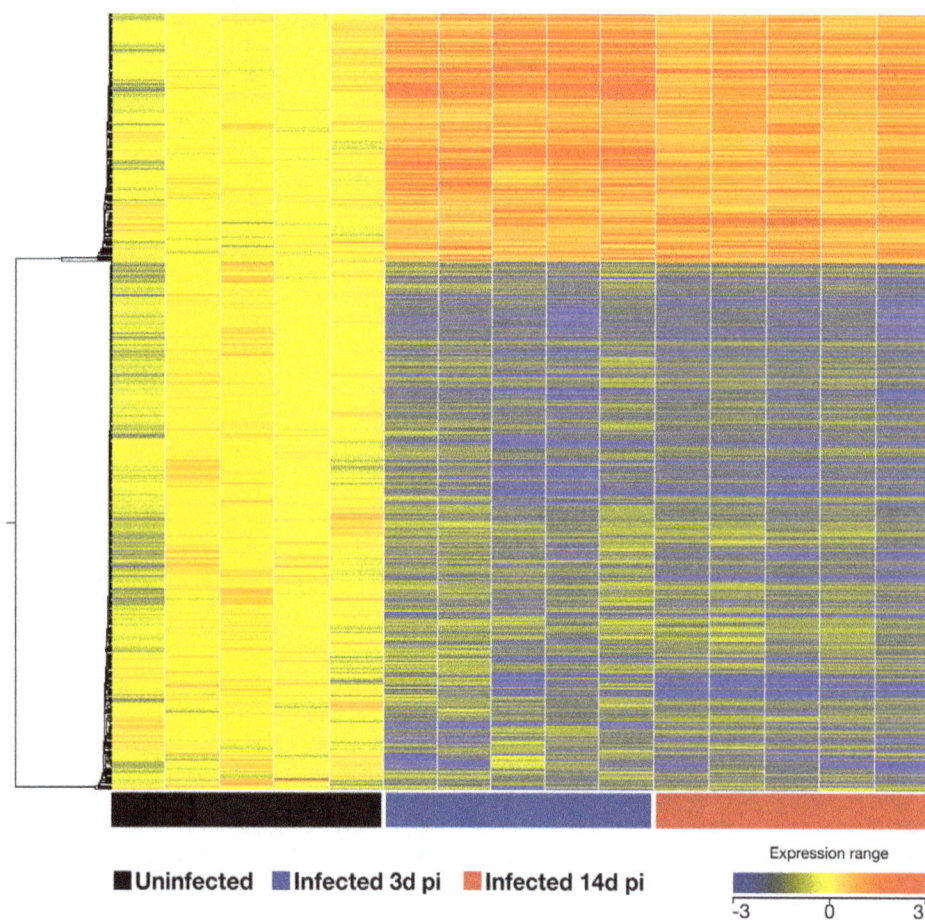

Figure 1. Spleen gene signature after 3 and 14 days after infection with *M. bovis*. The global transcriptional response in spleen cells of mice infected with *M. bovis* was compared to responses in uninfected mice. Genes were considered significantly modulated when their corrected p-values were below 0.05 with more than 2-fold change of expression at both time points. After 3 and 14 days post-infection (blue square and red squares, respectively at the bottom of graph), the mice were euthanized and their splenocytes were stimulated in vitro for 3 days with M7 protein pool (*see Materials and Methods*). Black squares: Naïve control mice. Unsupervised hierarchical cluster was performed using a centroid linkage with a Person centered measure showing that 618 of these genes were modulated at both time points (see table S1 for list of these genes, with genes significantly modulated at both time points highlighted in bold).

Table 1. Expression of the most up-regulated genes found in the murine model in cattle using PBMC from uninfected (bTb-free, n = 9) and naturally with *M. bovis* infected cows (bTb, n = 11).

Gene Name	Gene Symbol	Mouse data Lung	Bovine PBMC data bTb Free Mean ± SEM of Log(FC)	bTb Mean ± SEM of Log(FC)	p-value
		14 days p.i.			
Interferon gamma	IFN-γ	82.54	0.068±0.30	2.122±0.19	<0.0001*
Interlukin-22	IL-22	74.15	0.125±0.32	2.215±0.20	0.0002*
Chemokine (C-X- motif) ligand 9	Cxcl9	23.8	0.149±0.24	2.492±0.26	<0.0001*
Interleukin-17A[a]	IL-17A	NA	0.509±0.33	1.73±0.13	0.0052
Chemokine (C-X- motif) ligand 10	Cxcl10	22.13	0.079±0.19	1.626±0.28	0.0004*
Lymphocyte-activation gene 3	Lag3	12.11	0.436±0.31	0.228±0.18	0.582
Signal transducer and activator of transcription 1	Stat1	3.15	0.234±0.11	0.466±0.17	0.3746
Granzyme B	GzmB	5.84	−0.167±0.19	−0.242±0.09	0.7249
Interferon regulatory factor	Irf4	4.25	0.275±0.21	0.200±0.13	0.7664
Interferon gamma inducible protein 47	Ifi47	4.14	0.008±0.02	0.089±0.17	0.7964
Interleukin-17 receptor E receptor	IL-17RE	3.99	0.567±0.36	−0.285±0.32	0.1638
		Spleen			
		3 days p.i. 14 days p.i.			
Granzyme A	GzmA	21.27 26.58	−0.232±0.35	1.245±0.23	0.0029*
Acetylgalactosamin transferase 3	Galnt3	19.21 13.34	−0.167±0.19	−0.242±0.09	0.7249
Adenosine deaminase	Ada	18.42 12.09	−0.641±0.12	−0.669±0.26	0.9366
Killer cell lectin-like receptor subfamily K member 1	Klrk1	5.02 4.81	1.206±0.59	−0.058±0.39	0.1141

The data are represented as mean (± SEM) fold changes in expression after stimulation of PBMC with bovine PPD-B. Significance level for comparison of results in bTb-free and infected animals: p -value≤0.0033 (*).
[a]Used as positive control.
NA, not applicable.

(77 genes, p-value = 8.2E−15) and Hematological System Development and Function (76 genes, p-value = 8.2E−15) (Figure 3B).

In antigen-stimulated splenocytes at 3 and 14 days p.i. we found statistically significant modulation of genes associated with the following dominant canonical pathways contained genes associated with T cell receptor Signalling (3 days p.i.: −log[p-value] = 5.65E+00 and ratio = 1.65E−01; 14 days p.i.: −log[p-value] = 7.8E00 and ratio = 1.93E−01) and iCOS-iCOSL Signaling in T Helper Cells (3 days p.i.: −log[p-value] = 4.83E00 and ratio = 1.39E−01; 14 days p.i.: −log[p-value] = 6.84E00 and ratio = 1.64E−01) (Figure 4A). Statistically significant modulation of genes of the following networks was also observed: Inflammatory Response (3 days p.i.: 175 genes, p-value = 7.51E−23; 14 days p.i.: 194 genes, p-value = 4.35E−33), Cellular Growth and Proliferation (3 days p.i.: 278 genes, p-value = 1.73E−22; 14 days p.i. : 289 genes, p-value = 2.51E−31), Hematological System Development and Function (3 days p.i.: 219 genes, p-value = 7.51E−23; 14 day p.i.: 235 genes, p-value = 2.51E−31), Tissue Morphology (3 days p.i. : 130 genes, p-value = 7.51E−23; 14 days p.i.: 142 genes, p-value = 1.59E−06), and Cell Death (3 days p.i.: 210 genes, p-value = 2.47E−19; 14 days p.i.: 227 genes, p-value = 2.09E−28) (Figure 4B).

Interestingly, when the networks and pathways associated with infection at the 14 days p.i. time point were compared between lung and spleen, the genes enriched in these pathways showed up-regulated expression in lung cells. In contrast, the same networks and pathways in spleen cells were enriched for genes whose expression was down-regulated. For example; whilst in the lungs the inflammatory response network is mainly represented by up-regulated genes, down-regulated genes dominate in the same network in spleen cells. Similarly, up-regulated genes were enriched in the T helper cell differentiation canonical pathway in lungs from infected mice, but in spleens the genes enriched in the same canonical pathway were predominantly regulated genes (Figure 5A and B).

Validation of differential gene expression in natural infected cattle by qPCR

Our principal translational objective was the identification of biomarkers with potential application for blood-based ante-mortem diagnosis of bTb in cattle. Based on our previous results [10,11], we hypothesized that results obtained in our mouse model could guide the selection of such markers for cattle. Thus, we evaluated the expression of a selection of genes most strongly up-regulated in the mouse experiments described above (Table 1) in cattle using PBMC from uninfected and cattle naturally infected with *M. bovis*. Apart from genes expressed in the lung of infected mice (14 days p.i.), we also selected genes from the murine spleen that were up-regulated both early and late after infection (3 and 14 days p.i.). IL17A was included as positive control as it had been shown previously to be associated with infected cattle [10,12,13]. RNA was prepared from PBMC cultures stimulated with PPD-B and the expression of these genes evaluated by qRT-PCR. The results are shown in Table 1. Five

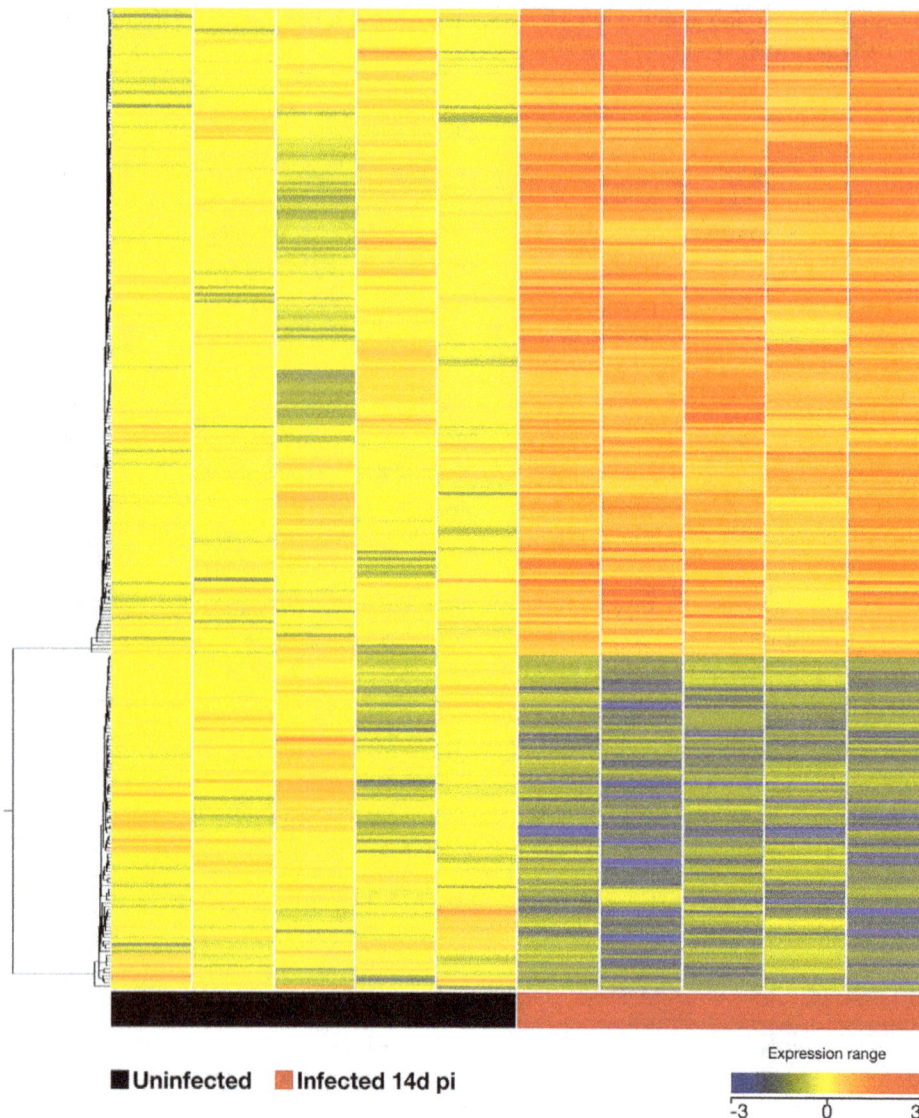

Figure 2. Pulmonary gene signature after 14 days after infection with *M. bovis*. The global transcriptional response in the lung of mice infected with *M. bovis* was compared the response of uninfected mice. Genes were considered significant when their correct p-value were below 0.05 with more than 2-fold change of expression. After 14 days post-infection the mice were euthanized and their lung cells were stimulated in vitro for 3 days with M7 protein pool (*see Materials and Methods*). Unsupervised hierarchical cluster was performed using a centroid linkage with a Person centered measure showing that 282 of these genes were modulated (see table S2 for list of these genes).

of the 14 genes selected based on the murine transcriptome analyses described above were found to be also significantly up-regulated in bovine PBMC from infected animals compared to naïve controls. The most highly modulated genes were those encoding IFN-γ, IL22, CXCL9, CXCL10, and GzmA (Table 1). The other 9 genes studied were not significantly modulated in bovine PBMC from infected animals (Table 1). The gene encoding for IL17A was also expressed stronger in bTb infected cattle compared to TB-free cows, although its expression was not quite statistically significant (P = 0.0052, Table 1).

When we compared the expression of the genes encoding IFN-γ, IL22, CXCL9, CXCL10, GzmA, and IL17A, we did not find correlations between their expression the disease severity described by the pathology scores [14] assigned after post *mortem* examinations of the infected cattle (data not shown). However, this study was not designed primarily to correlate expression levels with disease severity and we therefore acknowledge that its

statistical power was not sufficient to avoid type 2 errors. Larger animal numbers, including experimentally infected cattle need to be tested to validate this hypothesis in greater details.

In a final set of experiments we determined the phenotype of the bovine T cell subset(s) that transcribed the genes for IL22, IL17A and GzmA. IFN-γ in this system is exclusively produced by CD4+ T cells (Vordermeier, unpublished data) and was used as control. Highly enriched CD4+, CD8+ and TCRγδ+ (γδ+) T cell subset populations were isolated by FACS sorting and co-cultured in the presence of CD14+ monocytes were as APC and PPD-B. The expression of these genes was determined 24 hours later by qRT-PCR. The results (Fig. 6) demonstrated that ifn-γ and il22 were expressed by bovine CD4+ T cells. However, whilst il17A was also predominantly expressed by CD4+ cells; CD8+ and γδ+ T cells also expressed some il17A albeit an order of magnitude less. Granzyme A expression could be detected in both CD4+ and CD8+ T cell subsets (Figure 6).

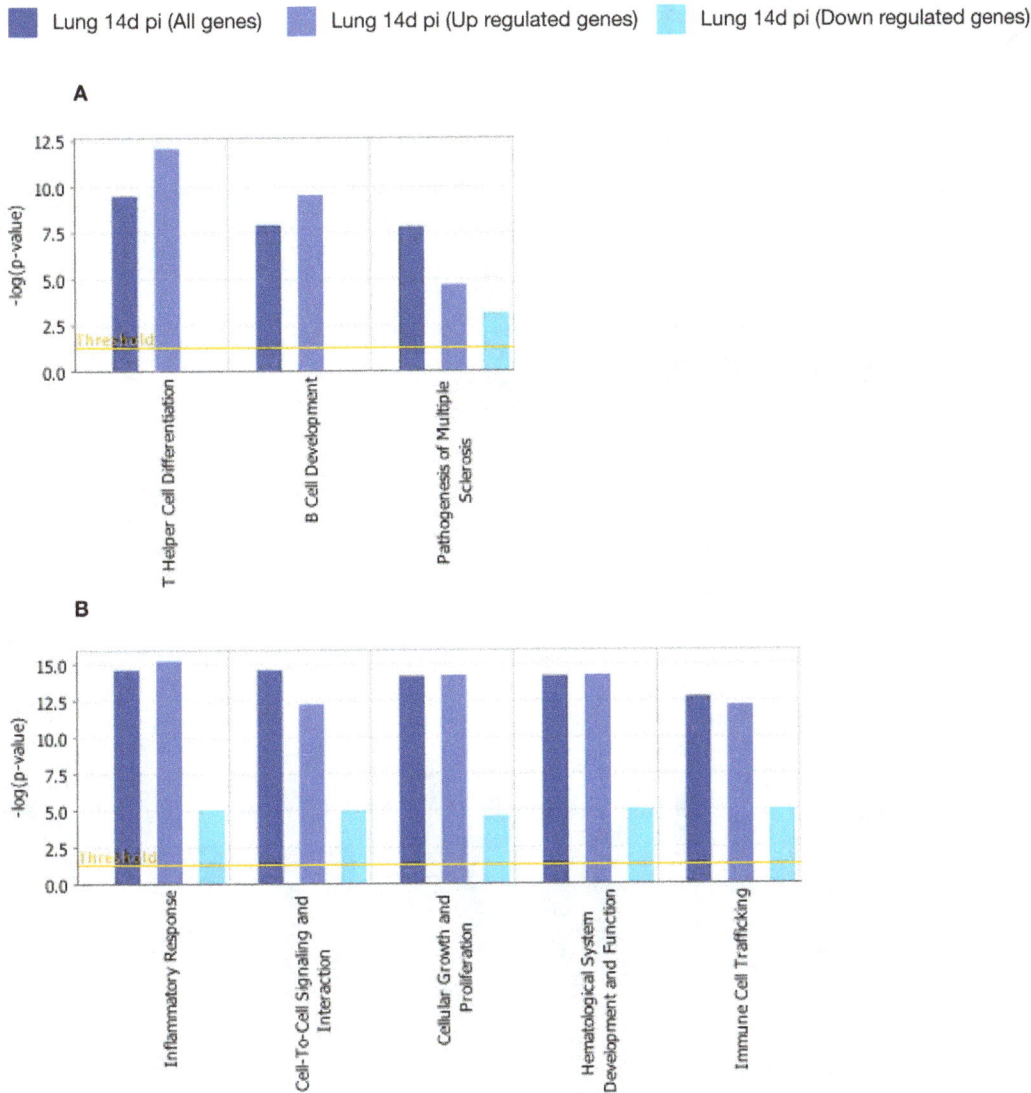

Figure 3. Functional networks (A) and canonical pathways (B) most significantly modulated in lung cells 14 days after *M. bovis* infection. Visualization of the trend and significance in the regulation of each network and pathway. Dark blue: all genes represented in a network. Light blue: genes that were up-regulated in a network. Cyan: gene those were down-regulated in a network. Fisher's exact test threshold value of p≤0.05.

Discussion

BTb remains an economically import disease of livestock species and improved diagnostic tests would benefit the implementation of control strategies. Transcriptomics approaches have been used to identify gene expression profiles to define biomarkers of TB in mice, primates and humans in different infection conditions. Several recent publications have reviewed these studies [15,16]. Likewise, studies in cattle, aiming to determine gene expression profiling, have been reviewed by Waters *et. al.* [17] focusing on *ex vivo studies and* macrophage infection. Yet, the interaction between host and *M. bovis*, which result in bTb, remains poorly characterized in cattle. The definition of such biomarkers induced after infection could have impact on the rational design of novel diagnostic approaches. We have used the advantages of the murine model (cheap, relatively short experimental periods, availability of reagents, detailed genome annotation) to study the host transcriptome after *M. bovis* infection. As we hypothesised our

analysis has lead to the validation in cattle of a number of biomarkers found in the murine system which include the genes encoding IL22, IL17A and Gzm A. PPD-B was used to stimulate bovine PBMC because it is the standard antigen used to diagnose bTb in livestock. In contrast, a protein cocktail (M7) was used to stimulate mouse lymphocytes because PPD-B is a poor antigen to stimulate murine responses despite the presence of these proteins in PPD-B (Hogarth *et al.*, unpublished observation). The reasons underlying this discrepancy in antigenic activity between the two species are not clear at present. Furthermore, the objective was to define bovine biomarkers applicable to routine ante-mortem blood based bTb diagnosis in cattle. Therefore, we targeted our analysis to peripheral blood as the only practical sample that can be collected readily from cattle in the field.

Interestingly, we could not validate in cattle the over-expression of all genes that we prioritised based on the mouse experiments. This could be due to the fact that we studied peripheral blood responses in cattle, whilst the mouse studies concentrated on

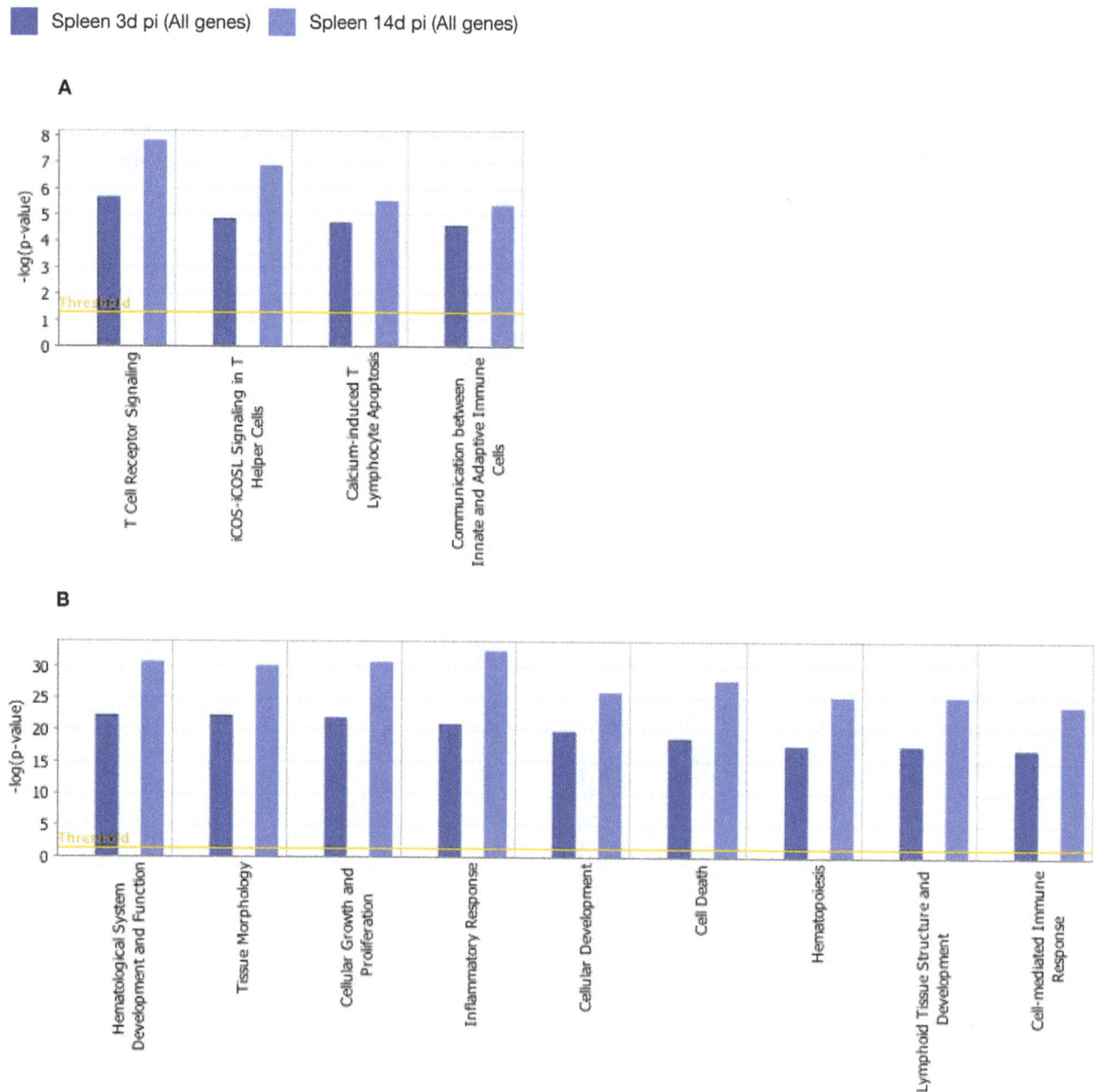

Figure 4. Functional networks (A) and canonical pathways (B) most significantly modulated in spleen cells 3 and 14 days after *M. bovis* infection. Visualization of the trend and significance in the regulation of each network and pathway are shown. Specific networks and pathways after 3 (dark blue bars) or 14 days p.i. (light blue bars) are indicated. Fisher's exact test threshold value of p≤0.05.

tissues (lung and spleen). In addition, the infection status is likely different between the two species populations studied: Murine responses were assessed relatively early after infection, whilst the time of infection in the cattle studied cannot be defined as these animals were naturally infected and are likely composed of a very heterogeneous group. It is therefore possible that not all responses found at the tissue sites of infection are reflected in the blood. However, our results demonstrated the value of the mouse system to guide the study of gene expression in cattle.

Our data also suggested that the networks and pathways associated both in lungs and spleen with infection at the 14 days p.i. time point showed up-regulated expression in the lung whilst the same networks and pathways in spleen cells were enriched for

genes whose expression was down-regulated. This could be explained by sequestration of particular cell populations into the lungs as principal site of infection as we previously proposed [18]. As our principal objective was to define bovine biomarkers useful for the ante-mortem diagnosis of bTb in cattle, we concentrated on the validation of potential markers that were strongly up-regulated in spleen and lung cells to allow the assessment of the widest selection of markers possible. In addition to their over-expression in mice, we also selected genes for validation in the bovine system on those whose products would have the potential to be detected by antibody-based assay systems such as ELISA. This lead therefore to the prioritisation of markers such as chemokines and cytokines.

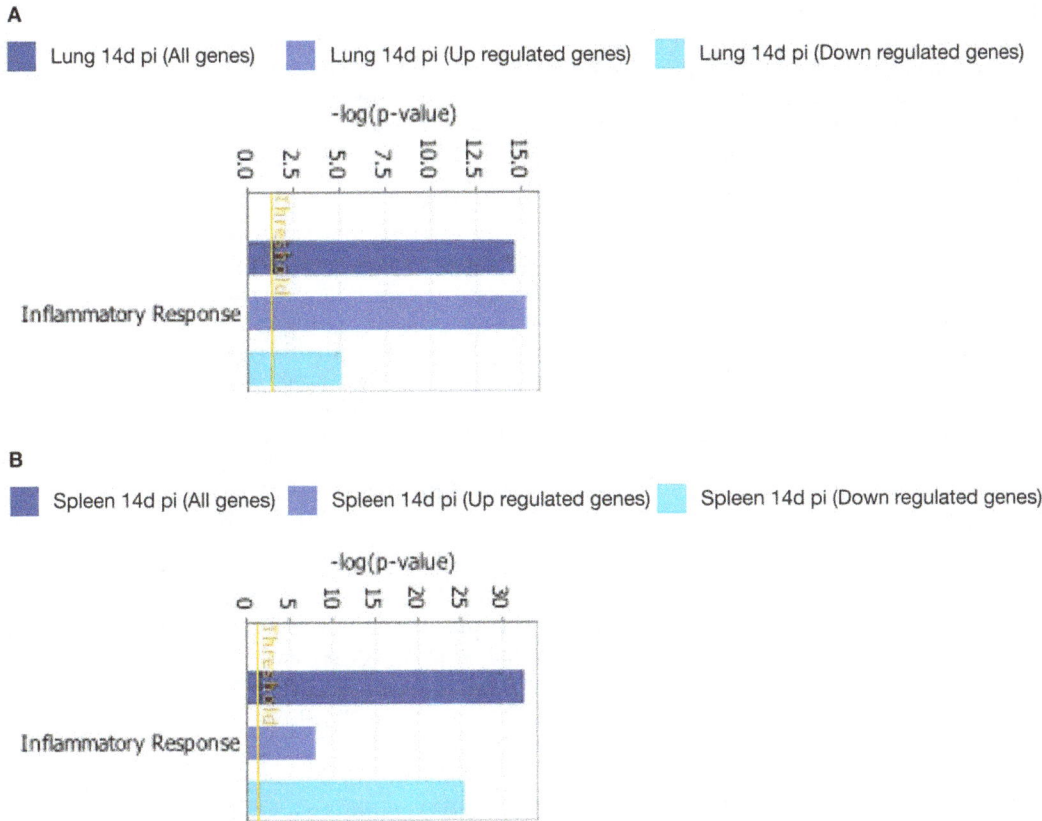

Figure 5. Induction of the inflammatory response network in lung (A) and spleen (B) cells at 14 days p.i. Dark blue: all genes enriched in this network. Light blue: genes that were up-regulated in this network. Cyan: gene those were down-regulated in this network.

IL-22 belongs to the IL-10 cytokine family and is produced by NK cells, mast cells, and T cells, especially Th17 and Th22 cells. It is involved in the antimicrobial defence of mucosal surfaces including in the airway by promoting innate immunity to bacterial infection. IL-22 has been shown to induce genes encoding antimicrobial proteins, β-defensins, S100 calcium binding proteins and to up-regulate the expression of chemokine (ccl1, cxcl5 and cxcl9) and cytokine genes (il-6 and g-csf). Furthermore, the functional consequences of IL-22/IL22R signalling can be potentiated by IL-17A/F and TNF-α in order to promote the expression of many of the genes encoding molecules involved in host defence in the lung [19]. The specific role of IL-22 in *M. tuberculosis* infection remains undefined, although it has been reported that IL-22 did not have a significant role in host protection and granuloma formation in mice [20,21]. In contrast, the production of IL-22 by human NK cells or addition of recombinant IL-22 to infected macrophages enhanced phagolysosomal fusion and reduces growth of *M. tuberculosis* [22]. In addition, CD4+ T effector cells bearing membrane-bound IL-22 (IL22+ CD4+ T cells) significantly reduced intracellular *M. tuberculosis* replication in macrophages isolated from rhesus macaques [23]. Whether IL-22 contributes to control TB at the site of infection is unknown. Nevertheless, active TB is associated with lower frequencies of IL17+ and IL22+ CD4+ T cells in peripheral blood [24]. In contrast, we have also demonstrated elevated expression of IL22 in lymph nodes from infected cattle (Aranday-Cortes et al., unpublished).

The role of IL17A in human tuberculosis has been described (reviewed in [25,26]. Although IL-17 might not play an equally important role in protection against mycobacterial infections as IFN-γ [27], recent studies have shown that IL-17 mediates an inflammatory response through granulopoiesis and consequent neutrophil accumulation. This may be required for protective immunity in the early stage of infection but could also become detrimental if its production remains high during later stages of disease [28]. In addition, IL-17 is reported to play an essential role

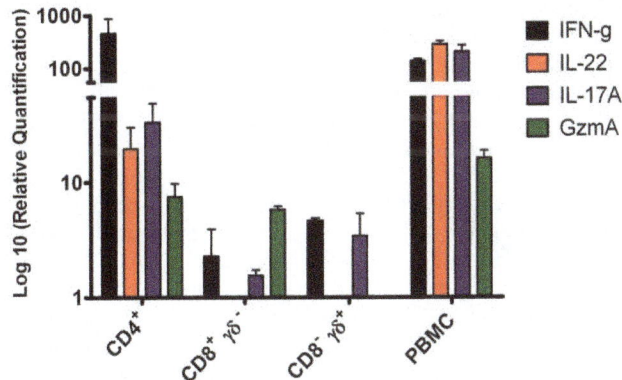

Figure 6. Phenotypic analysis of bovine T cell subsets that expressed the genes encoding for IL22, IL17a and GzmA. Highly purified CD4+, CD8+, and CD8−/TCRδ+ T cell populations were isolated by FACS sorting and the mRNA expression of these genes was determined after stimulation with PPD-B. Results are presented as mean fold increase compared to media control values ± SEM.

in the formation of granulomas in mice infected with BCG [29] and reduced Th17 CD4 T cell numbers are associated with PPD-induced impaired cytokine response in patients with HIV [30]. IL-17 producing γδ T cells were increased in patients with active pulmonary tuberculosis [31]. Interestingly, we have recently described a role for IL17A in the protective immune responses against bTb in cattle after BCG and BCG/viral subunit prime-boost experiments both in cattle [10] and mice [11]. In cattle its expression was up-regulated in protected animals after vaccination but before challenge and can therefore be defined as predictor of protection [10]. In this study we now also define it as a marker of disease progression in cattle and mice. Our data therefore are in agreement with an earlier report by Blanco et al. [13] who reported that il-17 expression was positively associated with pathology in cattle. Thus, our observations also support the notion that IL-17A is involved both in immune processes leading to protection or immunopathology of tuberculosis.

Granzyme A is the most abundant of the cytotoxic granules released by cytotoxic T cells (CTL) and NK cells. It can induce cell death independently of caspase activation [32,33] and T cells can reduce intracellular growth of *M. tuberculosis* by perforin and Fas/Fas ligand independent mechanism even in IFN-γ and TNF-α deficient mouse models [34,35]. One hypothesis which explains these observations, is that Th17/Th22 T cells may play a role in the pulmonary inflammatory response post-infection, by helping to elicit a pathogenic inflammatory response involving the activation of CTL. A similar relationship between TH17 cells and CD8$^+$ CTL has been described in tumour immunology [36].

Whilst it is acknowledged that IL-17A and IL-22 are produced not only by CD4$^+$ T cells, but also by CD8$^+$ and γδ T cells (as well as NK, NKT and non-T cells, which were not evaluated in this study) [37,38,39,40,41], our data demonstrated that both cytokines were predominantly expressed by CD4$^+$ T cells with a minor il-17A response also attributable to γδ T cells. It is therefore tempting to speculate that the responding bovine CD4$^+$ T cells belong to Th17 and/or Th22 subsets comparable to those described in other species [42,43]. Granzyme A was expressed equally in CD4$^+$ and CD8$^+$ which is suggestive of the induction of CTL of both T cell subsets following bTb infection of cattle.

Comparison between spleen samples obtained at 3 and 14 days p.i. and lungs samples at 14 days p.i. demonstrated that 32 genes were significantly modulated in all three sets of samples (Tables S1 and S2, genes highlighted with asterisk). Interestingly, only 4/32 genes were up-regulated (ubiquitin, lymphocyte antigen 6 complex, fmrd4 and ccr5). CCR5 is a chemokine receptor that binds CCL3, CCL4 and CCL5. The interaction between CCR5 and CCL5 may play an early protective role in limiting *M. tuberculosis* growth by recruiting T-cells, NK and macrophages to the lungs [44]. Further, reduction in number and frequency of Th1/Th17 CCR5$^+$ T cells was associated with reduced IFN-γ and IL-2 PPD responses in HIV-infected patients [30]. In contrast, severe TB in juvenile rhesus monkeys was associated with the up-regulation of ccr5 (as well as il-22 and other inflammatory cytokines and receptors) [45]. Thus, its precise role in tuberculosis is therefore unclear to-date.

Chemokines such as CXCL10 have been used as additional read-outs for blood-based IFN-γ release assays of human tuberculosis [46,47]. Its application increased overall test sensitivity compared to IFN-γ alone [48]. Measuring cxcl9 and cxcl10 expression by qRT-PCR has also been reported as potential platform to increase diagnostic sensitivity in human tuberculosis [49]. It is therefore interesting that we could show up-regulation of both of these genes also in murine lung cells and in bovine PBMC. Further validation of our results in cattle will determine whether

these, or the other genes validated in cattle such as il-22 or their protein products, will increase the accuracy of blood-based diagnostic tests for bTb when applied alongside IFN-γ release assays. However, the biomarkers identified in our study have so far been prioritised only based on their increased gene expression levels. Confirmation of their increased production at the protein level will be needed to turn them into valid diagnostic tests for bTb. Development of such antibody-based detection systems is now part of the process of translating our findings into practical such as ELISA-based, diagnostic tests for bTb.

In conclusions, we have shown that biomarkers defined in the murine system can be used to guide the analysis of biomarkers of disease in cattle. Further, we have prioritised a number of cytokines and chemokines as potential additional diagnostic markers for the blood based ante-mortem diagnosis of bTb to improve traditional IFN-γ release assays.

Materials and Methods

Ethics

This study and all procedures were approved by the Animal Health and Veterinary Laboratories Agency (AHVLA) Animal Use Ethics Committee (UK Home Office PCD 70/6905) and performed under appropriate personal and project licences within the conditions of the Animals (Scientific Procedures) Act 1986. All animals were housed in appropriate biological containment facilities at the AHVLA.

Animals

Mice. Female BALB/C mice were obtained from SPF facilities at Charles River Laboratories, Margate, UK.

Cattle. Heparinized blood samples were obtained from 11 naturally infected single intradermal comparative tuberculin test (SICTT)-positive reactors from herds know to have bTb. Infection was confirmed by the presence of visible pathology at post-mortem and the culture of *M. bovis* from tissues from these animals according to previously described procedures [14]. *Uninfected controls*: Heparinized blood sample were obtain from 9 SICTT-negative animals from bTb-free herds. They were also negative in the standard Bovigam IFN-γ release assay (Prionics, Switzerland).

Antigens

Cattle. Purified protein derivative from *M. bovis* (PPD-B, Prionics, Switzerland) was used in culture at 10 µg/ml for stimulating bovine Peripheral blood mononuclear cells (PBMC). Staphylococcal enterotoxin B (SEB, Sigma-Aldrich, UK) was used as a positive control at 1 µg/ml.

Mice. Antigen cell culture stimulations in mice were performed using an equal pool of seven secreted, immunogenic recombinant mycobacterial proteins (Rv1886c, Rv3019c, Rv3763, Rv3804c, [Lionex GmbH, Germany] Rv0251, Rv0287 and Rv0288 [Proteix s.r.o., Czech Republic]) common to *M. bovis* and BCG, referred here as M7 protein cocktail. We have previously shown that M7 induced strong and representative T cell responses in both vaccinated and infected mice [18]. Each protein was used at final concentration of 2 µg/ml in 3-day culture. Concanavalin A (Sigma-Aldrich) was used as a positive control at 5 µg/ml for murine cells.

Mycobacterial challenge

Mycobacterium bovis isolate AF2122/97 was grown to mid log phase in Middlebrook 7H9 broth supplemented with 4.16 g/L pyruvic acid, 10% (v/v) oleic acid, albumin, dextrose, and catalase (OADC) and 0.05% (v/v) Tween 80, subsequently stored at

−80°C, was used for all virulent challenges. Two groups of 5 mice each were challenged with approx 600 CFU via the intranasal route [50]. At days 3 and 14 post challenge five mice per group were euthanized and spleens and lungs harvested aseptically.

Cell isolation

Spleen and lung cells were prepared by as described previously [18] and suspended at 5×10^6/ml spleen cells and 5×10^5/ml lung cells. After stimulation, cells were washed ($300 \times g$, 5 min at room temperature) and supernatants removed. One ml of Trizol (Invitrogen, Paisley, UK) was then added and the cell lysates were stored at −80°C.

Bovine PBMC. PBMC were isolated from heparinized blood by Histopaque-1077 (Sigma-Aldrich) gradient centrifugation. Cells were resuspended at 1×10^6/ml in tissue culture medium (RPMI 1640 [Sigma-Aldrich] supplemented with 10% fetal calf serum [Sigma-Aldrich], nonessential amino acids [Sigma-Aldrich], 100 U/ml penicillin and 100 µg/ml streptomycin sulfate) and incubated overnight with PPD-B or SEB in 24-well tissue culture plates (Life Technologies, UK). The following day, plates were centrifuged ($300 \times g$, 5 min at room temperature) and the supernatant was removed. One ml of Trizol was then added and the cell lysates were stored at −80°C.

RNA extraction from bovine PBMC

Total RNA was extracted from PBMCs using TRIzol according to the protocol recommended by the manufacturer. Turbo DNA-free (Ambion, Huntingdon, UK) was used to remove genomic DNA contamination. The purity and concentration of RNA were evaluated by NanoDrop 1000 (Thermo Scientific, Horsham, UK). RNA with a ratio of A260/A280 ≥ 1.7 was used for the RT-qPCR validation study.

Cell Sorting

Cell sorting was performed using a Beckman Coulter MoFlo Astrios instrument. Bovine PBMCs were stained and sorted according to expression of the bovine T-cell surface markers CD4, CD8 and γδ TCR. The anti-bovine CD8 antibody (clone CC63) was supplied directly conjugated to Fluorescein isothiocyanate (AbD-Serotec, Kidlington, UK), whilst the anti-bovine CD4 antibody (clone CC8, AbD-Serotec) was custom conjugated to R-Phycoerythrin (Invitrogen). The anti-TcR-δ antibody (clone GB21A, VMRD, Pullman, WA) was used in the primary staining reaction as an unconjugated antibody and then labelled in a secondary staining reaction using an isotype specific anti-mouse IgG2b antibody directly conjugated to Alexa Fluor 633 (Invitrogen). Staining reactions were performed at 4°C for 15 minutes. CD14-positive cells were isolated using magnetic beads (Miltenyi Biotech, Bisley, UK) as described previously [51] and used as antigen-presenting cells. The purities of the sorted T cell populations were >99.% for CD4$^+$CD8$^-$ cells; >96% for TcR-δ$^+$ CD8$^-$ cells and >99.0% for TcR-δ$^-$ CD8$^+$ cells. In the assays, 1×10^6 sorted T cell populations were incubated for 24 h with 1×10^5 APC in 24-well plates in the presence of PPD-B and RNA processed as described above.

Murine RNA preparation and microarray hybridization

Spleen and lung cells were collected into Trizol and stored at −80°C until further processing. RNA was isolated from spleen and lung cells derived from control and infected mice using standard RNA extraction protocols (Miltenyi Biotech). The quality of RNA samples was assessed using the Agilent 2100 Bioanalyzer platform (Agilent Technologies, UK). All RNA samples revealed

acceptable RNA Integrity Number (RIN) values of between 7.4 and 9.6. For the linear T7-based amplification step, 0.06 µg– 0.5 µg of each total RNA samples was used as starting material. To produce Cy3-labeled cDNA, RNA samples were amplified and labeled using the Agilent Low RNA Input Linear Amp Kit (Agilent Technologies) following the manufacturer's protocol. Yields of cRNA and the dye-incorporation rate were measured in a ND-1000 Spectrophotometer (Thermo Scientific). In general, control samples were labeled with Cy3 and experimental samples were labeled with Cy5. The hybridization procedure was performed according to the Agilent 60-mer oligo microarray processing protocol using the Agilent Gene Expression Hybridization Kit. Briefly, 825 ng Cy3- and Cy5-labeled fragmented cDNA in hybridization buffer was hybridized overnight (17 hours, 65°C) to Agilent Whole Mouse Genome Oligo Microarrays 4x44K using Agilent's recommended hybridization chamber and oven. Finally, microarrays were washed once with $6 \times$ SSPE buffer (3.6 M NaCl, 0.2 M NaH$_2$PO$_4$, 0.02 M EDTA pH 7.4) contaning 0.005% N-lauroylsarcosine for 1 min at room termperature followed by a second wash with preheated $0.06 \times$ SSPE buffer (37°C) containing 0.005% N-lauroylsarcosine for 1 min. The last washing step was performed with acetonitrile for 30 seconds.

Normalization, filtering procedures and data analysis

Fluorescence signals of the hybridized Agilent Microarrays were detected using Agilent's Microarray Scanner System. Agilent's Feature Software (FES) was used to read out and process microarray image files. The software determines feature intensities (including background subtraction), rejects outliers and calculates statistical confidences. For determination of differential gene expression FES derived output data files were further analyzed using GeneSpring GX 11.5 (Agilent Technologies). After baseline transformation to mean of control samples (spleen and lung from uninfected mice), we decided to focus on those genes that reliably change their expression, then we filtered the microarrays following three conditions: 1) *Filter by value*. Genes that do not have normalized signal intensity values of more than −0.5 and 0.5 were disregarded. 2) *Filter by flags*. All the genes with flags values present in at least 100% of the values in any 1 out of the 3 conditions were considered. 3) Filter by percentile. All the genes with raw signal intensity values between 25 and 100 in any 1 out of the 3 conditions were also considered. Finally, all the genes in coincidence between filtering by flags group and filtering by percentile group were kept for statistical analysis.

After filtering, parametric analysis of variance was applied to compare mean expression levels in each analysis. Data were considered significant when the Benjamini Hochberg false discovery rate (FDR) for the comparison under analysis was <0.05, and the significance level was <0.05. In order to focus on highly regulated genes, we also restricted the majority of the analysis to genes with changes in expression levels of at least 2.0-fold change (FC) in all the conditions. All data set can be downloaded from Gene Expression Omnibus public data base at www.ncbi.nml.nih.gov/geo/ with the GEO accession number GSE33058.

Lists of genes resulting from these analyses were submitted to Ingenuity Pathway Analysis (IPA; Ingenuity® Systems, USA, www.ingenuity.com). In order to identify the most significant functional networks (biological functions and diseases) and canonical pathways related to each comparison, the analysis was performed using the following strategy: A core analysis was performed with all the genes with p≤0.05 and fold change ≥2 for each comparison; then for the same comparisons a core analysis was performed only considering those genes that showed p≤0.05

and were at least 2 fold up-regulated. Further and independently a last core analysis was performed for those genes with p≤0.05 that were at least 2-fold down-regulated. Finally, these analyses were compared. Fisher's exact test with a threshold value of p≤0.05 was used in all the analyses. The rationale behind this strategy is to visualize the trend and significance in the regulation for each network and pathway. Thus, we show three columns for each comparison: one showing all the genes related to a specific network and pathway, followed by two extra columns showing how the networks and pathways are enriched by up- or down-regulated genes.

Reverse transcriptase and quantitative Real-time PCR validation

cDNA from PBMCs was synthesized from total RNA samples using random primers and reverse transcription with SuperScript III Vilo reverse transcriptase following the manufacturers protocol (Applied Biosystem, Paisley, UK). cDNA from cell sorting was synthesized using μMACS One-step cDNA Kit (Miltenyi Biotec) following manufacturers instructions. Transcripts were quantified by qPCR with Fast SYBR Green master mix (Applied Biosystem) following manufactures conditions. qPCR analysis was performed using the ABI 7500 Fast Real Time PCR System (Applied Biosystem) in triplicate from media control, PPD-B and SEB-stimulated PBMCs cDNA. The fold increase was calculated by comparison with the expression of endogenous controls genes SDHA and G3PDH using the $2^{-\Delta\Delta ct}$ calculation [52].

Statistical analysis

Responses between cattle naturally infected with *M. bovis* and naïve controls were analysed by Student's t-test on log transformed data using Prism (Graph Pad, USA). To control for type I errors due to multiple comparison, the Bonferroni's correction for multiple tests was applied and the significance level set at p<0.003.

Supporting Information

Table S1   Significant modulation of spleen cell genes early after 3 days p.i. (1109) and at later time-point of 14 days p.i. (1134). Genes in bold (618) were modulated at both time points. Ns = no significant expression at this time point. The genes marked with (*) result common after comparison between spleen samples after 3 and 14 days p.i. and lungs samples after 14 days p.i. with M. bovis showed expression of (32).

Table S2   Significant modulation of spleen cell genes early after 3 days p.i. (1109) and at later time-point of 14 days p.i. (1134). Genes in bold (618) were modulated at both time points. Ns = no significant expression at this time point. The genes marked with (*) result common after comparison between spleen samples after 3 and 14 days p.i. and lungs samples after 14 days p.i. with M. bovis showed expression of (32).

Acknowledgments

We would like to acknowledge our colleagues in the AHVLA Animal Services Unit for their dedication to animal welfare. We would also like to thank AHVLA field staff for their assistance in recruiting naturally infected cattle.

Author Contributions

Conceived and designed the experiments: EAC PJH HMV. Performed the experiments: EAC PJH DAK AOW BVR. Analyzed the data: EAC PJH HMV. Wrote the paper: EAC PJH AL HMV.

References

1. Thoen C, Lobue P, de Kantor I (2006) The importance of Mycobacterium bovis as a zoonosis. Vet Microbiol 112: 339–345.
2. Schiller I, Oesch B, Vordermeier HM, Palmer MV, Harris BN, et al. (2010) Bovine tuberculosis: a review of current and emerging diagnostic techniques in view of their relevance for disease control and eradication. Transbound Emerg Dis 57: 205–220.
3. Gormley E, Doyle MB, Fitzsimons T, McGill K, Collins JD (2006) Diagnosis of Mycobacterium bovis infection in cattle by use of the gamma-interferon (Bovigam) assay. Vet Microbiol 112: 171–179.
4. Wood PR, Jones SL (2001) BOVIGAM: an in vitro cellular diagnostic test for bovine tuberculosis. Tuberculosis (Edinb) 81: 147–155.
5. Lalvani A, Millington KA (2008) T Cells and Tuberculosis: Beyond Interferon-gamma. J Infect Dis 197: 941–943.
6. Jones GJ, Pirson C, Hewinson RG, Vordermeier HM (2010) Simultaneous measurement of antigen-stimulated interleukin-1 beta and gamma interferon production enhances test sensitivity for the detection of Mycobacterium bovis infection in cattle. Clin Vaccine Immunol 17: 1946–1951.
7. Hogarth PJ, Logan KE, Vordermeier HM, Singh M, Hewinson RG, et al. (2005) Protective immunity against Mycobacterium bovis induced by vaccination with Rv3109c–a member of the esat-6 gene family. Vaccine 23: 2557–2564.
8. Chegou NN, Black GF, Kidd M, van Helden PD, Walzl G (2009) Host markers in QuantiFERON supernatants differentiate active TB from latent TB infection: preliminary report. BMC Pulm Med 9: 21.
9. Flynn JL, Chan J, Triebold KJ, Dalton DK, Stewart TA, et al. (1993) An essential role for interferon gamma in resistance to Mycobacterium tuberculosis infection. J Exp Med 178: 2249–2254.
10. Vordermeier HM, Villarreal-Ramos B, Cockle PJ, McAulay M, Rhodes SG, et al. (2009) Viral booster vaccines improve Mycobacterium bovis BCG-induced protection against bovine tuberculosis. Infect Immun 77: 3364–3373.
11. Aranday Cortes E, Kaveh D, Nunez-Garcia J, Hogarth PJ, Vordermeier HM (2010) Mycobacterium bovis-BCG vaccination induces specific pulmonary transcriptome biosignatures in mice. PLoS ONE 5: e11319.
12. Vordermeier HM, Cockle PC, Whelan A, Rhodes S, Palmer N, et al. (1999) Development of diagnostic reagents to differentiate between Mycobacterium bovis BCG vaccination and M. bovis infection in cattle. Clin Diagn Lab Immunol 6: 675–682.

13. Blanco FC, Bianco MV, Meikle V, Garbaccio S, Vagnoni L, et al. (2011) Increased IL-17 expression is associated with pathology in a bovine model of tuberculosis. Tuberculosis (Edinb) 91: 57–63.
14. Vordermeier HM, Chambers MA, Cockle PJ, Whelan AO, Simmons J, et al. (2002) Correlation of ESAT-6-specific gamma interferon production with pathology in cattle following Mycobacterium bovis BCG vaccination against experimental bovine tuberculosis. Infect Immun 70: 3026–3032.
15. Walzl G, Ronacher K, Hanekom W, Scriba TJ, Zumla A (2011) Immunological biomarkers of tuberculosis. Nat Rev Immunol 11: 343–354.
16. Zarate-Blades CR, Silva CL, Passos GA (2011) The impact of transcriptomics on the fight against tuberculosis: focus on biomarkers, BCG vaccination, and immunotherapy. Clin Dev Immunol 2011: 192630.
17. Waters WR, Palmer MV, Thacker TC, Davis WC, Sreevatsan S, et al. (2011) Tuberculosis immunity: opportunities from studies with cattle. Clin Dev Immunol 2011: 768542.
18. Kaveh DA, Bachy VS, Hewinson RG, Hogarth PJ (2011) Systemic BCG immunization induces persistent lung mucosal multifunctional CD4 T(EM) cells which expand following virulent mycobacterial challenge. PLoS ONE 6: e21566.
19. Sonnenberg GF, Fouser LA, Artis D (2011) Border patrol: regulation of immunity, inflammation and tissue homeostasis at barrier surfaces by IL-22. Nat Immunol 12: 383–390.
20. Wilson MS, Feng CG, Barber DL, Yarovinsky F, Cheever AW, et al. (2010) Redundant and pathogenic roles for IL-22 in mycobacterial, protozoan, and helminth infections. J Immunol 184: 4378–4390.
21. Yao S, Huang D, Chen CY, Halliday L, Zeng G, et al. (2010) Differentiation, distribution and gammadelta T cell-driven regulation of IL-22-producing T cells in tuberculosis. PLoS Pathog 6: e1000789.
22. Dhiman R, Indramohan M, Barnes PF, Nayak RC, Paidipally P, et al. (2009) IL-22 produced by human NK cells inhibits growth of Mycobacterium tuberculosis by enhancing phagolysosomal fusion. J Immunol 183: 6639–6645.
23. Zeng G, Chen CY, Huang D, Yao S, Wang RC, et al. (2011) Membrane-bound IL-22 after de novo production in tuberculosis and anti-Mycobacterium tuberculosis effector function of IL-22+ CD4+ T cells. J Immunol 187: 190–199.
24. Scriba TJ, Kalsdorf B, Abrahams DA, Isaacs F, Hofmeister J, et al. (2008) Distinct, specific IL-17- and IL-22-producing CD4+ T cell subsets contribute to the human anti-mycobacterial immune response. J Immunol 180: 1962–1970.

25. Khader SA, Bell GK, Pearl JE, Fountain JJ, Rangel-Moreno J, et al. (2007) IL-23 and IL-17 in the establishment of protective pulmonary CD4+ T cell responses after vaccination and during Mycobacterium tuberculosis challenge. Nat Immunol 8: 369–377.

26. Khader SA, Cooper AM (2008) IL-23 and IL-17 in tuberculosis. Cytokine 41: 79–83.

27. Wozniak TM, Saunders BM, Ryan AA, Britton WJ (2010) Mycobacterium bovis BCG-specific Th17 cells confer partial protection against Mycobacterium tuberculosis infection in the absence of gamma interferon. Infect Immun 78: 4187–4194.

28. Nandi B, Behar SM (2011) Regulation of neutrophils by interferon-{gamma} limits lung inflammation during tuberculosis infection. J Exp Med 208: 2251–2262.

29. Okamoto Yoshida Y, Umemura M, Yahagi A, O'Brien RL, Ikuta K, et al. (2010) Essential role of IL-17A in the formation of a mycobacterial infection-induced granuloma in the lung. J Immunol 184: 4414–4422.

30. Clark S, Page E, Ford T, Metcalf R, Pozniak A, et al. (2011) Reduced T(H)1/T(H)17 CD4 T-cell numbers are associated with impaired purified protein derivative-specific cytokine responses in patients with HIV-1 infection. J Allergy Clin Immunol 128: 838–846, e835.

31. Peng MY, Wang ZH, Yao CY, Jiang LN, Jin QL, et al. (2008) Interleukin 17-producing gamma delta T cells increased in patients with active pulmonary tuberculosis. Cell Mol Immunol 5: 203–208.

32. Anthony DA, Andrews DM, Watt SV, Trapani JA, Smyth MJ (2010) Functional dissection of the granzyme family: cell death and inflammation. Immunol Rev 235: 73–92.

33. Lieberman J (2010) Granzyme A activates another way to die. Immunol Rev 235: 93–104.

34. Canaday DH, Wilkinson RJ, Li Q, Harding CV, Silver RF, et al. (2001) CD4(+) and CD8(+) T cells kill intracellular Mycobacterium tuberculosis by a perforin and Fas/Fas ligand-independent mechanism. J Immunol 167: 2734–2742.

35. Gallegos AM, van Heijst JW, Samstein M, Su X, Pamer EG, et al. (2011) A gamma interferon independent mechanism of CD4 T cell mediated control of M. tuberculosis infection in vivo. PLoS Pathog 7: e1002052.

36. Martin-Orozco N, Muranski P, Chung Y, Yang XO, Yamazaki T, et al. (2009) T helper 17 cells promote cytotoxic T cell activation in tumor immunity. Immunity 31: 787–798.

37. Hamada H, Garcia-Hernandez Mde L, Reome JB, Misra SK, Strutt TM, et al. (2009) Tc17, a unique subset of CD8 T cells that can protect against lethal influenza challenge. J Immunol 182: 3469–3481.

38. Lockhart E, Green AM, Flynn JL (2006) IL-17 production is dominated by gammadelta T cells rather than CD4 T cells during Mycobacterium tuberculosis infection. J Immunol 177: 4662–4669.

39. O'Brien RL, Roark CL, Born WK (2009) IL-17-producing gammadelta T cells. Eur J Immunol 39: 662–666.

40. Roark CL, Simonian PL, Fontenot AP, Born WK, O'Brien RL (2008) gammadelta T cells: an important source of IL-17. Curr Opin Immunol 20: 353–357.

41. Witte E, Witte K, Warszawska K, Sabat R, Wolk K (2010) Interleukin-22: a cytokine produced by T, NK and NKT cell subsets, with importance in the innate immune defense and tissue protection. Cytokine Growth Factor Rev 21: 365–379.

42. Duhen T, Geiger R, Jarrossay D, Lanzavecchia A, Sallusto F (2009) Production of interleukin 22 but not interleukin 17 by a subset of human skin-homing memory T cells. Nat Immunol 10: 857–863.

43. Sallusto F, Lanzavecchia A (2009) Human Th17 cells in infection and autoimmunity. Microbes Infect 11: 620–624.

44. Vesosky B, Rottinghaus EK, Stromberg P, Turner J, Beamer G (2010) CCL5 participates in early protection against Mycobacterium tuberculosis. J Leukoc Biol 87: 1153–1165.

45. Qiu L, Huang D, Chen CY, Wang R, Shen L, et al. (2008) Severe tuberculosis induces unbalanced up-regulation of gene networks and overexpression of IL-22, MIP-1alpha, CCL27, IP-10, CCR4, CCR5, CXCR3, PD1, PDL2, IL-3, IFN-beta, TIM1, and TLR2 but low antigen-specific cellular responses. J Infect Dis 198: 1514–1519.

46. Whittaker E, Gordon A, Kampmann B (2008) Is IP-10 a better biomarker for active and latent tuberculosis in children than IFNgamma? PLoS ONE 3: e3901.

47. Ruhwald M, Petersen J, Kofoed K, Nakaoka H, Cuevas LE, et al. (2008) Improving T-cell assays for the diagnosis of latent TB infection: potential of a diagnostic test based on IP-10. PLoS ONE 3: e2858.

48. Ruhwald M, Dominguez J, Latorre I, Losi M, Richeldi L, et al. (2011) A multicentre evaluation of the accuracy and performance of IP-10 for the diagnosis of infection with M. tuberculosis. Tuberculosis (Edinb) 91: 260–267.

49. Kasprowicz VO, Mitchell JE, Chetty S, Govender P, Huang KH, et al. (2011) A molecular assay for sensitive detection of pathogen-specific T-cells. PLoS ONE 6: e20606.

50. Logan KE, Gavier-Widen D, Hewinson RG, Hogarth PJ (2008) Development of a Mycobacterium bovis intranasal challenge model in mice. Tuberculosis (Edinb) 88: 437–443.

51. Vordermeier M, Ameni G, Glass EJ (2011) Cytokine responses of Holstein and Sahiwal zebu derived monocytes after mycobacterial infection. Trop Anim Health Prod.

52. Livak KJ, Schmittgen TD (2001) Analysis of relative gene expression data using real-time quantitative PCR and the 2(−Delta Delta C(T)) Method. Methods 25: 402–408.

9

Transmission of MRSA between Companion Animals and Infected Human Patients Presenting to Outpatient Medical Care Facilities

Jorge Pinto Ferreira[1,2]*, Kevin L. Anderson[1], Maria T. Correa[1], Roberta Lyman[1], Felicia Ruffin[2], L. Barth Reller[2], Vance G. Fowler Jr.[2]

1 Department of Population Health and Pathobiology (PHP), North Carolina State University (NCSU) College of Veterinary Medicine, Raleigh, North Carolina, United States of America, 2 Department of Infectious Diseases, Duke University School of Medicine, Durham, North Carolina, United States of America

Abstract

Methicillin-resistant *Staphylococcus aureus* (MRSA) is a significant pathogen in both human and veterinary medicine. The importance of companion animals as reservoirs of human infections is currently unknown. The companion animals of 49 MRSA-infected outpatients (cases) were screened for MRSA carriage, and their bacterial isolates were compared with those of the infected patients using Pulsed-Field Gel Electrophoresis (PFGE). Rates of MRSA among the companion animals of MRSA-infected patients were compared to rates of MRSA among companion animals of pet guardians attending a "veterinary wellness clinic" (controls). MRSA was isolated from at least one companion animal in 4/49 (8.2%) households of MRSA-infected outpatients vs. none of the pets of the 50 uninfected human controls. Using PFGE, patient-pets MRSA isolates were identical for three pairs and discordant for one pair (suggested MRSA inter-specie transmission p-value = 0.1175). These results suggest that companion animals of MRSA-infected patients can be culture-positive for MRSA, representing a potential source of infection or re-infection for humans. Further studies are required to better understand the epidemiology of MRSA human-animal inter-specie transmission.

Editor: Tara C. Smith, University of Iowa, United States of America

Funding: This work was supported in part by the National Institutes of Health (NIH) K24AI093969-01 and R01 AI068804. Dr. Ferreira's stipend was partially supported by Fulbright program, a not-for-profit organization. No additional external funding was received for this study. The funders had no role in study design, data collection and analysis, decision to publish, or preparation of the manuscript.

Competing Interests: Dr. Vance G. Fowler has received or has pending grants from NIH, Astellas, Cubist, Inhibitex, Merck, Theravance, Cerexa, Pfizer, Novartis, Advanced Liquid Logic; has received royalties from UpToDate; has been paid for development of educational presentations by Astellas, Merck, Pfizer, Targanta, Theravance, Wyeth, Novartis, Vertex, Medimmune; has served as a consultant for Astellas, Cubist, Inhibitex, Johnson & Johnson, Shire, Leo Pharmaceuticals, Merck, NovaDigm, Medicines Company, Baxter, Biosynexus, Inimex, Galderma; has received honoraria from Arpida, Astellas, Cubist, Inhibitex, Merck, Pfizer, Targanta, Theravance, Wyeth, Ortho-McNeil, Novartis & Vertex Pharmaceuticals; and has served on an advisory committee and on a speaker's bureau for Cubist. There are no patents, products in development or marketed products related to this study to declare.

* E-mail: jmferrei@ncsu.edu

Introduction

The epidemiology of methicillin-resistant *Staphylococcus aureus* (MRSA) is dynamic [1,2]. First identified in the 1960s, MRSA was initially considered a nosocomial pathogen. Beginning in the late 20th century, a specific clone of MRSA, known as USA300, emerged as a leading cause of community-acquired infection [3–5]. Recently, another strain of MRSA, Sequence Type 398 (ST-398), has been shown to be strongly associated with livestock [6], accounting for up to 20% of all human cases of MRSA infection in the Netherlands [7].

During this time, a growing number of reports have described probable transmission of *S. aureus* and MRSA, in particular, between humans and companion animals [8–13]. Little is known, however, about the potential role of companion animals in the transmission of MRSA to humans. For example our understanding regarding direction of transmission, persistence of colonization, rate of animal-human transmission, inter-specie transmission risk factors, animal population or breeds with increased risk to be carriers of MRSA and the significance of companion animals as reservoirs for human MRSA infections are all incomplete.

In the current study, we sought to investigate the significance of pets/companion animals as sources of MRSA infection or re-infection for human outpatients by evaluating MRSA transmission between MRSA-infected outpatients and their companion animals. Our results suggest that this reservoir might be more significant than currently considered.

Materials and Methods

Ethics Statement

This cross-sectional study was a collaboration between Duke University School of Medicine and North Carolina State University College of Veterinary Medicine and was approved by Institutional Review Boards (CR1_Pro00018484; 1417-10) and Animal Care and Use Committees (A-329-09-11; 10-054-B) at both participating institutions.

Ascertainment of Cases and Control Groups

Between January and May 2010, MRSA-positive patients seen as outpatients at a large southeastern United States hospital were identified. Other inclusion criteria were an age of 18 years or older, ability to speak in English and residence within a 50 miles radius from the hospital. The health care providers of the patients meeting these criteria were contacted by study personnel to obtain permission to contact the individuals. If the health care provider consented, patients were contacted by phone to determine if they had companion animals. If patients lived with companion animals and consented (in written form) to participate in the study, a household visit was scheduled to obtain nasal swabs from the animals to determine their MRSA status. A short questionnaire was given to the animal guardians on the day of the visit. The goal of this questionnaire was to identify inter-specie transmission risk factors. Forty nine patients, 76 dogs, 25 cats and 3 hamsters were included in the study population. Thirteen adult (older than eighteen) family members (of the 49 human cases) voluntarily participated in this study, answering the questionnaire and self-collecting nasal swabs to determine their MRSA status.

Companion animals presenting to a veterinary institution wellness clinic and their guardians served as a control population. Animals were voluntarily taken to this clinic mainly for prophylactic vaccinations, being otherwise generally healthy. The control population included 50 people and 45 dogs and 30 cats.

We used contingency tables to assess the associations between case/control status and the exposure/demographic variables. Counts, percentages and odds ratios were calculated to quantitate the strengths of these associations and the statistical significance was determined with Fisher's exact test. Statistical analysis was performed with SAS 9.2 (SAS Institute, Cary, NC, USA).

Microbiological identification of MRSA isolates

The clinical human MRSA isolates from the patients were collected from the Clinical Microbiology Laboratory of the medical school integrated in this project and stored ($-80°C$) until required for additional use.

Staphylococcus spp. identification was performed in accordance with routine laboratory techniques, including typical colony morphology, gram stain, catalase and coagulase tests. *S. aureus* and *S. pseudintermedius* diagnosis was confirmed by multiplex PCR [14]. Resistance to oxacillin and cefoxitin was determined using standard disk diffusion [15]. *S. aureus* isolates were classified as MRSA if the inhibition zone was less than or equal to 21 mm for cefoxitin or less than or equal to 10 mm for oxacillin [15]. Oxacillin was used to determine susceptibility of the *S. pseudintermedius* isolates. When the inhibition zone was less than or equal to 17 mm, they were considered resistant.

mecA PCR was performed on the human and animal MRSA isolates [16].

Genetic relatedness was evaluated by use of pulsed field gel electrophoresis (PFGE) and *spa* typing, as previously described [17,18].

Results

A total of 49 MRSA-infected outpatients (cases) and 50 uninfected (human) controls participated in the study. The animal case population was larger than the control population (total of 107 vs 75 animals) and included more dogs than the animal control population (76 vs. 45).

Four out of the 49 (8.2%) human cases with culture-confirmed MRSA infections lived with a companion animal (2 dogs, 1 cat, 1 hamster) from which MRSA was isolated. One of the patients diagnosed with MRSA lived with a methicillin-resistant *Staphylococcus pseudintermedius* (MRSP) positive dog.

No MRSA or MRSP was found in the 13 family members of the MRSA-infected patients that voluntarily participated in this study, or in the 50 humans or 75 animals of the control population.

Using PFGE, three of the human-animal MRSA pairs were identical and one was discordant (figure 1). Three of the four human-animal MRSA isolates pairs were classified as *spa* type 2 and clonal complex 5 (table 1).

Table 2 presents the results of the univariable analysis (based on the questionnaire answers) of the variables potentially associated with MRSA carriage and human-animal transmission. The ones that were significantly different between cases and controls are highlighted.

Discussion

Our results provide further evidence into the potential significance of companion animals as a source of infection and/or re-infection of humans/outpatients. These findings are particularly important, as MRSA is the most common identifiable cause of soft tissue infection in the US [3] and it is estimated that about 75 million dogs and 88 million cats are owned in the US [19]. Because companion animals are increasingly seen and treated as family members by their guardians [20], the opportunity for transmission between humans and pets is only likely to increase. Our results are consistent with previous reports. Weese *et al.* (2006) studied the transmission of MRSA in veterinary clinics and in the households, after the identification of a MRSA positive animal. These authors described 6 cases. MRSA was isolated from 16% (14/88) of household contacts or veterinary personnel and in all of the 6 cases it was possible to find at least one human isolate identical to the animal (initial) one [21]. More recently, Faires *et al.* evaluated both the rate of MRSA transmission from infected animals to humans and vice-versa. When the MRSA-infected animal was initially identified, at least one MRSA-colonized person was identified in over one-quarter (6/22; 27.3%) of the study households. By contrast, only one of the 8 (12.5%) study households of MRSA-infected humans contained a MRSA-colonized pet [22]. By evaluating about 5 times the number of MRSA-infected humans as Faires *et al.* and finding a similar companion animal MRSA colonization rate (~8%), the current study externally validates the findings of the previous study. Our results clearly demonstrate that MRSA transmission between infected patients and companion animals occurs. Such transmission between humans and animals has been previously implicated as potential cause of recurrent MRSA infections [8–13]. Previous publications have described cases where human MRSA could not be linked with traditional MRSA sources in the community or health care facilities [23]. This challenges the accepted epidemiology of MRSA and suggests that there are currently unrecognized/unknown sources of MRSA. Finding 5 out of 8 (62.5%) MRSA isolates that were not identical to any of the most common (and previously described by the Centers for Disease Control (CDC)) Hospital Acquired (HA) or Community Acquired (CA) MRSA clones seems to reinforce this idea.

Not finding MRSA in any of the humans or animals of the control population was surprising. Veterinarians have been described as a professional group with increased risk of carrying MRSA [7,24]. Different prevalence studies have found very diverse prevalence values in small/companion animals [25–28]. To our knowledge, prevalence in companion animals has never been determined in North Carolina, which makes it hard to evaluate the absence of MRSA in the animal control population.

Our study has limitations. Finding MRSA in both outpatients and their companion animals is suggestive of inter species transmission of this agent. However, we can only speculate about transmission and there is the possibility that both parts became infected from different sources. Direction of transmission also

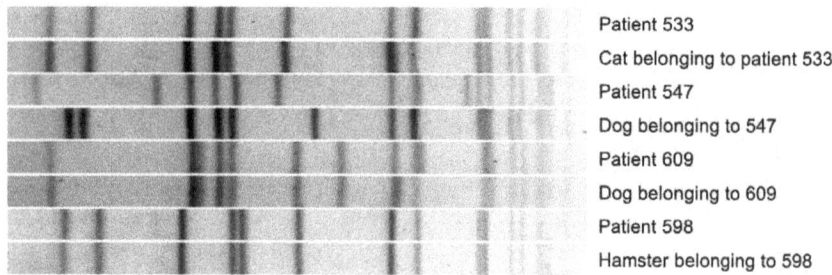

Figure 1. PFGE comparison of human and animal MRSA pairs.

cannot be determined. Finding 3 concordant human-animal MRSA pairs is not statistically significant (p = 0.1175) considering a reasonable significance level and therefore a larger sample size should be considered in future studies. The most ideal control population would have been the one formed by outpatients diagnosed with methicillin sensitive *Staphylococcus aureus* (MSSA) living with companion animals, with the same number of both humans and animals in the study and control populations (a 1:1 ratio). Using the population of animals and their guardians that attended a wellness clinic was, therefore, a convenient, involving less costs and more readily available choice. We still believe, however, that this gave us an estimate of the prevalence of MRSA co-existence at the household level in healthy humans and animals in the general population. The average time between a MRSA outpatient identification (control) and sampling/swabbing of its companion animals was approximately one month, so there is a possibility that some colonized animals were missed [22].

Other Staphylococcus spp. trans-infection

The primary goal of this project was to study human-animal MRSA transmission. Increased attention has, at the same time, been given by the scientific community to other *Staphylococcus* species (spp.) inter-specie transmission [29–32]. More recently, a novel staphylococcus has been identified: *Staphylococcus pseudintermedius* [33]. Since *S. pseudintermedius* is coagulase positive, the possibility of misdiagnosis in clinical microbiology laboratories is possible and has to be taken into consideration [31,34]. Our finding of a human infected with MRSA living with an MRSP animal should be investigated in future projects. The exchange of

genetic material between different species of staphylococci has been repeatedly reported and emphasized [32,35,36] and its significance for human infections is currently unknown.

Challenges and future research

One of the most challenging aspects of this project was the enrollment of patients. Of the 557 patients diagnosed with MRSA during our study at the medical school hospital integrated in this project, 231 would match our inclusion criteria and only 49 were enrolled (response rate of approximately 21% (49/231)).Reasons for this included: difficulty in reaching the health care providers and patients, the non-existence of companion animals in the household, residences being outside the 50 mile radius, the inexistence of financial compensation to the participants, and patient or medical team declining participation.

Future research should focus on the dynamics of transmission. Longitudinal studies with multiple samplings of animals and humans will be critical in addressing questions regarding direction of transmission and duration of colonization. Obtaining an IRB permission for the enrollment and sampling of children would be important, as MRSA is known to be more prevalent in younger kids [37]. Environmental samples should also be taken at the household level to identify other potential sources of reinfection. Staphylococcus diagnostic protocols should be carefully reviewed to make sure that the recently discovered coagulase positive staphylococci are included in the differential diagnosis list. Staphylococci should be characterized at the molecular level with different techniques (PFGE, multiplex PCR, multi locus sequence typing, *spa* typing) to allow a better comparison with different studies and traceability of the isolates origin.

Table 1. Summary of the classification of the MRSA isolates, using *spa* typing.

patient : animal pair	CDC classification	*spa* typing	clonal complex	Pair similarity	Specific risk factor(s)
patient 533 cat 533	USA 100 USA 100	type 2 type 2	cc 5 cc 5	identical	patient was cancer survivor and had been hospitalized in the previous year; animal was allowed to move freely in house
patient 547 dog 547	USA 300 not a common CDC-designated isolate	type 1 type176	cc 8 cc 5	Non identical	patient had been hospitalized in the previous year and animal was allowed to move freely in the house
patient 598 hamster 598	not a common CDC-designated isolate not a common CDC-designated isolate	type 2 type 2	cc 5 cc 5	identical	patient with diabetes, organ transplant, renal insufficiency and depression that had been hospitalized in the previous year; animal with open sores
patient 609 dog 609	not a common CDC-designated isolate not a common CDC-designated isolate	type 2 type 2	cc 5 cc 5	identical	patient was a healthcare worker and animal was allowed to move freely in the house

Table 2. Univariable analysis (based on the questionnaire answers) of the variables potentially associated with MRSA carriage and human-animal transmission.

Variable	Cases (n ; %)	Controls (n ; %)	OR	95% CI
Do you have a FM who is HCW?				
Yes	7 (14.28%)	17 (34%)		
No	42 (85.71%)	33 (66%)	0.32	[0.12, 0.87]
Do you have a FM who is a veterinarian?				
Yes	1 (2.27%)	9 (18%)		
No	43 (97.72%)	41 (82%)	0.11	[0.01, 0.87]
Are there children in the household?				
Yes	**22 (44.9%)**	**8 (16%)**		
No	**27 (55.1%)**	**42 (84%)**	**4.28**	**[1.67, 10.98]**
Has a FM been treated with AB in the past year?				
Yes	22 (44.9%)	14 (29.79%)		
No	27 (55.1%)	33 (70.21%)	1.92	[0.83, 4.45]
Has a FM been diagnosed with MRSA in the past year?				
Yes	**8 (16.33%)**	**1(2.04%)**		
No	**41 (83.67%)**	**48 (97.96%)**	**9.37**	**[1.12, 78.05]**
Were you hospitalized in the past year?				
Yes	**15 (31.25%)**	**4 (8%)**		
No	33 (68.75%)	46 (92%)	**5.23**	**[1.59, 17.18]**
Have you been diagnosed with a disease or take medication that affects your immune condition?				
Yes	**28 (57.14%)**	**3 (6%)**		
No	**21 (42.86%)**	**47 (94%)**	**20.89**	**[5.71, 76.42]**
Are you a HCW?				
Yes	8 (16.33%)	3 (6%)		
No	41 (83.67%)	47 (94%)	3.06	[0.76, 12.29]
Aware of recent (past month) contact with person or animals MRSA positive?				
Yes	7 (14.29%)	5 (10%)		
No	42 (85.71%)	45 (90%)	1.5	[0.44, 5.09]
Were you treated with any AB in the past year?				
Yes	**38 (77.55%)**	**18 (36%)**		
No	**11 (22.45%)**	**32 (64%)**	**6.14**	**[2.53, 14.89]**
Do any of your animals have current sores?				
Yes	7 (14.28%)	6 (12%)		
No	42 (85.71%)	44 (88%)	1.22	[0.34, 3.51]
Were any of your animals hospitalized in the past year?				
Yes	5 (10.20%)	6 (12%)		
No	44 (89.80%)	44 (88%)	0.83	[0.26, 3.25]
Are any of your animals allowed to go outdoors?				
Yes	24 (48.98%)	11 (22%)		
No	25 (51.02%)	39 (78%)	3.4	[0.71, 4.07]
Are any of your animals allowed to move freely in the house?				
Yes	36 (74%)	46 (92%)		
No	13 (26%)	4 (8%)	0.24	[0.16, 1.79]
Are any of the animals allowed to lick human faces?				
Yes	21 (42.86%)	37 (74%)		
No	28 (57.14%)	13 (26%)	0.26	[0.24, 1.31]
Are any of the animals allowed to sleep where humans sleep?				

Table 2. Cont.

Variable	Cases (n ; %)	Controls (n ; %)	OR	95% CI
Yes	31 (63.27%)	37 (74%)		
No	18 (36.73%)	13 (26%)	0.61	[0.34, 1.90]
Do you have contact with your animals everyday?				
Yes	42 (85.71%)	45 (88.89%)		
No	7 (14.29%)	5 (11.11%)	1.5	[0.35, 4.05]

The ones that were significantly different between cases and controls are highlighted. "Don't know" or "missing" answers were excluded from the analysis. Legend: FM = family member; HCW = health care worker; AB = antibiotic.

Conclusions

Nearly 8% of MRSA outpatients lived with a MRSA pet. When faced with chronic and or recurrent MRSA cases, physicians should consider the possibility of household pets as MRSA source. Patients should be informed of this possibility. Unnecessary close contact should be avoided and heightened hygiene practices should be instituted. Sampling/swabbing of all the human and animals in a household seems appropriate to identify unrecognized sources and break potential cycles of reinfection especially in cases involving immunocompromised patients. It is critical that medical and veterinary institutions partner and collaborate in researching this topic. The legal/institutional approval that regulates this type of partnerships should be expedited to encourage them. MRSA epidemiology is a perfect example of an infectious disease agent whose control requires a "One Health" approach.

Acknowledgments

The authors would like to acknowledge the Clinical Microbiology Laboratory staff of Duke medical school that partnered in this project for their help with the recovery of the human MRSA isolates and continuous support, availability and collaboration in this project; Lawrence Park, for his assistance with statistical analysis and Thomas Rude for his assistance with laboratory analysis involving the human samples.

Author Contributions

Conceived and designed the experiments: JPF KLA MTC LBR VGF. Performed the experiments: JPF RL. Analyzed the data: JPF KLA MTC VGF. Contributed reagents/materials/analysis tools: KLA LBR VGF. Wrote the paper: JPF KLA MTC RL FR LBR VGF.

References

1. Karchmer AW, Bayer AS (2008) Methicillin-resistant *Staphylococcus aureus*: An evolving clinical challenge. Clin Infect Dis Jun 1;46 Suppl 5: S342–3.
2. Blanc DS, Petignat C, Wenger A, Kuhn G, Vallet Y, et al. (2007) Changing molecular epidemiology of methicillin-resistant *Staphylococcus aureus* in a small geographic area over an eight-year period. Journal of Clinical Microbiology 45(11): 3729–36.
3. Moran GJ, Krishnadasan A, Gorwitz RJ, Fosheim GE, McDougal LK, et al. (2006) Methicillin-resistant *S. aureus* infections among patients in the emergency department. N Engl J Med Aug 17;355(7): 666–74.
4. King MD, Humphrey BJ, Wang YF, Kourbatova EV, Ray SM (2006) Emergence of community-acquired methicillin-resistant *Staphylococcus aureus* USA 300 clone as the predominant cause of skin and soft-tissue infections. Ann Intern Med Mar 7;144(5): 309–17.
5. Daum RS (2007) Clinical practice. Skin and soft-tissue infections caused by methicillin-resistant *Staphylococcus aureus*. N Engl J Med Jul 26;357(4): 380–90.
6. Smith TC, Pearson N (2011) The emergence of *Staphylococcus aureus* ST398. Vector Borne Zoonotic Dis 11(4): 327–39. Epub 2010 Oct 6.
7. van Loo I, Huijsdens X, Tiemersma E, de Neeling A, van de Sande-Bruinsma N (2007) Emergence of methicillin-resistant *Staphylococcus aureus* of animal origin in humans. Emerg Infect Dis Dec;13(12): 1834–9.
8. Scott GM, Thomson R, Malone-Lee J, Ridgway GL (1988) Cross-infection between animals and man: Possible feline transmission of *Staphylococcus aureus* infection in humans? J Hosp Infect Jul;12(1): 29–34.
9. Cefai C, Ashurst S, Owens C (1994) Human carriage of methicillin-resistant *Staphylococcus aureus* linked with pet dog. Lancet Aug 20;344(8921): 539–40.
10. Manian FA (2003) Asymptomatic nasal carriage of mupirocin-resistant, methicillin-resistant *Staphylococcus aureus* (MRSA) in a pet dog associated with MRSA infection in household contacts. Clin Infect Dis Jan 15;36(2): e26–8.
11. van Duijkeren E, Wolfhagen MJ, Box AT, Heck ME, Wannet WJ, et al. (2004) Human-to-dog transmission of methicillin-resistant *Staphylococcus aureus*. Emerg Infect Dis Dec;10(12): 2235–7.
12. van Duijkeren E, Wolfhagen MJ, Heck ME, Wannet WJ (2005) Transmission of a panton-valentine leucocidin-positive, methicillin-resistant *Staphylococcus aureus* strain between humans and a dog. J Clin Microbiol Dec;43(12): 6209–11.
13. Baptiste KE, Williams K, Willams NJ, Wattret A, Clegg PD (2005) Methicillin-resistant staphylococci in companion animals. Emerg Infect Dis Dec;11(12): 1942–4.
14. Sasaki T, Tsubakishita S, Tanaka Y, Sakusabe A, Ohtsuka M (2010) Multiplex-PCR method for species identification of coagulase-positive staphylococci. J Clin Microbiol 48(3): 765–9.
15. Wayne PA (2008) Clinical and Laboratory Standards Institute. Performance standards for antimicrobial susceptibility testing: Twentieth informational supplement.
16. Lee JH (2006) Occurrence of methicillin-resistant *Staphylococcus aureus* strains from cattle and chicken, and analyses of their *mec*A, *mec*R1 and *mec*I genes. Vet Microbiol Apr 16;114(1–2): 155–9.
17. Centers for Disease Control and Prevention (C.D.C.), Department of Health and Human Services, Washington, DC (2001) Oxacillin-resistant *Staphylococcus aureus* on PulseNet (OPN): Laboratory protocol for molecular typing of *S. aureus* by pulsed field gel electrophoresis (PFGE).
18. Mathema B, Mediavilla J, Kreiswirth BN (2008) Sequence analysis of the variable number tandem repeat in *Staphylococcus aureus* protein A gene: Spa typing. Methods Mol Biol 431: 285–305.
19. Oehler R, Velez A, Mizrachi M, Lamarche J, Gompf S (2009) Bite-related and septic syndromes caused by cats and dogs. The Lancet Infectious Diseases 9(7): 439.
20. Guardabassi L, Schwarz S, Lloyd DH (2004) Pet animals as reservoirs of antimicrobial-resistant bacteria. J Antimicrob Chemother Aug 54(2): 321–32.
21. Weese JS, Dick H, Willey BM, McGeer A, Kreiswirth BN, et al. (2006) Suspected transmission of methicillin-resistant *Staphylococcus aureus* between domestic pets and humans in veterinary clinics and in the household. Vet Microbiol Jun 15;115(1–3): 148–55.
22. Faires M, Tater K, Weese JS (2009) An investigation of methicillin-resistant *Staphylococcus aureus* colonization in people and pets in the same household with an infected person or infected pet. J Am Vet Med Assoc 235(5): 540.
23. Silbergeld EK, Davis M, Leibler JH, Peterson AE (2008) One reservoir: Redefining the community origins of antimicrobial-resistant infections. Med Clin North Am Nov;92(6): 1391,40.
24. Hanselman BA, Kruth SA, Rousseau J, Low DE, Willey BM (2006) Methicillin-resistant *Staphylococcus aureus* colonization in veterinary personnel. Emerg Infect Dis Dec;12(12): 1933–8.
25. Loeffler A, Pfeiffer DU, Lindsay JA, Magalhaes RJ, Lloyd DH (2010) Prevalence of and risk factors for MRSA carriage in companion animals: A survey of dogs, cats and horses. Epidemiol Infect Oct 14: 1–10.
26. Boost MV, O'Donoghue MM, James A (2008) Prevalence of *Staphylococcus aureus* carriage among dogs and their owners. Epidemiol Infect Jul;136(7): 953–64.
27. Loeffler A, Boag AK, Sung J, Lindsay JA, Guardabassi L (2005) Prevalence of methicillin-resistant *Staphylococcus aureus* among staff and pets in a small animal referral hospital in the UK. J Antimicrob Chemother Oct;56(4): 692–7.

28. Lilenbaum W, Nunes EL, Azeredo MA (1998) Prevalence and antimicrobial susceptibility of staphylococci isolated from the skin surface of clinically normal cats. Lett Appl Microbiol Oct;27(4): 224–8.

29. van Duijkeren E, Kamphuis M, van der Mije IC, Laarhoven LM, Duim B (2011) Transmission of methicillin-resistant *Staphylococcus pseudintermedius* between infected dogs and cats and contact pets, humans and the environment in households and veterinary clinics. Vet Microbiol 150(3–4): 338–43.

30. Van Hoovels L, Vankeerberghen A, Boel A, Van Vaerenbergh K, De Beenhouwer H (2006) First case of *Staphylococcus pseudintermedius* infection in a human. J Clin Microbiol 44(12): 4609–12.

31. Chuang C, Yang Y, Hsueh P, Lee P (2010) Catheter-related bacteremia caused by *Staphylococcus pseudintermedius* refractory to antibiotic-lock therapy in a hemophilic child with dog exposure. J Clin Microbiol 48(4): 1497–8.

32. Frank L, Kania S, Kirzeder E, Eberlein L, Bemis D (2009) Risk of colonization or gene transfer to owners of dogs with meticillin-resistant *Staphylococcus pseudintermedius*. Vet Dermatol 20(5–6): 496.

33. Devriese LA, Vancanneyt M, Baele M, Vaneechoutte M, De Graef E (2005) *Staphylococcus pseudintermedius* sp. nov., a coagulase-positive species from animals. Int J Syst Evol Microbiol Jul;55(Pt 4): 1569–73.

34. van Duijkeren E, Houwers DJ, Schoormans A, Broekhuizen-Stins MJ, Ikawaty R (2008) Transmission of methicillin-resistant *Staphylococcus intermedius* between humans and animals. Vet Microbiol Apr 1;128(1–2): 213–5.

35. Leonard FC, Markey BK (2008) Methicillin-resistant *Staphylococcus aureus* in animals: A review. Vet J Jan;175(1): 27–36.

36. Lloyd DH (2007) Reservoirs of antimicrobial resistance in pet animals. Clin Infect Dis Sep 1;45 Suppl 2: S148–52.

37. Sanders RC, Jr., Diokno RM, Romero J (2011) MRSA infections in children. J Ark Med Soc 107(13): 288–90.

10

Commutability of Possible External Quality Assessment Materials for Cardiac Troponin Measurement

Shunli Zhang[1,2], Jie Zeng[1], Chuanbao Zhang[1], Yilong Li[3], Haijian Zhao[1], Fei Cheng[1,2], Songlin Yu[4], Mo Wang[1,2], Wenxiang Chen[1]*

1 Beijing Hospital and National Center for Clinical Laboratories, Ministry of Health, Beijing, China, 2 Chinese Academy of Medical Sciences and Peking Union Medical College, Beijing, China, 3 Department of Laboratory Medicine, Beijing Hospital, Ministry of Health, Beijing, China, 4 Department of Laboratory Medicine, Peking Union Medical College Hospital, Beijing, China

Abstract

Background: The measurement of cardiac troponin is crucial in the diagnosis of myocardial infarction. The performance of troponin measurement is most conveniently monitored by external quality assessment (EQA) programs. The commutability of EQA samples is often unknown and the effectiveness of EQA programs is limited.

Methods: Commutability of possible EQA materials was evaluated. Commercial control materials used in an EQA program, human serum pools prepared from patient samples, purified analyte preparations, swine sera from model animals and a set of patient samples were measured for cTnI with 4 assays including Abbott Architect, Beckman Access, Ortho Vitros and Siemens Centaur. The measurement results were logarithm-transformed, and the transformed data for patient samples were pairwise analyzed with Deming regression and 95% prediction intervals were calculated for each pair of assays. The commutability of the materials was evaluated by comparing the logarithmic results of the materials with the limits of the intervals. Matrix-related biases were estimated for noncommutable materials. The impact of matrix-related bias on EQA was analyzed and a possible correction for the bias was proposed.

Results: Human serum pools were commutable for all assays; purified analyte preparations were commutable for 2 of the 6 assay pairs; commercial control materials and swine sera were all noncommutable; swine sera showed no reactivity to Vitros assay. The matrix-related biases for noncommutable materials ranged from −83% to 944%. Matrix-related biases of the EQA materials caused major abnormal between-assay variations in the EQA program and correction of the biases normalized the variations.

Conclusion: Commutability of materials has major impact on the effectiveness of EQA programs for cTnI measurement. Human serum pools prepared from patient samples are commutable and other materials are mostly noncommutable. EQA programs should include at least one human serum pool to allow proper interpretation of EQA results.

Editor: John Calvert, Emory University, United States of America

Funding: This study was supported by research grants from the National High Technology Research and Development Program of China (863 Program) (No. 2011AA02A102 and No. 2011AA02A116). The funders had no role in study design, data collection and analysis, decision to publish, or preparation of the manuscript.

Competing Interests: The authors have declared that no competing interests exist.

* Email: wchen@bjhmoh.cn

Introduction

The measurement of cardiac troponin (cTn) has become an important clinical laboratory measurement because of its central role in the diagnosis of acute myocardial infarction (MI) [1]. Both cTnT and cTnI are specific and sensitive biomarkers of myocardial injury with necrosis. Currently, all cTnT assays are produced by a single manufacturer and assay results are comparable, whereas cTnI assays are produced by various manufacturers and the results are variable [2,3]. This variability is undesirable for clinical use of the important biomarker and efforts are being made toward standardization of cTnI measurements [2,4,5].

Identification of variability of measurement results between assays and surveillance of the effectiveness of standardization is best accomplished through external quality assessment (EQA) (or proficiency testing) programs that use commutable samples [6–8]. EQA is now a common practice in laboratory medicine and nearly all clinical laboratories (assays) regularly participate in EQA programs; the samples used in EQA programs need to be commutable or the commutability needs to be known, otherwise the purpose of evaluating the comparability of different assays will not be fulfilled [9,10]. However, for practical reasons, most current cTnI EQA programs use processed materials with unknown commutability and the interpretation of EQA results is often difficult. Our cardiac marker EQA programs using commercial control materials have shown between-assay discrepancies in cTnI results that are very different from that in the cut-off values (the 99th percentiles) of the assays (internal data and will be presented in this report), suggesting major noncommutability of the control materials. If this is the case, the magnitude of the noncommutability of the materials needs to be known and, when necessary and possible, more suitable materials need to be used in the EQA program.

Materials most likely to be commutable would be serum pools prepared according to the CLSI C37A guideline [11] which describes a rigorous protocol for the collection of blood from donors and the preparation of genuine serum pools for cholesterol. The C37A protocol has been validated or used in investigations to produce commutable samples for several other analytes [8], but it would hardly be applicable to the preparation of samples for cTnI measurement because detectable cTnI is primarily seen in MI patients. The best available approach to obtain materials likely to be commutable would be the use of leftover patient samples [8]. The commutability of such samples for cTnI measurement has been suggested [5,12]. Because of the sample volume required in an EQA program, the preparation of the patient sample pools would involve a series of steps such as collecting, freezing storage, thawing, pooling, filtering, aliquoting, and re-freezing. Commutability of so-prepared materials for cTnI measurement has not been studied.

The use of patient samples, though possible, still poses significant difficulties especially in collecting samples in sufficient volume and with appropriate analyte concentrations. Combination of patient samples with more easily available materials that have acceptable commutability might be a practical approach for the EQA of cTnI. Other sources of possible EQA materials for cTnI may include purified analyte spiked in a serum matrix and animal sera. It has been reported that a cTn TIC complex purified from human heart tissue has reasonable commutability, though not totally commutable, among cTnI assays [5,13]. A Standard Reference Material (SRM 2921) has been prepared from the TIC complex by NIST [14]. It has also been reported that cTnIs in big mammals share high homology with human cTnI and shows adequate responses to human cTnI assays [15,16]. Among cTnIs in species, swine cTnI seems to have the most similar cross-reactivity to human cTnI antibodies [17]. The degree of commutability of these materials is currently unknown.

To interpret our EQA results and analyze the impact of noncommutability of samples on EQA programs, and in search for possible EQA materials for cTnI, in this study we evaluated the commutability of the control materials used in our EQA program, frozen serum pools prepared from patient samples, the NIST SRM 2921 diluted with human serum and swine sera from MI model animals.

Materials and Methods

The study was a commutability study carried out according to a protocol as described in the CLSI C53A guideline [18]. The study involved measurement of prepared materials together with a set of individual patient samples with different cTnI assays. The mathematical relationships among the results of different assays for the prepared materials were compared with that for patient samples.

Ethics Statement

The study involved use of leftover patient samples and animal serum samples. The leftover patient samples were all de-identified during the collection. It was also ensured that appropriate amount of serum was collected from each patient sample so that a certain

Table 1. Assay group means and inter-laboratory CVs of cTnI measurements in the 2013 EQA program.

Assay	N[a]	Mean, ng/ml					CV, %				
		L1[b]	L2[b]	L3[b]	L4[b]	L5[b]	L1[b]	L2[b]	L3[b]	L4[b]	L5[b]
Access	126	0.04	0.69	3.16	0.50	2.17	25.0	17.4	16.8	18.0	18.4
Architect	60	0.16	6.56	32.59	5.02	22.74	18.8	7.9	8.3	8.0	6.8
Centaur	63	0.07	1.64	9.43	1.10	5.65	14.3	11.6	12.6	10.9	12.0
Vitros	13	0.08	3.35	18.58	2.65	12.39	12.5	3.6	6.2	4.2	4.5

[a]Number of laboratories.
[b]EQA material level 1 through 5.

Table 2. Patient serum sample cTnI concentrations and measurement CVs with different assays.

Assay	cTnI concentration, median (range), ng/ml	Within-run CV, median (range), %	Total CV[a], %
Access	1.475 (0.026~25.472)	5.9 (0.5–14.5)	4.9
Architect	1.735 (0.016–23.534)	2.5 (0.1–13.2)	2.2
Centaur	2.198 (0.033–41.285)	2.2 (0.0–15.1)	5.1
Vitros	1.522 (0.027–23.944)	1.0 (0.0–11.8)	1.3

[a]Estimated from measurement results of patient serum pool level 4.

volume was left for possible repetition of measurement. The use of patient samples in the present study has been reviewed and approved by the Ethics Committee of Beijing Hospital, Ministry of Health. The animal serum samples were stored swine sera from model MI animals that had been used in a previous study. The animals were induced with MI to test the effect of a traditional medicine (extracts of *salvia miltiorrhiza* and *carthamus tinctorius*) on post-MI coronary microcirculation. The study was conducted at the Research Center for Coronary Heart Disease, Fuwai Hospital and had been approved by the ethics committee of the institution.

Individual Patient Samples

The individual patient samples used for the commutability study were leftover patient serum samples collected from the clinical laboratories of Beijing Hospital and Tongren Hospital. De-identified patient samples with measurable cTnI values (with a Beckmann Access assay at Beijing Hospital or a Siemens Centaur

assay at Tongren Hospital) and sufficient leftover sample volume (sufficient for measurement in triplicate with 4 assays) were collected. A total of 75 samples were collected from 71 patients (36–92 years of age, 55 males) who were either admitted to the hospitals because of symptoms of suspected myocardial ischemia or hospitalized with diagnosed MI. Each of the samples was split into 4 aliquots and frozen at −86°C. All the samples were collected, aliquoted and frozen within 30 hours after blood drawn.

Prepared Materials

Materials evaluated for commutability in the study included control materials used in our 2013 EQA program, frozen serum pools prepared from leftover patient samples, SRM preparations made by diluting the SRM 2921 with human serum and swine sera from MI model animals.

EQA materials. The EQA materials used in our 2013 cardiac marker EQA program were Bio-Rad Liquichek Cardiac

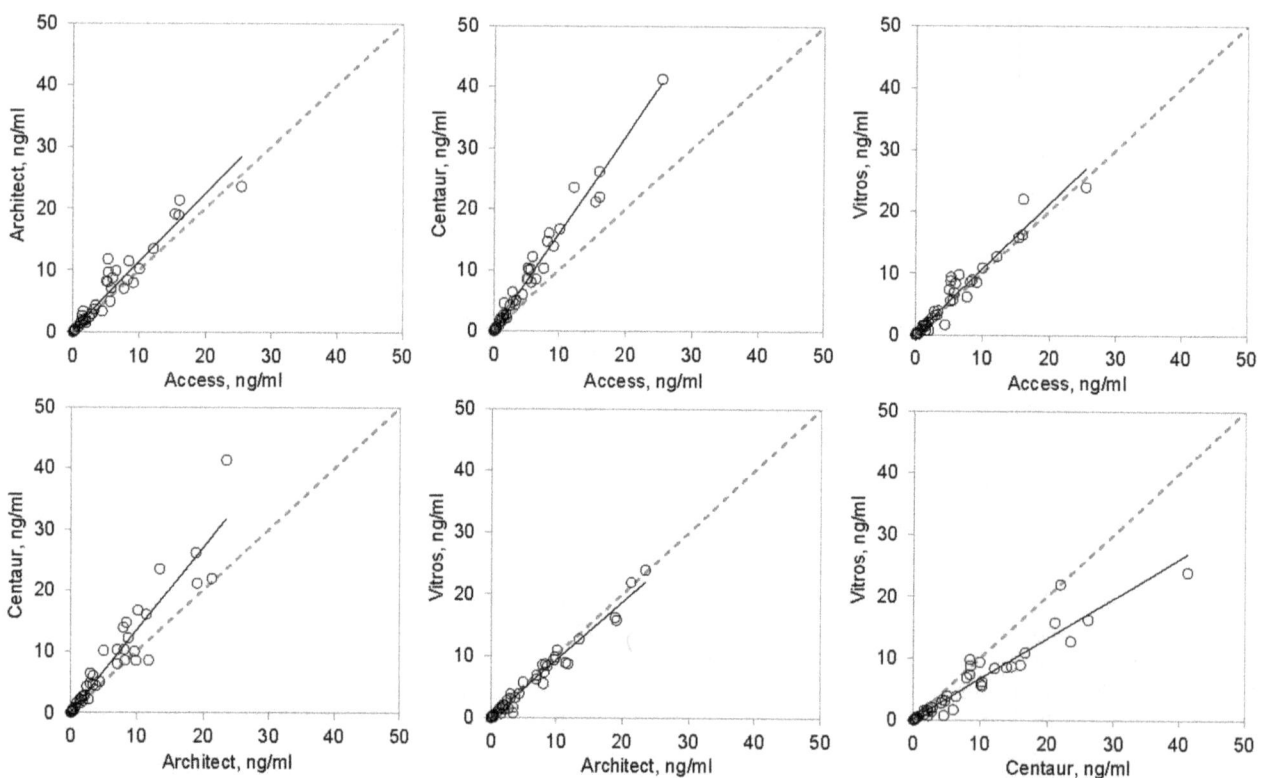

Figure 1. Scatter plots of cardiac troponin I (cTnI) concentrations measured with different assays. The cTnI concentrations of 61 patient samples were measured in triplicate with 4 assays including Abbott Architect (Architect), Beckman Access (Access), Ortho Vitros (Vitros) and Siemens Advia Centaur (Centaur). The means of the triplicates with different assays were pairwise plotted. The solid lines are trend lines and the dashed are the equality (y = x) lines.

Table 3. Between-assay correlations of measurement results for patient samples.

Assay pair (x–y)	Slope (95% CI)[a]	Intercept (95% CI)[a]	r[b]
Access-Architect	1.183 (1.099~1.264)	−0.005 (−0.018~0.008)	0.967
Access-Centaur	1.624 (1.523~1.684)	−0.020 (−0.045~−0.001)	0.989
Access-Vitros	1.068 (1.042~1.122)	0.017 (0.003~0.030)	0.974
Architect-Centaur	1.379 (1.223~1.447)	−0.023 (−0.047~0.006)	0.956
Architect-Vitros	0.957 (0.898~0.994)	0.015 (−0.001~0.026)	0.988
Centaur-Vitros	0.676 (0.631~0.732)	0.031 (0.013~0.052)	0.961

[a]Passing-Bablok slopes and intercepts expressed as mean and 95% confidence interval (CI).
[b]Pearson correlation coefficient.

Markers Plus Control LT control materials. Five levels of the materials (EQA L1-5) selected from Lots 23541, 23542, 23543, 29791 and 29792 were used for the program. Two levels (EQA L2 and L4) were evaluated as representatives for commutability.

Human serum pools. The human serum pools were also prepared from leftover patient serum samples collected from the two Hospitals. Possible volumes of leftover samples with cTnI values higher than 1 ng/ml (Beckmann Access assay or Siemens Centaur assay) were collected into tubes and frozen at −86°C every day. During a period of about 2 months, a total volume of approximately 200 ml of serum comprising 120 patient samples were obtained. The frozen aliquots of serum were thawed, pooled and tested for cTnI with Siemens Centaur CP assay. These primary pools were then diluted with a normal human serum pool, which was previously prepared and frozen-stored, to produce 5 patient serum pools (HSP L1-5) with cTnI values (Siemens Centaur CP assay) of approximately 8, 4, 2, 0.2 and 0.04 ng/ml, respectively. The pools were thoroughly mixed, filtered through 0.22 μm membranes, aliquoted in 0.8 ml into 2-ml cryogenic vials and stored at −86°C.

SRM preparations. Two levels of SRM preparations (SRM L1 and L2) were prepared by a serial dilution of SRM 2921 with a normal human serum pool. The cTnI concentrations of the preparations calculated from the assigned value [13] were 14.08 and 1.14 ng/ml, respectively. The preparations were aliquoted and frozen at −86°C.

Swine sera. Two cTnI positive swine sera were obtained as gifts from the Research Center for Coronary Heart Disease, Cardiovascular Institute & Fuwai Hospital, Chinese Academy of Medical Sciences. The sera were prepared from blood samples taken from model animals with MI induced by a balloon occlusion of the left anterior descending artery.

Measurement of the Samples and Materials

The individual patient samples and prepared materials were measured with 4 cTnI assays including Abbott Architect (Architect), Beckman Access (Access), Ortho Vitros (Vitros) and Siemens Advia Centaur (Centaur). The cut-off values (99th percentiles) of the assays indicated in the assay instructions were 0.028, 0.04, 0.034 and 0.04 ng/ml, and the reportable ranges 0.01–50, 0.01–100, 0.012–80 and 0.006–50 ng/ml, respectively. The measurements were performed by the Abbott Shanghai Laboratory (Architect) and clinical laboratories of Beijing Hospital (Access and Centaur) and Beijing Haidian Hospital (Vitros). A detailed measurement protocol was prepared and understood by all the laboratories. The samples and materials were so labeled that the prepared materials were interspersed between patient samples. The whole set of samples was divided into 3 subsets for

measurements in 3 days. Patient serum pool level 4 was included in each subset for the estimation of within-laboratory total CV. The samples were shipped on dry ice to laboratories outside the Hospital. On the day of measurement in each laboratory, a subset of samples were allowed to stand at room temperature for 30–60 minutes for thawing and mixed for 30 minutes on a hematology mixer. The samples were briefly centrifuged to collect the sample volumes which were fairly sufficient for the measurements. The samples were measured in triplicate and the order of measuring samples was reversed between the replicates. Calibrations were performed every day.

Data Analysis

Individual patient samples with measured cTnI concentrations out of any of the reportable ranges of the 4 assays were excluded for data analysis. Twelve such samples were excluded, eight of which were too low to be detectable with the Vitros assay and four were too high with the Centaur assay. One sample had incomplete data for the Vitros assay and another showed an exceptionally high value with the Access assay and these two samples were also excluded. The remaining 61 samples were used for the analysis of between-assay correlations and the evaluation of the commutability of prepared materials. The between-assay slopes and intercepts for the 6 assay pairs formed by the 4 assays were estimated with Passing-Bablok regression on the basis of the mean values of the triplicate measurements. The Pearson correlation coefficients were also calculated. For commutability evaluation, the measurement results were logarithm-transformed because of the heteroscedasticity of the data. The transformed data were analyzed with Deming regression and 95% prediction intervals were calculated for each pair of assays, using formulas given in the CLSI C53A document [18]. The commutability of the prepared materials was evaluated by comparing the logarithms for the materials with the limits of the intervals. For the estimation of matrix-related biases for noncommutable materials, the predicted logarithms were back-transformed and relative differences of measured values from predicted values were calculated. The Passing-Bablok regressions were performed with Analyse-it and all other analyses with Microsoft Excel.

Results

Results from EQA program

Our institution (National Center for Clinical Laboratories) as a national EQA provider distributes 5 samples biannually to applicant laboratories for the EQA of cardiac markers. The samples used have been commercial control materials. For the first EQA event in 2013, 418 laboratories using 32 assays participated

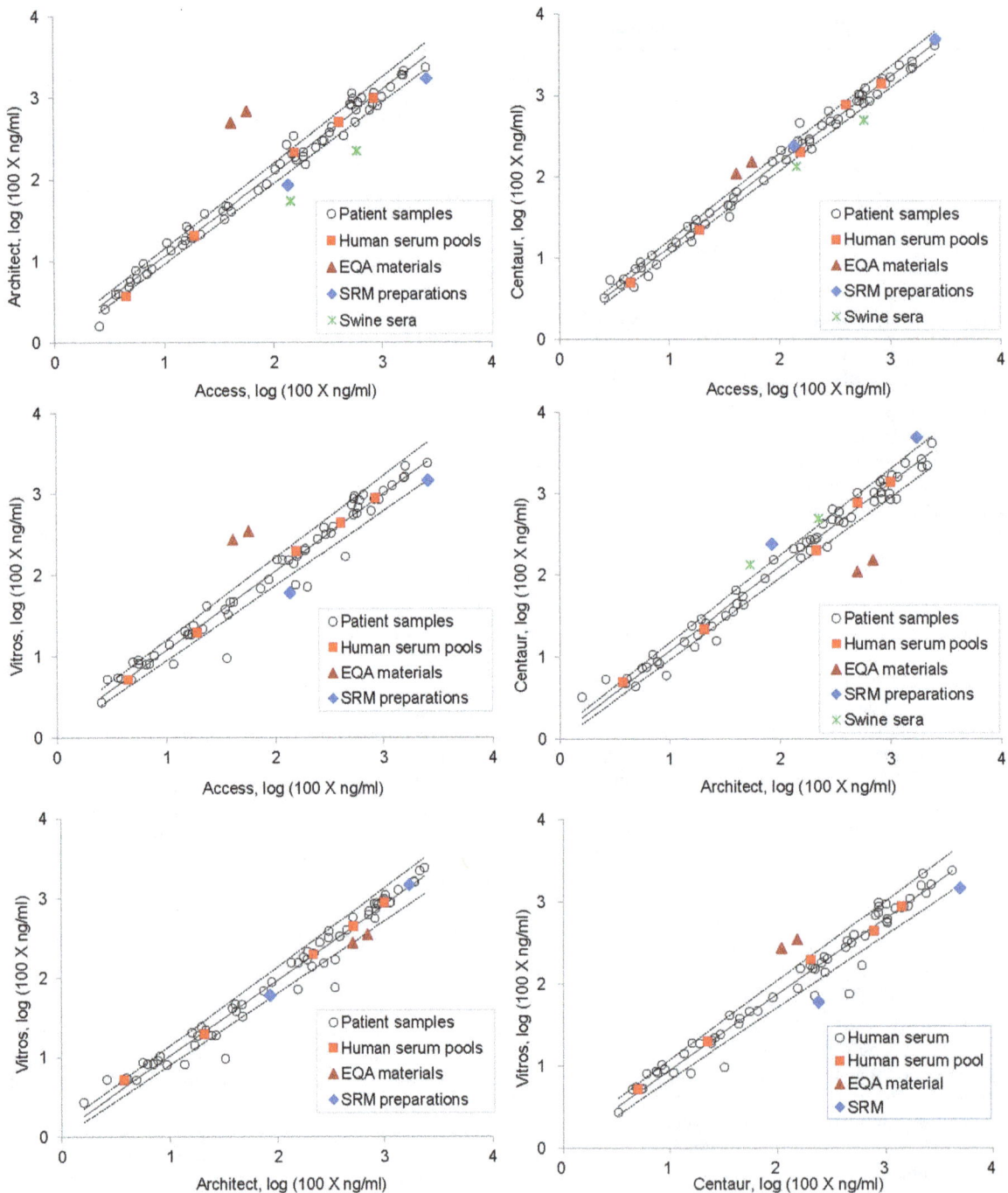

Figure 2. Commutability of prepared materials for cardiac troponin I (cTnI) measurement. Prepared materials (control materials used in our 2013 EQA program, frozen serum pools prepared from leftover patient samples, SRM preparations made by diluting the SRM 2921 with human serum and swine sera from MI model animals) together with a set of patient samples were measured for cTnI with 4 assays including Abbott Architect (Architect), Beckman Access (Access), Ortho Vitros (Vitros) and Siemens Advia Centaur (Centaur). The measurement results were logarithm-transformed and results for patient samples obtained with different assays were pairwise analyzed with Deming regression and 95% prediction intervals were calculated for each pair of assays. Prepared materials with measurement results (transformed) outside the prediction intervals are considered noncommutable. The solid lines are the regression lines and dashed are the limits of the prediction intervals.

in the program. The major participant assays were Access (126 user laboratories), Centaur (63), Architect (60) and Vitros (13). **Table 1** shows the assay peer group means and inter-laboratory CVs of cTnI measurements with the assays. The peer group means varied approximately 2 to 10 fold. The inter-laboratory CVs were also variable.

Measurement Results for Patient Samples

In the present study, we measured patient samples with the 4 assays for the purpose of evaluating the commutability the EQA materials and other materials. The medians and ranges of the measured cTnI concentrations and measurement precisions for the patient samples are shown in **Table 2**. The median cTnI

Table 4. Measurement results for patient serum pools, EQA materials, SRM materials and swine sera.

Assay	Human serum pools					EQA materials		SRM preparations		Swine sera	
cTnI concentration, ng/ml	L1	L2	L3	L4	L5	L2	L4	L1	L2	L1	L2
Access	8.41	4.05	1.56	0.19	0.04	0.57	0.41	25.80	1.36	5.79	1.43
Architec	9.89	5.02	2.14	0.21	0.04	6.87	4.97	17.11	0.85	2.23	0.54
Centaur	13.98	7.70	2.03	0.22	0.05	1.52	1.09	48.91	2.39	4.94	1.34
Vitros	8.86	4.41	1.97	0.20	0.05	3.45	2.71	14.72	0.60	ND[a]	ND[a]

[a]Not detectable.

concentrations of the 61 samples obtained with different assays varied from 1.475 ng/ml to 2.198 ng/ml. The ranges of cTnI concentrations were approximately 1000-fold wide (e.g. 0.026~25.472 ng/ml for Access assay) and the standard deviations of the triplicate measurements were evidently proportional to the concentration levels. The median within-run CVs for the assays were between 1.0% and 5.9% and the within-laboratory total CVs as estimated from the results of human serum pool level 4 ranged from 1.3% to 5.1%.

The between-assay correlations of measurement results for the patient samples were further analyzed with pair-wise regressions. Because of the heteroscedasticity and the wide range of the data, Passing-Bablok regression was used for the estimation of slopes and intercepts of the assay pairs. The Pearson correlation coefficients were also calculated to get approximate indications of the linearity. The Passing-Bablok slopes and intercepts and the Pearson correlation coefficients are shown in **Table 3**. The slopes varied from 0.676 to 1.624 among the assay pairs. Though all the intercepts analytically seemed to be negligible, 3 of the 6 assay pairs showed intercepts that might be significantly different from 0. The Pearson correlation coefficients ranged from 0.956 to 0.989. The scatter plots for the assay pairs illustrating the linearity and the distribution of the data are presented in **Figure 1**.

Commutability of Prepared Materials

The cTnI concentrations of the prepared materials (human serum pools, EQA materials, SRM preparations and swine sera) measured with different assays are listed in **Table 4**. Also because of the heteroscedasticity and the wide range of the data, logarithm transformation and Deming regression were used for the commutability evaluation. Commutability of the materials among different assays is shown in **Figure 2** and summarized in **Table 5**. The human serum pools were all commutable for all the assays. The SRM preparations were commutable for 2 of the 6 assay pairs. The EQA materials and the swine sera were all noncommutable for all the assays and the swine sera showed no reactivity to Vitros assay. To estimate the magnitude of the noncommutability of the materials, matrix-related biases were calculated (see the Materials and Methods section) for the noncommutable materials (**Table 6**). The matrix-related biases for the EQA materials ranged from −83% to 944%, the SRM preparations from −65% to 124%, and the swine sera from −68% to 99% (with the exclusion of Vitros assay).

The matrix-related biases of the EQA materials definitely caused abnormal between-assay variations in the EQA program. **Figure 3A** shows normalized cTnI levels (values relative to the all-assay mean) of the EQA materials (level 1~5, calculated from Table 1 data) in comparison with that of the human serum pools (from Table 4). Between-assay variations on the EQA materials were much larger (CV of ~80%) than that on the human serum pools (CV of ~20%). Correction for the matrix-related biases was tried. The normalized cTnI values of EQA material level 2 and human serum pool level 3, which were the respective medians of the 5 levels of the 2 categories of samples, were compared and correction factors were calculated for each assay by dividing the human serum pool value by the EQA material value. The factors were applied to all EQA values and the between-assay variations became similar to that on human serum pools as shown in **Figure 3B**.

Discussion

Assays for cTnI measurement have evolved several generations and improved considerably in respects of analytical sensitivity,

Table 5. Commutability of patient serum pools, EQA materials, SRM preparations and swine sera.

Assay pair (x–y)	Patient serum pools	EQA materials	SRM preparations	Swine sera
Access-Architect	1	0	0	0
Access-Centaur	1	0	1	0
Access-Vitros	1	0	0	0
Architect-Centaur	1	0	0	0
Architect-Vitros	1	0	1	0
Centaur-Vitros	1	0	0	0

"1" and "0" denote commutable and noncommutable, respectively.

precision and between-assay variation [2,3]. The improvement will continue as more efforts are being made toward standardization of cTnI measurement [2,4,5]. The performance of cTnI measurement is most conveniently monitored through EQA programs. For EQA programs to fulfill this purpose, however, EQA materials need to be commutable or to be of known commutability [8].

There have been very few studies on the commutability of materials for cTnI measurement [5,13]. Candás-Estébanez et al [19] reported apparently different measurement precisions on control materials and plasma samples measured with a cTnI measurement system. Information on the commutability of possible EQA materials is basically lacking. In this study, we evaluated the commutability of commercial control materials, human serum pools prepared from patient samples, purified analyte preparations and model animal serum samples, which would represent major possible sources of EQA materials. The study showed that only human serum pools were commutable among major cTnI assays and all other materials were variously noncommutable with matrix-related biases ranging from −83% to 944% (**Figure 2**, **Table 5** and **Table 6**).

The commutability of human serum pools has been suggested by their ability to harmonize measurement results of different assays [5,12]. The commutability may also be assumed because the pools can be considered averaged patient samples. However, preparation of the pools requires multiple treatments of patient samples and it is important to test whether the treatments, especially the freeze-thawing, diluting with normal serum, filtering and prolonged storage at various temperatures, causes alterations in the analyte or its matrix that influence the measurement. This study demonstrates that cTnI is resistant to the treatments and commutable sample materials can be prepared from leftover patient samples.

The measurement of cTnI seems to be especially susceptible to commutability influences. In this study, swine sera showed no reactivity to one assay, and matrix-related biases as high as ∼10 fold were observed on the control materials, and even the SRM preparations, the analyte of which is human troponin complex, showed matrix-related biases of up to ∼2 fold (**Table 6**). The causes of the noncommutability are complicated and related to both the measurement principles of the assays and nature of the analyte and its matrix [3]. Current cTnI assays are sandwich type immunoassays using monoclonal capture and detection antibodies. Different assays may use different combinations of antibodies with various specificities and affinities to the cTnI molecule. It is known that serum cTnI is subject to posttranslational modifications, such as proteolytic degradation and phosphorylation, and complexations with other molecules (e.g., TnC, heparin, heterophile antibodies, and cTnI specific autoantibodies) in the circulation [3]. For this and probably other reasons, the cTnI analytes in the prepared materials may be different from patient serum cTnI, depending on the origin and the history of processing of the materials. Animal cTnI may also be different in primary structure [15,16]. Furthermore, the matrixes of the control materials and the swine sera would apparently be different from that of patient serum. All these differences may influence different assays to varying degrees and the observed noncommutability would be a reflection of the variable influences.

The complexity of cTnI measurement would also be reflected by the between-assay correlations of measurement results of

Table 6. Matrix-related biases for noncommutable materials.

Assay pair (x–y)	Commutability-related bias, %					
	EQA materials		SRM preparations		Swine sera	
	L2	L4	L1	L2	L1	L2
Access-Architect	931	944	−47	−47	−68	−68
Access-Centaur	83	85			−48	−39
Access-Vitros	439	483	−42	−59	NR[a]	NR[a]
Architect-Centaur	−83	−83	109	124	71	99
Architect-Vitros	−41	−37			NR[a]	NR[a]
Centaur-Vitros	209	231	−46	−65	NR[a]	NR[a]

[a]No reactivity of swine sera to Vitros assay.

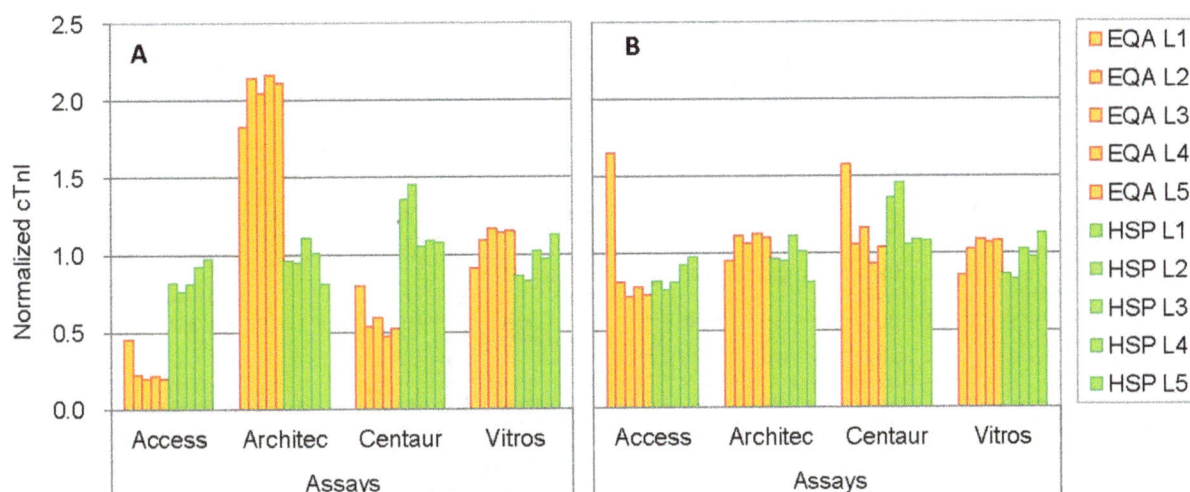

Figure 3. Between-assay variations on EQA materials before (A) and after (B) correction for matrix-related biases. The cTnI concentrations of 5 levels of EQA materials (EQA L1~5) for different assays from a EQA program were normalized by dividing each assay group mean by the all-assay mean and the normalized values for EQA materials were compared with that for human serum pools (also 5 levels, HSP L1~5). Between-assay variations on the EQA materials were much larger (CV of ~80%) than that on the human serum pools (CV of ~20%) because of matrix-related biases (A). The variations became similar when the biases were corrected (B).

patient samples (**Figure 1** and **Table 3**). Relatively large scatters and low Pearson correlation coefficients of the data were observed on the assay pairs.

The noncommutability of the control materials caused exceptional between-assay variations in our EQA programs (**Table 1** and **Figure 3A**). The matrix-related biases on the materials ranged from −83% to 944% (**Table 6**). Without this information, the EQA results could hardly be interpreted and might lead to erroneous conclusions regarding the comparability of the assays.

EQA programs should ideally use commutable sample materials. Based on the results of this study and other available information [2–5,12,13], human serum pools prepared from patient samples seem currently to be the only commutable materials for cTnI measurement. EQA programs desirably distribute multi-level samples that cover a large part of the measurement ranges of assays. Obviously, it is difficult to prepare all the EQA materials from patient samples. Theoretically, EQA programs can also use sample materials of known commutability. However, commutability is highly material and assay specific and it is almost impossible to test the materials with all contemporary assays for all EQA events. A practical approach may be a combination of human serum pools with other more easily available materials. An EQA program includes at least one human serum pool that has an analytically relevant cTnI value, and uses other materials for all other intended sample levels. The EQA process itself serves as a "commutability study" at the same time and the matrix-related biases can be reasonably corrected by applying factors to the assay peer group means as described in the Results section and shown in **Figure 3B**. Similar approaches have also been proposed in previous reports [8]. This correction is obviously based on an assumption that the matrix-related biases are proportional and thus the materials should be of the same origin. The noncommutability of the materials would also need to be reasonable, or the inter-laboratory CV for the peer groups may not be reliable. For this purpose, human troponin TIC complex diluted with human serum would be possible candidates based on this study. The usefulness of swine serum materials is uncertain and depends on monoclonal antibodies used in future assays.

It should also be noted that the ideal EQA is that in which, besides the use of commutable samples, the values of the samples are assigned with a reference method or an accepted protocol so that all the routine assays can be evaluated against "true values" [8]. This has actually been realized for some clinical chemistry analytes, such as cholesterol, creatinine, and HbA1c. International organizations are working on the reference measurement of cTnI [20,21] and accuracy-based EQA for cTnI may be expected in the future.

A major limitation of the study is that only 4 assays were used for the commutability evaluations. This is mainly because of the available volume of individual patient samples. It is very difficult to get sufficient volume of individual samples for measurement in triplicate with more assays. Another limitation is that the patient samples were frozen before analysis. This is related to the availability of sufficient number of fresh cTnI positive samples with sufficient leftover volumes. It took about 2 months to collect the 75 samples in 2 hospitals. The commutability of human serum pools demonstrated in the study may imply the acceptability of the use of frozen samples.

In conclusion, commutability of EQA materials has major impact on the effectiveness of EQA programs for cTnI measurement. Human serum pools prepared from patient samples are commutable and other materials are mostly noncommutable. EQA programs for cTnI should include at least one human serum pool to allow proper interpretation of EQA results.

Acknowledgments

We are most grateful to Abbott Diagnostics (Shanghai), Beckman Coulter (Shanghai), Ortho Clinical Diagnostics (Shanghai) and Siemens Healthcare Diagnostic (Shanghai) for their kind technical supports. We thank Dr. Jing Yao at Fuwai Hospital for providing the swine sera.

Author Contributions

Conceived and designed the experiments: SZ JZ CZ WC. Performed the experiments: SZ JZ. Analyzed the data: SZ JZ CZ FC SY WC. Contributed reagents/materials/analysis tools: SZ YL HZ FC MW. Wrote the paper: SZ WC.

References

1. Thygesen K, Alpert JS, Jaffe AS, Simoons ML, Chaitman BR, et al. (2012) Third universal definition of myocardial infarction. Circulation 126: 2020–2035.
2. Tate JR, Bunk DM, Christenson RH, Katrukha A, Noble JE, et al. (2010). Standardization of cardiac troponin I measurement: past and present. Pathology 42: 402–408.
3. Apple FS, Collinson PO. (2012) Analytical characteristics of high-sensitivity cardiac troponin assays. Clin Chem 58: 54–61.
4. Panteghini M, Bunk DM, Christenson RH, Katrukha A, Porter RA, et al. (2008) Standardization of troponin I measurements: an update. Clin Chem Lab Med 46: 1501–1506.
5. Christenson RH, Duh SH, Apple FS, Bodor GS, Bunk DM, et al. (2006) Towards standardization of cardiac troponin I measurements. Part II: Assessing commutability of candidate reference materials and harmonization of cardiac troponin I assays. Clin Chem 52: 1685–1692.
6. Miller WG, Myers GL, Gantzer M, Kahn SE, Schönbrunner ER, et al. (2011) Roadmap for harmonization of clinical laboratory measurement procedures. Clin Chem 57: 1108–1117.
7. Tate JR, Johnson R, Barth J, Panteghini M (2014) Harmonization of laboratory testing - Current achievements and future strategies. Clin Chim Acta 432: 4–7.
8. Miller WG, Jones GRD, Horowitz GL, Weykamp C (2011) Proficiency testing/ external quality assessment: current challenges and future directions. Clin Chem 57: 1670–1680.
9. Miller WG, Myers GL, Rej R (2006) Why commutability matters. Clin Chem 52: 553–554.
10. Miller WG, Myers GL (2013) Commutability still matters. Clin Chem 59: 1291–1293.
11. CLSI (1999) Preparation and validation of commutable frozen human serum pools as secondary reference materials for cholesterol measurement procedures; approved guideline. CLSI document C37-A. Wayne (PA): CLSI.
12. Tate JR, Heathcote D, Koerbin G, Thean G, Andriske D, et al. (2002) The harmonization of cardiac troponin I measurement is independent of sample time collection but is dependent on the source of calibrator. Clin Chim Acta 324: 13–23.
13. Christenson RH, Duh SH, Apple FS, Bodor GS, Bunk DM, et al. (2001) Standardization of cardiac troponin I assays: round robin of ten candidate reference materials. Clin Chem 47: 431–437.
14. Bunk DM, Welch MJ (2006) Characterization of a new certified reference material for human cardiac troponin I. Clin Chem 52: 212–219.
15. Apple FS, Murakami MM, Ler R, Walker D, York M (2008) Analytical characteristics of commercial cardiac troponin I and T immunoassays in serum from rats, dogs, and monkeys with induced acute myocardial injury. Clin Chem 54: 1982–1989.
16. O'Brien PJ, Landt Y, Ladenson JH (1997) Differential reactivity of cardiac and skeletal muscle from various species in a cardiac troponin I immunoassay. Clin Chem 43: 2333–2338.
17. HyTest Ltd (2014) Markers of Cardiovascular Diseases and Metabolic Syndrome. http://www.hytest.fi/news/102012/troponin-i-assay-development.
18. CLSI (2010). Characterization and qualification of commutable reference materials for laboratory medicine; approved guideline. CLSI document C53-A. Wayne (PA): CLSI.
19. Candás-Estébanez B, Cano-Corres R, Dot-Bach D, Valero-Politi J (2012) Lack of commutability between a quality control material and plasma samples in a troponin I measurement system. Clin Chem Lab Med 50: 2237–2238.
20. Noble JE, Bunk DM, Christenson RH, Cole KD, He HJ, et al. (2010) Development of a candidate secondary reference procedure (immunoassay based measurement procedure of higher metrological order) for cardiac troponin I: I. Antibody characterization and preliminary validation. Clin Chem Lab Med 48: 1603–1610.
21. He HJ, Lowenthal MS, Cole KD, Bunk D, Wang L (2011) An immunoprecipitation coupled with fluorescent Western blot analysis for the characterization of a model secondary serum cardiac troponin I reference material. Clin Chim Acta 412: 107–111.

11

Rhinoceros Feet Step Out of a Rule-of-Thumb: A Wildlife Imaging Pioneering Approach of Synchronized Computed Tomography-Digital Radiography

Gabriela Galateanu[1]*[◑], **Robert Hermes**[1◑], **Joseph Saragusty**[1], **Frank Göritz**[1], **Romain Potier**[2], **Baptiste Mulot**[2], **Alexis Maillot**[3], **Pascal Etienne**[4], **Rui Bernardino**[5], **Teresa Fernandes**[5], **Jurgen Mews**[6], **Thomas Bernd Hildebrandt**[1]

1 Department of Reproduction Management, Leibniz Institute for Zoo and Wildlife Research, Berlin, Germany, 2 ZooParc de Beauval, Saint-Aignan, France, 3 Parc zoologique d'Amnéville, Amnéville-les-Thermes, France, 4 Parc zoologique de La Barben (Pélissane), La Barben, France, 5 Hospital Veterinário, Jardim Zoológico de Lisboa, Lisbon, Portugal, 6 Clinical Application Research Center, Toshiba Medical Systems Europe, Zoetermeer, The Netherlands

Abstract

Currently, radiography is the only imaging technique used to diagnose bone pathology in wild animals situated under "field conditions". Nevertheless, while chronic foot disease in captive mega-herbivores is widely reported, foot radiographic imaging is confronted with scarcity of studies. Numerous hindrances lead to such limited numbers and it became very clear that the traditional perspective on bone imaging in domestic animals based on extensive studies and elaborated statistical evaluations cannot be extrapolated to their non-domestic relatives. For these reasons, the authors initiated a multi-modality imaging study and established a pioneering approach of synchronized computed tomography (CT) and digital radiography (DR), based on X-ray projections derived from three-dimensional CT reconstructed images. Whereas this approach can be applied in any clinical field, as a case of outstanding importance and great concern for zoological institutions, we selected foot bone pathologies in captive rhinoceroses to demonstrate the manifold applications of the method. Several advances were achieved, endowing the wildlife clinician with all-important tools: prototype DR exposure protocols and a *modus operandi* for foot positioning, advancing both traditional projections and, for the first-time, species-related radiographic views; assessment of radiographic diagnostic value for the whole foot and, in premiere, for each autopodial bone; together with additional insights into radiographic appearance of bone anatomy and pathology with a unique, simultaneous CT-DR correlation. Based on its main advantages in availing a wide range of keystone data in wildlife imaging from a limited number of examined subjects and combining advantages of CT as the golden standard method for bone diseases' diagnostic with DR's clinical feasibility under field conditions, synchronized CT-DR presents a new perspective on wildlife's health management. With this we hope to provide veterinary clinicians with concrete imaging techniques and substantial diagnostic tools, which facilitate straightforward attainment and interpretation of field radiography images taken worldwide.

Editor: Antonio Gonzalez-Bulnes, INIA, Spain

Funding: These authors have no support or funding to report.

Competing Interests: None of the authors of this paper has a financial or personal relationship with other people or organizations that could inappropriately influence or bias the content of this paper. Although seven of the authors are employed by commercial entities (RP and BM: ZooParc de Beauval, France; AM: Parc zoologique d'Amnéville, France; PE: Parc zoologique de La Barben, France; RB and TF: Hospital Veterinário, Jardim Zoológico de Lisboa, Portugal; JM: Toshiba Medical Systems Europe, The Netherlands).

* Email: galateanu@izw-berlin.de

◑ These authors contributed equally to this work.

Introduction

Diagnostic imaging in domestic animals has a long-established pedestal on a plethora of published data supported by huge numbers (tens of thousands) of examined subjects. Not so is the situation for their wild counterparts. To illustrate this present and huge discrepancy, we purposely chose the most frequently applied imaging procedure in large animals, foot radiography, and compared between the most studied large mammals on land, the horse, as a representative for domestic animals, and the elephant, as a representative for wild animals. The only foot radiographic studies with indicated numbers of subjects found in *Elephantidae* (n = 4) included, in total, 15 elephants, with the largest number being 11 individuals per study [1,2,3,4]. Nonetheless, an identical number of *Equidae* foot radiographic studies (n = 4), elected from 216 currently recorded publications, included 995 horses, with the largest number being 523 subjects per study [5,6,7,8].

All-important hindrances lead to such scarce numbers of radiographic studies in wild animals, especially mega-herbivores. Among them can be mentioned: difficulty in access to free-ranging or captive wild animals [9], their untamed disposition implying serious risks in approaching them [10,11], temporal constraints and survival risks imposed by prerequisite sedation and/or general anesthesia [12,13,14], tendency to disguise any sign of disease or clinical symptoms until late stages when they cannot be concealed any longer [15,16], and difficulty of performing and interpreting radiographic examinations under "field conditions" [17]. These numbers decrease further in two additional circumstances. One condition is radiographic positioning intricacy due to massive body size of mega-vertebrates [18,19]. The other situation is the intrinsic value of endangered wild animals, some of them being "the last of their kind", as can be seen in rhinoceroses [20,21,22,23,24,25,26,27,28,29]. Under these circumstances, any procedures that necessitate physical restraint, handling, transportation, sedation and/or general anesthesia will require a profound clinical justification, and thus are rarely performed. These challenges account for radiologic under-diagnosis of foot pathology in large-sized mammals [30].

Yet, chronic foot disease in captive herbivores is widely reported [10,31,32]. Remarkable evidence suggesting that foot osteopathology in hoofed mammals is more widespread, severe and diverse than previously thought [30,33] should force us to rethink of radiographic diagnosis in captive mega-herbivores as routine examination to be incorporated into their health management. At any rate, apart from the elephant [2,18,19,34], radiographic techniques, imaging protocols, and radiographic interpretation of foot bone anatomy and/or pathology in mega-vertebrates have not been established to date.

It became very clear that the traditional perspective on bone imaging in domestic animals based on extensive studies and elaborated statistical evaluations cannot be extrapolated to their non-domestic relatives. A new imaging strategy for assessment of different pathologies in wild animals became imperative and it is thus called for.

On this account, the authors initiated a comprehensive study, based on multi-modality imaging. We established a pioneering approach of synchronized computed tomography (CT) and digital radiography (DR), providing a new perspective on wildlife management. Whereas this approach can be applied in any clinical field, as a case in point, we selected one disease of outstanding importance: foot bone pathologies in wild animals. For this reason, synchronized CT-DR is demonstrated here using rhinoceros feet to show the manifold applications of the method. With this we hope to provide veterinary clinicians with concrete imaging techniques and substantial diagnostic tools which will facilitate straightforward implementation and interpretation of field radiographic images from rhinoceros feet taken worldwide. Without such advances, wildlife imaging will remain under the rule-of-thumb, now prevailing by necessity.

Materials and Methods

Ethics Statement

The four rhinoceroses (two Southern white and two Indian) included in our study were captive animals from the following zoological gardens: Parc zoologique d'Amnéville, France; Parc zoologique de La Barben (Pélissane), France; ZooParc de Beauval, France; and Jardim Zoológico de Lisboa, Portugal. Southern white rhinoceros is listed under the IUCN the Red List of Endangered Species as Near Threatened and the Indian rhinoceros is listed as Vulnerable. These animals either died (rhinoceros 4: metastasized adenocarcinoma) or were euthanized due to chronic, non-resolvable health issues and subsequent animal welfare reasons, following internal decision-making process in the respective zoos (rhinoceros 1: foot epidermoid carcinoma with 3rd grade lameness; rhinoceros 2: generalized chronic ulcerative dermatitis; rhinoceros 3: chronic pododermatitis and recumbency without movement). The euthanasia procedures were performed in conformity with the international guidelines for euthanasia in non-domestic species,

specifically for mega-vertebrates [35]. In accordance with these guidelines, animals were first immobilized with etorphine hydrochloride to achieve full recumbent anesthesia. Euthanasia was then achieved by intravenous administration of a barbiturate.

No animal work was involved at any stage in the process and all samples (distal feet) were collected after the unrelated death of the animals. The zoos were approached upon our learning of the animals' death and gave their permission to use the feet for this study, in the context of mandatory *post mortem* examination and disease diagnosis. This *post mortem* diagnostic study was in accordance with the guidelines of the Internal Committee of Ethics and Animal Welfare of the Leibniz Institute for Zoo and Wildlife Research as stipulated under approval number 2006-01-02.

Rhinoceroses

Ten distal limbs (five front and five hind legs) obtained *post mortem* from four captive rhinoceroses, were used for this study (Table 1). The rhinoceroses were of two species: Southern white rhinoceros (*Ceratotherium simum simum*) and greater one-horned, or Indian, rhinoceros (*Rhinoceros unicornis*). Distal limb encompassed the autopodium (and its related soft-tissue structures) represented by the hand (manus) or foot (pes), being composed of podial elements (carpus/tarsus), metapodials (metacarpus/metatarsus) and phalanges [36].

Rhinoceros 1 (Southern white rhinoceros) presented a medial, large tumefaction on its hind left foot, diagnosed histologically as epidermoid carcinoma. Rhinoceros 3 (Indian rhinoceros) suffered from chronic pododermatitis in all four limbs for many years. Rhinoceroses 2 (Southern white rhinoceros) and 4 (Indian rhinoceros) had no reported foot disease. Rhinoceroses 1 and 3 were euthanized due to foot related disorders and rhinoceros 2 was euthanized and rhinoceros 4 died due to other, unrelated, pathologies.

The legs of the two Southern white rhinoceroses were sectioned above the carpal and tarsal joints (included). Except for the hind foot of rhinoceros 4, Indian rhinoceroses' legs were sectioned at the level of carpal and, respectively, tarsal joints (partially included). Therefore, the total number of bones included in this study was 257 instead of 278.

Computed tomographic data acquisition and imaging

Computed tomographic data was acquired from all ten distal limbs using a high-resolution, 128-slice scanner (Aquilion CX, Toshiba Medical Systems Cooperation, Tochigi, Japan). Settings for the CT helical scan protocol were: 120 kV, 100–300 mA, 0.6 s rotation time, helical pitch HP 41.0 and 0.5 mm acquisition slice thickness. Reconstruction protocols included two soft tissue reconstructions (body-standard and body-sharp) and a high-resolution reconstruction algorithm for bones. The reconstruction slice thickness/slice interval of both was set to 1/0.8 mm and 0.5/0.25 mm.

Vitrea workstation with ViTREA 2 version 4.0 medical diagnostic software (Vital Images Inc., Minnetonka, MN, USA) provided the tools for two-dimensional (2D) and three-dimensional (3D) processing and analysis of the CT images. Among these tools, volume-rendering software, simultaneous imaging of specific anatomical and pathological structures of interest using a combination of 2D orthogonal Multi-Planar Reconstructions (MPR) and 3D images; a virtual cutting function in combination with 2D and 3D segmentation allowed us to focus on the region of interest. A wide variety of clinical viewing protocols and fine adjustment of visualization parameters, e.g. adjustments of threshold and transparency settings enhanced the diagnostic

Table 1. Rhinoceroses.

Rhinoceroses	Species	Gender	Age (Years)	Feet
Rhinoceros 1	*Ceratotherium simum simum*	Male	38	HL
Rhinoceros 2	*Ceratotherium simum simum*	Male	38	FR, FL, HL
Rhinoceros 3	*Rhinoceros unicornis*	Female	24	FR, FL, HR, HL
Rhinoceros 4	*Rhinoceros unicornis*	Female	34	FL, HR

Ceratotherium simum simum- Southern white rhinoceros, *Rhinoceros unicornis-* Indian rhinoceros, FR - front right, FL - front left, HR - hind right, HL - hind left autopodium.

quality of the images. Oblique and curved MPRs were required in order to delineate several lesions with a complex 3D architecture.

Synchronized computed tomography and digital radiography

Fully rendered volumetric (3D) CT images were acquired from all ten feet. Based on a predefined sectional plane of the object, synchronized X-ray projections were calculated and generated by applying specialized software tools on the image console.

For each foot, eight 3D CT images (45° apart) equivalent to eight standard radiographic views were generated. In order to simulate DR views, the acquired CT datasets were used to generate renderings from 8 different viewing directions for each foot. Thus, each 3D CT image was transformed into a synchronized digital radiographic image (Synch DR), in total eighty Synch DR images for all ten feet (Fig.1).

The standardized nomenclature for radiographic projections in veterinary medicine was used [37,38]. The projections performed, indicating point-of-entry to point-of-exit direction of the primary X-ray beam, were four orthogonal projections: dorso-palmar (plantar) [DPa(l)], palmaro (plantaro)-dorsal [Pa(l)D], medio-lateral [ML], latero-medial [LM], and four oblique projections: dorsomedial-palmaro (plantaro) lateral [DM-Pa(l)LO], dorsolateral-palmaro (plantaro) medial [DL-Pa(l)MO], palmaro (plantaro) medial-dorsolateral [Pa(l)M-DLO] and palmaro (plantaro) lateral-dorsomedial [Pa(l)L-DMO]. For simplification reasons, "P" was used for either Pa (palmar) or Pl (plantar), when it was not relevant if it is front or hind foot.

Windowing and leveling of each Synch DR were further adjusted in order to obtain the best radiographic quality in terms of resolution, contrast and noise. These Synch DR images were designated as gold standard images and were used as reference in establishing the most accurate positioning and appropriate exposure parameters for direct digital radiography (DR).

Direct digital radiography

Traditional DR was conducted on all nine distal limbs from rhinoceroses 2, 3 and 4, using a mobile x-ray unit (Mobi X-Ray, SEDECAL, Madrid, Spain) and Canon CXDI-1 image plate (Canon CXDI-1 System Digital Radiography; CANON Europe N.V. Medical Products Division, Amstelveen, The Netherlands).

Different radiographic projections were achieved by maintaining the X-ray generator and image plate in the same position, while rotating the foot. The foot was positioned parallel to and in the nearest proximity of the image plate.

An optimal exposure chart was established showing the relationship between different radiographic views and the exposure values: miliampere (mA), kilovolt peak (kVp), time (s), at a constant source-to-film or focus-to-film distance (FFD) of 100 cm.

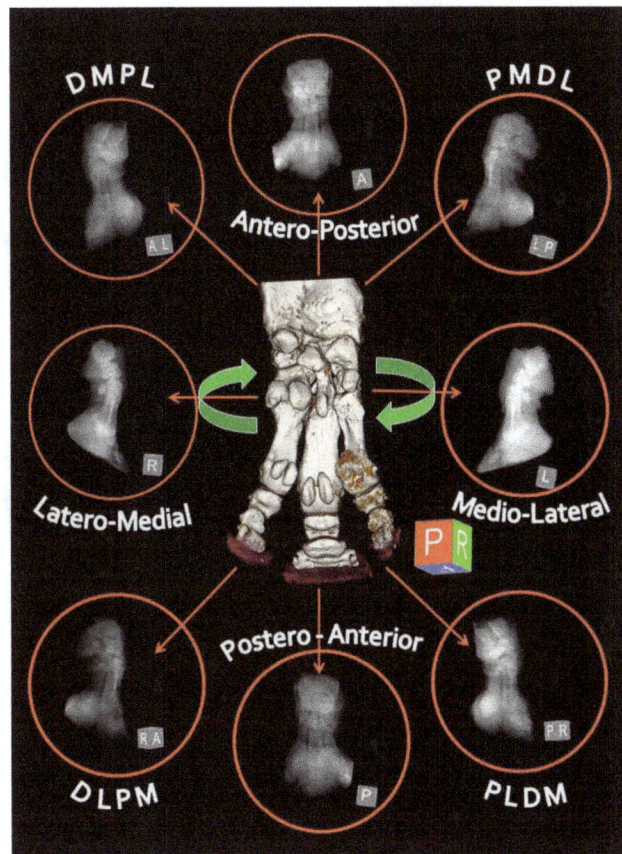

Figure 1. Principle of method in synchronized computed tomography (CT)-digital radiography (DR). Digital radiographic images are calculated and generated from fully rendered, tri-dimensional (3D) CT images. Standard orthogonal (n=4) and oblique (n=4) radiographic views (45° apart) are shown here using as example the left front distal limb of Southern white rhinoceros 2. The abbreviations used represent the oblique projections characterized by the point-of-entry to point-of-exit direction of the primary X-ray beam: DMPL [dorsomedial-palmarolateral], PMDL [palmaromedial-dorsolateral], PLDM [palmarolateral-dorsomedial], and DLPM [dorsolateral-palmaromedial].

Different anatomical landmarks and radiographic planes were investigated to nominate reference indicators for foot positioning and the outcome is presented in the "Results" section.

For each foot, eight radiographic views were performed in accordance with the gold standard Synch DR images established before. Seventy-two DR were thus assessed for depiction of bone anatomy and pathology.

Digital radiographic evaluation

Two criteria were investigated in each radiographic view:

a) Number of bones that were discernible at a diagnostic value (presented as percentage from the total number of foot's bones);

b) Perceptible radiographic details of each bone estimated with a 5-point radiographic rating scale. The following values were used, from 1 to 5: 1 = deficient (many bones superimposed and no detail), 2 = inadequate (three or more bones superimposed, poor detail), 3 = satisfactory (two bones superimposed, but relatively good detail), 4 = good (minimal or partial superimposition, good detail), 5 = excellent (minimal superimposition, very good detail).

Diagnostic value of every radiographic view was assessed solely for each bone and, by summation, entirely for the whole foot.

Conventional analogic radiography

Sixteen plain or analog radiographs (AR) of all feet, including four radiographic views per foot were performed and manually developed in rhinoceros 3, using a HF 300 X-ray unit (GmbH Gierth), X-Omat radiographic cassette, Kodak Lanex Medium Screen and Kodak T-Mat L/RA radiographic films. The exposure parameters were: 40 mA, 76 kVp, 0.06 s for all projections of hind feet and medio-lateral projection of front feet; 40 mA, 74 kVp, 0.06 s for the rest of front feet's projections, all at a constant FFD of 80 cm.

Statistical analysis

Statistical analysis was performed using PASW Statistics 18 (formerly SPSS, IBM Inc., Chicago, IL). The Chi-square goodness-of-fit exact test was used to test whether the observed proportions for categorical variables differ from the hypothesized equal distribution.

Rhinoceros 1 suffered from epidermoid carcinoma on the only limb available from this animal. As this tumor may have been the cause for at least some of the osteopathologies found in this foot and thus may have biased the statistical analysis, we have also analyzed our data after excluding this animal. Results indicate no biasing effect of rhinoceros 1 as none of the comparisons changed in a way that alter our findings (data not shown). Results are therefore shown for all four rhinoceroses combined.

A P-value <0.05 was considered statistically significant for all statistical tests.

Results

Reference radiographic techniques

Exposure parameters (mAs, kVp) were similar for both Southern white and Indian rhinoceroses, with no differences between front and hind feet, as can be seen in the proposed technique chart (Fig. 2). The highest exposure factors were required for the ML/LM views, whereas the lowest exposure was entailed for PD/DP views. Oblique views called for intermediary exposure parameters. An alternative exposure chart is also proposed, applying a longer exposure time. The main advantages of this alternative protocol are lower kVp and higher mA, leading to an improved bone imaging (Fig. S1). Additionally, in this variant, all oblique and DP/PD orthogonal projections could be performed with identical exposure.

The most reliable anatomical landmark found in both Indian and Southern white rhinoceros was the toenail of the third (central) digit. Radiographic projections obtained at angles of 45°, or multiples of it, from the reference dorsal mid-line passing through the central toenail, were as follows: DP —45°— DM-PL —45°— ML — 45°— PM-DL — 45°— PD — 45°— PL-DM — 45°— LM —45°— DL-PM — 45°— DP (Fig. 1).

Specifically for digits, Synch DR revealed that, in order to achieve minimal bone super-imposition, projection angles must have different values in rhinoceroses than the traditional projections known from domestic radiography. Starting with DP view, these were the optimal angles for the front foot: DPa —20°— DM-PaL —60°— ML — 70°— PaM-DL — 30°— PaD — 20°— PaL-DM — 70°— LM —60°— DL-PaM — 30°— DPa (Fig. 3 and Fig. S2-8). Starting with DP view, these were the optimal angles for the hind foot: DPl —20°— DM-PlL —70°— ML — 70°— PlM-DL — 20°— PlD — 20°— PlL-DM — 70°— LM —70°— DL-PlM — 20°— DPl. By comparison, rhinoceroses' specific projection angles revealed higher numbers of detected digits' osteopathologies than the traditional angles, in all feet.

Radiographic diagnostic value

Except for the first carpal row in Indian rhinoceroses (not included), radiographic detail value of each bone per radiographic view was identical for Southern white and Indian rhinoceroses (Fig. 4, 5). Likewise, the number (percentage) and, respectively, radiographic detail of autopodial bones as a unit per view were identical for Southern white and Indian rhinoceroses (Fig.6, 7). Additionally, in Southern white and Indian rhinoceroses, the radiographic projection with the highest diagnostic value for both front and hind feet was the PD view (Fig.6, 7).

Comparison of the diagnostic value (depicted bones' number and detail) of different radiographic views revealed dissimilar patterns between front and hind feet (Fig.6, 7). The most valuable views in terms of number of depicted bones, represented as percentage from the total number of autopodial bones, were PaD (83.3%), DPa (75%), PaL-DMO (75%), for the front foot and PlD (90%), DL-PlMO (90%), PlM-DLO (90%), for the hind foot. The most valuable views in terms of radiographic detail, represented as total units in 5-point radiographic scale, were PaD (44), DPa (42), PaL-DMO (41), for the front foot and PlD (40), DPl (38), PlM-DLO (38), for the hind foot.

Distinctly, there was not always a direct relationship between the two parameters (number and discernible detail) for a specific foot's radiographic view. As a case in point, for the hind foot, PlD, DL-PlMO, and PlM-DLO views provide information about the same number of bones (90% discernible bones), but the radiographic detail is higher on PlD view (40 points in the rating scale), followed by PlM-DLO (38 points in the rating scale) and DL-PlMO (34 points in the rating scale).

Additionally, no relationship was found between the diagnostic values for the whole autopodium and for any specific bone. For example, first carpal bone was very well visualized (5 in the rating scale) in DM-PaLO view, but indiscernible (1 in the rating scale) in PaM-DLO view, though both projections had the same overall diagnostic value (66.66% discernible bones and 38 points in the rating scale).

Bone anatomy and pathology in computed tomographic imaging

Computed tomographic images depicted both bone anatomy and pathology (Fig. 8). A total of 257 autopodial bones were investigated in this study. Among them, 69 bones (26.8%) at 117 sites in all Indian and Southern white rhinoceroses presented pathological changes. These comprised of a large spectrum of lesions including cortical sclerosis (Fig. S9), proliferative new bone formation and bone remodeling (Fig. S10) with loss of normal shape (33/117; 28.2%), intra- and periarticular mineralized bodies or bony fragments (27/117; 23.1%; Fig. S11), fractures (19/117; 16.2%; Fig. S12), periosteal proliferation (continuous and interrupted; 19/117; 16.2%; Fig. S13), osteolysis and bone rarefaction

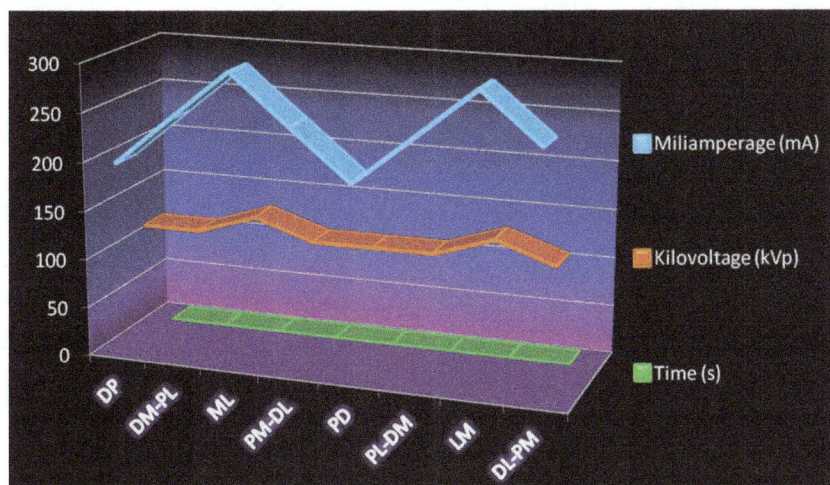

Figure 2. Radiographic exposure chart for front and hind feet in both Southern white and Indian rhinoceroses. On the horizontal axis are the eight radiographic views and the vertical axis shows the exposure values of: milliampere (mA), kilovolt peak (kVp) and time (s) for each projection at a constant source-to-film, or focus-to-film, distance (FFD) of 100 cm. Standard radiographic views were: DP [dorso-palmar (plantar)], DM-PL [dorsomedial-palmaro (plantaro) lateral], ML [medio-lateral], PM-DL [palmaro (plantaro) medial-dorsolateral], PD [palmaro (plantaro)-dorsal], PL-DM [palmaro (plantaro) lateral-dorsomedial]; LM [latero-medial], DL-PM [dorsolateral-palmaro (plantaro) medial].

(13/117; 11.1%). Enlargement of the linear radiolucent areas along the distal border of the distal phalanx termed "vascular channels", and changes in the trabecular pattern were also found. Bone cystic formation (n = 4) and ankylosis (n = 2) were the rarest osteopathologies. Concomitant presence of several lesions was similar in appearance to end stage degenerative joint disease (DJD), osteoarthrosis and/or osteoarthritis. Of the 117 sites with bone pathologies, significantly more were situated in the front limbs than in the hind limbs (n = 72 vs. n = 45, respectively; Chi-square = 6.231, P = 0.016). Comparison between the medial and

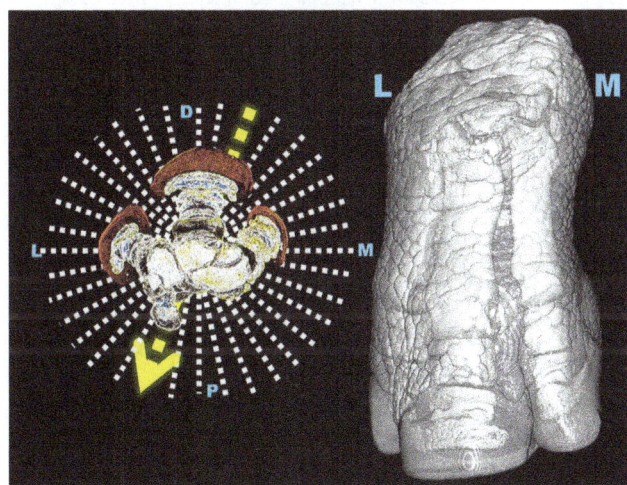

Figure 3. Rhinoceroses' species-related radiographic views. Dorsomedial-palmarolateral (DMPL) 20° oblique view performed at a projection angle of 20° from the dorsal mid-plane (arrow) allows a better visualization of all digits than the traditional DMPL 45° oblique view. Positioning technique is demonstrated on tri-dimensional computed tomographic (3D CT) image of Indian rhinoceros 3 right front foot (right side image) and schematically represented using a cross-sectional CT image (left side image). Semi-transparent 3D CT imaging protocol was employed to show both foot's exterior aspect and the underlying bony structures.

lateral digits revealed a higher prevalence of osteopathologies on the medial digit in the hind (n = 18 vs. n = 7; Chi-square = 4.840, P = 0.043) but not in the front (n = 27 vs. n = 20; Chi-square = 1.043, P = 0.382) limbs. The third or middle digit was less affected than the medial digit in the hind limbs (n = 18 vs. n = 5; Chi-square = 7.348, P = 0.011) as well as in the front limbs (n = 27 vs. n = 11; Chi-square = 6.737, P = 0.014). When prevalence of osteopathologies per digit was compared for both front and hind limbs combined, there were more osteopathologies in the medial digit (n = 45) when compared to the lateral digit (n = 27; Chi-square = 4.500, P = 0.044) or the middle digit (n = 16; Chi-square = 13.787, P = 0.00026). While the medial digit presented more osteopathologies when compared to the lateral digit, this was not the case when the middle, or third, digit was compared to the lateral one. No difference was found in either front or hind limbs or if both front and hind feet were combined when prevalence of osteopathologies was compared between the middle and lateral digits. The only difference found between the medial and lateral digits when osteopathologies' prevalence was compared was in the occurrence of periosteal reaction (n = 13 vs. n = 3, respectively; Chi-square = 6.250, P = 0.021). There were also more periosteal reaction (n = 13 vs. n = 1; Chi-square = 10.286, P = 0.00183) and bone remodelling (n = 15 vs. n = 1; Chi-square = 12.250, P = 0.00052) in the medial digit when compared to the middle digit. The digits (including metapodial, phalangeal and sesamoidal bones) were by far the most prevalent site for osteopathologies, presenting more osteopathologies than in the podial elements (carpus and tarsus) combined (n = 88 vs. n = 29; Chi-square = 29.752, P<0.00001). Of the digital elements, the phalanges constituted 77.2% of the lesions, metapodials 15.9% of the lesions, and proximal sesamoids 6.8% of the lesions. Within the digits, the highest prevalence of osteopathologies (54.4% of the lesions) was in the third phalanx (n = 37, with 19 lesions in the hind legs and 18 in the front legs), more than the second phalanx (n = 17; Chi-square = 7.407, P = 0.0091) or the first phalanx (n = 14; Chi-square = 10.373, P = 0.00177). There was no difference in osteopathologies prevalence between the first and second phalanges. The carpal and tarsal bones presented a wide variety of pathologies

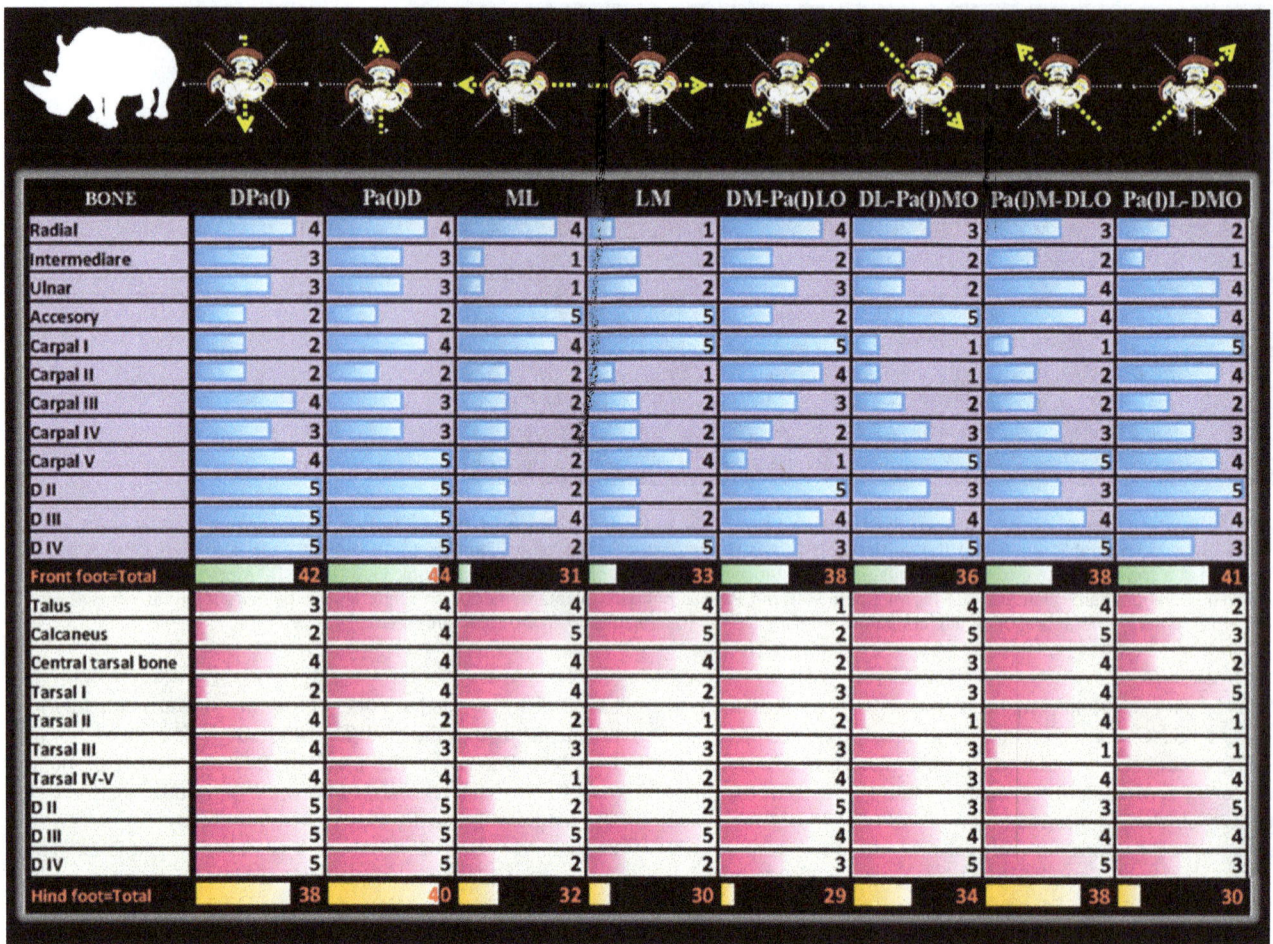

BONE	DPa(l)	Pa(l)D	ML	LM	DM-Pa(l)LO	DL-Pa(l)MO	Pa(l)M-DLO	Pa(l)L-DMO
Radial	4	4	4	1	4	3	3	2
Intermediare	3	3	1	2	2	2	2	1
Ulnar	3	3	1	2	3	2	4	4
Accesory	2	2	5	5	2	5	4	4
Carpal I	2	4	4	5	5	1	1	5
Carpal II	2	2	2	1	4	1	2	4
Carpal III	4	3	2	2	2	2	2	2
Carpal IV	3	3	2	2	2	3	3	3
Carpal V	4	5	2	4	1	5	5	4
D II	5	5	2	2	5	3	3	5
D III	5	5	4	2	2	4	4	4
D IV	5	5	2	5	3	5	5	3
Front foot=Total	42	44	31	33	38	36	38	41
Talus	3	4	4	4	1	4	4	2
Calcaneus	2	4	5	5	2	5	5	3
Central tarsal bone	4	4	4	4	2	3	4	2
Tarsal I	2	4	4	2	3	3	4	5
Tarsal II	4	2	2	1	2	1	4	1
Tarsal III	4	3	3	3	3	3	1	1
Tarsal IV-V	4	4	1	2	4	3	4	4
D II	5	5	2	2	5	3	3	5
D III	5	5	5	5	4	4	4	4
D IV	5	5	2	2	3	5	5	3
Hind foot=Total	38	40	32	30	29	34	38	30

Figure 4. One-criterion diagnostic value of traditional (45° and multiples of 45° projection angles) radiographic views. Radiographic diagnostic value per view was calculated by summation of the perceptible radiographic detail assessed with a 5-point rating scale for each autopodial bone of front and, respectively, hind feet in Southern white rhinoceros. Standard radiographic views are schematically represented on the top row. Abbreviations: digits II, III, IV [D II, D III, D IV]; views: dorso-palmar (plantar) [DPa(l)], palmaro (plantaro)-dorsal [Pa(l)D], medio-lateral [ML], latero-medial [LM], and four oblique projections: dorsomedial-palmaro (plantaro) lateral [DM-Pa(l)LO], dorsolateral-palmaro (plantaro) medial [DL-Pa(l)MO], palmaro (plantaro) medial-dorsolateral [Pa(l)M-DLO] and palmaro (plantaro) lateral-dorsomedial [Pa(l)L-DMO].

such as fractures, focal osteolysis, enthesiophytosis, osteophytosis, cortical osteogenesis, bone remodeling, and ankylosis.

Bone anatomy and pathology in digital radiographic imaging

Synchronized CT-DR depicted radiographic aspect of both normal anatomy (Fig. 9) and bone pathology (Fig. 10; Figs. S9-S13). Digital and conventional radiographic images gave clear information on numerous bone lesions as: specific fractures, ankylosis, osteolysis, extensive new bone proliferation, bone fragments or mineralized bodies, severe periosteal reaction, bone remodeling etc. Nevertheless, other lesions detected in CT images could not be depicted by digital or conventional radiographs (osseous fissure lines, small or subchondral bone fractures, fractures with a complicated 3D architecture, mild periosteal reaction, minor bone remodeling, and cortical sclerosis).

Discussion

Need for a novel approach in large wild animals' imaging

Computed tomography, as the golden standard for bone imaging [39,40,41], can be performed in very large animals merely on excerpts and only *post mortem* [19,42,43,44]. This *ex situ* examination encounters several challenges related to harvesting, storage and transportation procedures. The only *ante mortem*, *in situ* imaging technique available to date for veterinary clinicians working under field conditions is radiography. Due to difficulties in approaching non-domestic animals, and especially mega-vertebrates, many diagnostic procedures are simply not done, overlooked, or performed too late.

Chronic foot disease, a devastating disorder generally thought to be confined to soft tissues, is widely reported [32,45,46] and a subject of concern for many zoological gardens owing to its severe impact on animal's general health [47,48,49]. Bearing in mind that the future for some species might be only in captivity, the importance of eradicating chronic foot disease never became as important as in captive wild animals. Hitherto, clinicians lacked the diagnostic imaging tools, namely radiographic techniques and protocols, as well as reference documentation regarding radiographic interpretation of both normal anatomy and pathology. In our opinion, the assumption as if chronic foot disease is due to soft tissue issues and the scarcity of data on foot bone pathology [50,51,52,53] are due to lack of radiographic assessment. Therefore, recognizing the importance of looking at this area of

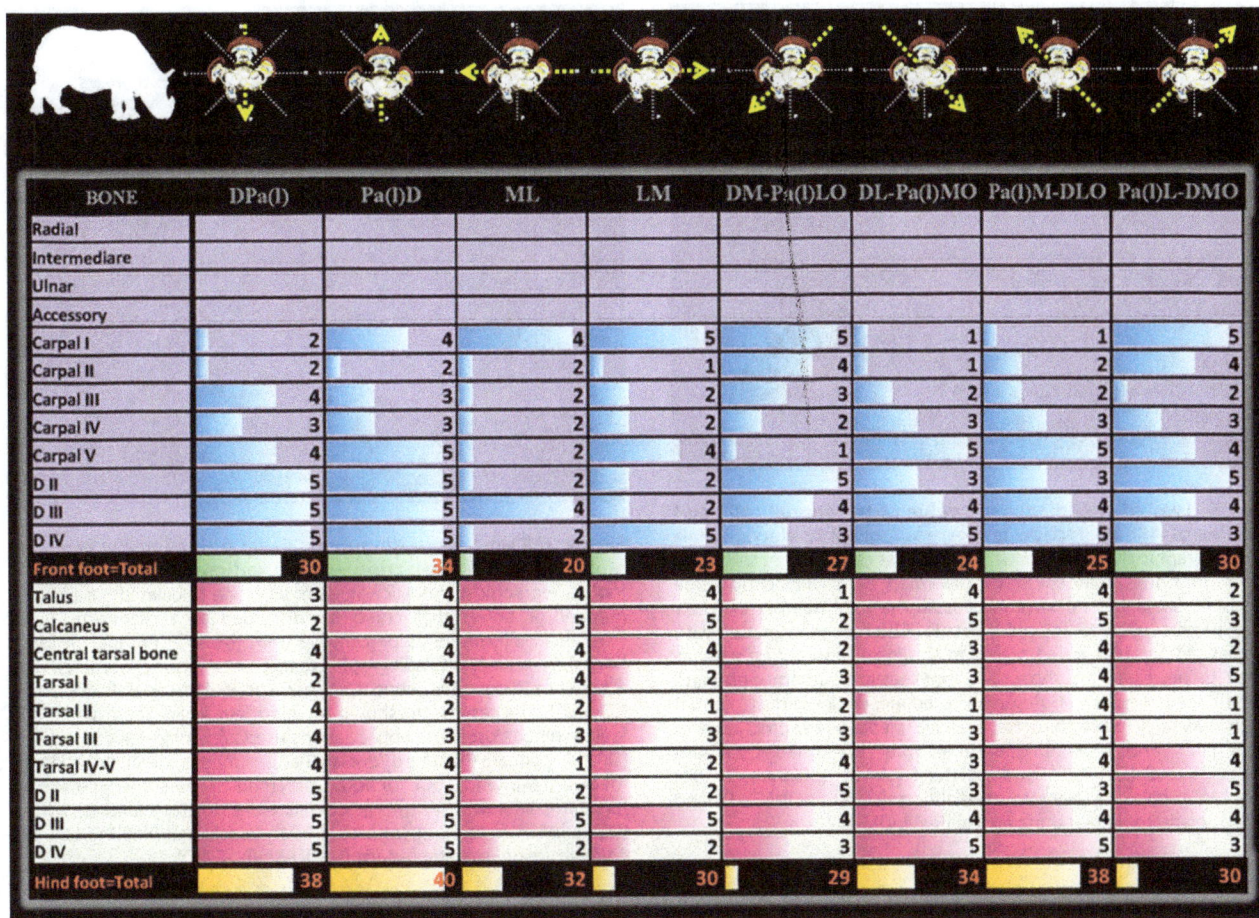

BONE	DPa(l)	Pa(l)D	ML	LM	DM-Pa(l)LO	DL-Pa(l)MO	Pa(l)M-DLO	Pa(l)L-DMO
Radial								
Intermediare								
Ulnar								
Accessory								
Carpal I	2	4	4	5	5	1	1	5
Carpal II	2	2	2	1	4	1	2	4
Carpal III	4	3	2	2	3	2	2	2
Carpal IV	3	3	2	2	2	3	3	3
Carpal V	4	5	2	4	1	5	5	4
D II	5	5	2	2	5	3	3	5
D III	5	5	4	2	4	4	4	4
D IV	5	5	2	5	3	5	5	3
Front foot=Total	30	34	20	23	27	24	25	30
Talus	3	4	4	4	1	4	4	2
Calcaneus	2	4	5	5	2	5	5	3
Central tarsal bone	4	4	4	4	2	3	4	2
Tarsal I	2	4	4	2	3	3	4	5
Tarsal II	4	2	2	1	2	1	4	1
Tarsal III	4	3	3	3	3	3	1	1
Tarsal IV-V	4	4	1	2	4	3	4	4
D II	5	5	2	2	5	3	3	5
D III	5	5	5	5	4	4	4	4
D IV	5	5	2	2	3	5	5	3
Hind foot=Total	38	40	32	30	29	34	38	30

Figure 5. One-criterion diagnostic value of traditional (45° and multiples of 45° projection angles) radiographic views. Radiographic diagnostic value per view was calculated by summation of the perceptible radiographic detail assessed with a 5-point rating scale for each autopodial bone of front and, respectively, hind feet in Indian rhinoceroses. Standard radiographic views are schematically represented on the top row. Abbreviations: digits II, III, IV [D II, D III, D IV]; views: dorso-palmar (plantar) [DPa(l)], palmaro (plantaro)-dorsal [Pa(l)D], medio-lateral [ML], latero-medial [LM], and four oblique projections: dorsomedial-palmaro (plantaro) lateral [DM-Pa(l)LO], dorsolateral-palmaro (plantaro) medial [DL-Pa(l)MO], palmaro (plantaro) medial-dorsolateral [Pa(l)M-DLO] and palmaro (plantaro) lateral-dorsomedial [Pa(l)L-DMO].

science anew, we confronted it from a different, non-invasive perspective: imaging diagnosis. To this end, a pioneering approach of synchronized computed tomography and digital radiography was instituted [54,55,56]. Reported technical impediments (scarce number of animals, positioning intricacy, etc) have been met with success and the knowledge achieved can be used as a valuable groundwork for future radiographic studies.

Tools offered by synchronized computed tomography and digital radiography

The main advantage of Synch CT- DR is its capability to provide a wide range of keystone data in wildlife imaging from a limited number of examined subjects. Additionally, it combines the advantages of CT as the golden standard method for bone diseases' diagnostic with DR's clinical feasibility under field conditions. Several advances were achieved from this pioneering approach, providing the wildlife clinician with all-important tools:

a) Prototype digital radiographic exposure protocols and a *modus operandi* for foot positioning, advancing both traditional projections and first-time, species-related radiographic views;

b) Radiographic diagnostic value for the whole foot and, in premiere, for each autopodial bone;

c) Additional insights into radiographic appearance of bone anatomy and pathology with a unique CT-DR correlation.

Reference radiographic techniques

It is indisputable that dissimilar radiographic techniques will lead to reporting inconsistency, and any comparison of the already scarce data will therefore be impossible. Conversely, use of a consistent technique will facilitate case consultations and comparative, inter-institutional imaging studies.

This study was designed to identify the relevant radiographic views and proper exposure parameters for accurate depiction of normal anatomy and pathological changes in the rhinoceros foot.

Several aspects must be taken into consideration, as follows. Hoof's preparation is of the utmost importance in eliminating several artifacts and producing radiographs of diagnostic quality [57]. Considering the uniqueness of each X-ray generator and detector combination, clinicians need to develop their own techniques for obtaining good radiographic quality [58]. Presented exposure charts are offered as reference. Adjustment of these techniques should be made, taking into consideration the animal's weight and size, foot's condition and the pathology involved (bone versus soft tissue). Bearing in mind the large size of the rhinoceros,

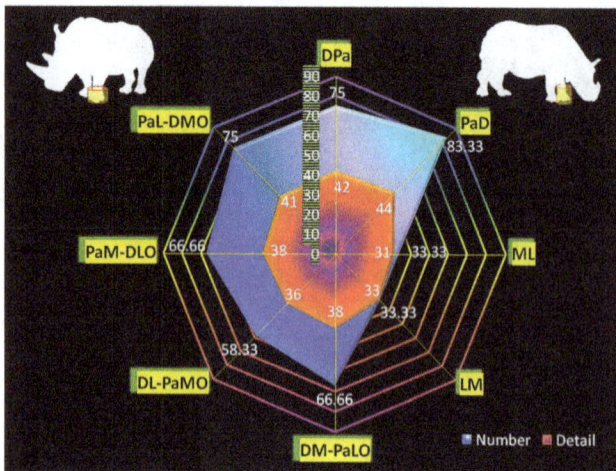

Figure 6. Two-criteria diagnostic value of traditional (45° and multiples of 45° projection angles) radiographic views. Whole foot radiographic diagnostic value per view was calculated based on: a) number of bones that could be discerned at a diagnostic value ("Number", presented as percentage from the total number of foot's bones); b) perceptible radiographic details of each bone estimated with a 5-point radiographic rating scale and summated for all foot's bones ("Detail"). The results are shown for front feet in Southern white and Indian rhinoceroses. The abbreviations used are: dorso-palmar (plantar) [DPa(l)], palmaro (plantaro)-dorsal [Pa(l)D], medio-lateral [ML], latero-medial [LM], and four oblique projections: dorsomedial-palmaro (plantaro) lateral [DM-Pa(l)LO], dorsolateral-palmaro (plantaro) medial [DL-Pa(l)MO], palmaro (plantaro) medial-dorsolateral [Pa(l)M-DLO] and palmaro (plantaro) lateral-dorsomedial [Pa(l)L-DMO].

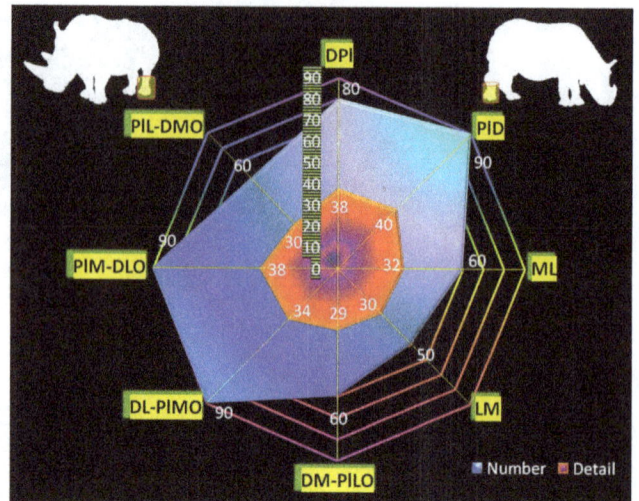

Figure 7. Two-criteria diagnostic value of traditional (45° and multiples of 45° projection angles) radiographic views. Whole foot radiographic diagnostic value per view was calculated based on: a) number of bones that could be discerned at a diagnostic value ("Number", presented as percentage from the total number of foot's bones); b) perceptible radiographic details of each bone estimated with a 5-point radiographic rating scale and summated for all foot's bones ("Detail"). The results are shown for hind feet in Southern white and Indian rhinoceroses. The abbreviations used are: dorso-palmar (plantar) [DPa(l)], palmaro (plantaro)-dorsal [Pa(l)D], medio-lateral [ML], latero-medial [LM], and four oblique projections: dorsomedial-palmaro (plantaro) lateral [DM-Pa(l)LO], dorsolateral-palmaro (plantaro) medial [DL-Pa(l)MO], palmaro (plantaro) medial-dorsolateral [Pa(l)M-DLO] and palmaro (plantaro) lateral-dorsomedial [Pa(l)L-DMO].

positioning for various studies should be performed by rotating a portable radiographic unit (X-ray beam) and the image plate at required angles corresponding to each projection. Beam-plate angles of 90° were used, but other angles should be investigated because they may reveal more appropriate projections, as it was found in horses [59,60] and, very recently, in elephants [61]. Projection angles of 45° between different radiographic views will give detailed foot evaluation. Nevertheless, this study showed that species dependent anatomical variations must be taken into account. Due to rhinoceros' special foot anatomy, traditional positioning using, as accurate landmarks, specific anatomical structures could not be applied. Distinctive features responsible for difficulty in visualization and palpation of any anatomical landmark include: considerable skin thickness, distal leg's bulk and cylindrical shape, massive central foot pad, digits' largest part (metapodials and first phalanges) included into compact soft tissue mass and, especially, the asymmetric arrangement of the medial and lateral digits in the front foot. Therefore, foot positioning was performed taking as reference line the dorsal aspect of the mid-sagittal plane (perpendicular on and passing through the middle of the third digit). The central (third digit) toenail was used as anatomical landmark. New radiographic views were established for a better visualization of the rhinoceros' digits while avoiding or minimizing superimposition of the large sesamoids on the metapodial and phalangeal elements. Distinctive anatomy of rhinoceros' front foot, with medial metacarpus (Mc II) being rotated inwardly along its vertical axis and positioned more palmary in comparison with the central metacarpal bone (Mc III), accounted for the differences encountered on projection angles between front and hind legs.

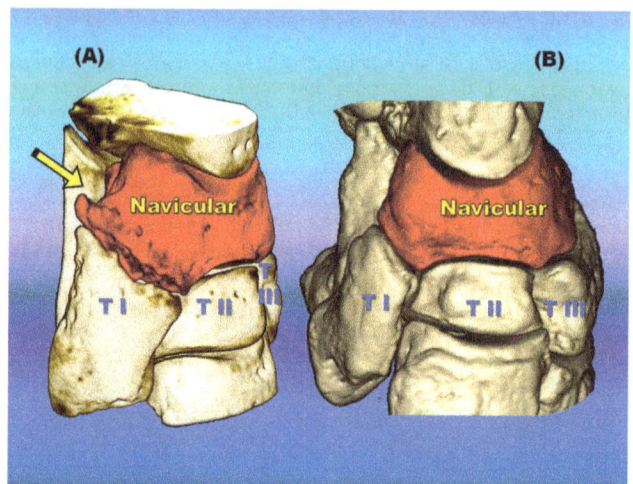

Figure 8. Left navicular (central tarsal bone, CTB) comparative imaging in two Southern white rhinoceroses. Tri-dimensional computed tomographic (3D CT) images of CTB allowed comparison of multiple bone pathologies (A) in rhinoceros 1 with normal anatomical aspect (B) in rhinoceros 2. Encountered osteopathologies are: cortical osteogenesis represented by massive, unstructured new bone production and remodelling, with a beak-like formation oriented plantaro-medially (arrow). Additionally (A), the articular surface between CTB and first tarsal bone (TI) is highly irregular, characterized by decreased joint space width and articular bone proliferation that bridges the contiguous bones (ankylosis). The second (TII) and the third (TIII) tarsal bones are within normal limits on both rhinoceroses (A, B).

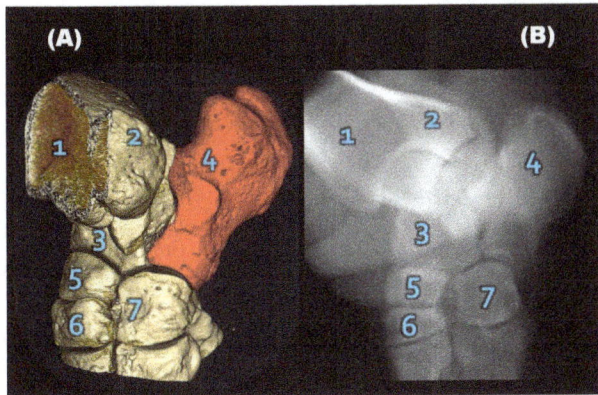

Figure 9. Tarsal normal anatomy depicted in Southern white rhinoceros 2 left hind foot by (A) computed tomography (CT) and (B) synchronized digital radiography (Synch DR). This projection (B) allows the best visualization of calcaneus (highlighted on CT image A) with minimal superimposition of other bony elements. The abbreviations used are: 1-tibia, 2- fibula, 3- talus, 4- calcaneus, 5-navicular, 6-tarsal III, and 7- tarsal IV bones.

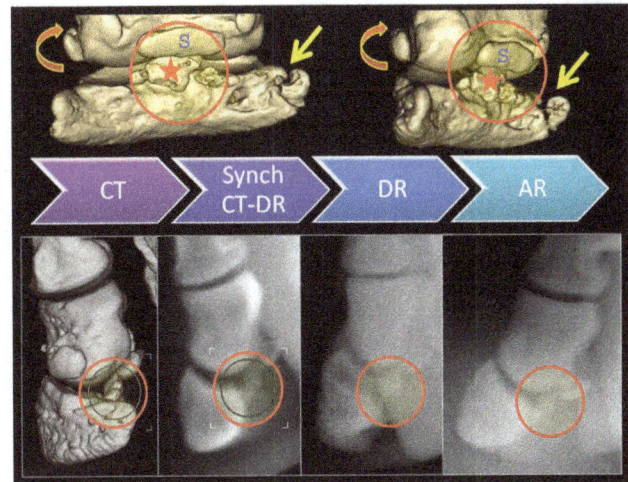

Figure 10. Multi-modality imaging diagnosis of bone pathology in Indian rhinoceros 1. Fractured bony fragments (circle and star) of the distal phalanx of the left front central digit are imaged ventral to the central small sesamoid (S) by means of: analog radiography (AR), digital radiography (DR), computed tomography (CT), and synchronized CT-DR (Synch CT-DR). Uppermost CT images reveal additional osteopathologies: the second phalanx - dorso-lateral fracture with a displaced fragment (curved arrow); the third phalanx - complete fracture of the medial palmar process (*processus palmaris medialis*, straight arrow).

Radiographic diagnostic value

Unlike articulations between long bones, carpal and tarsal joints are considerably polyostotic, with complex 3D general architecture and complicated, multi-facet bone geometry. For these reasons, an accurate evaluation of these joints requires multiple radiographic views. Most commonly, eight radiographs per foot, with four orthogonal and four oblique projections are insufficient for reliable podial assessment, frequently necessitating additional views: hyperflexion, hyperextension, adduction, abduction, skyviews etc. Unlike their domestic relatives, these all-inclusive standard procedures are difficult to perform in wild animals due to the need for sedation or anesthesia, and temporal and positioning intricacies. Thus, the clinician will benefit from an exhaustive knowledge of the diagnostic potential of each radiographic view, making possible the establishment of high-priority views to start with. The present study endows with data on diagnostic value of each radiographic projection, in general, and for each autopodial bone in particular (excepting first carpal row in Indian rhinoceroses, not included). A comparative study of segregated first row carpal bones revealed minimal morphologic differences between Southern white and Indian rhinoceroses. Therefore, the radiographic diagnostic values were extrapolated from Southern white to Indian rhinoceroses for radial, intermediary, ulnar and accessory carpal bones.

Multi-modality comparative imaging study

The results of our study indicate that bone lesions were present in both Indian and Southern white rhinoceros species. Reported bone pathology comprises a wide spectrum of lesions affecting a large number of autopodial bones. It was encountered in rhinoceroses with soft tissue tumour or with known chronic foot disease (rhinoceroses 1, 3) and, most surprisingly, in a Southern white rhinoceros (rhinoceros 2) and an Indian rhinoceros (rhinoceros 4) that showed no discernible clinical signs of foot afflictions. Possible origins, prevalence and distribution of foot bone pathology were discussed previously [30].

This study allowed a comparison of radiographic findings obtained with CT, DR and AR. Despite superimposition of a 3D structure (bones) on a 2D plane [39], conventional and digital radiography are sensitive in depiction of different bone patholo-

gies. Above all, one result is worth specific mentioning: the conventional radiographs were able to depict excellent bone details, regardless of being manually developed. Nevertheless, minor lesions (numerous in rhinoceros 4) or even more extensive lesions surrounded by multiple bones could not be depicted. These findings are in concordance with previous published data in horses [40,41,62,63], reinforcing the conclusion that CT is very useful for diagnosis of subtle bone lesions when radiography remains inconclusive [64], yet in rhinoceroses, being applied only *post mortem*.

Conclusions

Far from being a wild dream, imaging in wild animals has been advancing in fits comprehending that improved knowledge of radiologic diagnosis is important for animals' welfare. Our study makes known by what means synchronized computed tomography- digital radiography provides manifold diagnostic tools, a novel perspective and major advances in wildlife's diagnostic imaging.

Putting all together, it is highly recommended that foot radiographic examination became a standard diagnostic technique and, ideally, also a periodic monitoring tool in captive wild animals. Radiographic investigations counted as highly diagnostic and non-invasive procedures should be relied upon when developing the most appropriate wildlife management and conservation strategies.

Supporting Information

Figure S1 Additional radiographic exposure chart for front and hind feet in both Southern white and Indian rhinoceroses. On the horizontal axis are the eight radiographic views and the vertical axis shows the exposure values of: milliampere (mA), kilovolt peak (kVp) and time (s) for each projection at a constant source-to-film or focus-to-film distance

(FFD) of 100 cm. Standard radiographic views were: DP [dorso-palmar (plantar)], DM-PL [dorsomedial-palmaro (plantaro) lateral], ML [medio-lateral], PM-DL [palmaro (plantaro) medial-dorsolateral], PD [palmaro (plantaro)-dorsal], PL-DM [palmaro (plantaro) lateral-dorsomedial]; LM [latero-medial], DL-PM [dorsolateral-palmaro (plantaro) medial].

Figure S2 Dorso-palmar (DP) orthogonal view performed at a projection angle of 0° from the dorsal mid-plane (arrow). Positioning technique is demonstrated on three-dimensional computed tomographic (3D CT) images of Indian rhinoceros 3 right front foot (right side image) and schematically represented using a cross-sectional CT image (left side image). Semi-transparent 3D CT imaging protocol was employed to show both foot's exterior aspect and the underlying bony structures.

Figure S3 Medio-lateral (ML) 80° view performed at a projection angle of 80° from the dorsal mid-plane (arrow) allows a better visualization of all digits than the traditional ML 90° orthogonal view. Positioning technique is demonstrated on three-dimensional computed tomographic (3D CT) images of Indian rhinoceros 3 right front foot (right side image) and schematically represented using a cross-sectional CT image (left side image). Semi-transparent 3D CT imaging protocol was employed to show both foot's exterior aspect and the underlying bony structures.

Figure S4 Palmaromedial-dorsolateral (PMDL) 150° oblique view performed at a projection angle of 150° from the dorsal mid-plane (arrow) allows a better visualization of all digits than the traditional PMDL 135° oblique view. Positioning technique is demonstrated on three-dimensional computed tomographic (3D CT) images of Indian rhinoceros 3 right front foot (right side image) and schematically represented using a cross-sectional CT image (left side image). Semi-transparent 3D CT imaging protocol was employed to show both foot's exterior aspect and the underlying bony structures.

Figure S5 Palmaro-dorsal (PD) 180° orthogonal view performed at a projection angle of 180° from the dorsal mid-plane (arrow) is identical with the traditional DMPL 180° orthogonal view. Positioning technique is demonstrated on three-dimensional computed tomographic (3D CT) images of Indian rhinoceros 3 right front foot (right side image) and schematically represented using a cross-sectional CT image (left side image). Semi-transparent 3D CT imaging protocol was employed to show both foot's exterior aspect and the underlying bony structures.

Figure S6 Palmarolateral-dorsomedial (PLDM) 200° oblique view performed at a projection angle of 200° from the dorsal mid-plane (arrow) allows a better visualization of all digits than the traditional PLDM 225° oblique view. Positioning technique is demonstrated on three-dimensional computed tomographic (3D CT) images of Indian rhinoceros 3 right front foot (right side image) and schematically represented using a cross-sectional CT image (left side image). Semi-transparent 3D CT imaging protocol was employed to show both foot's exterior aspect and the underlying bony structures.

Figure S7 Latero-medial (LM) 270° orthogonal view performed at a projection angle of 270° from the dorsal mid-plane (arrow) is identical with the traditional LM 270° orthogonal view. Positioning technique is demonstrated on three-dimensional computed tomographic (3D CT) images of Indian rhinoceros 3 right front foot (right side image) and schematically represented using a cross-sectional CT image (left side image). Semi-transparent 3D CT imaging protocol was employed to show both foot's exterior aspect and the underlying bony structures.

Figure S8 Dorsolateral-palmaromedial (DLPM) 330° oblique view performed at a projection angle of 330° from the dorsal mid-plane (arrow) allows a better visualization of all digits than the traditional DLPM 315° oblique view. Positioning technique is demonstrated on three-dimensional computed tomographic (3D CT) images of Indian rhinoceros 3 right front foot (right side image) and schematically represented using a cross-sectional CT image (left side image). Semi-transparent 3D CT imaging protocol was employed to show both foot's exterior aspect and the underlying bony structures.

Figure S9 Osteolysis and bone rarefaction (circle) in rhinoceros 2 left front foot on the distal metacarpal bone and first phalanx of the second (medial) digit. These pathologies are visualized by synchronized computed tomography (A) and digital radiography (B).

Figure S10 Proliferative new bone formation and bone remodeling anatomy (circle) depicted in Southern white rhinoceros 2 right front foot-palmar aspect (P) by (A) computed tomography (CT) and (B) synchronized digital radiography (Synch DR).

Figure S11 Intra-articular bony fragment showed in (A) computed tomography (CT) and (B) synchronized digital radiography (Synch DR) of Indian rhinoceros 1 left front foot. This bony fragment (circle) has smooth margins and is situated on the lateral aspect of the central digit between the metacarpus and the first phalanx.

Figure S12 Bone pathology (circle) demonstrated in left tarsal joint in rhinoceros 1 by means of (A) synchronized digital radiography (Synch DR) and (B) computed tomography (CT). Left central tarsal bone (CTB) fractures are concealed by new bone production and, therefore, undetectable on three-dimensional CT images, but visible on Synch DR images. At the level of these fractures, CTB distalo-medial aspect reveals a mixed pattern of trabecular focal bone loss (osteolysis) and cortical osteogenesis represented by massive, unstructured new bone production and remodeling, with a beak-like formation oriented plantaro-medially, hook-shaped (circle). Additionally, the articular surface between CTB and first tarsal bone (TI) is highly irregular, characterized by decreased joint space width, articular bone proliferation that bridges the contiguous bones (ankylosis), erosion and lysis of the articular cartilage and underlying bone (asterisk).

Figure S13 Periosteal proliferation demonstrated in rhinoceros 1 left hind foot, on the lateral aspect of the second metatarsal bone (circle) by (A) computed tomog-

raphy (CT) and (B) synchronized digital radiography (Synch DR).

Acknowledgments

The authors are grateful for the support granted by the staff of the Parc Zoologique d'Amnéville, Parc Zoologique de La Barben and ZooParc de Beauval, all in France and of the Jardim Zoológico de Lisboa, Portugal.

Author Contributions

Conceived and designed the experiments: GG RH JS FG JM TBH. Performed the experiments: GG JM RP BM. Analyzed the data: GG JS TBH FG JM RH. Contributed reagents/materials/analysis tools: AM PE RP BM RB TF. Wrote the paper: GG JS RH TBH. Critically reviewed and commented on the manuscript: FG AM PE RP BM RB TF JM.

References

1. Kaulfers C, Geburek F, Feige K, Knieriem A (2010) Radiographic imaging and possible causes of a carpal varus deformity in an Asian elephant (*Elephas maximus*). Journal of Zoo and Wildlife Medicine 41: 697–702.

2. Hittmair KM, Vielgrader HD (2000) Radiographic diagnosis of lameness in African elephants (*Loxodonta africana*). Veterinary Radiology & Ultrasound 41: 511–515.

3. Siegal-Willott J, Isaza R, Johnson R, Blaik M (2008) Distal limb radiography, ossification, and growth plate closure in the juvenile Asian elephant (*Elephas maximus*). Journal of Zoo and Wildlife Medicine 39: 320–334.

4. Gage LJ, Fowler ME, Pascoe JR, Blasko D (1997) Surgical removal of infected phalanges from an Asian elephant (*Elephas maximus*). Journal of Zoo and Wildlife Medicine 28: 208–211.

5. Honnas CM, O'Brien TR, Linford RL (1988) Distal phalanx fractures in horses. Veterinary Radiology 29: 98–107.

6. Kaser-Hotz B, Ueltschi G (1992) Radiographic appearance of the navicular bone in sound horses. Veterinary Radiology & Ultrasound 33: 9–17.

7. Eksell P, Uhlhorn H, Carlsten J (1999) Evaluation of different projections for radiographic detection of tarsal degenerative joint disease in icelandic horses. Veterinary Radiology & Ultrasound 40: 228–232.

8. Hampson BA, de Laat MA, Mills PC, Walsh DM, Pollitt CC (2013) The feral horse foot. Part B: radiographic, gross visual and histopathological parameters of foot health in 100 Australian feral horses. Australian Veterinary Journal 91: 23–30.

9. Wobeser GA (1994) Investigation and Management of Disease in Wild Animals. New York: Plenum Press. 265 p.

10. Zuba JR (2012) Hoof disorders in nondomestic artiodactylids. In: Fowler ME, Miller RE, editors. Zoo and Wild Animal Medicine, Current Therapy. St. Louis, Missouri: Elsevier Saunders. pp. 619–627.

11. Fowler ME (2006) Physical restraint and handling. In: Fowler ME, Mikota SK, editors. Biology, Medicine, and Surgery of Elephants. Ames, IA, USA: Blackwell Publishing. pp. 75–90.

12. Raath JP (1999) Anesthesia of white rhinoceroses. In: Fowler ME, Miller RE, editors. Zoo and Wild Animal Medicine, Current Therapy. St. Louis, Missouri: W. B. Saunders Company. pp. 556–561.

13. Ebedes H, Raath JP (1999) Use of tranquilizers in wild herbivores. In: Fowler ME, Miller RE, editors. Zoo and Wild Animal Medicine, Current Therapy. St.Louis, Missouri: W. B. Saunders Company. pp. 575–585.

14. Fowler ME (2010) Restraint and Handling of Wild and Domestic Animals. 3rd ed. Ames. IA, USA: Wiley-Blackwell. pp. 343–354.

15. Adelman JS, Martin LB (2009) Vertebrate sickness behaviors: Adaptive and integrated neuroendocrine immune responses. Integrative and Comparative Biology 49: 202–214.

16. Hart BL (2011) Behavioural defences in animals against pathogens and parasites: parallels with the pillars of medicine in humans. Philosophical Transactions of the Royal Society B: Biological Sciences 366: 3406–3417.

17. Farrow CS (2009) Veterinary Diagnostic Imaging: Birds, Exotic Pets and Wildlife. 1st ed. Maryland Heights, MO, USA: Mosby, Inc. pp. 346–359.

18. Siegal-Willott JL, Alexander A, Isaza R (2012) Digital Radiography of the Elephant Foot. In: Fowler ME, Miller RE, editors. Zoo and Wild Animal Medicine, Current Therapy. St. Louis, Missouri: Elsevier Saunders. pp. 515–523.

19. Gage L (2006) Radiology. In: Fowler ME, Mikota SK, editors. Biology, Medicine, and Surgery of Elephants.Ames, IA, USA: Blackwell Publishing. pp. 192–197.

20. Emslie R (2012) *Ceratotherium simum*. In: IUCN 2012. IUCN Red List of Threatened Species. Version 2012.2

21. Emslie R (2012) *Diceros bicornis*. In: IUCN 2012. IUCN Red List of Threatened Species. Version 2012.2

22. van Strien NJ, Manullang B, Sectionov IW, Khan MKM, Sumardja E, et al. (2008) *Dicerorhinus sumatrensis*. In: IUCN 2012. IUCN Red List of Threatened Species. Version 2012.2

23. van Strien NJ, Steinmetz R, Manullang B, Sectionov IW, Han KH, et al. (2008) *Rhinoceros sondaicus*. In: IUCN 2012. IUCN Red List of Threatened Species. Version 2012.2

24. Rookmaaker LC (1998) The Rhinoceros in Captivity. The Hague, The Netherland: SPB Academic Publishing bv. 115 p.

25. Versteege L (2012) 2011 European Studbook White Rhino (*Ceratotherium Simum*). Hilvarenbeek, The Netherland: Safaripark Beekse Bergen. 194 p.

26. von Houwald F, Pagan O (2012) Greater One-Horned or Indian Rhinoceros *Rhinoceros unicornis* Linné 1758, International Studbook 2011. Basel, Switzerland: Basel Zoo. 63 p.

27. Kock RA, Garnier J (1993) Veterinary management of three species of rhinoceroses in zoological collections In: Ryder OA, editor. Rhinoceros Biology and Conservation: Proceedings of an International Conference. San Diego, CA: San Diego Zoological Society. pp. 325–345.

28. Talukdar BK, Emslie R, Bist SS, Choudhury A, Ellis S, et al. (2008) *Rhinoceros unicornis*. In: IUCN 2012. IUCN Red List of Threatened Species. Version 2012.2

29. Biddle R, Pilgrim M (2012) Eastern Black rhino EEP *Diceros bicornis michaeli*, European Studbook 2011. Chester, UK: Chester Zoo. 36 p.

30. Galateanu G, Hildebrandt TB, Maillot A, Etienne P, Potier R, et al. (2013) One small step for rhinos, one giant leap for wildlife management- imaging diagnosis of bone pathology in distal limb. PLoS One 8: e68493.

31. Schmitt DL (2003) Proboscidea (Elephants). In: Fowler ME, Miller RE, editors. Zoo and Wild Animal Medicine. St. Louis, MO: Saunders. pp. 541–549.

32. Miller RE (2003) Rhinoceridae (Rhinoceroses). In: Fowler ME, Miller RE, editors. Zoo and Wild Animal Medicine. St. Louis, MO: Saunders. pp. 558–569.

33. Galateanu G, Hermes R, Göritz F, Szentiks CA, Wibbelt G, et al. (2013) An extensive study: Diagnostic imaging of normal anatomy and pathology in hoofed mammal's distal limb; 2013 8–11 May, 2013; Vienna, Austria. pp. 26 (Abstract).

34. Gage LJ (1999) Radiographic techniques for the elephant foot and carpus. In: Fowler ME, Miller RE, editors. Zoo and Wild Animal Medicine, Current Therapy. St. Louis, Missouri: W. B. Saunders Company. pp. 517–520.

35. Atkinson MW (2006) Megavertebrates. In: Bear CK, editor. Guidelines for the Euthanasia of Nondomestic Animals. Yulee, FL, USA: Amerian Association of Zoo Veterinarians. pp. 89–93.

36. Liem KF, Bemis WE, Walker Jr WF, Grande L (2001) Functional Anatomy of the Vertebrates: An Evolutionary Perspective. Belmont, CA: Thomason Brooks/Cole. 703 p.

37. Shively MJ (1988) Synonym equivalence among names used for oblique radiographic views of distal limbs. Veterinary Radiology 29: 282–284.

38. Smallwood JE, Shively MJ, Rendano VT, Habel RE (1985) A standardized nomenclature for radiographic projections used in veterinary medicine. Veterinary Radiology 26: 2–9.

39. Seeram E (2009) Computed Tomography: Physical Principles, Clinical Applications, and Quality Control. St. Louis, MI, USA: Saunders Elsevier. 536 p.

40. Bergman H-J, Saunders J (2011) Equine fractures. In: Schwarz T, Saunders J, editors. Veterinary Computed Tomography. Chichester, UK: Wiley-Blackwell. pp. 457–462.

41. Bergman H-J, Saunders J (2011) Equine upper limbs (carpus, tarsus, stifle). In: Schwarz T, Saunders J, editors. Veterinary Computed Tomography. Chichester, UK: Wiley-Blackwell. pp. 483–501.

42. Hutchinson JR, Delmer C, Miller CE, Hildebrandt T, Pitsillides AA, et al. (2011) From flat foot to fat foot: Structure, ontogeny, function, and evolution of elephant "sixth toes". Science 334: 1699–1703.

43. Hutchinson JR, Miller C, Fritsch G, Hildebrandt T (2008) The Anatomical Foundation for Multidisciplinary Studies of Animal Limb Function: Examples from Dinosaur and Elephant Limb Imaging Studies. In: Endo H, Frey R, editors. Anatomical Imaging, Towards a New Morphology. Tokyo: Springer. pp. 23–38.

44. Galateanu G, Göritz F, Szentiks CA, Hildebrandt TB (2013) Diagnostic imaging of normal anatomy and pathology in giraffe's distal limb; 2013 8–11 May, 2013; Vienna, Austria. pp. 127.

45. Strauss G, Seidel B (1982) Pododermatis purulenta beim Panzernashorn (*Rhinoceros unicornis*) - ein Fallbericht. Internationalen Symposiums über die Erkrankungen der Zootiere 24. Veszprém, Hungary: Akademie Verlag. pp. 177–181.

46. von Houwald FF (2001) Foot problems in Indian Rhinoceroses (*Rhinoceros unicornis*) in zoological gardens: Macroscopic and microscopic anatomy, pathology, and evaluation of the causes [Doctorate]. Zurich: Universität Zürich. 104 p.

47. Roocroft A, Oosterhuis J (2001) Foot care for captive elephants. In: Csuti B, Sargent EL, Bechert US, editors. The Elephant's Foot: Prevention and Care of Foot Conditions in Captive Asian and African Elephants. : Iowa State University Press. pp. 21–52.

48. Fowler ME (2006) Foot Disorders. In: Fowler ME, Mikota SK, editors. Biology, Medicine, and Surgery of Elephants. Ames, IA: Blackwell Publishing. pp. 271–290.

49. West G (2006) Musculoskeletal System. In: Fowler ME, Mikota SK, editors. Biology, Medicine, and Surgery of Elephants. Ames, IA: Blackwell Publishing. pp. 263–270.

50. Greer M, Greer JK, Gillingham J (1977) Osteorathritis in selected wild mammals. Proceedings of the Oklahoma Academy of Sciences 57: 39–43.

51. Wallach JD (1967) Degenerative arthritis in a black rhinoceros. Journal of the American Veterinary Medical Association 151: 887–889.

52. Flach EJ, Walsh TC, Dodds J, White A, Crowe OM (2003) Treatment of osteomyelitis in a greater one-horned rhinoceros (*Rhinoceros unicornis*); 28 May - 01 June; Rome, Italy. pp. 1–7.

53. Harrison TM, Stanley BJ, Sikarskie JG, Bohart G, Ames NK, et al. (2011) Surgical amputation of a digit and vacuum-assisted-closure (V.A.C.) management in a case of osteomyelitis and wound care in an Eastern black rhinoceros (*Diceros bicornis michaeli*). Journal of Zoo and Wildlife Medicine 42: 317–321.

54. Galateanu G, Hildebrandt TB, Maillot A, Godefroy A, Hermes R (2012) Rhinoceros feet make the first step: A synchronized computed tomography and digital radiography; 2012 16–19 May, 2012; Bussolengo, Italy. pp. 142.

55. Galateanu G, Potier R, Hildebrandt TB, Maillot A, Godefroy A, et al. (2012) Rhinoceros foot step out of a rule-of-thumb: A synchronized computed tomography and digital radiography; 2012 26–31 August, 2012; Bursa, Turkey. pp. 40.

56. Galateanu G, Hildebrandt TB, Hermes R (2013) New clinical tools in rhinoceroses' management: imaging diagnosis applying synchronized computed tomography and digital radiography; 2013 8–11 May, 2013; Vienna, Austria. pp. 128.

57. Starrak GS (1996) Radiology corner equine foot radiography—hoof preparation. Veterinary Radiology & Ultrasound 37: 116–117.

58. Kirberger RM (1999) Rradiograph quality evaluation for exposure variables—a review. Veterinary Radiology & Ultrasound 40: 220–226.

59. Uhlhorn H, Ekman S, Haglund A, Carlsten J (1998) The accuracy of the dorsoproximal-dorsodistal projection in assessing third carpal bone sclerosis in standardbred trotters. Veterinary Radiology & Ultrasound 39: 412–417.

60. Uhlhorn H, Eksell P (1999) The dorsoproximal-dorsodistal projection of the distal carpal bones in horses: An evaluation of different beam-cassette angles. Veterinary Radiology & Ultrasound 40: 480–485.

61. Mumby C, Bouts T, Sambrook L, Danika S, Rees E, et al. (2013) Validation of a new radiographic protocol for Asian elephant feet and description of their radiographic anatomy. Veterinary Record In Press.

62. Rose PL, Seeherman H, O'Callaghan M (1997) Computed tomographic evaluation of comminuted middle phalangeal fractures in the horse. Veterinary Radiology & Ultrasound 38: 424–429.

63. Peterson PR, Bowman KF (1988) Computed tomographic anatomy of the distal extremity of the horse. Veterinary Radiology 29: 147–156.

64. Ruohoniemi M, Tervahartiala P (1999) Computed tomographic evaluation of finnhorse cadaver forefeet with radiographically problematic findings on the flexor aspect of the navicular bone. Veterinary Radiology & Ultrasound 40: 275–281.

12

Hospital and Community Ampicillin-Resistant *Enterococcus faecium* Are Evolutionarily Closely Linked but Have Diversified through Niche Adaptation

Marieke J. A. de Regt[1]*, Willem van Schaik[1], Miranda van Luit-Asbroek[1], Huberta A. T. Dekker[1], Engeline van Duijkeren[2], Catherina J. M. Koning[3], Marc J. M. Bonten[1], Rob J. L. Willems[1]

1 Department of Medical Microbiology, University Medical Center Utrecht, Utrecht, the Netherlands, 2 Department of Infectious Diseases and Immunology, Faculty of Veterinary Medicine, Utrecht University, Utrecht, the Netherlands, 3 Department of Internal Medicine, University Hospital Maastricht, Maastricht, the Netherlands

Abstract

Background: Ampicillin-resistant *Enterococcus faecium* (ARE) has emerged as a nosocomial pathogen. Here, we quantified ARE carriage in different community sources and determined genetic relatedness with hospital ARE.

Methods and Results: ARE was recovered from rectal swabs of 24 of 79 (30%) dogs, 11 of 85 (13%) cats and 0 of 42 horses and from 3 of 40 (8%) faecal samples of non-hospitalized humans receiving amoxicillin. Multi-locus Sequence Typing revealed 21 sequence types (STs), including 5 STs frequently associated with hospital-acquired infections. Genes previously found to be enriched in hospital ARE, such as IS16, orf903, orf905, orf907, were highly prevalent in community ARE (≥79%), while genes with a proposed role in pathogenesis, such as *esp*, *hyl* and *ecbA*, were found rarely (≤5%) in community isolates. Comparative genome analysis of 2 representative dog isolates revealed that the dog strain of ST192 was evolutionarily closely linked to two previously sequenced hospital ARE, but had, based on gene content, more genes in common with the other, evolutionarily more distantly related, dog strain (ST266).

Conclusion: ARE were detected in dogs, cats and sporadically in healthy humans, with evolutionary linkage to hospital ARE. Yet, their accessory genome has diversified, probably as a result of niche adaptation.

Editor: Niyaz Ahmed, University of Hyderabad, India

Funding: Willem van Schaik was funded through the Nederlandse Organisatie voor Wetenschappelijk Onderzoek [NWO-VENI grant 916.86.044]. The funders had no role in study design, data collection and analysis, decision to publish, or preparation of the manuscript.

Competing Interests: The authors have declared that no competing interests exist.

* E-mail: mjaderegt@gmail.com

Introduction

Enterococcus faecium is a common inhabitant of the gastrointestinal tract of humans and animals, frequently causing opportunistic infections in critically ill patients. During the 1980s, the incidence of infections caused by ampicillin-resistant *E. faecium* (ARE) rapidly increased in the U.S., followed by an epidemic rise of vancomycin-resistant *E. faecium* (VRE) in the 1990s [1–2]. Nowadays, more than 90% of *E. faecium* recovered from healthcare associated infections in the U.S. are ampicillin-resistant and 80% are vancomycin-resistant [3]. In Europe, the majority of nosocomial invasive *E. faecium* isolates are resistant to ampicillin and VRE infection rates are increasing in several countries [4].

Molecular epidemiological studies based on Multi-locus Sequence Typing (MLST) revealed that the vast majority of *E. faecium* isolates causing clinical infections and nosocomial outbreaks belong to a globally dispersed polyclonal subpopulation, genotypically different from *E. faecium* strains colonizing healthy humans and animals in the community [5]. These so-called hospital *E. faecium* strains, which have been collectively termed Clonal Complex 17 (CC17), are characterized by ampicillin and ciprofloxacin resistance and are specifically enriched with over one

hundred genes, including genes encoding for antibiotic resistance and factors with a putative role in colonization and/or virulence [5–8]. Recent studies have indicated that isolates from CC17 are not strictly clonally related and that there is considerable genetic diversity among these isolates indicating that they most probably do not constitute a single clonal complex [9].

Until recently, ARE were recovered only sporadically from animals and humans outside the nosocomial environment [10–11], rendering resistance against ampicillin a highly specific marker for the hospital *E. faecium* subpopulation. Yet, colonization with *E. faecium* resistant to ampicillin was recently reported among Danish and English dogs [12]. In this report, 76% of the colonized dogs carried ARE isolates with sequence types (STs) that are among the most common ARE lineages causing nosocomial infections. The observed overlap in prevailing STs between dog and infectious ARE isolates, raises the important question whether dogs, and perhaps also other community sources, may serve as a reservoir for ARE colonization and infections in hospitalized patients.

In this study, we extended the search for potential community ARE resources by screening domestic animals including dogs, cats and horses for ARE carriage. In addition, we have tested faecal samples from human volunteers, after exposure to selective antibiotic pressure, for ARE. Recovered community ARE were compared to the known hospital ARE reservoir by MLST, and by performing genetic and phenotypic assays examining antimicrobial susceptibility, ampicillin resistance mechanisms and the presence of genes putatively involved in virulence and/or colonization. Finally, two representative canine ARE isolates were selected for high-quality draft whole genome sequencing allowing a comparative genome analysis with previously sequenced *E. faecium* strains from human origin.

Materials and Methods

Samples

To study the occurrence of ARE colonization in non-clinical settings, samples were collected from different Dutch community sources. Rectal swabs were taken from 79 dogs from different regions of the Netherlands and from 42 horses from various stables in the province of Utrecht. In cats, the prevalence of ARE colonization was investigated by taking a swab from faecal samples of 85 cats that were sent to the Utrecht University Faculty of Veterinary Medicine for clinical evaluation for various reasons. Since the animal sampling in this study was minimally invasive and not incriminating nor harmful for the participating animals, ethical approval was not deemed necessary. Yet, all owners, gave verbal informed consent for sampling their pets. In addition, faecal samples from 40 healthy human volunteers, collected as part of a previously described clinical trial which was approved by the medical ethics committee of the University Hospital Maastricht, The Netherlands and for which all volunteers gave written informed consent [13], were screened for ARE-colonization. During this trial all participants received 500 mg of oral amoxicillin twice daily for seven days. To observe whether the use of selective antibiotics induced *in vivo* selection of ARE three faecal samples per participant, collected before (at day 0), during (at day 7) and after (at day 14) antibiotic treatment, were screened for ARE.

Microbiology and genotyping

The human faecal samples were frozen in a 1:4 glycerol-peptone dilution at $-20°C$ [13]. Rectal swabs and faecal samples were analyzed for the presence of ARE by inoculating 10 ml of Enterococcosel Enrichment Broth (Becton Dickinson, Cockeysville, MD) supplemented with aztreonam (75 mg/L) with rectal swabs or with 500 µl of the faecal dilution. These enrichment cultures were incubated for 48 hours at 37°C. The samples were subsequently cultured on Enterococcosel Agar plates (Becton Dickinson) supplemented with ampicillin (16 mg/L) for 48 hours. For each ARE-positive sample, one colony was picked for further analyses. All ARE were genotyped using Multi Locus Sequence Typing (MLST) [14] to determine the clonal relatedness among the obtained ARE and with the known nosocomial reservoir.

Antimicrobial susceptibility

MICs for ampicillin, vancomycin, gentamicin, ciprofloxacin, tetracycline, erythromycin and imipenem were determined in all isolated ARE strains using the Clinical and Laboratory Standards Institute (CLSI) broth dilution method. Strains were classified susceptible, intermediate or resistant for each antimicrobial, based on breakpoints defined by the CLSI or by the European Committee on Antimicrobial Susceptibility Testing (EUCAST; www.eucast.org).

DNA sequence analysis of *pbp5*

In hospital ARE high-level ampicillin resistance has been linked to mutations in the 3′ region of the *pbp5* gene [15]. To assess whether ampicillin resistance in community strains is caused by the same mechanism, a DNA sequence analysis of *pbp5* was performed. Total DNA was obtained from all recovered ARE as described before [16]. Generated sequences were compared with a *pbp5* gene reference sequence (GenBank accession no X84860).

Detection of putative virulence genes and DNA elements specifically enriched in hospital and community isolates

By Southern blot analysis, all ARE strains were screened for the presence of the putative virulence genes *esp*, *hyl*, *sgrA*, *ecbA*, *acm*, *sagA*, *pilA* (*fms21*), *pilB* (*ebpC*fm), *orf903* (*fms11*), *orf905* (*fms19*), *orf907* (*fms16*) [6,17], all encoding for adhesins, the gene *orf1481* [18], which is located on a previously identified putative metabolic island, and the IS-element *IS16* [7] using the probes depicted in Table 1 [12]. Of these genes and elements, *esp*, *hyl*, *sgrA*, *ecbA*, *orf903–907* (*fms11*, *16* and *19*), *orf1481* and IS16 have previously been described as being enriched in hospital ARE [5–8,17,19–20]. In addition, interruption of *acm* by IS256 was determined by PCR, as the presence of *IS256* in *acm* is negatively associated with hospital ARE [19]. *E. faecium* E1162, an ampicillin resistant blood isolate from a hospitalized patient, and E135, an ampicillin-susceptible faecal isolate from a non-hospitalized person, were included as positive and negative controls, respectively [21].

Putative virulence genes that were found to be less prevalent among the recovered community isolates than previously reported in hospital ARE, were subjected to further analysis. In community isolates with STs frequently observed among nosocomial ARE infections and outbreaks (ST16, ST18, ST19, ST78 and ST192), obtained from this study and the study of Damborg et al. [12], the prevalence of *esp*, *hyl*, *sgrA*, *ecbA* and *orf1481* was compared with the occurrence of these genes in hospital ARE isolates with similar STs, using Fisher's Exact test in SPSS 15.0 (SPSS Inc. Chicago, IL, USA). For this comparison hospital ARE strains were recovered from the MLST database (http://efaecium.mlst.net/, queried March 2010) and completed with isolates and additional data extracted from articles retrieved from Medline, that linked the aforementioned STs with the presence of one or more of the genes of interest [22–32].

The presence of the genes Efm4452_1561/EfmE4453_1839 and EfmE4452_1566/EfmE4453_1835, which are both contained on a putative mobile genetic element with a predicted role in the breakdown, transport and metabolism of xylopolysaccharides was determined by PCR (see table 1 for primer sequences).

Genome analysis of two dog isolates

Two representative canine ARE isolates from this study, E4452 and E4453, were selected for whole genome analysis. Chromosomal DNA was isolated as described previously [9] and sequenced on the Illumina Genome Analyzer IIx with a read length of 50 nt according to the manufacturer's protocol. A total of 5056696 and 7397885 matched reads were obtained for E4452 and E4453, respectively, resulting in $91\times$ and $131\times$ genome coverage. Assembly and annotation of the genomes was performed using the CLCbio Genomic Workbench version 3.7 (CLCbio, Aarhus, Denmark). Annotations were subsequently manually curated. The Whole Genome Shotgun projects of strains E4452 and E4453 have been deposited at DDBJ/EMBL/GenBank under the accession AEDZ00000000 and AEOU00000000.

Phylogenomic analysis of *E. faecium* was performed using the amino acid sequences of a set of 500 orthologous proteins of

Table 1. Oligonucleotide sequences.

Gene	Probe name	Oligonucleotide sequence (5′→3′)
esp	esp14F	AATTGATTCTTTAGCATCTGG
	esp12R	AGATTTCATCTTTGATTCTTGG
hyl	hylF	GAGTAGAGGAATATCTTAGC
	hylR	AGGCTCCAATTCTGT
sgrA	sgrAF	AATGAACGGGCAAATGAG
	sgrAR	CTTTTGTTCCTTAGTTGGTATGA
ecbA	ecbAF	GCAGTTTACAATGGTGTGAAGCAA
	ecbAR	CGGCTAATGAGTATTTGTCGTTCC
orf903	903F	TCAACGGACATACCATACCA
	903R	TCAGTTGGATTCCATGTGAT
orf905	905F	GTGACAGATTCATCTAATCAT
	905R	TCATTTTATTTCCCTCCTATTG
orf907	orf907F	GTGACCGGTTTTGATGAAAAC
	orf907R	TTAAGCTTCTGTTTCTTGATGGC
acm	acmF1	GATTTTTGAGATGATGATATAGTAG
	acmR4	GTATCTTCAGGTAGCATGTCTCC
pilA	pilAF	TGCTGATTTTGTTGGTATTTCG
	pilAR	GGCGTTCCTGAAGAGAACTCT
pilB	pilBF	GTGTTTGCAGAGGAGACAGC
	pilBR	GACAGAATAATTTACTGGGTCG
sagA	sagAF	CATGCTGACAGCAAAGTCA
	sagAR	AGAAGCACGCGAACAAGCA
orf1481	1481F	GTTTATCAACATGCTAGCCCA
	1481R	GCCAATGAGTTAGATGTAGCC
IS16	IS16F	AGCGGTGCGAATGATACCGC
	IS16R	CTTCCGATTCGCCGTCTTGAAC
EfmE4452_1561	1561F	CATCGGTACAAGCGGAGTTT
	1561R	TTCCGTTTTCAATGTGACGA
EfmE4452_1565	1565F	ATTGTTCGTGCCGGAGATAC
	1565R	GATGATCCCATTCCATTTGC

identical length that occur in E4452, E4453 and seven *E. faecium* genomes that were previously sequenced [9]. These sequences were aligned and concatenated using Geneious Pro 4.8.4 and subsequently phylogentic reconstruction was inferred using the Neighbor-Joining method, including bootstrapping with 1000 iterations. To determine differences in gene content between isolates, pairwise comparisons on the set of annotated proteins using BLAT [33] version 33×5 were performed. Proteins were scored as conserved between two strains when bi-directional hits with an amino acid identity ≥90% covering ≥50% of both protein sequences could be identified.

Results

ARE carriage

In the cross-sectional screening of different domestic animals, 24 (30%) of 79 dogs, 11 (13%) of 85 cats and none of 42 horses were colonized with ARE. Of the 24 colonized dogs, two lived together in one household while four shared their home with another non-colonized dog. There was no epidemiological link between the colonized cats. One dog was colonized with two morphologically

different strains, which were both included for further analysis. ARE was isolated from faecal samples of three (7.5%) of 40 healthy human volunteers that had received oral amoxicillin. In two participants ARE was isolated after antibiotic use (in one at day seven and in the other at both day seven and fourteen). In one participant ARE was only detected in the faecal sample taken before the start of amoxicillin administration.

MLST

MLST analysis of 39 community ARE strains revealed 21 different STs, including eight new STs (Table 2). ST266 was isolated most frequently and was found in both cats and dogs and in one human volunteer. Comparison with the international *E. faecium* MLST database revealed that four of the recovered 21 STs have been previously cultured from dogs. Eleven of the 21 STs have been isolated from hospitalized patients before, of which nine were associated with clinical infections. Two STs were previously cultured from non-hospitalized persons and three from livestock. MLST analysis revealed that the two colonized dogs sharing a household carried different STs (ST192 and ST373). The two morphologically different strains recovered from a single dog did not have identical STs (ST266 and ST274).

Antimicrobial susceptibility and *pbp5*

All 39 isolates displayed high-level resistance to ampicillin, with MICs ranging from 64 to >512 μg/ml, and resistance to imipinem, with MICs ranging from 8 to 256 μg/ml. In addition, 35 (90%) and 30 (77%) isolates were resistant to tetracycline (MICs ranging from 16 to >64 μg/ml) and erythromycin(all MICs>32 μg/ml), respectively. All isolates were susceptible to vancomycin. High-level resistance to gentamicin (MIC>128 μg/ml) was present in two (5%) strains and high-level resistance to ciprofloxacin (MIC>64 μg/ml), which is associated with hospital ARE [34], was observed in only three (1 dog, 2 cats) isolates. Mutations in the C-terminal region of *pbp5* identical to those previously found in hospital ARE and which are linked to high-level ampicillin resistance [15] were found in all strains (Table 3). In total, 10 different *pbp5* alleles, based on the depicted polymorphisms, were identified. Although the recovered alleles were shared by strains with several STs, *pbp5* allele polymorphisms were highly conserved within isolates with identical STs. For example, 11 of the 12 isolates with ST266, recovered from dogs, cats and a human volunteer had *pbp5* allele 8.

Prevalence of putative virulence genes and DNA elements enriched in hospital isolates

The genes *orf903* (fms11), *orf905* (fms19), *orf907* (fms16), were highly prevalent in community ARE isolates. This was also the case for IS16, which previously has been shown to be enriched in hospital ARE (Table 4) [7,35]. Other genes previously found to be enriched among hospital isolates were found in about half (*sgrA, orf1481*) or only in a few (*esp, hyl, ecbA*) of the community isolates [6,8,17–18]. When community strains with STs regularly involved in nosocomial infections and outbreaks (i.e. ST16, ST18, ST19, ST78 and ST192), recovered from this study (n = 7) and the study of Damborg et al. (n = 37) [12], were compared with hospital ARE isolates with similar STs recovered from the online MLST database (n = 377) or from literature (n = 60) [22–32], *esp, hyl* and *sgrA* were significantly underrepresented in the community strains compared to the hospital strains, while this was not the case for *ecbA* and *orf1481* (Table 5). Integration of IS256 in *acm*, previously suggested to be indicative for community-origin of strains [19], was only found in three isolates. *pilA, pilB, acm,* and

Table 2. Multilocus sequence types (STs) of recovered ARE isolates and previous occurrence among other sources.

ARE isolates current study		No. of isolates with identical ST in MLST database[a] per source						
		Hospital[b]	Community[c]					Total
ST	Frequency (source)	HAI	CS	LS	D	C		All
16	1 (D)	47	-	-	-	-		72
18	1 (C)	103	1	1	-	-		114
19	2 (D)	7	-	-	5	-		12
78	1 (C)	139	1	-	16	-		168
128	1 (D)	1	-	-	-	-		1
148	1 (D)	-	-	1	-	-		1
168	2 (D)	3	-	-	-	-		3
192	2 (D)	56	-	-	8	-		64
264	1 (C)	1	-	-	-	-		1
266	12 (6x C, 5x D, 1x H)	2	-	-	10	-		12
274	4 (1 x C, 3x D)	1	-	-	-	-		1
373	1 (D)	1	-	-	-	-		1
393	1 (H)	-	-	1	-	-		1
453	1 (D)	-	-	-	-	-		-
454	1 (D)	-	-	-	-	-		-
455	1 (D)	-	-	-	-	-		-
456	2 (D, H)	-	-	-	-	-		-
457	1 (D)	-	-	-	-	-		-
458	1 (D)	-	-	-	-	-		-
459	1 (D)	-	-	-	-	-		-
477	1 (C)	-	-	-	-	-		-

[a]http://efaecium.mlst.net/ queried March 2010;
[b]HAI = hospital-associated isolates (i.e., clinical isolates, hospital surveillance, hospital outbreak);
[c]CI = clinical isolate; CS = Community human surveillance; LS = Livestock; D = dogs; C = cats.

Table 3. Polymorphisms in the C-terminal region of *pbp5*[a].

Allele	Source[b] ST	426	461	462	466	466'	470	476	477	485	496	497	499	525	546	558	582	586	629	MIC range
Reference X84860		M	Q	V	S	x	H	A	L	M	N	F	A	E	N	A	G	V	E	
1	D (5x) 19 (2x), 454, 455, I 457	-	-	-	-	-	Q	-	-	-	K	-	T	D	-	-	-	-	V	128–256
2	D (2x) 168 (2x)	-	-	-	-	-	Q	-	-	**T**	K	-	T	D	-	-	-	L	V	128–256
3	D (4x), C (1x) 274 (4x), 458	-	K	-	-	S	Q	-	-	A	K	-	T	D	-	-	-	L	V	≥512
4	D (3x), H (1x) 16, 148, 373, 393	-	K	-	-	S	Q	-	-	A	K	-	T	D	-	-	-	-	V	≥512
5	D (1x), H (1x) 456 (2x)	-	-	-	D	S	Q	-	-	A	K	-	T	D	-	-	-	L	V	>512
6	C (2x) 477, 266	-	-	-	D	S	Q	S	M	-	K	L	T	D	-	-	-	L	V	>512
7	C (1x) 264	-	-	-	D	S	Q	S	-	-	K	L	T	D	-	-	-	-	V	256
8	C (6x), D (9x), H (1x) 18, 192 (2x), 266 (11x), 453, 459	-	-	-	-	S	Q	-	-	A	K	-	T	D	-	-	-	-	V	≥512
9	D (1x) 128	-	-	-	-	S	Q	-	-	**T**	K	-	T	D	-	-	-	-	V	64
10	C (1x) 78	-	-	A	-	S	Q	-	-	A	K	-	T	D	T	T	S	-	V	>512

[a]Amino acid mutations that contribute to ampicillin resistance are indicated in bold [15]. The one-letter abbreviation code is used to denote the amino acids. The – sign indicates no change in amino acid compared to the reference allele.
[b]Source (and frequency) of the isolates carrying a particular allele: D = dog; C = cat; H = human.

Table 4. Prevalence of putative virulence genes.

Gene[a]	No. of isolates (%)	Source[b]
Adhesins		
esp	1 (3)	C
hyl	2 (5)	C
sgrA	17 (44)	C, D
ecbA	2 (5)	C, D
orf903	32 (82)	C, D, H
orf905	32 (82)	C, D, H
orf907	32 (82)	C, D, H
acm	39 (100)	C, D, H
pilA	35 (90)	C, D, H
pilB	38 (97)	C, D, H
sagA	39 (100)	C, D, H
Sugar metabolism		
orf1481	19 (49)	C, D
IS-elements		
IS16	31 (79)	C, D, H
IS256 in acm	3 (8)	C, D, H
Community specific genes tentatively involved in sugar metabolism		
EfmE4452_1561	28 (72)	C, D, H
EfmE4452_1565	28 (72)	C, D, H

[a]The genes acm, pilA, pilB and sagA are prevalent among all E. faecium strains; the genes EfmE4452_1561 and EfmE4452_1565 are uniquely present in community ARE isolates (this paper). All other genes are specifically enriched among hospital isolates [5,7–8,18–19,52].
[b]Source of the isolates carrying a particular gene: D = dog; C = cat; H = human.

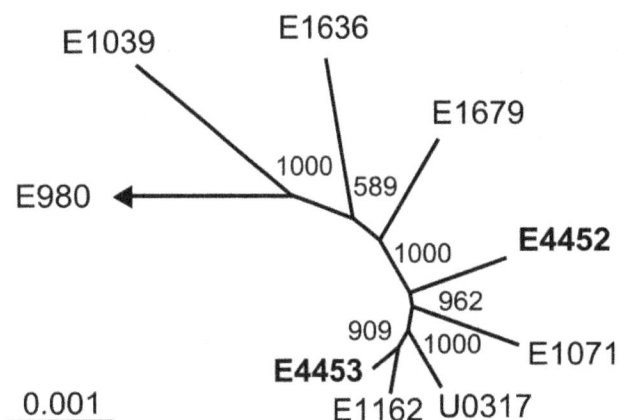

Figure 1. Phylogenomic analysis of canine E. faecium strains E4452 and E4453. Unrooted neighbor-joining tree of E. faecium based on the concatenated alignments of 500 orthologous proteins (containing 15168 residues). Bootstrap values are based on 1000 permutations.

sagA were found in 90% or more of the isolates, which is in concordance with earlier observations that these genes are ubiquitously present in E. faecium [19–20,36].

Genome analysis of E. faecium E4452 and E4453

To further characterize the evolutionary links between community and hospital E. faecium strains, we determined draft genome sequences of two canine E. faecium strains (strain codes E4452 and E4453) that were isolated as part of this study. These strains were isolated in August 2008 from two dogs that were kept separate from each other in different households. According to

MLST these strains were assigned to ST266 (E4452) and ST192 (E4453). Both these STs are common among dog strains and may therefore be representative for a significant proportion of dog-associated E. faecium strains. In this study 12 of 37 dog strains had ST266 and two ST192, while in the study of Damborg ST266 and ST192 were the third and fourth most common dog ST, respectively (Table 2) [12]. Draft genome sequences of these isolates were determined using Illumina sequencing technology, which, in combination with novel assembly methods, has previously been used to successfully sequence genomes of bacteria [37–38] to the draft stage.

De novo assemblies for both strains resulted in draft genome sequences of E4452 and E4453 containing 2.77 Mbp and 2.82 Mbp, in 268 and 374 contigs, respectively. Contig N50s were 18110 bp and 13956 bp, for E4452 and E4453 respectively. Phylogenomic analysis of the dog strains from this study showed that E4453 (ST192) is relatively closely related to strains E1162 (ST17) and U0317 (ST78) (Figure 1). This is in agreement with the MLST results since ST192 is a single locus variant of ST78 and a double locus variant of ST17. The same analysis demonstrates that strain E4452 (ST266), which based on its MLST profile is not closely related to ST17 and ST78 (3–4 different loci), is more distantly related to the clinical isolates E1162 and U0317 based on phylogenomics.

Table 5. Comparison community and hospital isolates with similar STs (ST16, ST18, ST19, ST78 and ST192).

Gene	Community isolates (n = 37)[a]		Hospital isolates (n = 437)[b]		p-value[c]
	tested, n	presence gene, n (%)	tested, n	presence gene, n (%)	
esp	37	1 (3)	433	314 (73)	<0.001
hyl	37	1 (3)	51	24 (47)	<0.001
sgrA	36	15 (42)	23	23 (100)	<0.001
ecbA	36	18 (50)	23	16 (70)	0.18
orf1481	7	7 (100)	21	20 (95)	0.99

[a]includes 7 isolates(1x ST16, 1x ST18, 2x ST19, 1x ST78, 2x ST192) recovered in this study and 30 (6x ST19, 16x ST78, 8x ST192) isolates recovered by Damborg et al. [12];
[b]includes 377 isolates (60x ST16, 97x ST18, 7x ST19, 160x ST78, 53x ST192) present in the MLST database at March 16, 2010 and 60 isolates (2x ST16, 9x ST18, 49x ST78) described in literature [22–32];
[c]Fisher's Exact test.

Interestingly, gene content comparisons between the clinical isolates E1162 and U0317 and the canine strains E4452 and E4453 reveal that the clinical isolates have more genes in common with each than with the two *E. faecium* strains from dogs and, *vice versa*, that the strains from dogs have more genes in common with each other than with the clinical isolates (Table 6). This indicates that there are genes and genetic elements that are specific for either the canine or the clinical strains. Indeed, we were able to identify 32 genes that were shared by both canine *E. faecium* strains but which were absent from all other 28 *E. faecium* strains for which the genome sequence was publicly available in December 2010 (Table 7). None of the strains of which the genomes were previously sequenced have been isolated from dogs. The genes that are unique to the two *E. faecium* strains from dogs include a number of genes that are putatively located on mobile genetic elements (plasmids and/or conjugative transposons) and which have a predicted role in the breakdown, transport and metabolism of xylopolysaccharides. PCR analysis on two of the unique canine genes, *EfmE4452_1561* and *EfmE4452_1565* (Table 7), contained on the putative xylopolysaccharides breakdown, transport and metabolism cluster, demonstrated that both genes were concomitantly present in 28 (72%) of the 39 recovered community ARE isolates, including 18 (72%) of 25 canine, eight (73%) of 11 feline and, interestingly, two (67%) of three human isolates with STs that were also carried by dogs (Table 4). Notably, none of these two genes are present in any of the 28 *E. faecium* genome sequences that were publicly available in November 2011. Most of these genome sequences have been determined from clinical isolates, indicating that this element is relatively scarce in hospital-acquired strains. The incongruence between phylogenomic analysis based on conserved protein sequences from the core genome and genomic relatedness based on gene content strongly indicates that niche-specific adaptation of the accessory genome has occurred in *E. faecium* isolates that inhabit the gastrointestinal tracts of dogs.

Discussion

The rapid emergence of ARE as important nosocomial pathogen during the last two decades is thought to be the result of intra- and inter-hospital transmission of a relatively limited number of clones with a genetic make-up favouring colonisation, infection and subsequent transmission among hospitalized patients [6]. Possibly, influx of ARE from the community also contributes to its emergence in hospitals, since ARE have been recovered from community sources. In the past decade, ARE carriage was found to be prevalent among dogs and/or cats in Italy, Belgium, Portugal and the U.S. [39–42]. Furthermore, ARE had also been isolated from canine urinary tract infections and feline surgical site infections in the U.S. and Switzerland, respectively [43–44].

Table 6. Number of shared Coding Sequences (CDS) between canine *E. faecium* isolates E4452 and E4453 and clinical *E. faecium* isolates E1162 and U0317[a].

Strains	E4452	E4453	E1162	U0317
E4452	**2715**	2234	2108	2133
E4453		**2823**	2208	2145
E1162			**2694**	2268
U0317				**2965**

[a]The total number of CDS in each genome sequence is indicated in bold.

However, since none of these studies determined the genotypic background of ARE isolates, their descent and potential linkage to hospital clones remains unknown. A potential genetic link between ARE in animals and the hospital setting was proposed in 2009 by Damborg and co-workers who described widespread ARE carriage among English and Danish dogs and showed that most of these isolates belong to clones associated with nosocomial infections [12].

Here we present evidence of genotypic concordance, based on MLST, between hospital and community ARE. This demonstrates that community and hospital ARE isolates are evolutionarily linked. The question is whether evolutionary linkage between hospital and community ARE also implies epidemiological linkage, i.e. cross-transmission between the two reservoirs. Evidently, the ARE population recovered from the community is not an exact copy from the circulating reservoir in Dutch hospitals. Eight of the 21 STs found in the community have, up till now, never been reported to colonize or infect patients (http://efaecium.mlst.net/) and the *esp*, *hyl* and *sgrA* genes, which were previously implicated in *E. faecium* virulence, are underrepresented in these community strains. This denotes a significant discrepancy in accessory gene content between hospital and community ARE that includes putative virulence and antimicrobial resistance genes, and indicates that if zoonotic transfer of ARE occurs, it only occurs infrequently.

Phylogenomic analysis of two dog strains from this study and seven previously sequenced *E. faecium* genomes derived from humans [9] only strengthens this notion. Based on its core genome, the ST192 dog isolate was found to be relatively closely related to the two previously sequenced clinical strains (E1162 and U0317) [9]. This leads to the conclusion that on an evolutionary time scale this particular canine isolate is related to the isolates that are currently causing the majority of clinical infections. Congruent with MLST analysis, the ST266 dog strain was more distantly related to the clinical isolates, indicating that not all ampicillin-resistant isolates from the community are closely related to ampicillin-resistant clinical isolates. Yet, when comparing the gene content of these strains, the two dog strains had more genes in common with each other than with the clinical isolates. A number of genes appeared to be specific for either the strains from dogs or the clinical isolates. For example, both E1162 and U0317 carry a 64–68 kb pathogenicity island (ICEEfm1) that contains the *esp* gene [9,45–46], which is involved in biofilm formation [21] and infections in a mouse model [47–48]. Both canine *E. faecium* strains E4452 and E4453 are lacking ICEEfm1 and indeed so far *esp* has not been found among ampicillin-resistant canine isolates. On the other hand, 32 genes including a cluster of genes involved in the breakdown, transport and metabolism of xylopolysaccharides, were uniquely present in the dog strains while being absent in all of the other 28 *E. faecium* genome sequences that are currently publicly available were found. This cluster contains a gene annotated as a β-xylosidase which is homologous to genes from *Enterococcus gallinarum* (67% amino acid identity) and *Roseburia intestinalis* (65% amino acid identity), a common anaerobic xylanolytic gut commensal [49]. This finding suggests that *E. faecium* strains from dogs have acquired a genetic element that enable the metabolism of xylose-containing oligo- and polysaccharides. These sugars, which originate from plant materials, are commonly found in commercial dog foods [50] and may thus reflect a metabolic adaptation of *E. faecium* to the canine (and possibly feline) gastrointestinal tract, especially since the majority of the recovered community isolates carried at least two of the genes contained on this element. From three of the 40 healthy human volunteers ARE could be isolated and in two of them only

Table 7. Genes from canine *E. faecium* strains E4452 and E4453 which are absent from 28 other *E. faecium* genome sequences[a].

E4452 locus tags	E4453 locus tags	Annotation
EfmE4452_0533	EfmE4453_2272	hypothetical protein
EfmE4452_0534	EfmE4453_2271	hypothetical protein
EfmE4452_0535	EfmE4453_2270	putative mobilization protein
EfmE4452_0537	EfmE4453_2268	hypothetical protein
EfmE4452_0538	EfmE4453_2267	hypothetical protein
EfmE4452_0539	EfmE4453_2266	hypothetical protein
EfmE4452_0540	EfmE4453_2265	replication initiator protein
EfmE4452_0553	EfmE4453_0769	hypothetical protein
EfmE4452_0595	EfmE4453_1802	hypothetical protein
EfmE4452_0597	EfmE4453_1800	hypothetical protein
EfmE4452_1556	EfmE4453_1844	putative ATP-binding protein
EfmE4452_1557	EfmE4453_1843	related to integrase of Tn552
EfmE4452_1558	EfmE4453_1842	Resolvase/integrase Bin
EfmE4452_1560	EfmE4453_1840	toxin-antitoxin system, toxin component, MazF family
EfmE4452_1561	EfmE4453_1839	D-xylulose kinase
EfmE4452_1563	EfmE4453_1837	transporter permease
EfmE4452_1564	EfmE4453_1836	ABC transporter
EfmE4452_1565	EfmE4453_1835	beta-1,4-xylosidase
EfmE4452_1566	EfmE4453_1834	xylose isomerase
EfmE4452_1567	EfmE4453_2638	xylose operon repressor
EfmE4452_1568	EfmE4453_2637	conserved hypothetical protein
EfmE4452_1773	EfmE4453_0609	heavy metal translocating P-type ATPase
EfmE4452_2486	EfmE4453_2323	hypothetical protein
EfmE4452_2488	EfmE4453_0817	conjugative transposon protein
EfmE4452_2492	EfmE4453_0822	conjugative transposon protein
EfmE4452_2493	EfmE4453_0823	conjugative transposon protein
EfmE4452_2494	EfmE4453_0825	hypothetical protein
EfmE4452_2495	EfmE4453_0826	conjugative transposon protein
EfmE4452_2496	EfmE4453_0827	NLP/P60 family protein, putative cell wall hydrolase
EfmE4452_2500	EfmE4453_0830	hypothetical protein

[a]black lines indicate that genes are located on different contigs in the draft genome sequences.

after oral administration of amoxicillin followed by enrichment cultures. One of the volunteers carried a ST that was previously isolated from a clinical infection, but that did not belong to one of the major clones (STs 16, 17, 18, 78, 117, 192, 202, 203) now frequently encountered in hospitals world-wide (http://efaecium.mlst.net/). The low ARE colonization prevalence among healthy humans in the community and the absence of ARE clones currently dominating the nosocomial epidemiology supports the hypothesis that, in hospitalized patients, endogenous selection only plays a minor role in ARE acquisition, relative to cross-transmission [12,51]. Interestingly, two human volunteers were colonized with STs that were also isolated from domestic animals, including ST266 which was most frequently found among colonized dogs and cats. Moreover, the accessory genome of these human and animal strains was indistinguishable, including the presence of at least two of the newly identified, unique community genes, that are putatively located on the genetic element with a predicted role in the breakdown, transport and metabolism of xylopolysaccharides. This finding suggests that ARE may occasionally be transferred between humans and pets.

Up till now, we can only speculate on why ARE frequently colonize the feline and canine intestinal tract. In humans, ARE colonization is rarely found without prior exposure to selective antibiotics (Table 2) [10–11], and when this is not different for domestic animals it would imply that the intestinal microbiota of these pets is frequently challenged by antibiotics, either through therapeutic intake or via other unknown routes. Another possibility is that dogs and cats represent the natural ecological niche for ARE, which makes that they more easily reside (in higher quantities) in the canine and feline than in the human intestinal tract. Perhaps, the mutations in *pbp5* which confer ampicillin resistance in clinical isolates, may even represent the natural *E. faecium* phenotype in the gastrointestinal tract of dogs and cats. If true, this would imply that nosocomial ARE clones have originated and evolved from the animal reservoir. Yet, we cannot rule out the possibility that community and hospital ARE share a common ancestor of other origin, or, that the canine and feline isolates represent early evolutionary descendents of hospital ARE, who in time have lost genetic properties in the absence of selective forces imposed by the nosocomial environment.

In this study, we have demonstrated that the nosocomial and the community reservoir of ARE, present in patients, dogs, cats and sporadically in healthy humans, are evolutionarily linked but that niche separation and adaptation has driven clones onto different evolutionary trajectories resulting in sequential acquisition or loss of adaptive elements including virulence and antimicrobial resistance traits due to selective forces imposed by either the hospital or community environment. This may imply that *E. faecium* hospital clones have originated and evolved from the animal reservoir and that sequential events of zoonotic transfer may have contributed to the diversity in genetic background and accessory genome observed among the polyclonal ARE subpopulation that successfully resides in the nosocomial setting.

Author Contributions

Conceived and designed the experiments: MR WS RW MB. Performed the experiments: MR WS ED MvL-A HD CK. Analyzed the data: MR WS RW. Contributed reagents/materials/analysis tools: MR WS RW ED MvL-A HD CK. Wrote the paper: MR WS RW MB.

References

1. Grayson ML, Eliopoulos GM, Wennersten CB, Ruoff KL, De Girolami PC, et al. (1991) Increasing resistance to beta-lactam antibiotics among clinical isolates of Enterococcus faecium: a 22-year review at one institution. Antimicrob Agents Chemother 35: 2180–2184.
2. Murray BE (2000) Vancomycin-resistant enterococcal infections. N Engl J Med 342: 710–721.
3. Hidron AI, Edwards JR, Patel J, Horan TC, Sievert DM, et al. (2008) NHSN annual update: antimicrobial-resistant pathogens associated with healthcare-associated infections: annual summary of data reported to the National Healthcare Safety Network at the Centers for Disease Control and Prevention, 2006–2007. Infect Control Hosp Epidemiol 29: 996–1011.
4. Werner G, Coque TM, Hammerum AM, Hope R, Hryniewicz W, et al. (2008) Emergence and spread of vancomycin resistance among enterococci in Europe. Euro Surveill 13.
5. Willems RJ, Top J, van Santen M, Robinson DA, Coque TM, et al. (2005) Global spread of vancomycin-resistant Enterococcus faecium from distinct nosocomial genetic complex. Emerg Infect Dis 11: 821–828.
6. Willems RJ, van Schaik W (2009) Transition of Enterococcus faecium from commensal organism to nosocomial pathogen. Future Microbiol 4: 1125–1135.
7. Leavis HL, Willems RJ, van Wamel WJ, Schuren FH, Caspers MP, et al. (2007) Insertion sequence-driven diversification creates a globally dispersed emerging multiresistant subspecies of E. faecium. PLoS Pathog 3: e7.
8. Willems RJ, Homan W, Top J, van Santen-Verheuvel M, Tribe D, et al. (2001) Variant esp gene as a marker of a distinct genetic lineage of vancomycin-resistant Enterococcus faecium spreading in hospitals. Lancet 357: 853–855.
9. van Schaik W, Top J, Riley DR, Boekhorst J, Vrijenhoek JE, et al. (2010) Pyrosequencing-based comparative genome analysis of the nosocomial pathogen Enterococcus faecium and identification of a large transferable pathogenicity island. BMC Genomics 11: 239.
10. Biavasco F, Foglia G, Paoletti C, Zandri G, Magi G, et al. (2007) VanA-type enterococci from humans, animals, and food: species distribution, population structure, Tn1546 typing and location, and virulence determinants. Appl Environ Microbiol 73: 3307–3319.
11. Top J, Willems R, Blok H, de Regt M, Jalink K, et al. (2007) Ecological replacement of Enterococcus faecalis by multiresistant clonal complex 17 Enterococcus faecium. Clin Microbiol Infect 13: 316–319.
12. Damborg P, Top J, Hendrickx AP, Dawson S, Willems RJ, et al. (2009) Dogs are a reservoir of ampicillin-resistant Enterococcus faecium lineages associated with human infections. Appl Environ Microbiol 75: 2360–2365.
13. Koning CJ, Jonkers DM, Stobberingh EE, Mulder L, Rombouts FM, et al. (2008) The effect of a multispecies probiotic on the intestinal microbiota and bowel movements in healthy volunteers taking the antibiotic amoxycillin. Am J Gastroenterol 103: 178–189.
14. Homan WL, Tribe D, Poznanski S, Li M, Hogg G, et al. (2002) Multilocus sequence typing scheme for Enterococcus faecium. J Clin Microbiol 40: 1963–1971.
15. Rice LB, Bellais S, Carias LL, Hutton-Thomas R, Bonomo RA, et al. (2004) Impact of specific pbp5 mutations on expression of beta-lactam resistance in Enterococcus faecium. Antimicrob Agents Chemother 48: 3028–3032.
16. Top J, Schouls LM, Bonten MJ, Willems RJ (2004) Multiple-locus variable-number tandem repeat analysis, a novel typing scheme to study the genetic relatedness and epidemiology of Enterococcus faecium isolates. J Clin Microbiol 42: 4503–4511.
17. Hendrickx AP, Willems RJ, Bonten MJ, van Schaik W (2009) LPxTG surface proteins of enterococci. Trends Microbiol 17: 423–430.
18. Heikens E, van Schaik W, Leavis HL, Bonten MJ, Willems RJ (2008) Identification of a novel genomic island specific to hospital-acquired clonal complex 17 Enterococcus faecium isolates. Appl Environ Microbiol 74: 7094–7097.
19. Nallapareddy SR, Singh KV, Okhuysen PC, Murray BE (2008) A functional collagen adhesin gene, acm, in clinical isolates of Enterococcus faecium correlates with the recent success of this emerging nosocomial pathogen. Infect Immun 76: 4110–4119.
20. Sillanpaa J, Prakash VP, Nallapareddy SR, Murray BE (2009) Distribution of genes encoding MSCRAMMs and Pili in clinical and natural populations of Enterococcus faecium. J Clin Microbiol 47: 896–901.
21. Heikens E, Bonten MJ, Willems RJ (2007) Enterococcal surface protein Esp is important for biofilm formation of Enterococcus faecium E1162. J Bacteriol 189: 8233–8240.
22. Billstrom H, Top J, Edlund C, Lund B (2009) Frequent occurrence of multidrug-resistant CC17 Enterococcus faecium among clinical isolates in Sweden. J Appl Microbiol.
23. Bonora MG, Olioso D, Lo Cascio G, Fontana R (2007) Phylogenetic analysis of vancomycin-resistant Enterococcus faecium genotypes associated with outbreaks or sporadic infections in Italy. Microb Drug Resist 13: 171–177.
24. Brilliantova AN, Kliasova GA, Mironova AV, Tishkov VI, Novichkova GA, et al. Spread of vancomycin-resistant Enterococcus faecium in two haematological centres in Russia. Int J Antimicrob Agents 35: 177–181.
25. Hsieh YC, Lee WS, Ou TY, Hsueh PR. Clonal spread of CC17 vancomycin-resistant Enterococcus faecium with multilocus sequence type 78 (ST78) and a novel ST444 in Taiwan. Eur J Clin Microbiol Infect Dis 29: 25–30.
26. Khan MA, van der Wal M, Farrell DJ, Cossins L, van Belkum A, et al. (2008) Analysis of VanA vancomycin-resistant Enterococcus faecium isolates from Saudi Arabian hospitals reveals the presence of clonal cluster 17 and two new Tn1546 lineage types. J Antimicrob Chemother 62: 279–283.
27. Klare I, Konstabel C, Mueller-Bertling S, Werner G, Strommenger B, et al. (2005) Spread of ampicillin/vancomycin-resistant Enterococcus faecium of the epidemic-virulent clonal complex-17 carrying the genes esp and hyl in German hospitals. Eur J Clin Microbiol Infect Dis 24: 815–825.
28. Lee WG, Lee SM, Kim YS (2006) Molecular characterization of Enterococcus faecium isolated from hospitalized patients in Korea. Lett Appl Microbiol 43: 274–279.
29. Libisch B, Lepsanovic Z, Top J, Muzslay M, Konkoly-Thege M, et al. (2008) Molecular characterization of vancomycin-resistant Enterococcus spp. clinical isolates from Hungary and Serbia. Scand J Infect Dis 40: 778–784.
30. Panesso D, Reyes J, Rincon S, Diaz L, Galloway-Pena J, et al. Molecular Epidemiology of Vancomycin-Resistant Enterococcus faecium: A Prospective, Multicenter Study in South American Hospitals. J Clin Microbiol.
31. Werner G, Klare I, Fleige C, Witte W (2008) Increasing rates of vancomycin resistance among Enterococcus faecium isolated from German hospitals between 2004 and 2006 are due to wide clonal dissemination of vancomycin-resistant enterococci and horizontal spread of vanA clusters. Int J Med Microbiol 298: 515–527.
32. Zhu X, Zheng B, Wang S, Willems RJ, Xue F, et al. (2009) Molecular characterisation of outbreak-related strains of vancomycin-resistant Enterococcus faecium from an intensive care unit in Beijing, China. J Hosp Infect 72: 147–154.
33. Kent WJ (2002) BLAT-the BLAST-like alignment tool. Genome Res 12: 656–664.
34. Leavis HL, Willems RJ, Top J, Bonten MJ (2006) High-level ciprofloxacin resistance from point mutations in gyrA and parC confined to global hospital-adapted clonal lineage CC17 of Enterococcus faecium. J Clin Microbiol 44: 1059–1064.
35. Werner G, Fleige C, Geringer U, van Schaik W, Klare I, et al. (2011) IS element IS16 as a molecular screening tool to identify hospital-associated strains of Enterococcus faecium. BMC Infect Dis 11: 80.
36. Sillanpaa J, Nallapareddy SR, Prakash VP, Qin X, Hook M, et al. (2008) Identification and phenotypic characterization of a second collagen adhesin, Scm, and genome-based identification and analysis of 13 other predicted MSCRAMMs, including four distinct pilus loci, in Enterococcus faecium. Microbiology 154: 3199–3211.
37. Beres SB, Carroll RK, Shea PR, Sitkiewicz I, Martinez-Gutierrez JC, et al. (2010) Molecular complexity of successive bacterial epidemics deconvoluted by comparative pathogenomics. Proc Natl Acad Sci U S A 107: 4371–4376.
38. Harris SR, Feil EJ, Holden MT, Quail MA, Nickerson EK, et al. (2010) Evolution of MRSA during hospital transmission and intercontinental spread. Science 327: 469–474.
39. Jackson CR, Fedorka-Cray PJ, Davis JA, Barrett JB, Frye JG (2009) Prevalence, species distribution and antimicrobial resistance of enterococci isolated from dogs and cats in the United States. J Appl Microbiol 107: 1269–1278.
40. Moyaert H, De Graef EM, Haesebrouck F, Decostere A (2006) Acquired antimicrobial resistance in the intestinal microbiota of diverse cat populations. Res Vet Sci 81: 1–7.

Hospital and Community Ampicillin-Resistant Enterococcus faecium Are Evolutionarily Closely Linked...

105

41. Ossiprandi MC, Bottarelli E, Cattabiani F, Bianchi E (2008) Susceptibility to vancomycin and other antibiotics of 165 Enterococcus strains isolated from dogs in Italy. Comp Immunol Microbiol Infect Dis 31: 1–9.

42. Rodrigues J, Poeta P, Martins A, Costa D (2002) The importance of pets as reservoirs of resistant Enterococcus strains, with special reference to vancomycin. J Vet Med B Infect Dis Vet Public Health 49: 278–280.

43. Boerlin P, Eugster S, Gaschen F, Straub R, Schawalder P (2001) Transmission of opportunistic pathogens in a veterinary teaching hospital. Vet Microbiol 82: 347–359.

44. Simjee S, White DG, McDermott PF, Wagner DD, Zervos MJ, et al. (2002) Characterization of Tn1546 in vancomycin-resistant Enterococcus faecium isolated from canine urinary tract infections: evidence of gene exchange between human and animal enterococci. J Clin Microbiol 40: 4659–4665.

45. Leavis H, Top J, Shankar N, Borgen K, Bonten M, et al. (2004) A novel putative enterococcal pathogenicity island linked to the esp virulence gene of Enterococcus faecium and associated with epidemicity. J Bacteriol 186: 672–682.

46. Top J, Sinnige JC, Majoor EA, Bonten MJ, Willems RJ, et al. (2011) The recombinase IntA is required for excision of esp-containing ICEEfm1 in Enterococcus faecium. J Bacteriol 193: 1003–1006.

47. Leendertse M, Heikens E, Wijnands LM, van Luit-Asbroek M, Teske GJ, et al. (2009) Enterococcal surface protein transiently aggravates Enterococcus faecium-induced urinary tract infection in mice. J Infect Dis 200: 1162–1165.

48. Sava IG, Heikens E, Kropec A, Theilacker C, Willems R, et al. (2010) Enterococcal surface protein contributes to persistence in the host but is not a target of opsonic and protective antibodies in Enterococcus faecium infection. J Med Microbiol 59: 1001–1004.

49. Chassard C, Goumy V, Leclerc M, Del'homme C, Bernalier-Donadille A (2007) Characterization of the xylan-degrading microbial community from human faeces. FEMS Microbiol Ecol 61: 121–131.

50. Council NR Nutrient requirements of dogs and cats. National Academies Press; 2006.

51. de Regt MJ, van der Wagen LE, Top J, Blok HE, Hopmans TE, et al. (2008) High acquisition and environmental contamination rates of CC17 ampicillin-resistant Enterococcus faecium in a Dutch hospital. J Antimicrob Chemother 62: 1401–1406.

52. Hendrickx AP, van Luit-Asbroek M, Schapendonk CM, van Wamel WJ, Braat JC, et al. (2009) SgrA, a nidogen-binding LPXTG surface adhesin implicated in biofilm formation, and EcbA, a collagen binding MSCRAMM, are two novel adhesins of hospital-acquired Enterococcus faecium. Infect Immun 77: 5097–5106.

13

A Comparison of Portable Ultrasound and Fully-Equipped Clinical Ultrasound Unit in the Thyroid Size Measurement of the Indo-Pacific Bottlenose Dolphin

Brian C. W. Kot*, Michael T. C. Ying, Fiona M. Brook

Department of Health Technology and Informatics, The Hong Kong Polytechnic University, Hung Hom, Hong Kong SAR, China

Abstract

Measurement of thyroid size and volume is a useful clinical parameter in both human and veterinary medicine, particularly for diagnosing thyroid diseases and guiding corrective therapy. Procuring a fully-equipped clinical ultrasound unit (FCUS) may be difficult in most veterinary settings. The present study evaluated the inter-equipment variability in dolphin thyroid ultrasound measurements between a portable ultrasound unit (PUS) and a FCUS; for both units, repeatability was also assessed. Thyroid ultrasound examinations were performed on 15 apparently healthy bottlenose dolphins with both PUS and FCUS under identical scanning conditions. There was a high level of agreement between the two ultrasound units in dolphin thyroid measurements (ICC = 0.859–0.976). A high intra-operator repeatability in thyroid measurements was found (PUS: ICC = 0.854–0.984, FCUS: ICC = 0.709–0.954). As a conclusion, no substantial inter-equipment variability was found between PUS and FCUS in dolphin thyroid size measurements under identical scanning conditions, supporting further application of PUS for quantitative analyses of dolphin thyroid gland in both research and clinical practices at aquarium settings.

Editor: Justin David Brown, University of Georgia, United States of America

Funding: This project was funded by The Hong Kong Polytechnic University Research Studentship (G5556 RGGH). The funders had no role in study design, data collection and analysis, decision to publish, or preparation of the manuscript.

Competing Interests: The authors have declared that no competing interests exist.

* E-mail: briankot@yahoo.co.uk

Introduction

Ultrasound is a non-invasive, real-time imaging tool that provides high resolution images for soft tissue characterization, and allows repeatable measurements. 2-D ultrasound has a prominent role in evaluating the morphology of the thyroid gland in humans [1–3] and companion animals [4–7]. The mammalian thyroid gland is critical in regulating metabolic functions including cardiac rate and output, lipid catabolism, skeletal growth, and production of oxygen and heat. Environmental contaminants and local environmental influences have been implicated in thyroid hormone imbalances [8] and development of morphological and histological abnormalities [9–11] leading to calf mortality [12]. To the best of our knowledge, the formal literature is devoid of any reference to the diagnosis of thyroid abnormalities in living dolphins. In order to accurately diagnose and assess thyroid abnormalities in live animals, reliable methods of assessing the thyroid morphology must be developed so that corrective therapy can be undertaken.

In human medicine, the thyroid volume is a useful clinical measure, particularly in the diagnosis of thyroid diseases and accurate determination of the iodine-131 dosage used in radioiodine therapy for hyperthyroidism. Volume measurement of each lobe is usually estimated using the ellipsoid equation [13] i.e. volume = $\pi/6 \times$ craniocaudal $\times$ mediolateral $\times$ dorsoventral dimensions and its derivatives using the cross-sectional area [14]. Recently, efforts have been made to establish a standardized scanning protocol in evaluating the morphology of the thyroid gland in a group of Indo-Pacific bottlenose dolphins using a fully-equipped clinical ultrasound unit (FCUS) with 3-D ultrasound capabilities [15]. Using these equations [13,14], 4 ultrasound thyroid volume measurement methods (Methods A–D) were developed, in which 13 linear and 5 cross-sectional measurements were undertaken in the dolphin thyroid study. Since serial ultrasound measurements of the dimensions of thyroid gland have been proven to be useful in identifying thyroid diseases and monitoring treatment response [1,16,17], assessment of the aforementioned dimensions of the dolphin thyroid gland is essential, in addition to the thyroid volume itself.

Access to a FCUS, as well as 3-D ultrasound equipment, may be limited at zoological and aquarium settings. Procuring a FCUS is not always feasible in most veterinary settings due to its high start-up and maintenance cost. In addition, its bulkiness makes it unfavourable in various captive animal settings. A portable ultrasound unit (PUS) equipped with basic ultrasound functions for veterinary medicine has a comparatively lower cost that is affordable for most zoological and aquarium settings. Ultrasound studies conducted in various veterinary clinical settings, as well as wildlife research projects, have been mostly performed with different PUSs [18,19]. However, the miniaturization of the PUS is believed to create compromises in function, and there are concerns regarding the image quality in these smaller and less expensive units. In view of the presently extensive applications of PUS in veterinary imaging, from being a diagnostic tool for routine clinical check-up of a range of species, to conducting disease screening, conservation projects, commercial services, herd management and clinical research, it is important to evaluate the inter-equipment variability between the PUS and FCUS in terms of direct linear measurements as well as cross-sectional areas of specific planes, which are essential parameters for volume measurement of an interested organ. In addition, the intra-operator variability (repeatability) of the individual PUS and FCUS should be further examined under the same scanning conditions to ensure accurate assessments of the thyroid size in follow-up examinations throughout the course of treatment.

The aims of the present study were to evaluate the inter-equipment variability in dolphin thyroid ultrasound linear and cross-sectional area measurements between a PUS (Aloka SSD 900) and a FCUS (Philips HD 11) under identical scanning conditions, and to assess the repeatability of these measurements using both ultrasound units.

Methods

Subjects and Study Design

Fifteen *Tursiops aduncus* at Ocean Park, Hong Kong (5 males and 10 females) were included in the study. The mean age of the subjects was 15.1 years (range, 2–35 years). Diets consisted of different proportions of capelin, sardine, herring and squid, along with vitamin and mineral supplements. The subjects were apparently healthy with no recent history of illnesses, and were not receiving medication that could alter thyroid gland physiology during the time of the study. Serum concentrations of thyroxine (free [fT4] and total [tT4]), triiodothyronine (free [fT3], total [tT3]) were also determined on each individual subject and the values were all within normal ranges [20]. All dolphins involved in the study were trained to cooperate for neck ultrasound examination. Ultrasound images from each dolphin were taken on its thyroid using a PUS Aloka SSD 900 ultrasound unit in conjunction with a 5 MHz curvilinear transducer (Aloka Company Ltd., Tokyo, Japan) and a FCUS Philips HD 11 ultrasound unit in conjunction with a 5−2 MHz broadband curved array transducer (Philips Medical System, Bothell, Washington, 98021, USA).

Technical Differences between the PUS and the FCUS

The Aloka SSD 900 ultrasound unit is a miniaturized portable general imaging ultrasound unit that provides 256 shades of gray resolution and dynamic focus. This PUS is more portable than the FCUS because of its comparatively small size and low weight (13.6 kg). Similar to the FCUS, the PUS also offers a full range of measurement functions for clinical ultrasound examinations and incorporates super high density transducers to enhance imaging resolution.

Technical details of the PUS and the FCUS that may influence the thyroid linear and cross-sectional area measurements are listed (Table 1).

Thyroid Ultrasound Imaging and Measurement

Ultrasound measurements using both units were performed by the same operator (BK) and the operator was blinded to the linear and cross-sectional area measurements obtained from both units. There was a time interval of at least 30 minutes between measurements of the 2 sets of images from the same dolphin thyroid gland. Therefore, recall bias of the results for the same dolphin thyroid gland was avoided. The operator had more than 3 years of experience in performing dolphin thyroid ultrasound examinations. Standardized scanning protocol for dolphin thyroid gland was used in the present study [15]. Four 2-D ultrasound

Table 1. Technical details of the portable ultrasound unit (PUS) and the fully-equipped clinical ultrasound unit (FCUS).

Technical details	Ultrasound Machine	
	PUS	**FCUS**
Transducer frequency (MHz)	5	5–2
Frame rate (frames per second)	max 237	max 785
Gain setting	operator defined	operator defined
Grey scale	operator defined	operator defined
Persistence setting	4 settings	7 settings
Number of depth settings	11	30
Number of focus settings	4 user-selectable focal zones	4 user-selectable focal zones
Image resolution (axial resolution)	At 5 cm depth: 1 mm; At 11 cm depth: 1 mm	At 5 cm depth: 1 mm; At 11 cm depth: 1 mm
	At 5 MHz	At 4.25 MHz (centre frequency)
Image resolution (lateral resolution)	At 5 cm depth: 2 mm; At 11 cm depth: 4 mm	At 5 cm depth: 2 mm; At 11 cm depth: 4 mm
	At 5 MHz	At 4.25 MHz (centre frequency)

thyroid volume measurement methods (Methods A–D) were developed using the ellipsoid equation [13] i.e. volume $= \pi/6 \times$ craniocaudal $\times$ mediolateral $\times$ dorsoventral dimensions; and its derivatives using the cross-sectional area is shown (Table 2) [14]. Detailed linear and cross-sectional area measurements were undertaken as described below.

Methods A and B

Once the location of the thyroid gland was identified, the transducer was then moved cranially and caudally until the scan plane showing the maximum transverse dimension of the thyroid gland (TS_MAX) was obtained and the TS_MAX was then

Table 2. Equations of each method for calculating the thyroid volume.

Method	Equation for calculation of thyroid volume
A (2-D US[f])	$\pi/6 \times$ TS_MAX[a] $\times$ mean of craniocaudal dimension in 3 planes (LS_L[b], LS_MID[c] and LS_R[d]) $\times$ mean of dorsoventral dimension in 3 planes (LS_L[b], LS_MID[c] and LS_R[d])
B (2-D US[f])	$2/3 \times$ TS_MAX[a] $\times$ mean of cross-sectional area of 3 planes (LS_L[b], LS_MID[c] and LS_R[d])
C (2-D US[f])	$\pi/6 \times$ craniocaudal $\times$ mediolateral $\times$ dorsoventral
D (2-D US[f])	$2/3 \times$ craniocaudal $\times$ maximum cross-sectional area[e]
E (3-D US[g])	Calculated by in-built software (QLAB, Philips)

[a] The maximum transverse dimension of the thyroid gland.
[b] The maximum longitudinal scan plane of the left thyroid lobe.
[c] The longitudinal scan plane of the midline of the thyroid gland.
[d] The maximum longitudinal scan plane of the right thyroid lobe.
[e] $\pi/4 \times$ mediolateral $\times$ dorsoventral.
[f] Two-dimensional ultrasound.
[g] Three-dimensional ultrasound.

measured (Figure 1). The transducer was then rotated 90°, to show the longitudinal scan planes of the thyroid gland. A full survey of the thyroid gland was performed in the longitudinal scan with the transducer moved from the left lobe to the right lobe. Images of the three longitudinal scan planes were recorded (Figures 2, 3, 4): 1. scan plane showing the midline of the thyroid gland (LS_MID); 2. scan plane showing the maximum longitudinal dimension of the left lobe (LS_L); 3. scan plane showing the maximum longitudinal dimension of the right lobe (LS_R). In each longitudinal scan plane, the dorsoventral dimension, the craniocaudal dimension, and the cross-sectional area of the thyroid lobe were measured.

Methods C and D

The transducer was initially placed obliquely on one side of the thyroid gland and then the transducer was slightly rotated clockwise and anticlockwise until the image showing the longest axis of the thyroid lobe was identified and recorded. The long axis of the thyroid lobe was then measured (Figure 5). The transducer was then rotated 90° to show the cross-sectional image of the

thyroid lobe. A full survey of the cross-sectional image of the thyroid lobe was performed by scanning from the upper to lower poles of the thyroid gland. The scan plane showing the maximum cross-sectional area of the thyroid lobe was recorded, and the dorsoventral dimension, the mediolateral diameter and the cross-sectional area of the thyroid lobe were measured (Figure 6). The same scanning protocol was repeated for the contralateral thyroid lobe.

During the thyroid scanning with each ultrasound unit, time-gain-compensation and depth settings were adjusted to optimize image quality. For both ultrasound units, all measurements were performed using the electronic calipers. For the Aloka SSD 900 ultrasound unit, all images were recorded onto thermal printing paper, scanned and stored into digital format, while the images obtained by the Philips HD 11 were captured and stored digitally.

Statistical Analysis

To analyze the inter-equipment variability of both ultrasound units, different thyroid ultrasound linear and cross-sectional area

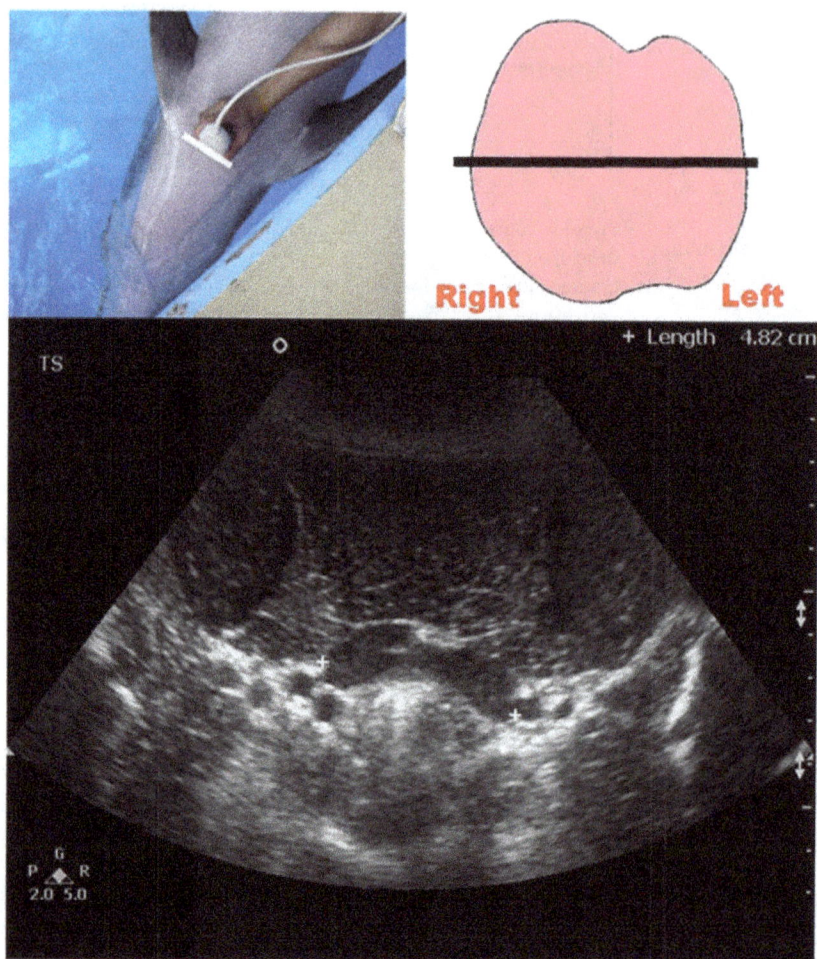

Figure 1. Ultrasound measurement of the maximum transverse dimension of the dolphin thyroid gland (TS_MAX). Top left picture shows the position of the transducer at the neck region. Top right picture shows the schematic diagram of the thyroid gland in a dorsal orientation with the straight line representing the position of the transducer. Bottom image shows a transverse grey scale sonogram of the thyroid gland of a bottlenose dolphin. Note the maximum transverse dimension of the thyroid gland is measured (calipers +).

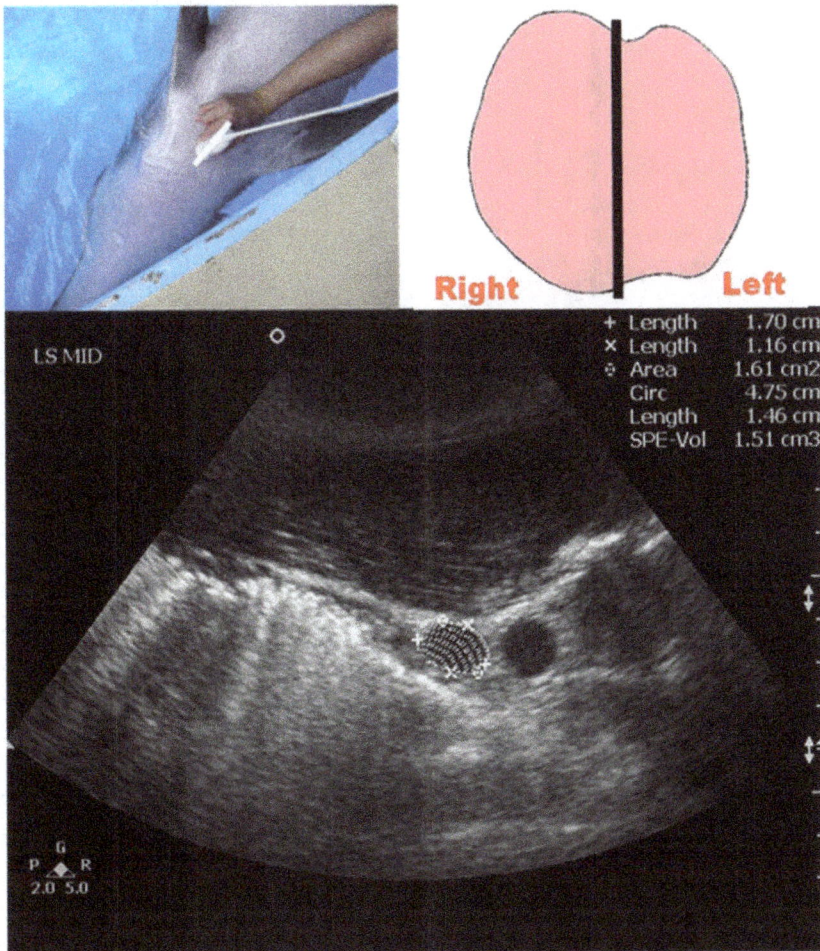

Figure 2. Ultrasound measurement of the longitudinal dimension of the dolphin thyroid gland at the midline (LS_MID). Top left picture shows the position of the transducer at the neck region. Top right picture shows the schematic diagram of the thyroid gland in a dorsal orientation with the straight line representing the position of the transducer. Bottom image shows a longitudinal grey scale sonogram of the thyroid gland of a bottlenose dolphin. Note the dorsoventral dimension (calipers x), the craniocaudal dimension (calipers +) and the cross-sectional area (dotted line) are measured respectively.

measurements were assessed by the intraclass correlation coefficient (ICC) and 95% confidence intervals (C.I.). In order to evaluate the intra-operator variability (repeatability) of the different thyroid ultrasound linear and cross-sectional area measurements, intraclass correlation coefficient (ICC) and 95% C.I. were also used to assess the level of agreement of the measurements in a single operator (BK). An ICC>0.7 is commonly used to indicate sufficient general reliability [21,22]. All statistical analyses were carried out using SPSS (SPSS for windows 16.0, SPSS Inc., Chicago, Illinois).

This study was licensed under the Animals Control of Experiments Ordinance, Cap 340, issued by the Department of Health of Hong Kong Special Administrative Region. All procedures were reviewed and approved by the Animal Subjects Ethics Sub-committee of the Hong Kong Polytechnic University and the Scientific Advisory Committee of Ocean Park Hong Kong.

Results

The inter-equipment variability of the different thyroid ultrasound linear and cross-sectional area measurements is

shown (Table 3). Overall, the ICC was 0.964 with 95% C.I. range of 0.889–0.988. Results demonstrated that the ICC values of all measurements were above 0.85, indicating correlations of over 85% between both ultrasound units. The cross-sectional area measurements yielded a higher inter-equipment reproducibility than the linear measurements. Overall, both ultrasound units yielded a high level of agreement in different thyroid ultrasound linear and cross-sectional area measurements.

The intra-operator variability (repeatability) of using the 2 ultrasound units in thyroid ultrasound linear and cross-sectional area measurements is shown (Table 4). Overall, the ICC was 0.974 with 95% C.I. range of 0.925–0.991 for the PUS and 0.962 with 95% C.I. range of 0.891–0.987 for the FCUS. The cross-sectional area measurements yielded a higher intra-operator repeatability than the linear measurements. Results demonstrated that both ultrasound units yielded a high intra-operator repeatability for all thyroid ultrasound linear and cross-sectional area measurements. Compared to the FCUS, the PUS showed a higher repeatability.

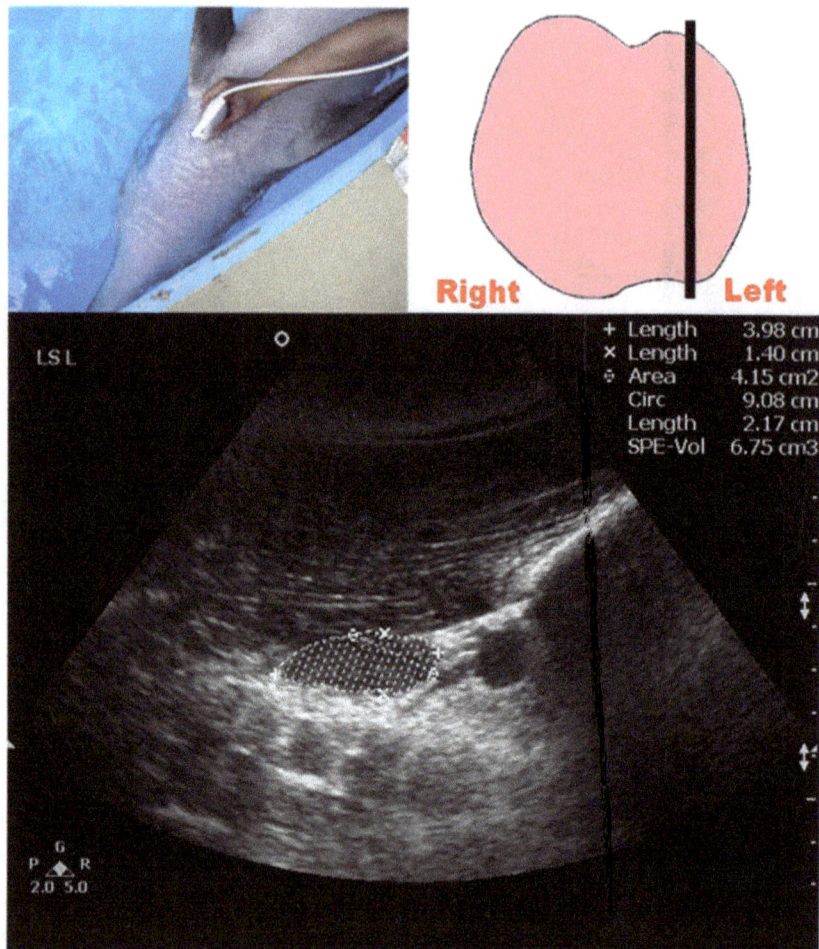

Figure 3. Ultrasound measurement of the maximum longitudinal dimension of the left thyroid lobe of a dolphin (LS_L). Top left picture shows the position of the transducer at the neck region. Top right picture shows the schematic diagram of the thyroid gland in a dorsal orientation with the straight line representing the position of the transducer. Bottom image shows a longitudinal grey scale sonogram of the left thyroid lobe of a bottlenose dolphin. Note the maximum longitudinal dimension of the left thyroid lobe is demonstrated, and the dorsoventral dimension (calipers x), the craniocaudal dimension (calipers +) and the cross-sectional area (dotted line) are measured respectively. The same ultrasound measurement of the maximum longitudinal dimension was repeated on the right thyroid lobe.

Discussion

Ultrasound is considered as a safe, non-invasive and well-tolerated imaging method in non-sedated animals [19]. Diagnostic ultrasound enables serial examinations to monitor the progress of clinical condition and treatment response. The results of the present study demonstrated that ultrasound is an effective and reliable tool for measuring thyroid parameters. To the best of our knowledge, there has been no previous research investigating dolphin thyroid measurements using 2 different ultrasound machines, therefore the current study reflects the potential of detecting changes that exceed measurement error, for clinical and research applications.

There was a high level of agreement between the 2 ultrasound units in dolphin thyroid measurements, with the ICC values ranging from 0.859 to 0.976. Theoretically, the reproducibility (ICC) has a maximum value of 1. In most papers, a reproducibility of 0.7 and higher for labeling methods or units is considered to be sufficient [21,22]. Thus, the results supported a high degree of

agreement between the PUS and FCUS to quantify dolphin thyroid volume.

Results of the present study demonstrated that both the PUS and FCUS had a high intra-operator repeatability in thyroid measurements, with the ICC values of the PUS ranging from 0.854 to 0.984, and the ICC values of the FCUS ranging from 0.709 to 0.954. These results supported that the measurements yielded by the PUS are not only comparable to that of the FCUS, but that each unit can be used to perform thyroid volume measurements in a consistent manner.

Overall, the inter-equipment and intra-operator variability was minimal due to a number of reasons. The presence of a well-defined capsulated thyroid gland improved visualization on ultrasound scanning, enabling a higher precision while performing linear and cross-sectional area measurements. Since the dolphin thyroid gland was situated at the thoracic inlet, midway between the insertions of the pectoral flippers, this minimized measurement variation caused by the effect of physiological activity such as heart beats and breathing during the scan. In the present study, a standard scanning protocol for the four 2-D ultrasound thyroid

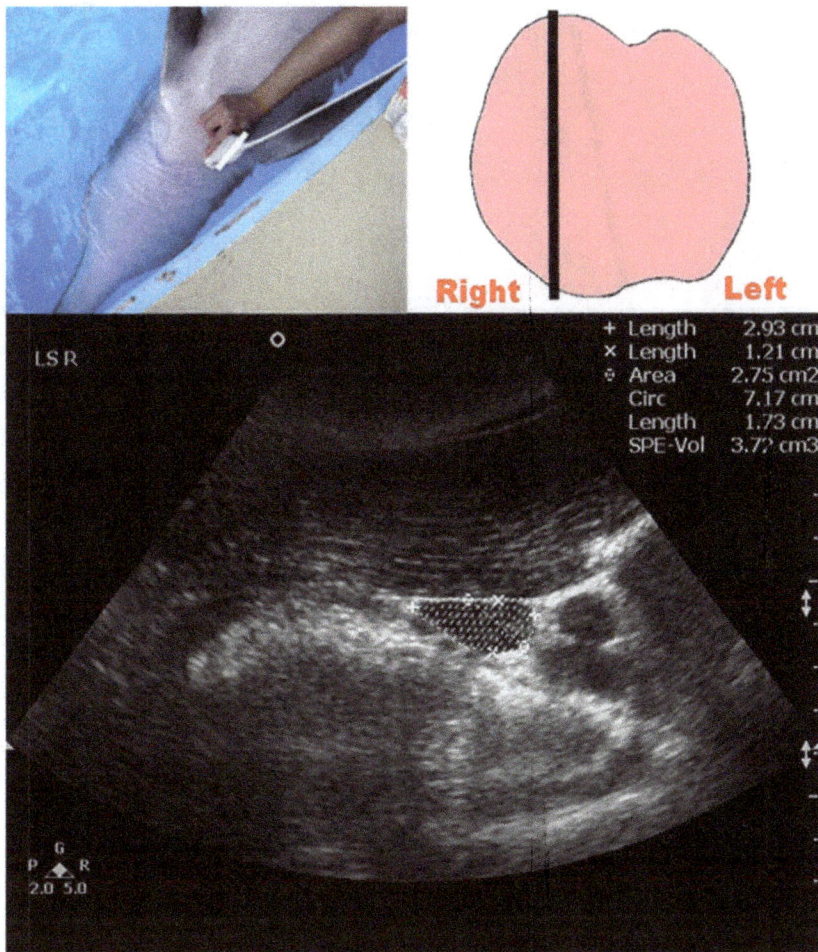

Figure 4. Ultrasound measurement of the maximum longitudinal dimension of the right thyroid lobe of a dolphin (LS_R). Top left picture shows the position of the transducer at the neck region. Top right picture shows the schematic diagram of the thyroid gland in a dorsal orientation with the straight line representing the position of the transducer. Bottom image shows a longitudinal grey scale sonogram of the right thyroid lobe of a bottlenose dolphin. Note the maximum longitudinal dimension of the right thyroid lobe is demonstrated, and the dorsoventral dimension (calipers x), the craniocaudal dimension (calipers +) and the cross-sectional area (dotted line) are measured respectively.

volume measurement methods was implemented, allowing the operator to have a clear and a precise sense of the procedures, facilitating the consistency of measurements during the ultrasound scanning. A single operator performed the present study enabling familiarity and greater experience with the established protocol. All dolphins involved in the study were trained to cooperate for neck ultrasound examination in a dorsal recumbence position, with their neck straightened and remaining still at the poolside. This prevented the distortion of the thyroid gland and thus allowed higher consistency with measurements during the ultrasound scanning.

These findings are in accordance with the results of the previous *in vivo* and *in vitro* studies which have incorporated ICC as a statistical test to assess agreement. A high correlation in the inter-operator and intra-operator measurements of the mean splenic length (ICC value of 0.89 and 0.94) has been previously identified [23]; similarly, a high correlation was also demonstrated in the inter-operator and intra-operator measurements of the cross-sectional area of the tibial nerve at the tarsal tunnel (ICC values ≥ 0.86) [24]. For inter-equipment variability, previous studies reported that measures obtained using both PUS and FCUS were not significantly different and were equally repeatable [25–27]. However, the direct comparisons must be treated with caution. Our present study focused on the agreement between the 2 compared ultrasound units, rather than the accuracy of the portable ultrasound unit itself. Comparison of dolphin thyroid volume measurement accuracy using the 2 captioned ultrasound units is not possible due to the lack of a standard of reference. In our previous study, 3-D ultrasound thyroid volume measured by the FCUS was compared with the 2-D ultrasound thyroid volume measurement with the identical ultrasound unit and settings [15]. 3-D ultrasound thyroid volume measurements cannot be used as the standard of reference in the present study, since 3-D ultrasound is a functional capability of the FCUS. The PUS measurements have a substantially different image quality, and thus would result in a bias in favour of the FCUS measurements. As such, instead of looking into the accuracy of both ultrasound units on their own, the present study investigated the agreement between these 2 ultrasound units (with the FCUS measurement accuracy validated in our previous study).

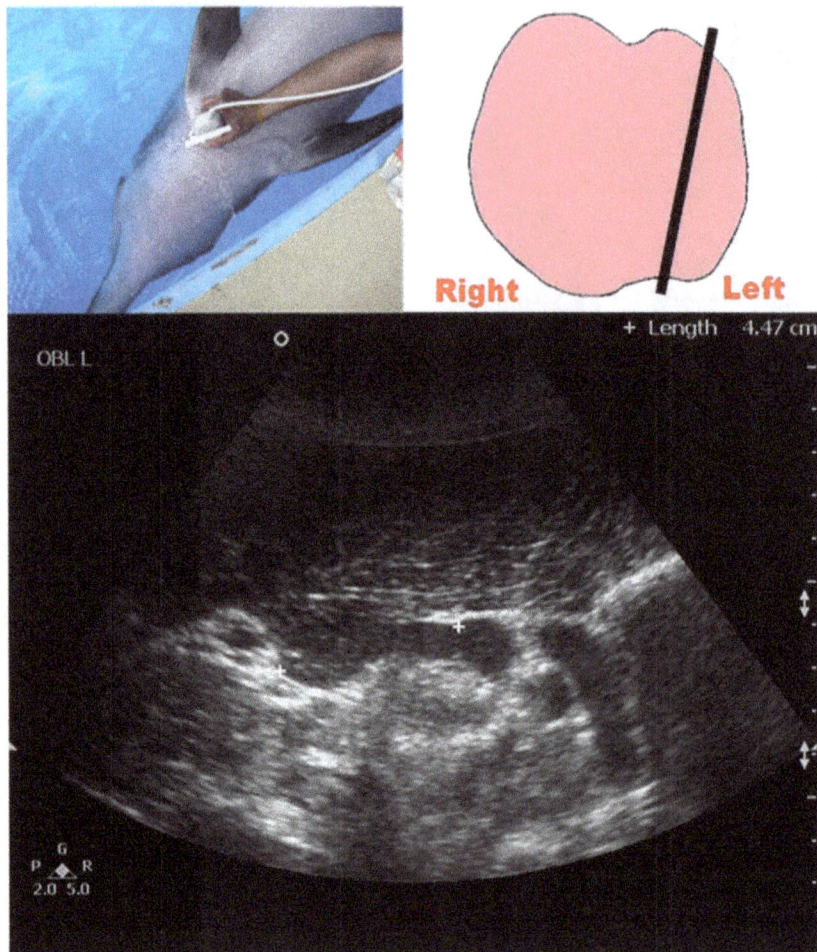

Figure 5. Ultrasound measurement of the long axis of the left thyroid lobe of a dolphin. Top left picture shows the position of the transducer at the neck region. Top right picture shows the schematic diagram of the thyroid gland in a dorsal orientation with the straight line representing the position of the transducer. Bottom image shows an oblique grey scale sonogram of the left thyroid lobe of a bottlenose dolphin. Note the long axis of the left thyroid lobe is measured (calipers +).

In the present study, the PUS yielded a higher intra-operator repeatability than the FCUS. Compared to the FCUS, the PUS has less precise calipers, limiting the measurements to 1 decimal place. In contrast, the FCUS gives the measurements to 2 decimal places, making it less prone to rounding error. This may give the PUS a higher intra-operator repeatability since the measurements had a higher degree of estimation with more measurements demonstrating absolute agreement.

The cross-sectional area measurements were found to have a higher inter-equipment reproducibility and intra-operator repeatability than that of the linear measurements. In a previous study, the cross-sectional area measurements of custom-made tissue phantoms had a higher inter- and intra-operator reliability than the linear measurements [28]. Additionally, the inter-operator variability for calculating thyroid volume was found to be statistically significant when using the formula with linear measurements, but was not statistically significant when using the formula with cross-sectional area measurements [14]. In the present study, for Methods A and B, the maximum cross-sectional area measurements from all 3 maximum longitudinal dimension scan planes yielded a higher reliability than the linear measurements (craniocaudal and

dorsoventral dimensions). However, there may be difficulties in consistently estimating the linear measurements on the maximum longitudinal dimension scan plan between the 2 ultrasound scans. Since the thyroid gland was not a true oval shaped structure for the measurement on the longitudinal planes in Methods A and B and the transverse planes in Methods C and D, the determination of maximum long axis dimension was highly subjective, which possibly resulted in a larger variation on the linear measurements. In contrast, the determination of the maximum cross-sectional area relied on manual free-hand tracing of the thyroid borders, which was considered to be a relatively easier and more straight-forward procedure, resulting in a higher reproducibility and repeatability on the measurements. The same issues applied for Methods C and D, in which the maximum cross-sectional area measurements in the scan plane 90 degrees to the craniocaudal dimension also yielded a higher reliability than the linear measurements (mediolateral and dorsoventral dimensions). Moreover, it is possible that there are different measurements of the craniocaudal and dorsoventral dimensions on the same image plane; however, the cross-sectional area based on the same image plane would not change, resulting in a higher reliability than the linear measurements.

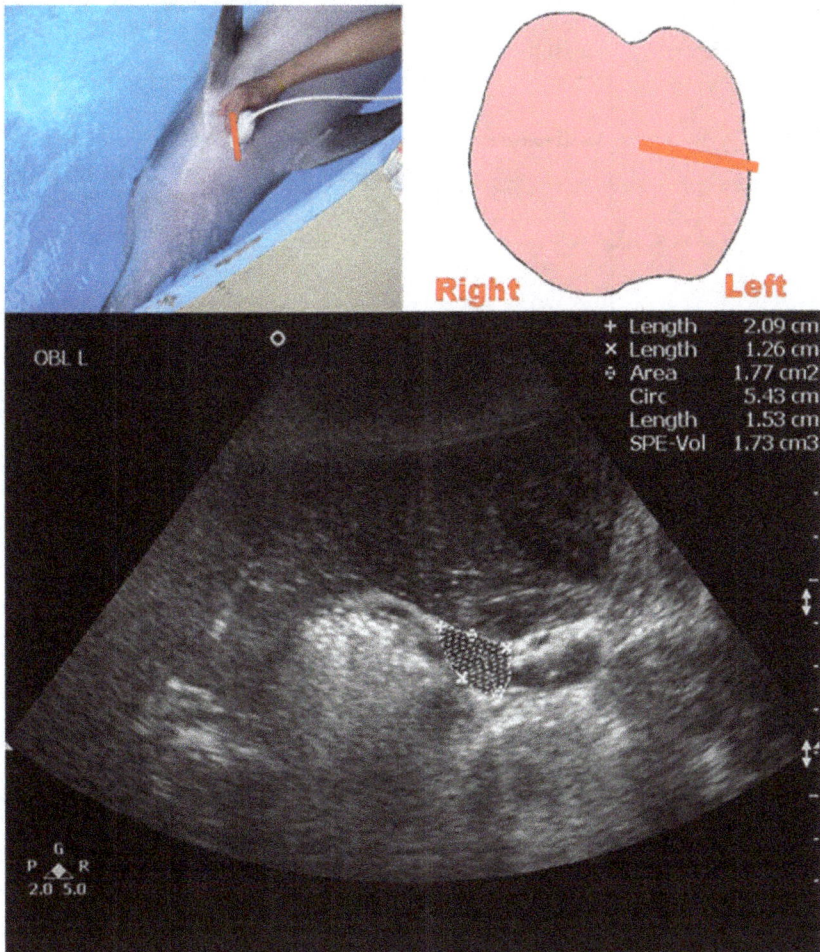

Figure 6. Ultrasound measurement of the maximum cross-sectional area of the left thyroid lobe of a dolphin. Top left picture shows the position of the transducer at the neck region. Top right picture shows the schematic diagram of the thyroid gland in a dorsal orientation with the straight line representing the position of the transducer. Bottom image shows an oblique grey scale sonogram of the left thyroid lobe of a bottlenose dolphin. Note the maximum cross-sectional area of the left thyroid lobe is demonstrated, and the dorsoventral dimension (calipers x), the mediolateral dimension (calipers +) and the cross-sectional area (dotted line) are measured respectively.

Even though this study has the undeniable merit of offering valuable insight into the agreement between the PUS and the FCUS in the application of dolphin thyroid measurements, there are some limitations. Due to the limited availability of multiple units, the number of unit representing in each category (PUS and FCUS) for comparison was restricted to one only. It may alter the results yielded using different units. Further studies in investigating the agreement with multiple units representing each category are suggested to minimize the intrinsic differences in the compared units. The transducers of the compared units were not in the identical frequency range. This is virtually unattainable since the FCUS in this study utilizes the latest transducer technology, which provides a broad range of frequencies rather than a single frequency emitted by the PUS compatible transducer. Image resolution may be degraded due to the frequency differences, and thus may affect the measurement accuracy. To minimize this difference in technology, the transducer frequency of the FCUS was set to the "middle to high" range between 5–2 MHz, which should be comparable to the 5 MHz used in the PUS transducer. With broad bandwidth transducers used in FCUS unit, the manipula-tion of transmit frequency bandwidth and received frequency bandwidth was allowed, which facilitated the operator to optimize image data to match the target requirement. 'Middle to high' frequency on the 5–2 MHz transducer of the FCUS unit was equivalent to 4.25 MHz centre frequency (3.5–5 MHz operational sensitivity). In addition, the issue of image quality comparison between the captioned ultrasound units had not been mentioned in the present study. According to a previous study, the image quality is undoubtedly a component of the diagnostic ability of a system, but is only one facet in determining an optimal system [29]. Although we believe that the measurement accuracy may possibly be affected by the different image quality yielded, the degree of influence should be insignificant in our case, due to the presence of a well-defined capsulated thyroid gland in the dolphin which allows for an accurate linear measurement on different thyroid dimensions. Despite the controversy in objectively defining the image quality [30,31], there is no doubt that differential diagnosis was confirmed when a more advanced clinical ultrasound unit was used, which inevitably produced higher quality ultrasound images for clinical diagnosis. Studies have

Table 3. Inter-equipment variability of the ultrasound thyroid linear and cross-sectional area measurements.

Measurement	ICC[k] (2,1)	95% C.I.[l] of ICC[k] (Lower - Upper)
Max TS[a]	0.969	0.896–0.990
L LS[b] (H[h])	0.907	0.752–0.967
L LS[b] (W[i])	0.915	0.766–0.971
L LS[b] (CSA[j])	0.934	0.821–0.977
Mid LS[c] (H[h])	0.939	0.829–0.979
Mid LS[c] (W[i])	0.938	0.801–0.980
Mid LS[c] (CSA[j])	0.976	0.894–0.993
R LS[d] (H[h])	0.958	0.818–0.987
R LS[d] (W[i])	0.933	0.813–0.977
R LS[d] (CSA[j])	0.949	0.648–0.987
L Obl[e] (L[g])	0.943	0.819–0.981
L Obl[e] (H[h])	0.936	0.824–0.978
L Obl[e] (W[i])	0.877	0.677–0.957
L Obl[e] (CSA[j])	0.949	0.859–0.982
R Obl[f] (L[g])	0.924	0.796–0.974
R Obl[f] (H[h])	0.859	0.638–0.950
R Obl[f] (W[i])	0.925	0.758–0.976
R Obl[f] (CSA[j])	0.959	0.884–0.986

[a]The maximum transverse dimension of the thyroid gland.
[b]The maximum longitudinal scan plane of the left thyroid lobe.
[c]The longitudinal scan plane of the left thyroid lobe.
[d]The maximum longitudinal scan plane of the right thyroid lobe.
[e]The oblique scan plane of the left thyroid lobe.
[f]The oblique scan plane of the right thyroid lobe.
[g]Length; craniocaudal dimension.
[h]Height; dorsoventral dimension.
[i]Width; mediolateral dimension.
[j]Cross-sectional area.
[k]Intraclass Correlation Coefficient.
[l]Confidence Interval.

Table 4. Intra-operator (repeatability) variability of the ultrasound thyroid linear and cross-sectional area measurements.

Measurement	PUS[m]		FCUS[n]	
	ICC[k] (3,1)	95% C.I.[l] of ICC[k] (Lower - Upper)	ICC[k] (3,1)	95% C.I.[l] of ICC[k] (Lower - Upper)
Max TS[a]	0.974	0.924–0.991	0.954	0.870–0.984
L LS[b] (H[h])	0.949	0.854–0.982	0.722	0.351–0.897
L LS[b] (W[i])	0.890	0.705–0.962	0.863	0.640–0.952
L LS[b] (CSA[j])	0.927	0.797–0.975	0.904	0.738–0.967
Mid LS[c] (H[h])	0.965	0.900–0.988	0.856	0.624–0.949
Mid LS[c] (W[i])	0.914	0.765–0.970	0.835	0.577–0.941
Mid LS[c] (CSA[j])	0.981	0.945–0.994	0.884	0.691–0.960
R LS[d] (H[h])	0.973	0.921–0.991	0.887	0.697–0.961
R LS[d] (W[i])	0.854	0.619–0.948	0.851	0.613–0.947
R LS[d] (CSA[j])	0.974	0.925–0.991	0.951	0.861–0.983
L Obl[e] (L[g])	0.984	0.952–0.994	0.867	0.650–0.953
L Obl[e] (H[h])	0.934	0.815–0.977	0.898	0.724–0.964
L Obl[e] (W[i])	0.928	0.800–0.975	0.878	0.676–0.957
L Obl[e] (CSA[j])	0.956	0.873–0.985	0.928	0.799–0.875
R Obl[f] (L[g])	0.950	0.857–0.983	0.939	0.829–0.979
R Obl[f] (H[h])	0.930	0.806–0.976	0.709	0.327–0.892
R Obl[f] (W[i])	0.896	0.720–0.964	0.802	0.508–0.929
R Obl[f] (CSA[j])	0.975	0.927–0.992	0.851	0.614–0.948

[a]The maximum transverse dimension of the thyroid gland.
[b]The maximum longitudinal scan plane of the left thyroid lobe.
[c]The longitudinal scan plane of the left thyroid lobe.
[d]The maximum longitudinal scan plane of the right thyroid lobe.
[e]The oblique scan plane of the left thyroid lobe.
[f]The oblique scan plane of the right thyroid lobe.
[g]Length; craniocaudal dimension.
[h]Height; dorsoventral dimension.
[i]Width; mediolateral dimension.
[j]Cross-sectional area.
[k]Intraclass Correlation Coefficient.
[l]Confidence Interval.
[m]Portable ultrasound unit.
[n]Fully-equipped clinical ultrasound unit.

suggested that PUS provides a significant benefit that can drastically alter the disposition and treatment in patients at Accident and Emergency Departments, Intensive Care Units, small-scale hospitals and remote location settings [30,32–34]. In view of the concerns raised from zoological and aquarium settings, a PUS could play an adequate role in improving a variety of veterinary procedures by providing a real-time, non-invasive clinical tool. Further studies in objectively evaluating the difference in image quality between the PUS and the FCUS in a zoological or aquarium setting are suggested to reinforce confidence of using PUS in veterinary medicine.

Conclusions

There was no substantial inter-equipment variability between PUS and FCUS in thyroid size measurements. Both systems had high intra-operator repeatability in thyroid size measurements, substantiating further application of PUS for quantitative analyses of dolphin thyroid gland in research and clinical practice at an aquarium setting, when FCUS is not available.

Acknowledgments

The authors thank the Marine Mammal Department of Ocean Park, Hong Kong for dolphin training and husbandry and Ocean Park Corporation for support of this project. Special thanks to Mr. Winson K. Chan for his editing of the revised manuscript.

Author Contributions

Conceived and designed the experiments: BCWK MTCY FMB. Performed the experiments: BCWK. Analyzed the data: BCWK. Contributed reagents/materials/analysis tools: BCWK. Wrote the paper: BCWK.

References

1. AIUM (2003) Practice Guideline for the performance of thyroid and parathyroid ultrasound examination. J Ultrasound Med 22: 1126–1130.

2. Hegedüs L (2001) Thyroid ultrasound. Endocrinol Metab Clin North Am 30: 339–360.

3. Khati N, Adamson T, Johnson KS, Hill MC (2003) Ultrasound of the thyroid and parathyroid glands. Ultrasound Q 19: 162–176.

4. Brömel C, Pollard RE, Kass PH, Samii VF, Davidson AP, et al. (2006) Comparison of ultrasonographic characteristics of the thyroid gland in healthy small-, medium-, and large-breed dogs. Am J Vet Res 67: 70–77.

5. Cartee RE, Finn Bodner ST, Gray BW (1993) Ultrasound examination of feline thyroid. JDMS 9: 323–326.

6. Reese S, Breyer U, Deeg C, Kraft W, Kaspers B (2005) Thyroid sonography as an effective tool to discriminate between euthyroid sick and hypothyroid dogs. J Vet Intern Med 19: 491–498.

7. Wisner ER, Mattoon JS, Nyland TG (2002) Neck. In: Nyland TG, Mattoon JS, eds. Small Animal Diagnostic Ultrasound. 2nd ed. Philadelphia: Saunders. pp 285–292.

8. Cowan DF, Tajima Y (2006) The thyroid gland in bottlenose dolphins (*Tursiops truncatus*) from the Texas Coast of the Gulf of Mexico: Normal structure and pathological changes. J Comp Pathol 135: 217–225.

9. Das K, Vossen A, Tolley K, Vikingsson G, Thron K, et al. (2006) Interfollicular fibrosis in the thyroid of the harbour porpoise: An endocrine disruption? Arch Environ Contam Toxicol 51: 720–729.

10. Mikaelian I, Labelle P, Kopal M, Dr Guise S, Martineau D (2003) Adenomatous hyperplasia of the thyroid gland in beluga whales (*Delphinapterus leucas*) from the St. Lawrence estuary and Hudson Bay, Quebec, Canada. Vet Pathol 40: 698–703.

11. Schumacher U, Zahler S, Heidemann G, Skirinisson K (1993) Histological investigations on the thyroid glands of marine mammals and the possible implications of marine pollution. J Wildl Dis 29: 103–108.

12. Garner MM, Shwetz C, Ramer JC, Rasmussen JM, Petrini K, et al. (2002) Congenital diffuse hyperplastic goiter associated with perinatal mortality in 11 captive-born bottlenose dolphins (*Tursiops truncatus*). J Zoo Wildl Med 33: 350–355.

13. Brunn J, Block U, Ruf G, Bos I, Kunze WP, et al. (1981) Volumetric analysis of thyroid lobes by real-time ultrasound. Dtsch Med Wochenschr 106: 1338–1340.

14. Shabana W, Peeters E, Verbeek P, Osteaux MM (2003) Reducing inter-observer variation in thyroid volume calculation using a new formula and technique. Eur J Ultrasound 16: 207–210.

15. Kot BCW, Ying MTC, Brook FM, Kinoshita RE (2011) Evaluation of 2-D and 3-D ultrasound in the assessment of the thyroid volume of the Indo-Pacific Bottlenose dolphin, *Tursiops aduncus*. J Zoo Wildl Med;In press.

16. Kot BCW, Ying MTC, Brook FM, Kinoshita RE, Cheng SCH, et al. (2011) Sonographic imaging of the thyroid gland and adjacent neck structures of the Indo-Pacific bottlenose dolphin, *Tursiops aduncus*. Am J Vet Res;In press.

17. Kot BCW, Ying MTC, Brook FM, Kinoshita RE, Dave K, et al. (2011) Sonographic evaluation of thyroid morphology during different reproductive events in female Indo-Pacific bottlenose dolphins, *Tursiops aduncus*. Mar Mamm Sci;In press.

18. Adams GP, Ward Testa J, Goertz CEC, Ream RR (2007) Ultrasonographic characterization of reproductive anatomy and early embryonic detection in the northern fur seal (*Callorhinus ursinus*) in the field. Mar Mamm Sci 23: 445–452.

19. King AM (2006) Development, advances and applications of diagnostic ultrasound in animals. Vet J 171: 408–420.

20. St. Aubin DJ (2001) Endocrinolgoy. In: Dieranf JA, Gulland FMD, eds. CRC Handbook of Marine Mammal Medicine. Boca Raton: CRC Press. pp 165–192.

21. Chien PFW, Khan KS (2001) Evaluation of a clinical test. II: Assessment of validity. Br J Obstet Gynaecol 108: 568–572.

22. Khan KS, Chien PFW (2001) Evaluation of a clinical test. I: Assessment of reliability. Br J Obstet Gynaecol 108: 562–567.

23. Li PS, Ying M, Chan KH, Chan PW, Chu KL (2004) The reproducibility and short-term and long-term repeatability of sonographic measurement of splenic length. Ultrasound Med Biol 30: 861–866.

24. Alshami A, Cairns C, Wylie B, Souvlis T, Coppieters M (2009) Reliability and size of the measurement error when determining the cross-sectional area of the tibial nerve at the tarsal tunnel with ultrasonography. Ultrasound Med Biol 35: 1098–1102.

25. Hing WA, Rome K, Cameron AFM (2009) Reliability of measuring abductor hallucis muscle parameters using two different diagnostic ultrasound machines. J Foot Ankle Res 2: 33–40.

26. Legerlotz K, Smith HK, Hing WA (2010) Variation and reliability of ultrasonographic quantification of the architecture of the medial gastrocnemius muscle in young children. Clin Physiol Funct Imaging 30: 198–205.

27. Magnussen CG, Fryer J, Venn A, Laakkonen M, Raitakari OT (2006) Evaluating the use of a portable ultrasound machine to quantify intima-media thickness and flow-mediated dilation: agreement between measurements from two ultrasound machines. Ultrasound Med Biol 32: 1323–1329.

28. Warner MB, Cotton AM, Stokes MJ (2008) Comparison of curvilinear and linear ultrasound imaging probes for measuring cross-sectional area and linear dimensions. J Med Eng Technol 32: 498–504.

29. Rosenthal MS (2005) Characterization of image system performance via diagnostic accuracy. Acad Emerg Med 12: 176–177.

30. Blaivas M, Brannam L, Theodoro D (2004) Ultrasound image quality comparison between an inexpensive handheld emergency department (ED) ultrasound machine and a large mobile ED ultrasound system. Acad Emerg Med 11: 778–781.

31. Shrimali V, Anand RS, Kumar V, Srivastav RK (2009) Medical feature based evaluation of structuring elements for morphological enhancement of ultrasonic images. J Med Eng Technol 33: 158–169.

32. Blaivas M, Kuhn W, Reynolds B, Brannam L (2005) Change in differential diagnosis and patient management with the use of portable ultrasound in a remote setting. Wilderness Environ Med 16: 38–41.

33. Ryan SM, Smith E, Sidhu PS (2002) Comparison of the SonoSite and Acuson 128/XP10 ultrasound machines in the 'bed-side' assessment of the post liver transplant patient. Eur J Ultrasound 15: 37–43.

34. Stamilio DM, McReynolds T, Endrizzi J, Lyons RC (2004) Diagnosis and treatment of a ruptured ectopic pregnancy in a combat support hospital during Operation Iraqi Freedom: case report and critique of a field-ready sonographic device. Mil Med 169: 681–683.

14

Longitudinal Study on Methicillin-Resistant *Staphylococcus pseudintermedius* in Households

Laura M. Laarhoven[1], Phebe de Heus[1], Jeanine van Luijn[1], Birgitta Duim[1], Jaap A. Wagenaar[1,2], Engeline van Duijkeren[1,3]*

1 Department of Infectious Diseases and Immunology, Faculty of Veterinary Medicine, Utrecht University, Utrecht, The Netherlands, 2 Central Veterinary Institute of Wageningen UR, Lelystad, The Netherlands, 3 Laboratory for Zoonoses and Environmental Microbiology, National Institute of Public Health and the Environment, Bilthoven, The Netherlands

Abstract

Methicillin-resistant *Staphylococcus pseudintermedius* (MRSP) is an emerging pathogen in dogs and has been found in Europe, Asia and North America. To date most studies are one-point prevalence studies and therefore little is known about the dynamics of MRSP in dogs and their surrounding. In this longitudinal study MRSP colonization in dogs and the transmission of MRSP to humans, contact animals and the environment was investigated. Sixteen dogs with a recent clinical MRSP infection were included. The index dogs, contact animals, owners and environments were sampled once a month for six months. Samples taken from the nose, perineum and infection site (if present) of the index cases and contact animals, and the nares of the owners were cultured using pre-enrichment. Index cases were found positive for prolonged periods of time, in two cases during all six samplings. In five of the 12 households that were sampled during six months, the index case was intermittently found MRSP-positive. Contact animals and the environment were also found MRSP-positive, most often in combination with a MRSP-positive index dog. In four households positive environmental samples were found while no animals or humans were MRSP-positive, indicating survival of MRSP in the environment for prolonged periods of time. Genotyping revealed that generally similar or indistinguishable MRSP isolates were found in patients, contact animals and environmental samples within the same household. Within two households, however, genetically distinct MRSP isolates were found. These results show that veterinarians should stay alert with (former) MRSP patients, even after repeated MRSP-negative cultures or after the disappearance of the clinical infection. There is a considerable risk of transmission of MRSP to animals in close contact with MRSP patients. Humans were rarely MRSP-positive and never tested MRSP-positive more than once suggesting occasional contamination or rapid elimination of colonization of the owners.

Editor: Tara C. Smith, University of Iowa, United States of America

Funding: This study was supported by a grant from the Royal Dutch Veterinary Association. The funders had no role in study design, data collection and analysis, decision to publish, or preparation of the manuscript.

Competing Interests: The authors have declared that no competing interests exist.

* E-mail: Engeline.van.duijkeren@rivm.nl

Introduction

Methicillin-resistant *Staphylococcus pseudintermedius* (MRSP) has recently emerged as a significant pathogen in companion animals [1]. Most infections caused by MRSP are skin infections such as pyoderma. Other infections such as otitis externa, (surgical) wound infections and urinary tract infections can also be associated with MRSP [1–4]. The predominant clone circulating in Europe with sequence type (ST) 71 often contains genes that confer resistance to multiple antimicrobials routinely used in small animal practice [5]. Human infections with MRSP have been described; however, this is very uncommon [6–9]. The prevalence of MRSP has recently been studied in various dog populations [2,10–12]. Rates vary widely among dogs in the community, 1.5%–4.5%, and among dogs at veterinary clinics, 2.1%–30% [10,11,13,14,15]. These cross-sectional studies have shown that MRSP is distributed worldwide. However, these studies only provide information from a single sampling. Little is known about the persistence of MRSP in dogs and their surrounding, including the humans and animals in close contact with the MRSP patient. It is often unclear if dogs or humans are actually colonized persistently or transiently or merely contaminated with MRSP. Investigations into long-term colonization with MRSP in dogs and humans are lacking, but are essential for the differentiation between short-term and long-term colonization and for a better understanding of the transmission of MRSP and the subsequent development of infection control measurements. The objectives of this study were to evaluate longitudinally MRSP colonization in dogs and to study the transmission to humans, contact animals and the environment.

Materials and Methods

Study design

Dogs with a recent clinical MRSP infection, which had been diagnosed at the Veterinary Microbiological Diagnostic Centre (VMDC), the Netherlands, between September 2009 and January 2010, were included in the study. During this period 27 patients had been identified at the VMDC and the owners were contacted after permission from their veterinarian. Sixteen (59%) owners agreed that their dogs, contact animals and the household members could be included. The main reason for owners to deny participation was that their veterinarian was not willing to participate in the study. Since March 2010, within seven months of the initial diagnosis of MRSP infection, the index cases, contact animals, owners and environment were sampled once a month for six months. Sampling was approved by the Medical Ethical Committee of Utrecht University (METC 09-399/C) and the Experimental Animal Committee (DEC 2009.II.10.093). All participants completed a written informed consent.

Sampling

Nasal and perineum swabs were taken each month from the index case and contact animals using a sterile cotton-wool swab (Cultiplast ®). If the index case had clinical signs of an infection, an additional swab was taken from the site of infection (e.g., the vertical ear canal or a skin lesion).

In addition, nasal swabs were taken from the owners and other household members.

In each household, three samples from the environment were taken each month using moist wipes (Sodibox, s1 kit Ringer's solution, France). These environmental wipes were taken from the sleeping place of the index case, the feeding place and one site not physically accessible to the animals, i.e. above a door or on a cabinet. A surface of approximately 20×20 cm was sampled. Each wipe was taken wearing new sterile gloves to prevent cross-contamination. First and last samples were taken by the researcher. The other samples were taken by the owners or the veterinarian and sent to the laboratory.

Microbiological analysis and genotyping

The swabs and wipes were analyzed individually using a pre-enrichment containing Mueller Hinton broth with 6.5% sodium chloride [16]. After overnight incubation at 37°C, 1 ml of the pre-enrichment was transferred into 9 ml selective enrichment of phenyl red mannitol broth with 75 mg/L aztreonam and 5 mg/L ceftizoxime (bioMérieux, Marcy-'l Etoile, France). After overnight incubation at 37°C, 10 µl of the selective enrichment broth was inoculated onto sheep blood agar (Biotrading, The Netherlands). Suspected colonies were identified as members of the *Staphylococcus intermedius* group (SIG) using standard techniques including colony morphology, tests for catalase, coagulase and API ID32 Staph (bioMérieux). *S. pseudintermedius* isolates were identified using PCR-restriction fragment length polymorphism (RFLP) assay based on the *Mbo*I-digestion pattern of a PCR-amplified internal fragment of the *pta* gene as described [17]. In addition, isolates were tested for the *mecA* gene [18]. The index dogs and contact animals were classified as MRSP-positive when one or more samples from the animal were MRSP-positive.

From each household the first and last MRSP isolates from the index case, the contact animal, the owner and the environment, if present, were genotyped. The MRSP isolates were typed with multilocus sequence typing (MLST), pulsed-field gel electrophoresis (PFGE), *spa* typing and SCC*mec* typing as previously described [19-24]. MLST targeting four genes: *agrD*, *cpn60*, *pta* and *tuf* was performed. The allele numbers and sequence types (ST) were assigned by comparison to allele sequences present in the NCBI nucleotide database and using the key table for MLST typing of *Staphylococcus intermedius* group (SIG) strains [19]. All novel allele sequences were assigned by the MLST database curator [5]. PFGE was performed using *Sma*I and *Cfr*9I digestion. PFGE was run for 24h at 5.6V/cm and with pulsed time ramping from 2 to 5 s [22]. *Spa* typing was performed according to described protocols [21,24], using the primers SPspaF (5'-AAGTAGTGATATTCTTGCT-3') and SPspaR (5'-CCAGGTTGAACGACATGCAT-3'). For determination of the

SCC*mec* elements, the SCC*mec* type II/III was detected with the primers described by Descloux et al. [23] and all other SCC*mec* types were detected with the multiplex assays described by Kondo et al. [20].

Results

Index cases

The 16 index dogs had pyoderma (n = 5), otitis externa (n = 5), post-operative wound infections (n = 4), non-surgical wound (n = 1) and rhinitis (n = 1). Two index dogs were sampled only once, because one of them was euthanized and the owner of the other dog did not longer want to participate in the study. Two index cases were sampled only three or five times respectively, because in the first case the dog had no longer clinical signs of infection and was repeatedly MRSP-negative and in the second case the owner went on a holiday for several months.

A total of 229 swabs were taken from the index dogs, of which 61 (26.6%) were found MRSP-positive (Table 1). The prevalence of MRSP in the index dogs from the first to the sixth sampling was 87.5% (14/16), 71.4% (10/14), 42.9% (6/14), 46.2% (6/13), 30.8% (4/13) and 58.3% (7/12) respectively. Of the 12 index dogs, that were sampled for six months, two dogs were continuously MRSP-positive, five dogs were intermittently MRSP-positive, four dogs became MRSP-negative during the six months and one dog was never found MRSP-positive after the initial MRSP-positive sample (Table S1). One dog (household 1) was found MRSP-positive more than one year after the initial sample. In 10 of the 12 dogs the clinical signs persisted during the study period of six months. One dog occasionally showed clinical signs and one dog did not show clinical signs during six months. The MRSP-positive sites of an index dog showed considerable variation during the samplings (Table S1).

MRSP was found on swabs from the perineum (n = 29), the infection site (n = 19) and the nose (n = 13) (Table 1).

Contact animals

Seven contact animals, six dogs and one cat, from seven households were included in the study. In six of these seven households MRSP-positive contact animals were found (Table S1). A total of 68 swabs were taken from the contact animals of which 13 (19.1%) were found MRSP-positive. The prevalence of MRSP in the contact animals from the first to the sixth sampling was 71.4% (5/7), 40.0% (2/5), 0% (0/5), 0% (0/5), 20% (1/5) and 50% (2/4), respectively. Generally, MRSP-positive contact animals were only found in combination with MRSP-positive index dogs. However, in one household the index dog became MRSP-negative while the contact animal was repeatedly MRSP-positive. In one household (household 16) the contact animal showed signs of an ear infection and was also sampled at the infection site in addition to the samples from nose and perineum. MRSP was cultured from swabs taken from the nose (n = 7), the perineum (n = 5) and on one of the swabs taken from the infection site of the contact animal in household 16 (Table 1).

Humans

Twenty-five persons living in the same household as the index dogs were included in the study. A total of 140 nasal swabs were taken of which five (3.6%) were found MRSP-positive (Table 1). In the first sampling, 3/25 (12.0%) humans from three different households were MRSP-positive. During the following four samplings no human nasal samples were MRSP- positive. In the last sampling 2/22 (10.0%) humans from the same household were MRSP-positive (Table S1). In this household the clinical condition

Table 1. Number of MRSP+ samples found at the different sampling sites.

	Number of samples	MRSP+ samples (%)	MRSP+ site	MRSP+ samples per site (%)
Index dogs	229	61 (26,2)	Nose	31 (21,3)
			Perineum	29 (47,5)
			Infection site	19 (31,2)
Contact animals	68	13 (19,1)	Nose	7 (53,8)
			Perineum	5 (38,5)
			Infection site	1 (7,7)
Humans	140	5 (3,57)	Nose	5
Environment	236	43 (18,2)	Feeding place	18 (41,9)
			Sleeping place	18 (41,9)
			Inaccessible place	7 (16,2)
Total	673	122 (18,1)		

of the index case had worsened and MRSP was also found in the index dog, the contact dog and the environment. After testing MRSP-positive, two of the five owners were re-tested repeatedly during the study period and none of the owners were tested MRSP-positive more than once. The other three owners were not re-tested, because in one household the index dog was euthanatized and in the other household the two owners were tested MRSP-positive only in the last sampling.

Environment

A total of 43/236 (18.2%) environmental samples were MRSP-positive (Table 1). Positive environmental wipes were found in 68.8% (11/16), 28.6% (4/14), 0% (0/14), 30.8% (4/13), 0% (0/13) and 41.7% (5/12) of the households in the first to sixth sampling respectively. In general, MRSP-positive environmental wipes were found in combination with MRSP-positive animals. However, in four households MRSP-positive environmental wipes were found during a sampling without MRSP-positive animals (Table S1). The feeding place was MRSP-positive in 11 households, the sleeping place in nine and the site not physically accessible to the animal in six households.

Genotyping results

In 12 households several MRSP isolates from different sampling times were available, in three households only isolates from the first sampling time were available, and in one household all samples were MRSP-negative. This resulted in a total of 60 isolates that were genotyped.

Genotype ST71-J-t02-II/III was the dominant type found in 8/16 (50%) households (Table 2). No ST71 strains were present in five households that instead harboured strains with ST29, 111, 115, 131 and 143, respectively. Also strains with different STs were found within two household (households 11 and 16) and strains that were non-typeable with PFGE using SmaI, but showed related banding patterns after digestion with Cfr9I, type Cfr1 and Cfr2, respectively (Table 2). Remarkable was the finding that spa typing further differentiated strains that were indistinguishable with MLST and PFGE. In three households, either spa types t02 and t05 (households 2 and 12) or spa types t02 and t06 (household 7) were found, although spa types (t02, t05 and t06) were considered to be closely related as they differed only in the total number of central r03 repeats (Table 2). SCCmec II/III was most frequently found and associated with isolates of ST71. SCCmec

type V was found in combination with ST115. Isolates with ST29, 111 and 143 contained non-typeable SCCmec cassettes, as none of the multiplex PCR assays amplified a product (Table 2).

Discussion

To our knowledge, this is the first study investigating the occurrence of MRSP within a household with a (former) canine MRSP patient in time. The sampling results of the sixteen different households showed considerable variation in the persistence of MRSP. Although two dogs were continuously MRSP-positive during six months, dogs could also be MRSP-positive intermittently, occasionally with up to three months between two MRSP-positive samplings.

On the one hand, dogs with clinical signs and a proven MRSP infection in the past were not always MRSP-positive. As selective culturing was used and different sites were sampled (nose and perineum), the possibility of a false-negative culture result was greatly reduced. On the other hand one dog was even MRSP-positive more than one year after the initial sampling showing that MRSP can persist in dogs. As this was a field study and dogs with different clinical conditions were included, different treatment regimens were applied to the index cases. This could have affected the presence of MRSP. Index cases, which became MRSP-negative, however, included both dogs with and without a treatment. The same MRSP genotype was found in dogs without clinical signs for several months, suggesting long-term colonization rather than transient colonization. Taken together, these results show that veterinarians should stay alert with (former) MRSP patients, even after repeated MRSP-negative cultures or after the disappearance of the clinical infection.

This field study was performed in a setting with MRSP patients from different veterinary clinics in the Netherlands. The clinical condition, household situation, and/or provided therapies could have contributed to the variation in the presence of MRSP. Moreover, the study was performed from March to October 2010, therefore potential seasonal influences, including allergen exposure could not be excluded.

In addition to external influences, animal specific factors could also have played a role in the prevalence and persistence of MRSP in some canine patients. With S. aureus several factors are known to influence the rate of nasal carriage in humans [25]. For S. pseudintermedius, studies on the risk factors for colonization are rare. The presence of skin lesions, previous hospitalization and previous

Table 2. Typing results of MRSP isolates.

Index	Sampling	Isolate from:	MLST	PFGE	Spa	SCCmec
1	1	index dog	71	J	t02	II/III
	4	environment	71	J	new	II/III
	6	index dog	71	J	t02	II/III
2	1	index dog	71	J	t02	II/III
	2	index dog	71	J	t05	II/III
3	1	index dog	29	Cfr1	t09	NT
	1	contact animal	29	Cfr1	t09	NT
	1	humans	29	Cfr1	t09	NT
	1	environment	29	Cfr1	t09	NT
	5	index dog	29	Cfr1	t09	NT
	6	contact animal	29	Cfr1	t09	NT
	6	environment	29	Cfr1	t09	NT
4	1	index dog	71	J	t02	II/III
	1	environment	71	J	t02	II/III
	2	index dog	71	J	t02	II/III
5	1	environment	131	J	no	NT
6	1	index dog	111	U	no	NT
	2	index dog	111	U	no	NT
	3	index dog	111	U	no	NT
	4	index dog	111	U	no	NT
	6	index dog	111	U	no	NT
7	1	index dog	71	J	t02	II/III
	1	environment	71	J	t02	II/III
	2	index dog	71	J	t02	II/III
	2	contact animal	71	J	t06	II/III
	6	index dog	71	J	t06	II/III
	6	environment	71	J	t02	II/III
8	1	index dog	115	Q	new	V
	1	contact animal	115	Q	new	V
	1	environment	115	Q	new	V
	6	index dog	115	Q	new	V
	6	contact animal	115	Q	new	V
	6	humans	115	Q	new	V
	6	environment	115	Q	new	V
9	1	index dog	71	J	t02	II/III
	1	environment	71	J	t02	II/III
	2	environment	71	J	t02	II/III
	4	index dog	71	J	t02	II/III
10	1	index dog	71	J	t02	II/III
	6	index dog	71	J	t02	II/III
11	1	index dog	71	J	t02	II/III
	1	contact animal	71	J	t02	II/III
	1	environment	29	Cfr2	t09	NT
12	1	index dog	71	Y	t02	II/III
	1	contact animal	71	Y	t05	II/III
	1	humans	71	Y	t02	II/III
	1	environment	71	Y	t02	II/III
13	1	index dog	143	G	no	NT
	1	humans	143	G	no	NT
	1	environment	143	G	no	NT

Table 2. Cont.

Index	Sampling	Isolate from:	MLST	PFGE	Spa	SCCmec
	6	index dog	143	G	no	NT
	6	environment	143	G	no	NT
14	1	index dog	71	J	t06	II/III
	1	environment	71	J	t06	II/III
	6	index dog	71	J	t06	II/III
	6	environment	71	J	t06	II/III
15	NA	NA	NA	NA	NA	NA
16	1	index dog	29	Cfr2	t09	NT
	1	contact animal	29	Cfr2	t09	NT
	1	environment	29	Cfr2	t09	NT
	2	environment	71	J	t02	II/III

NA: No MRSP-isolates available.
NT: non-typeable.

antimicrobial therapy have been identified as a risk factors for carriage [2,15,26].

Animals in close contact with MRSP patients were frequently found MRSP positive, which was also described in a one point prevalence study by van Duijkeren et al.[27].

MRSP-positive contact animals were usually found in combination with MRSP-positive index dogs. However, in one household the index dog became MRSP-negative while the contact dog was repeatedly tested MRSP-positive with the same genotype that was originally isolated from the index case. During the study this contact dog received antimicrobials and was submitted to an animal hospital for health issues not related to MRSP. As MRSP are multidrug resistant this may have favoured colonization. Generally, contact animals carried the same MRSP-genotype as the index case. Only in two households (7 and 12) the contact animal carried MRSP with a different, but closely related, *spa* type. It shows that there is a high risk of transmission of MRSP to animals in close contact with MRSP patients and that veterinarians and owners should be aware of this risk.

In contrast to contact animals, humans are rarely found MRSP-positive [27,28]. In this study five owners in four households were found MRSP-positive with four different sequence types (ST71, ST29, ST115, ST143). The MRSP-positive humans were found in combination with MRSP-positive index dogs showing clinical signs, contact animals and environmental samples indicating considerable exposure. After testing MRSP-positive, two of the five owners were tested repeatedly and they were not tested MRSP-positive more than once. Both owners were MRSP-positive with a rare genotype, namely ST29-*Cfr*1-t09-NT and ST143-G-no-NT respectively. No eradication therapy was performed. These results suggest occasional contamination or rapid elimination of colonization of the owners. However, in a recent study by Paul et al. [29] 5/128 small animal dermatologists were found MRSP-positive and two of them were re-tested one month later and both tested MRSP-positive again with an isolate with the same *spa*-type as in the initial screening. The authors suggest that MRSP with MLST ST71 and ST106 are more able to colonize humans. However, it is also possible that the veterinarians were re-infected as they have frequent contact with infected pets.

In the present study, the majority of MRSP-positive environmental samples were those in which there was physical contact with the index case, indicating that physical contact is an efficient way of MRSP-transmission. The study of van Duijkeren et al. [27] shows that the feeding and sleeping place are most often found MRSP-positive, which is in concordance with this study. In six households, however, MRSP was found at the site where no physical contact was possible with the index case or contact animal. In addition, physical contact of the owners with these sites was scarce, because of poor accessibility. Therefore potential transmission of MRSP from the owner's hands to these sites was unlikely. However, a considerable amount of dust was collected at these sites each month, which indicates that besides physical contact, dust particles play a role in the maintenance and distribution of MRSP.

The emergence of MRSP in Europe is thought to be mainly due to clonal spread of one major clonal lineage MLST ST71-*spa* t02-SCC*mec* II-III. An interesting finding from the present study was that several different MLST types were found (ST71, ST29, ST111, ST115, ST131 and ST143), although MLST ST71 predominated. In general, similar or indistinguishable MRSP isolates were found in patients, contact animals and environmental samples within the same household indicating transmission within the household. In three households containing MRSP strains with ST111, ST115 and ST143 the same strain was found during the first and sixth sampling and no other strains were found, showing an ongoing infection or re-infection of the index dog with the same MRSP strain for six months. The risk of re-infection with MRSP should be considered since studies on the survival of *S. aureus* in the environment have shown that the bacteria can survive for a considerable amount of time in dust and the same may hold true for MRSP [30]. Moreover, in four households MRSP-positive environment wipes were found while all animals and humans at that time were MRSP-negative. Occasionally different genotypes were found within one household and within one sampling. In three households (2, 7 and 12) isolates were found that only differed in *spa* type. The obtained *spa* types belonged to types t02, t05 and t06 that differed only in the presence or absence of a central r03 repeat, and may suggest modification of the *spa* repeats after introduction of MRSP to the household rather than

independent acquisition of different MRSP types. An argument in favor of this theory is that all isolates within these 3 households shared the same PFGE pattern, SCC*mec* cassettes and MLST type. However, the presence of multiple MRSP strains in one household should also be considered, as shown in two households (11 and 16) that harbored MRSP isolates with different STs. Studies have shown that different MRSP strains can coexist in one animal [26].

In conclusion, dogs infected with MRSP can become colonized with MRSP and remain MRSP-positive for prolonged periods of time. In addition, dogs can test MRSP-positive after repeated MRSP-negative samplings or after the disappearance of the clinical infection. MRSP is easily transmitted to contact animals and the environment, which both are occasionally MRSP-positive without the presence of an MRSP-positive index dog. The contact animals and the environment might be reservoirs for recurrent MRSP infections in the index case or new MRSP infections in other animals. Long-term colonization of dogs was found, but transmission to humans was rare and humans were never found MRSP-positive more than once, suggesting contamination instead of colonization with MRSP.

Acknowledgments

The authors thank the personnel of the veterinary clinics and the dog owners for their cooperation.

Author Contributions

Conceived and designed the experiments: LML PdH JvL BD JAW EvD. Performed the experiments: LML PdH JvL BD JAW EvD. Analyzed the data: LML PdH JvL BD JAW EvD. Contributed reagents/materials/analysis tools: LML PdH JvL BD JAW EvD. Wrote the paper: LML PdH JvL BD JAW EvD.

References

1. Weese J, van Duijkeren E (2010) Methicillin-resistant *Staphylococcus aureus* and *Staphylococcus pseudintermedius* in veterinary medicine. Vet Microbiol 140: 418–429.
2. Griffeth GC, Morris DO, Abraham JL, Shofer FS, Rankin SC (2008) Screening for skin carriage of methicillin-resistant coagulase-positive staphylococci and *Staphylococcus schleiferi* in dogs with healthy and inflamed skin. Vet Dermatol 19: 142–149.
3. Penna B, Varges R, Martins R, Martins G, Lilenbaum W (2010) In vitro antimicrobial resistance of staphylococci isolated from canine urinary tract infection. Can Vet J 51: 738–742.
4. Penna B, Varges R, Medeiros L, Martins GM, Martins RR, et al. (2010) Species distribution and antimicrobial susceptibility of staphylococci isolated from canine otitis externa. Vet Dermatol 21: 292–296.
5. Perreten V, Kadlec K, Schwarz S, Gronlund Andersson U, Finn M, et al. (2010) Clonal spread of methicillin-resistant *Staphylococcus pseudintermedius* in Europe and North America: an international multicentre study. J Antimicrob Chemother 65: 1145–1154.
6. Stegmann R, Burnens A, Maranta CA, Perreten V (2010) Human infection associated with methicillin-resistant *Staphylococcus pseudintermedius* ST71. J Antimicrob Chemother 65: 2047–2048.
7. Gerstadt K, Daly JS, Mitchell M, Wessolossky M, Cheeseman SH (1999) Methicillin-resistant *Staphylococcus intermedius* pneumonia following coronary artery bypass grafting. Clin Infect Dis 29: 218–219.
8. Kempker R, Mangalat D, Kongphet-Tran T, Eaton M (2009) Beware of the pet dog: a case of *Staphylococcus intermedius* infection. Am J Med Sci 338: 425–427.
9. Campanile F, Bongiorno D, Borbone S, Venditti M, Giannella M (2007) Characterization of a variant of the SCC*mec* element in a bloodstream isolate of *Staphylococcus intermedius*. Microb Drug Resist 13: 7–10.
10. Hanselman BA, Kruth S, Weese JS (2008) Methicillin-resistant staphylococcal colonization in dogs entering a veterinary teaching hospital. Vet Microbiol 126: 277–281.
11. Sasaki T, Kikuchi K, Tanaka Y, Takahashi N, Kamata S, et al. (2007) Methicillin-resistant *Staphylococcus pseudintermedius* in a veterinary teaching hospital. J Clin Microbiol 45: 1118–1125.
12. Ruscher C, Lubke-Becker A, Wleklinski CG, Soba A, Wieler LH, et al. (2009) Prevalence of methicillin-resistant *Staphylococcus pseudintermedius* isolated from clinical samples of companion animals and equidaes. Vet Microbiol 136: 197–201.
13. Hanselman BA, Kruth SA, Rousseau J, Weese JS (2009) Coagulase positive staphylococcal colonization of humans and their household pets. Can Vet J 50: 954–958.
14. Vengust M, Anderson ME, Rousseau J, Weese JS (2006) Methicillin-resistant staphylococcal colonization in clinically normal dogs and horses in the community. Lett Appl Microbiol 43: 602–606.
15. Nienhoff U, Kadlec K, Chaberny IF, Verspohl J, Gerlach G, et al. (2011) Methicillin-resistant *Staphylococcus pseudintermedius* among dogs admitted to a small animal hospital. Vet Microbiol 150: 191–197.
16. Graveland H, van Duijkeren E, van Nes A, Schoormans A, Broekhuizen-Stins M, et al. (2009) Evaluation of isolation procedures and chromogenic agar media for the detection of MRSA in nasal swabs from pigs and veal calves. Vet Microbiol 139: 121–125.
17. Bannoehr J, Franco A, Iurescia M, Battisti A, Fitzgerald JR (2009) Molecular diagnostic identification of *Staphylococcus pseudintermedius*. J Clin Microbiol 47: 469–471.
18. Francois P, Pittet D, Bento M, Pepey B, Vaudaux P, et al. (2003) Rapid detection of methicillin-resistant *Staphylococcus aureus* directly from sterile or nonsterile clinical samples by a new molecular assay. J Clin Microbiol 41: 254–260.
19. Bannoehr J, Ben Zakour NL, Waller AS, Guardabassi L, Thoday KL, et al. (2007) Population genetic structure of the Staphylococcus intermedius group: insights into agr diversification and the emergence of methicillin-resistant strains. J Bacteriol 189: 8685–8692.
20. Kondo Y, Ito T, Ma XX, Watanabe S, Kreiswirth BN, et al. (2007) Combination of multiplex PCRs for staphylococcal cassette chromosome mec type assignment: rapid identification system for mec, ccr, and major differences in junkyard regions. Antimicrob Agents Chemother 51: 264–274.

21. Moodley A, Stegger M, Ben Zakour NL, Fitzgerald JR, Guardabassi L (2009) Tandem repeat sequence analysis of staphylococcal protein A (*spa*) gene in methicillin-resistant *Staphylococcus pseudintermedius*. Vet Microbiol 135: 320–326.

22. Murchan S, Kaufmann ME, Deplano A, de Ryck R, Struelens M, et al. (2003) Harmonization of pulsed-field gel electrophoresis protocols for epidemiological typing of strains of methicillin-resistant *Staphylococcus aureus*: a single approach developed by consensus in 10 European laboratories and its application for tracing the spread of related strains. J Clin Microbiol 41: 1574–1585.

23. Descloux S, Rossano A, Perreten V (2008) Characterization of new staphylococcal cassette chromosome mec (SCC*mec*) and topoisomerase genes in fluoroquinolone- and methicillin-resistant *Staphylococcus pseudintermedius*. J Clin Microbiol 46: 1818–1823.

24. Ruscher C, Lubke-Becker A, Semmler T, Wleklinski CG, Paasch A, et al. (2010) Widespread rapid emergence of a distinct methicillin- and multidrug-resistant *Staphylococcus pseudintermedius* (MRSP) genetic lineage in Europe. Vet Microbiol 144: 340–346.

25. Kluytmans J, van Belkum A, Verbrugh H (1997) Nasal carriage of *Staphylococcus aureus*: epidemiology, underlying mechanisms, and associated risks. Clin Microbiol Rev 10: 505–520.

26. Fazakerley J, Williams N, Carter S, McEwan N, Nuttall T (2010) Heterogeneity of *Staphylococcus pseudintermedius* isolates from atopic and healthy dogs. Vet Dermatol 21: 578–585.

27. van Duijkeren E, Kamphuis M, van der Mije IC, Laarhoven LM, Duim B (2011) Transmission of methicillin-resistant *Staphylococcus pseudintermedius* between infected dogs and cats and contact pets, humans and the environment in households and veterinary clinics. Vet Microbiol 150: 338–343.

28. Hanselman BA, Kruth S, Rousseau J, Weese JS (2009) Coagulase positive staphylococcal colonization of humans and their household pets. Can Vet J 50: 954–958.

29. Paul NC, Moodley A, Ghibaudo G, Guardabassi L (2011) Carriage of methicillin-resistant *Staphylococcus pseudintermedius* in small animal veterinarians: indirect evidence of zoonotic transmission. Zoonoses Public Health doi:10.1111/j.1863-2378.2011.01398.x.

30. Wagenvoort JH, Sluijsmans W, Penders RJ (2000) Better environmental survival of outbreak vs. sporadic MRSA isolates. J Hosp Infect 45: 231–234.

15

Risk Factors of *Coxiella burnetii* (Q Fever) Seropositivity in Veterinary Medicine Students

Myrna M. T. de Rooij[1], Barbara Schimmer[2], Bart Versteeg[2,3], Peter Schneeberger[3], Boyd R. Berends[4], Dick Heederik[1], Wim van der Hoek[2], Inge M. Wouters[1]*

1 Division of Environmental Epidemiology, Institute for Risk Assessment Sciences, Utrecht, the Netherlands, 2 Centre for Infectious Disease Control, National Institute for Public Health and the Environment, Bilthoven, the Netherlands, 3 Department of Medical Microbiology and Infection Control, Jeroen Bosch Hospital, 's-Hertogenbosch, the Netherlands, 4 Division of Veterinary Public Health, Institute for Risk Assessment Sciences, Utrecht, the Netherlands

Abstract

Background: Q fever is an occupational risk for veterinarians, however little is known about the risk for veterinary medicine students. This study aimed to assess the seroprevalence of *Coxiella burnetii* among veterinary medicine students and to identify associated risk factors.

Methods: A cross-sectional study with questionnaire and blood sample collection was performed among all veterinary medicine students studying in the Netherlands in 2006. Serum samples (n = 674), representative of all study years and study directions, were analyzed for *C. burnetii* IgG and IgM phase I and II antibodies with an immunofluorescence assay (IFA). Seropositivity was defined as IgG phase I and/or II titer of 1:32 and above.

Results: Of the veterinary medicine students 126 (18.7%) had IgG antibodies against *C. burnetii*. Seropositivity associated risk factors identified were the study direction 'farm animals' (Odds Ratio (OR) 3.27 [95% CI 2.14–5.02]), advanced year of study (OR year 6: 2.31 [1.22–4.39] OR year 3–5 1.83 [1.07–3.10]) having had a zoonosis during the study (OR 1.74 [1.07–2.82]) and ever lived on a ruminant farm (OR 2.73 [1.59–4.67]). Stratified analysis revealed study direction 'farm animals' to be a study-related risk factor apart from ever living on a farm. In addition we identified a clear dose-response relation for the number of years lived on a farm with *C. burnetii* seropositivity.

Conclusions: *C. burnetii* seroprevalence is considerable among veterinary medicine students and study related risk factors were identified. This indicates Q fever as an occupational risk for veterinary medicine students.

Editor: Dario S. Zamboni, University of São Paulo, Brazil

Funding: The authors have no support or funding to report.

Competing Interests: The authors have declared that no competing interests exist.

* E-mail: i.wouters@uu.nl

Introduction

Q fever is a zoonotic disease caused by the bacterium *Coxiella burnetii* and is, apart from community outbreaks, known as an occupational disease of veterinarians, farmers and abattoir workers [1]. Symptomatic acute Q fever mainly presents as fever and headache, hepatitis, or pneumonia [2,3]. Moreover, infection with *C. burnetii* is asymptomatic in approximately 60% of those infected [2]. Many Q fever infections are not diagnosed because of the often mild and nonspecific clinical symptoms [4]. Acute Q fever, whether or not symptomatic, can develop into chronic Q fever [3]. Chronic Q fever generally presents as a culture-negative endocarditis or vascular infection with a high case fatality [3]. Another important long-term effect is Q fever fatigue syndrome, which occurs in 10 to 20% of all acute Q fever cases [5].

C. burnetii is a pathogenic bacterium which can infect mammals, birds and arthropods [1]. Transmission of *Coxiella* to humans occurs primarily through air via bioaerosols [6]. Furthermore humans can be infected by intake of contaminated milk or food, but these routes of transmission are of minor relevance [7]. The

Coxiella bacterium is known to have two antigenic stages: the virulent phase I variant and the avirulent phase II variant [8]. In the body, *C. burnetii* is controlled by the T-cell dependent immune system, resulting in the production of specific antibodies [2]. Immunoglobulin G (IgG) is primarily effective against phase II antigen, while Immunoglobulin M (IgM) targets both phase I and II antigens [2]. The level of IgM increases rapidly after infection, thus is considered to be a marker of recent infection, however it can persist for many months [9,10]. IgG levels increase a few weeks after infection, but remain detectable for years or even throughout life [5,9].

Before the large community outbreaks in the Netherlands starting in 2007, *C. burnetii* seroprevalence was 2.4% in a general population sample taken in 2006–2007 [11]. Furthermore the study showed that persons who kept ruminants or with occupational animal contact had a higher risk to be infected with *Coxiella* [11]. Serum samples collected in the Netherlands in November 2009 showed that more than half of the livestock veterinarians were seropositive [12]. A similarly high seroprevalence for *C. burnetii* in veterinarians has been reported in other studies, with prevalence ranging from approximately 20 to 50% [13,14]. Hence a substantial number of veterinarians become infected during their career, or possibly during their veterinary education. Veterinary medicine students perform similar activities as veterinarians during their study and likely have an increased risk to become infected with *C. burnetii* also. Yet, little is known about seroprevalence among veterinary students and the possible risk factors.

Few serological studies have been done among veterinary students, showing prevalence figures of *Coxiella* antibodies to range from 10 to 40% [15–17]. Valencia *et al* showed that students at the beginning of their first study year had a seroprevalence of 4.0% which was significantly lower compared to the 16.8% prevalence in the fifth year, implying a gradual increase in prevalence over the study periods [16]. However, studies reporting on the seroprevalence for *C. burnetii* covering the complete educational program and study duration are thus far missing. In univariate analysis some risk factors for seropositivity were identified in these studies, i.e. male gender, contact with ruminants, and study direction, although multivariate analyses were not carried out [16,17]. We thus performed a large-scale cross sectional study to determine the seroprevalence of *C. burnetii* among all veterinary medicine students studying in the Netherlands in the year 2006. All study years and study directions were included in order to identify the pattern in seroprevalence of antibodies against *C. burnetii* and to determine the associated study-related factors and other student characteristics.

Methods

Study design and population

The cross sectional design and study population have been described before by Samadi *et al* [18]. Briefly, all 1416 students, who were registered as a student of veterinary medicine in 2006 at Utrecht University, the only faculty of Veterinary Medicine in the Netherlands, were requested to participate. Students of all study phases were asked to fill in an online questionnaire and were invited to donate a blood sample of 20 ml for serological testing. Non-responders were sent maximally two reminders. Blood collection was performed in 2006 before the start of large community outbreaks of Q fever in the Netherlands in 2007–2009.

Ethics statement

The study protocol was approved by the Ethical Committee of the Utrecht University. All participants gave written informed consent prior to blood collection.

Questionnaire

Information was collected on participants' demographic and study related characteristics and on their smoking habits and health status. Regular contact with diverse animal species was asked for during different periods of childhood and adulthood. Information was gathered about a farm childhood, the number of years lived on a farm, farm type and the activities performed on the farm. Questions about health status addressed general health, clinical symptoms and self-reported zoonotic diseases.

Study related characteristics for veterinary medicine students in the Netherlands are affected by the structure of the veterinary curriculum with its variety of directions and theoretical/practical stages. Six months after the start of the study the veterinary curriculum divides into two main directions: 'individually kept animals' and 'farm animal health'. After the second study year, the curriculum subdivides further. The direction 'individually kept animals' is split into 'companion animals' and 'equine'. The

direction: 'farm animal health' is also split further in 'farm animals and veterinary public health' and 'veterinary scientific research'. The first two study years consist of theoretical courses. During the third and fourth year the content of the courses shifts gradually towards practical lessons, but the majority is still theoretical. Fifth-year students start to follow internships at all departments but with the emphasis on their own specialization. Students with the companion animal direction mostly encounter cats and dogs, students at the equine department focus on horses and students doing the farm animal health specialization encounter mainly cows, pigs, poultry, sheep and goats.

Detection of *C. burnetii* IgG and IgM

Sera were analyzed for phase I and phase II IgG antibodies against *C. burnetii* at the Regional Laboratory of Medical Microbiology and Infection Control of the Jeroen Bosch Hospital in Den Bosch, using an Immunofluorescence Assay (IFA) according to the manufacturer's protocol (Focus Diagnostics). Sera were tested in a dilution series starting from a 1:32 till a 1:4096 dilution. An antibody titer of 1:32 and above for either IgG I or II antibodies of a serum sample was defined seropositive. A positive IgG test was followed by determination of phase I and II IgM antibodies by IFA.

Statistical analysis

All statistical analyses were carried out using SPSS for Windows (version 16). Univariate regression analyses were performed to investigate the association between seropositivity and possible risk factors. Variables in univariate analysis associated with seropositivity ($p < 0.20$) were selected for multivariate logistic regression analyses. These variables were tested for multicollinearity and after assumptions were met, both forward and backward regression analyses were applied. The final multivariate model was obtained with the criteria of a p-value of less than 0.05 for the model and for each variable itself. Smoothed regression analysis was performed to assess the shape of the association between seropositivity and the number of years a student had lived on a farm.

Results

Response

In total, 965 of all the 1416 veterinary medicine students responded to the questionnaire (68.2%) of which 5 were excluded in further analyses. One student was excluded because the questionnaire was not completed and four others as they represented study specializations with intrinsic low numbers. Of the 960 students providing a questionnaire, 674 students provided a blood sample as well (47.6% of the total population). The division over the different study phases and study directions of the respondents is shown in Figure 1.

Participants' characteristics

Of the participants that completed the questionnaire, 80% were women (Table 1). The mean age was 24 years with a range from 18 to 47 years. A high number (51.1%) of the students reported previous or current regular contact with farm animals outside the veterinary curriculum. Furthermore 645 students (67.2%) had regular contact with horses and 97.6% of the students had regular contact with pets. Of the students 39.5% grew up in a rural area and 13.5% had ever lived on a farm. Demographic characteristics of students who did not provide blood were generally similar to those who did, except for borderline significance for having lived on a farm or in a village (Table 1). Of the students 130 reported to have had a zoonosis during their study of which were reported

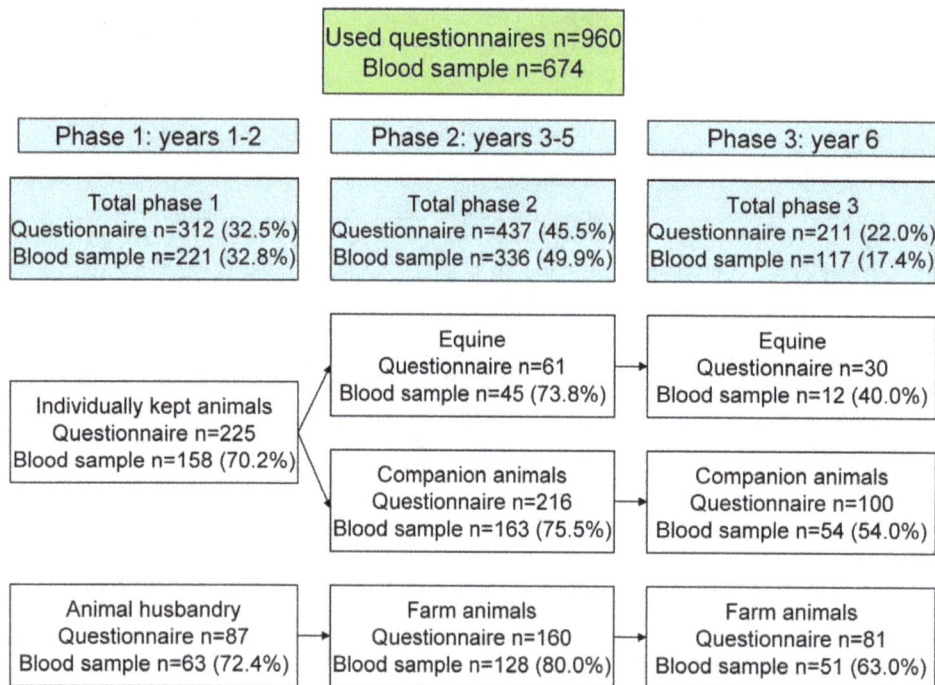

Figure 1. Numbers and percentages of participants per study direction and study phase.

most frequently: dermatophytosis (ringworm, 8.5%) and other fungal infections (5.5%, Table 2).

Serological results

Sera of 126 students (18.7%) were positive, with an IgG II titer ranging from 1:32 to 1:4096. Thirty percent (n = 38) of the students with a positive IgG II titer also had a positive IgG I titer ranging from 1:32 to 1:2084. There were no students with exclusive positive IgG I titers. Only sera with a positive IgG titer were tested for IgM antibodies. Of the IgG positives, 3% also had a positive IgM I with titers ranging from 1:32 to 1:256. While 19% of the IgG positives had also a positive IgM II indicating recent infection, with titers from 1:32 to >1:256. Seroprevalence showed an increase from study phase 1 (year 1–2) to phase 2 (year 3–5) and to phase 3 (year 6). Additionally, students mostly involved with farm animals had a much higher seroprevalence than those working with individually kept animals (Table 3).

Risk factor analyses

In the univariate analyses we identified variables associated with *C. burnetii* seropositivity as shown in Table 4. Male students were more often seropositive than females and seropositivity increased significantly with age per year. The study phase, study direction and whether or not internships were followed, were also associated. Moreover contact with cows, pigs, dogs and sheep was positively associated with seropositivity. Students who had lived on a farm were 2.9 times more likely to have *C. burnetii* antibodies. The risk was higher for having lived on a livestock breeding farm and was the highest for a ruminant farm. The risk for a positive serology significantly increased with each year the student had lived on the farm. The shape of this relationship was log-linear, implying that the risk for a positive serology significantly increased with each year the student had lived on the farm (p = 0.028; p-spline 2 df = 0.566; Figure 2). The following activities performed on the farm were associated with seropositivity: animal

nursing and work with liquid and/or solid manure. Students reporting to have had a zoonosis during their study had a higher chance of seropositivity. However none of the students reported to have had Q fever during their study (Table 2).General health status and specific clinical symptoms like cough, headache, unusually tired feeling, flu like symptoms and shortness of breath were not associated with seropositivity.

Ten variables were included in the initial multivariate regression model. In the final model the following were identified to be associated with seropositivity: having lived on a ruminant farm (OR 2.7), study direction 'farm animals' (OR 3.3), having had a zoonotic disease during study (OR 1.7) and duration of study (phase 2 (OR 1.8) and phase 3 (OR 2.3), (Table 5)).

We performed stratified analyses for students who had lived on a farm and those who did not, to investigate whether study direction remained an independent risk factor (Table 5). Results showed that the study direction 'farm animals' remained significantly associated with seropositivity for those who grew up on a farm (OR study direction = 4.9), as well as for those who did not (OR study direction = 3.3).

Discussion

In this cross-sectional study among Dutch veterinary students, we found a *C. burnetii* seroprevalence of 18.7% and identified several associated risk factors including study related factors. Only few studies have assessed zoonotic risks for veterinary medicine students. This is the first large-scale study that examined the seroprevalence for *Coxiella* among veterinary medicine students of all study years and directions. The overall observed seroprevalence was within the range of 10 to 40% reported in other studies for veterinary students of Spain, Brazil, California and Ohio [15–17].

The found prevalence is considerably lower than the prevalence of over 80% in Dutch livestock veterinarians sampled in 2009 [12]. The prevalence among these veterinarians might be slightly

Table 1. Descriptive characteristics (n (%) or stated otherwise) of the total study population and those who did and did not provide a blood sample.

Population characteristics	total	with blood	without blood
Number of students	960	674	286
Female	771 (80.3%)	540 (80.1%)	231 (80.8%)
Age, AM[a] (SD[b])	23.7 (3.7)	23.7 (3.6)	23.9 (3.8)
Weight (kg), AM[a] (SD[b])	68.5 (11.2)	68.3 (10.7)	69.1 (12.3)
Height (cm), AM[a] (SD[b])	174.6 (8.3)	174.4 (8.2)	175.2 (8.5)
Current smoker	103 (10.7%)	69 (10.2%)	34 (11.8%)
Past Smoker	86 (8.9%)	60 (8.9%)	26 (9.0%)
Regular contact[c] with animals besides the study:			
Horses	645 (67.2%)	451 (66.9%)	194 (67.8%)
Cows	312 (32.5%)	216 (32.0%)	96 (33.6%)
Pigs	136 (14.2%)	94 (13.9%)	42 (14.7%)
Sheep	275 (28.6%)	192 (28.5%)	83 (29.0%)
Poultry	307 (32.0%)	220 (32.6%)	87 (30.4%)
Goats	232 (24.2%)	166 (24.6%)	66 (23.1%)
Dogs	717 (74.7%)	507 (75.2%)	210 (73.4%)
Cats	712 (74.2%)	496 (73.6%)	216 (75.5%)
Rodents	715 (74.5%)	505 (74.9%)	210 (73.4%)
Birds	394 (41.0%)	283 (42.0%)	111 (38.8%)
Job with previous or current regular animal contact	439 (45.7%)	307 (45.5%)	132 (46.2%)
Growing up in rural area (village)[d]	379 (39.5%)	282 (41.8%)	97 (33.9%)
Farm childhood[e]	130 (13.5%)	100 (14.8%)	30 (10.5%)
Self reported zoonosis during VM[f]	190 (19.8%)	132 (19.6%)	58 (20.3%)
Self reported Q fever	0 (0%)	0 (0%)	0 (0%)
Positive Q fever status		126 (18.7%)	

[a]AM, Arithmetic Mean.
[b]SD, Standard Deviation.
[c]Previous or current regular contact (>once a week).
[d]Chi-square between providing and not-providing blood borderline significant with p = 0.07.
[e]Chi-square between providing and not-providing blood borderline significant with p = 0.08.
[f]VM, veterinary medicine.

higher than when sampling would have taken place in 2006, due to the environmental outbreaks starting in 2007. Conversely, other studies reported high seroprevalences of 20% and more for veterinarians in countries like the United States, Canada, Slovakia and Taiwan [13,14,19–21]. Comparing seroprevalences should however be done with caution, because different study populations and diagnostic tests applied might affect the outcomes. Recently, commercial IFAs and ELISAs have become available which are now predominantly used [22]. Despite this progress, there is still a wide interlaboratory variability due to different IgG and IgM cut-off levels applied [22]. There is no general consensus of the appropriate cut-off level as it depends on the population under study and the used antigen-preparation [23]. In this study IFA was used instead of ELISA because it is considered to be the reference method to study seroprevalence of *Coxiella* [24]. We chose a cut-off level of 1:32 instead of the 1:16 cut-off recommended by the manufacturer to increase specificity thus lowering the chance of false positives.

We found that students who grew up on a farm, especially on a ruminant farm, had a higher risk of being seropositive. All kinds of animals can be affected by *Coxiella* but ruminants are the most important reservoirs [25]. Furthermore almost all students performed at least one activity on the farm on which they had lived, for example more than 80% performed animal nursing. The shedding of *Coxiella* occurs primarily during aborting or parturition, thus likely occasions whereby students were often present [26,27]. A study in Spain among veterinary students documented working with ruminants as a risk factor and in Taiwan goat exposure was a risk factor for veterinarians [16,21].

The risk for a positive serology was found to significantly increase with each year the student had lived on a farm. The biological meaning of this is not known, as profound studies concerning exposure-response relations for *Coxiella* are lacking. Our finding might just reflect the increased probability to encounter *C. burnetii* exposure, as the risk for each exposure moment is constant given that one *Coxiella* organism entering the body is enough to cause disease [1]. On the other hand, our finding might be explained by a cumulative effect of long term exposure, suggesting that a threshold exposure should be met. Lastly, the level of exposure might be of importance as well: the persons who lived longer on a farm are more likely to have performed activities like animal nursing.

Students within the 'farm animals' direction had a three times higher risk to be seropositive than students from other directions.

Table 2. Overview of self-reported zoonotic diseases reported by veterinary medicine students (n = 960) during the veterinary medicine study.

Self reported zoonoses during VM[a]	Number (%)
Brucellosis	0 (0%)
Campylobacteriosis	10 (1.5%)
Cryptosporidiosis	0 (0%)
Ecthyma	9 (1.3%)
Giardiasis	1 (0.1%)
Cat scratch	3 (0.4%)
Leptospirosis	0 (0%)
Listeriosis	2 (0.3%)
Psittacosis	0 (0%)
Q fever	0 (0%)
Salmonellosis	8 (1.2%)
Dermatophytosis (ringworm)	57 (8.5%)
Other fungal infections	37 (5.5%)
Staphylococcus	5 (0.7%)
Toxoplasmosis	0 (0%)
VTEC	2 (0.3%)
Worminfection	13 (1.9%)

[a]VM, veterinary medicine.

The 'farm animal' direction itself includes regular contact with ruminants, but 'farm animal' students also often had contact with ruminants before or beside their study (Table 3). Furthermore the percentage of students with a farm childhood in this direction is considerably higher. Stratified analyses on farm childhood however showed study direction to be a risk factor also for those with a farm childhood, suggesting two independent effects, indicating also for these students the importance of their study for the development of seropositivity.

Longer study duration was associated with an increased likelihood for seropositivity. As mentioned before, the study has an increasing amount of practical lessons from the second study phase and onwards. Furthermore the last studyphase consists solely of internships whereby largely all veterinary activities are performed by the students. Thus, towards the end of the study the number of animal contact increases as well as the number of treatments executed. The treatment of cattle, swine and wildlife were previously reported as a risk factor for veterinarians [13]. Presumably, treatment of these species by students in their last phase can partly explain studyphase being a risk factor. In addition, by default students in later study phases are older likewise their possibility of becoming infected during their lifetime is higher [9]. Age as a risk factor was also found in a study amongst a Canadian general population and among U.S. veterinarians [13,19]. It could be argued that students in higher study phases have lived longer on a farm, and therefore are more likely to become seropositive. However, the average number of years students lived on a farm in study phase 1, 2 and 3 did not differ, being respectively 15.03, 14.84 and 16.75 years.

Table 3. Characteristics of students (n (%) or stated otherwise) who provided blood for the different study phases and by study direction.

Students study phase 1 (Year 1–2)	Farm animals	Individually kept animals
Number of students	63	158
Contact with ruminants outside VM[a]	44 (69.8%)	43 (27.2%)
Job with regular animal contact	29 (46.0%)	72 (45.6%)
Growing up in rural area (village)	38 (60.3%)	52 (32.9%)
Farm childhood	17 (27.0%)	16 (10.1%)
Positive *C. burnetii* status	15 (23.8%)	9 (5.7%)

Students study phase 2 (Year 3–5)	Farm animals	Companion animals	Horse
Number of students	128	163	45
Contact ruminants outside VM[a]	95 (74.2%)	48 (29.4%)	18 (40%)
Job with regular animal contact	57 (44.5%)	65 (39.9%)	29 (64.4%)
Growing up in rural area (village)	61 (47.7%)	59 (36.2%)	21 (46.7%)
Farm childhood	40 (31.2%)	10 (6.1%)	5 (11.1%)
Positive *C. burnetii* status	46 (35.9%)	19 (11.7%)	6 (13.3%)

Students study phase 3 (Year 6)	Farm animals	Companion animals	Horse
Number of students	51	54	12
Contact with ruminants outside VM[a]	27 (52.9%)	15 (27.8%)	6 (50%)
Job with regular animal contact	22 (43.1%)	27 (50.0%)	6 (50.0%)
Growing up in rural area (village)	24 (47.1%)	19 (35.2%)	8 (66.7%)
Farm childhood	7 (13.7%)	3 (5.6%)	2 (16.7%)
Positive *C. burnetii* status	19 (37.3%)	10 (18.5%)	2 (16.7%)

Note.
[a]Previous or current regular (>once a week) contact with ruminants outside the veterinary medicine curriculum.

Table 4. Univariate analysis of factors possibly associated with seropositivity for *Coxiella burnetii* among veterinary medicine students.

Variable	Odds Ratio (95% CI)	P-value
Male gender (n = 134 (19.9%))	1.74 (1.12–2.73)	0.018[b]
Age (per year)	1.10 (1.05–1.16)	0.000
Study direction farm animals (n = 242 (35.9%))	4.15 (2.76–6.22)	0.000[b]
Zoonotic disease during VM[a] (n = 132 (19.6%))	2.08 (1.34–3.24)	0.001[b]
Followed VM[a] internships (n = 171 (25.4%))	2.12 (1.41–3.21)	0.000
Regular contact with:		
Horses (n = 451 (66.9%))	1.13 (0.74–1.71)	0.601
Cows (n = 216 (32%))	2.39 (1.60–3.50)	0.000[b]
Pigs (n = 94 (13.9%))	1.72 (1.04–2.85)	0.045[b]
Sheep (n = 192 (28.5%))	1.73 (1.15–2.59)	0.009[b]
Poultry (n = 220 (32.6%))	1.29 (0.86–1.93)	0.246
Goats (n = 166 (24.6%))	1.35 (0.88–2.08)	0.207
Dogs (n = 507 (75.2%))	1.81 (1.10–3.01)	0.022[b]
Cats (n = 496 (73.6%))	0.96 (0.62–1.49)	0.911
Rodents (n = 505 (74.9%))	0.80 (0.52–1.24)	0.362
Birds (n = 283 (42.0%))	1.27 (0.86–1.88)	0.231
Former job with regular animal contact (n = 307 (45.5%))	0.91 (0.62–1.34)	0.692
Ever lived on a farm (n = 100 (14.8%))	2.86 (1.79–4.56)	0.000
Ever lived on a ruminant farm (n = 80 (11.9%))	3.78 (2.30–6.22)	0.000[b]
Ever lived on a livestock breeding farm (n = 67 (10.0%))	3.73 (2.18–6.31)	0.000
Years lived on a farm (per year)	1.07 (1.04–1.10)	0.024
Activities performed on the livestock farm:		
Animal nursing (n = 73 (82.0%))	4.40 (1.20–16.14)	0.022
Work with liquid and/or dry manure (n = 61 (68.5%))	3.23 (1.23–8.43)	0.017
Work with straw/hay (n = 75 (84.3%))	3.20 (0.86–11.94)	0.102
Plant nursing (n = 33 (37.1%))	1.61 (0.70–3.71)	0.291
Compared to currently in study phase 1		
Currently in study phase 2 (n = 336 (49.9%))	2.20 (1.34–3.62)	0.001[b]
Currently in study phase 3 (n = 117 (17.4%))	2.95 (1.64–5.34)	0.001[b]
Compared to town (15.000 to 80.000 inh) in childhood		
Grew up in a village (<15.000 inhabitants) (n = 282 (41.8%))	1.49 (0.97–2.29)	0.183
Grew up in a city (>80.000 inhabitants) (n = 110 (16.3%))	1.28 (0.72–2.27)	0.183
Compared to currently living in a student house		
Private house (n = 169 (25.1%))	1.45 (0.94–2.25))	0.218
Parental house n = 71 (10.5%))	0.95 (0.49–1.86)	0.218[b]
Compared to a none smoker		
Past smoker (n = 60 (8.9%))	1.11 (0.57–2.17)	0.898
Current smoker (n = 69 (10.2%))	1.13 (0.61–2.12)	0.898

Note.
[a]VM, veterinary medicine.
[b]Variables included in the multivariate analysis, other variables p<0.20 were excluded because of multicollinearity.

Students reporting zoonoses since the start of their study were more likely to be seropositive, although none of the 960 students reported to have had Q fever. Of the students 20% reported a zoonosis; most prevalent were ringworm and other fungal infections. A variety of fungi are known to be commensals of the animal skin, occasionally they can also be pathogenic either for animals or humans [28]. Students with frequent animal contact are presumably more exposed to several zoonotic pathogens [29].

Good hygiene is important for the prevention of these zoonoses [30]. Presumably zoonotic diseases were found to be a risk factor for *Coxiella* seropositivity because it reflects the students' amount of animal contact and hygiene practices. Whitney *et al* examined the use of personal protective equipment by veterinarians, whereby wearing always a lab coat and always a surgical mask were protective factors [13]. These findings indicate the probable benefit of strict hygienic measures. In contrast, recent findings

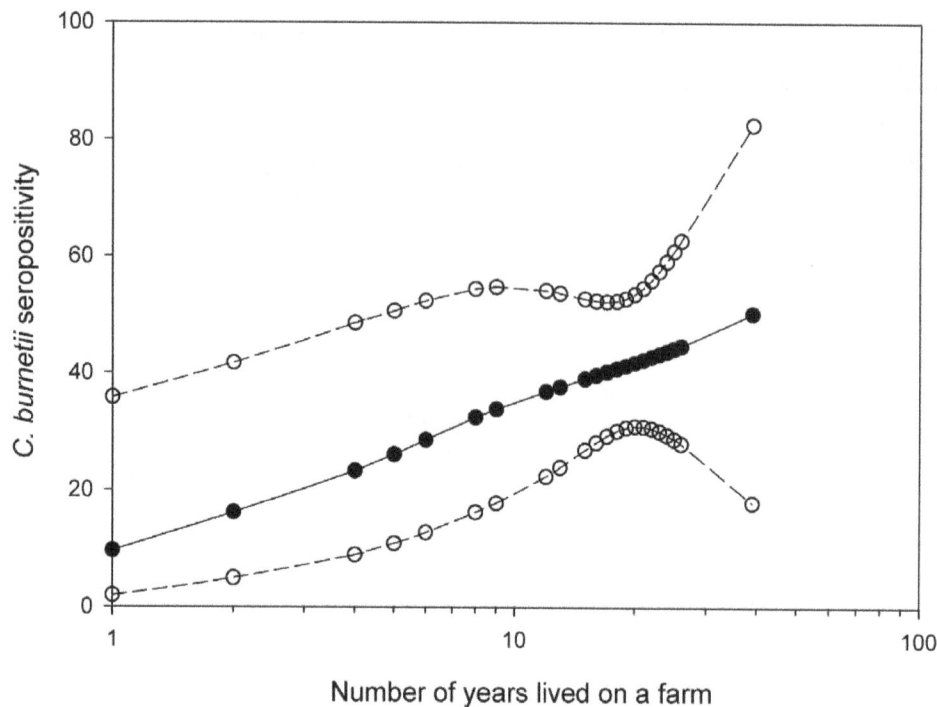

Figure 2. Association between *C. burnetii* seropositivity and number of years lived on a farm (p = 0.028, spline 2 d.f p = 0.586) for students who ever lived on a farm (n = 100). Open circles represent the 95% upper and lower confidence limits.

among culling workers showed seroconversion in around one out of five workers despite the use of personal protective equipment [31].

The seroprevalence of 18.7% for the Dutch veterinary students is high when compared to the seroprevalence of 2.4% for the general population in the Netherlands measured in the same time period, using the same methodology [11]. This indicates *C. burnetii* as a study or occupation related risk for veterinary students, as it also exists for veterinarians. It should be noted that 18.7% is the average prevalence in the study population. The risk for students in certain subgroups is considerably higher. For example the seroprevalence is 37.3% among students in the third study phase within the 'farm animals' direction. This overall prevalence of 18.7% is presumably a valid estimate for the general veterinary medicine student population, since about half of the total population provided a blood sample. The students who provided a blood sample showed to be only marginally different from the student population who did not.

The measurement series in the Netherlands revealed that the seroprevalence of students lies in between the prevalence observed in the general population and among veterinarians. However, students at the start of their study already had an increased seroprevalence of 10.9%. These students only have had theoretical courses; hence the increased seroprevalence can only be explained by other determinants, such as the frequent occurrence of a farm childhood in this population and the degree of ruminant contact prior to the start of their study. As could be expected, veterinary students have always been highly interested in animals. A large number of the students had regular contact with different animal species in childhood and around half of the students reported to have had a job with regular animal contact (Table 1). Students in the first phase within the 'farm animals' direction had a substantial higher seroprevalence (23.8%) than students in the 'individually kept animals' direction (5.7%, Table 3). This is likely a result of

previous contact with ruminants, as students with a farm childhood are more likely to choose for the 'farm animals' direction.

The risk factors identified comprised most of the risk factors found by several other studies both in open population and occupational settings. However, some other risk factors have been reported before, but could not be studied as the questionnaire did not include these items. An example is contact with pond water and knowledge of Q fever [13,21].

The implications of the high occurrence rate of seropositivity on students' health are not yet known. None of the students reported to have had Q fever. Q fever has a wide variety of non-specific symptoms and is often asymptomatic, so it is difficult to collect relevant information with a questionnaire over an extended period of time [2,3]. Poor recall might also have contributed to the low reported prevalence for Q fever. Furthermore the questionnaire was primarily based on the European Community Respiratory Health Survey questionnaire, and was not specifically directed to identify acute Q fever symptoms [32]. On the other hand, a high prevalence of self reported Q fever was not expected as as approximately 60% of Q fever infections are considered to be asymptomatic [4]. Both symptomatic and asymptomatic Q fever has been described to develop into chronic Q fever, although most information is available from symptomatic acute Q fever patients [3].Therefore research is needed to explore the risk for asymptomatic seroconverters of development into chronic Q fever.

This study raises the question whether specific measures have to be taken in this population to prevent development of *C. burnetii* infection. General protective measures may not be sufficient to protect students throughout their career. Therefore offering vaccination may be considered, like in Australia for personnel with high risk occupations [33], or yearly serological screenings as suggested for wool workers [34]. Moreover, in general, awareness about study related health risks should be strengthened. Knowl-

Table 5. Factors associated with *Coxiella burnetii* seropositivity obtained by multivariate analysis for all students and stratified by ever lived on a farm.

	All	Ever lived on a farm	
	OR (95% CI)	Yes (OR (95% CI))	No (OR (95% CI))
Study direction			
Farm animal health	3.27 (2.14–5.02)	4.86 (1.54–15.29)	3.32 (2.06–5.35)
Other direction	1.00	1.00	1.00
Study phase			
Phase 3 (Year 6)	2.31 (1.22–4.39)	0.43 (0.07–2.66)	3.16 (1.55–6.46)
Phase 2 (Year 3–5)	1.83 (1.07–3.10)	1.34 (0.46–3.94)	2.03 (1.09–3.79)
Phase 1 (Year 1–2)	1.00	1.00	1.00
Zoonotic disease during VM[a]			
Yes	1.74 (1.07–2.82)	7.23 (1.74–30.09)	1.34 (0.78–2.34)
No	1.00	1.00	1.00
Ever lived on ruminant farm			
Yes	2.73 (1.59–4.67)	-	-
No	1.00	-	-
Childhood municipality			
Village	-	0.53 (0.18–1.52)	1.53 (0.89–2.62)
City	-	-	2.18 (1.15–4.14)
Town		1.00	1.00

Note. Multivariate analysis for all students obtained with Forward and Backward logistic regression.
Stratified analysis obtained with Enter.
[a]VM, veterinary medicine.

edge regarding clinical symptoms of Q fever can improve referral to the occupational physician affiliated to the university and prevent development of chronic stages of disease.

To conclude, this is the first large-scale study that examined the seroprevalence for *C. burnetii* among veterinary medicine students across all study phases. It demonstrates a considerable *C. burnetii* seroprevalence among veterinary medicine students. Besides regular contact to ruminants outside the curriculum program, also study related factors were associated with seropositivity. This suggests the importance of Q fever as an occupational risk for veterinary medicine students. Interestingly, we demonstrated a log-linear relationship between the numbers of years lived on a farm and seropositivity. Since clinical Q fever illness was not self-reported further research is recommended to study the health implications of seropositivity. Overall, this study contributes to the knowledge and the awareness of Q fever as a risk for veterinary students in order to contribute to its prevention.

Acknowledgments

We are grateful to all participants without whom the study could not be conducted. We would like to thank Jamie Meekelenkamp of the Jeroen Bosch Hospital for the laboratory analyses. We also thank the dean of the Veterinary Medicine faculty and the department of student affairs for their cooperation when performing the study. Lot Bannink is acknowledged for coordinating the inclusion of the students.

Author Contributions

Conceived and designed the experiments: DH BRB IMW. Performed the experiments: MMTR BS BV PS WH IMW. Analyzed the data: MMTR IMW. Contributed reagents/materials/analysis tools: MMTR DH BS PS WH IMW. Wrote the paper: MMTR IW. Reviewed and commented on the manuscript: MMTR BS BV PS BRB DH WH IMW.

References

1. Madariaga MG, Rezai K, Trenholme GM, Weinstein RA (2003) Q fever: A biological weapon in your backyard. Lancet Infect Dis 3: 709–721.
2. Raoult D, Marrie TJ, Mege JL (2005) Natural history and pathophysiology of Q fever. Lancet Infect Dis 5: 219–226.
3. Parker NR, Barralet JH, Bell AM (2006) Q fever. Lancet 367: 679–688.
4. Maurin M, Raoult D (1999) Q fever. Clin Microbiol Rev 12: 518–553.
5. Sukocheva OA, Marmion BP, Storm PA, Lockhart M, Turra M, et al. (2010) Long-term persistence after acute Q fever of non-infective Coxiella burnetii cell components, including antigens. QJM 103: 847–863.
6. McQuiston JH, Childs JE (2002) Q fever in humans and animals in the United States. Vector Borne Zoonotic Dis 2: 179–191.
7. Woldehiwet Z (2004) Q fever (coxiellosis): Epidemiology and pathogenesis. Res Vet Sci 77: 93–100.
8. Heinzen RA, Hackstadt T, Samuel JE (1999) Developmental biology of Coxiella burnetii. Trends Microbiol 7: 149–154.

9. Dupont HT, Thirion X, Raoult D (1994) Q fever serology: Cutoff determination for microimmunofluorescence. Clin Diagn Lab Immunol 1: 189–196.
10. van der Hoek W, Meekelenkamp JC, Leenders AC, Wijers N, Notermans DW, et al. (2011) Antibodies against Coxiella burnetii and pregnancy outcome during the 2007–2008 Q fever outbreaks in the Netherlands. BMC Infect Dis 11: 44.
11. Schimmer B, Notermans DW, Harms MG, Reimerink JH, Bakker J, et al. (2012) Low seroprevalence of Q fever in the Netherlands prior to a series of large outbreaks. Epidemiol Infect Jan;140(1): 27–35. Epub 2011 Feb 16.
12. van Duynhoven Y, Schimmer B, van Steenbergen J, van der Hoek W. The story of human Q-fever in the Netherlands [Internet]. Netherlands: Ministry of Economic Affairs, Agriculture and Innovation. Available at http://english.minlnv.nl. Accessed 1 July 2011.
13. Whitney EA, Massung RF, Candee AJ, Ailes EC, Myers LM, et al. (2009) Seroepidemiologic and occupational risk survey for Coxiella burnetii antibodies among US veterinarians. Clin Infect Dis 48: 550–557.

14. Dorko E, Kalinova Z, Weissova T, Pilipcinec E (2008) Seroprevalence of antibodies to Coxiella burnetii among employees of the veterinary university in Kosice, eastern Slovakia. Ann Agric Environ Med 15: 119–124.

15. Schnurrenberger PR, Helwig JH, Bashe WJ, Jr. (1964) The incidence of zoonotic infections in veterinary students. J Am Vet Med Assoc 144: 384–386.

16. Valencia MC, Rodriguez CO, Punet OG, de Blas Giral I (2000) Q fever seroprevalence and associated risk factors among students from the veterinary school of Zaragoza, Spain. Eur J Epidemiol 16: 469–476.

17. Riemann HP, Brant PC, Franti CE, Reis R, Buchanan AM, et al. (1974) Antibodies to Toxoplasma gondii and Coxiella burneti among students and other personnel in veterinary colleges in California and Brazil. Am J Epidemiol 100: 197–208.

18. Samadi S, Spithoven J, Jamshidifard AR, Berends BR, Lipman L, et al. (2012) Allergy among veterinary medicine students in the Netherlands. Occup Environ Med 69: 48–55. Published Online First: 31 May 2011.

19. Marrie TJ, Pollak PT (1995) Seroepidemiology of Q fever in nova scotia: Evidence for age dependent cohorts and geographical distribution. Eur J Epidemiol 11: 47–54.

20. Marrie TJ, Fraser J (1985) Prevalence of antibodies to Coxiella burnetii among veterinarians and slaughterhouse workers in Nova Scotia. Can Vet J 26: 181–184.

21. Chang CC, Lin PS, Hou MY, Lin CC, Hung MN, et al. (2010) Identification of risk factors of Coxiella burnetii (Q fever) infection in veterinary-associated populations in southern Taiwan. Zoonoses Public Health 57: e95–101.

22. Raoult D (2009) Reemergence of Q fever after 11 september 2001. Clin Infect Dis 48: 558–559.

23. Abe T, Yamaki K, Hayakawa T, Fukuda H, Ito Y, et al. (2001) A seroepidemiological study of the risks of Q fever infection in Japanese veterinarians. Eur J Epidemiol 17: 1029–1032.

24. Blaauw GJ, Notermans DW, Schimmer B, Meekelenkamp J, Reimerink JH, et al. (2012) The application of an enzyme-linked immunosorbent assay or an immunofluorescent assay test leads to different estimates of seroprevalence of Coxiella burnetii in the population. Epidemiol Infect Jan;140(1): 36–41. Epub 2011 Feb 15.

25. Tissot-Dupont H, Amadei MA, Nezri M, Raoult D (2004) Wind in November, Q fever in December. Emerg Infect Dis 10: 1264–1269.

26. Sanchez J, Souriau A, Buendia AJ, Arricau-Bouvery N, Martinez CM, et al. (2006) Experimental Coxiella burnetii infection in pregnant goats: A histopathological and immunohistochemical study. J Comp Pathol 135: 108–115.

27. Hatchette T, Campbell N, Hudson R, Raoult D, Marrie TJ (2003) Natural history of Q fever in goats. Vector Borne Zoonotic Dis 3: 11–15.

28. Bond R (2010) Superficial veterinary mycoses. Clin Dermatol 28: 226–236.

29. Cascio A, Bosilkovski M, Rodriguez-Morales AJ, Pappas G (2011) The socio-ecology of zoonotic infections. Clin Microbiol Infect 17: 336–342.

30. National Association of State Public Health Veterinarians, Inc. (NASPHV) (2011) Compendium of measures to prevent disease associated with animals in public settings, 2011: National association of state public health veterinarians, inc. MMWR Recomm Rep 60: 1–24.

31. Whelan J, Schimmer B, Schneeberger P, Meelenkamp J, Ijff A, et al. (2011) Q fever among culling workers, the Netherlands, 2009–2010. Emerg Infect Dis 17(9): 1719–1723.

32. Burney PG, Luczynska C, Chinn S, Jarvis D (1994) The European community respiratory health survey. Eur Respir J 7: 954–960.

33. Tozer SJ, Lambert SB, Sloots TP, Nissen MD (2011) Q fever seroprevalence in metropolitan samples is similar to rural/remote samples in Queensland, Australia. Eur J Clin Microbiol Infect Dis Oct;30(10): 1287–93.

34. Wattiau P, Boldisova E, Toman R, Van Esbroeck M, Quoilin S, et al. (2011) Q fever in woolsorters, Belgium [letter]. Emerg Infect Dis Dec: [Epub ahead of print].

16

An Individual-Based Model of Transmission of Resistant Bacteria in a Veterinary Teaching Hospital

Neeraj Suthar[1], **Sandip Roy**[1,2], **Douglas R. Call**[1,3], **Thomas E. Besser**[1,3], **Margaret A. Davis**[1,4]*

1 Paul G. Allen School for Global Animal Health, College of Veterinary Medicine, Washington State University, Pullman, Washington, United States of America, **2** School of Electrical Engineering and Computer Science, College of Veterinary Medicine, Washington State University, Pullman, Washington, United States of America, **3** Dept. of Veterinary Microbiology and Pathology, College of Veterinary Medicine, Washington State University, Pullman, Washington, United States of America, **4** Dept. of Veterinary Clinical Sciences, College of Veterinary Medicine, Washington State University, Pullman, Washington, United States of America

Abstract

Veterinary nosocomial infections caused by antibiotic resistant bacteria cause increased morbidity, higher cost and length of treatment and increased zoonotic risk because of the difficulty in treating them. In this study, an individual-based model was developed to investigate the effects of movements of canine patients among ten areas (transmission points) within a veterinary teaching hospital, and the effects of these movements on transmission of antibiotic susceptible and resistant pathogens. The model simulates contamination of transmission points, healthcare workers, and patients as well as the effects of decontamination of transmission points, disinfection of healthcare workers, and antibiotic treatments of canine patients. The model was parameterized using data obtained from hospital records, information obtained by interviews with hospital staff, and the published literature. The model suggested that transmission resulting from contact with healthcare workers was common, and that certain transmission points (housing wards, diagnostics room, and the intensive care unit) presented higher risk for transmission than others (lobby and surgery). Sensitivity analyses using a range of parameter values demonstrated that the risk of acquisition of colonization by resistant pathogens decreased with shorter patient hospital stays ($P<0.0001$), more frequent decontamination of transmission points and disinfection of healthcare workers ($P<0.0001$) and better compliance of healthcare workers with hygiene practices ($P<0.0001$). More frequent decontamination of heavily trafficked transmission points was especially effective at reducing transmission of the model pathogen.

Editor: Alex Friedrich, University Medical Center Groningen, Netherlands

Funding: This work was entirely supported by the Paul G. Allen School for Global Animal Health, Washington State University, Pullman Washington. The funders had no role in study design, data collection and analysis, decision to publish, or preparation of the manuscript.

Competing Interests: The authors have declared that no competing interests exist.

* E-mail: madavis@vetmed.wsu.edu

Introduction

Antimicrobial resistance is a growing concern in modern health care settings as it increases morbidity, cost of treatment and mortality [1]. The prevalence of resistant bacteria in food animals may present a direct risk to public health [2,3] and companion animals may act as reservoirs of antimicrobial resistant bacteria that can be transmitted directly to people [4,5,6,7]. In human hospitals nosocomial infections cause approximately 90,000 deaths per year and an average of 5–10% of patients acquire nosocomial infections [8]. In veterinary hospitals the risk factors for nosocomial infections are similar to those in human healthcare settings. Lack of hand hygiene, use of invasive procedures, prolonged treatment and hospitalization and reliance on antimicrobials increase the risk of amplifying and transmitting antimicrobial resistant pathogens in veterinary hospitals [9,10]. *Escherichia coli* and *Klebsiella* spp. in particular have been strongly associated with urinary tract infections among human patients [11,12]. Canine cases of urinary tract infections caused by *E. coli* and *Klebsiella pneumoniae* are commonly diagnosed in veterinary settings and increasing numbers of antibiotic resistance cases in these bacterial species have made effective treatment more difficult [13].

Risk-based case control studies have shown that hospitalization is a serious risk factor for dogs becoming rectal carriers of multi-drug resistant (MDR) *E. coli* [14,15]. Dogs staying for over 6 days experience an increased risk of carrying MDR *E. coli* while those patients who had been hospitalized previously and/or had been treated with fluoroquinolones previously had higher probability of carrying MDR *E. coli* on arrival to the hospital. Veterinary hospitals may be the major source of resistant and MDR *E. coli* in horses [16]. Furthermore, increasing prevalence of MDR bacterial colonization of companion animals may have serious public health impacts [17].

Mathematical epidemic models have been applied to human hospital settings to analyze the risk factors associated with transmission of antibiotic resistant pathogens, to study associated molecular mechanisms and to evaluate control measures [18]. Three types of models have been commonly used to track nosocomial infections: deterministic models [19,20,21,22], stochastic models [23,24,25] and individual based models [26]. These models indicate that longer duration of treatment [26], delayed treatment and early breaks in treatment [27], reduced hospital staff [28], longer healthcare worker visits and larger populations of patients in the hospitals [29] increase the dissemination of antibiotic resistant bacteria while better hand hygiene compliance

[19] and combinatorial antibiotic therapy reduces this risk [27]. Horizontal gene transfer in the context of excessive antibiotic use can also lead to increased acquisition of antibiotic resistance, thereby potentially increasing the duration of antibiotic treatment and potential for treatment failure [30,31].

A model for veterinary settings has to account for the more frequent movement of the patients that is characteristic of these settings as compared to human hospitals. This movement is due, in part, to patient needs (e.g., environmental enrichment, walks for urination and defecation). Also, in veterinary settings there is reduced control over animal contacts with healthcare workers and surfaces due to petting, hand carriage of smaller animals, more proximity to the floor and defecation in cages. There are also important differences in housing and intensive care unit (ICU) arrangements. More canine patients can be accommodated in a much smaller veterinary hospital ICU by stacking their cages on top of each other as compared to the more spacious accommodation usually provided to human patients.

Published mathematical models for veterinary settings have been limited to deterministic approaches or regression analyses [32,33]. While these models and similar human models are useful for predicting risk factors and evaluating intervention measures, they do not take animal movements within the hospital into account. We developed an individual-based model (IBM) that tracks the movement of patients across the different points in the veterinary hospital where they come into contact with healthcare workers and various surfaces. This model improves on previous attempts to model nosocomial spread of antibiotic resistant pathogens by including variations in the rates of surface and healthcare worker contamination, routes of patient movement in the hospital, and other biologically relevant variables. We then use it to predict the probability of spread of antibiotic resistance under different control policies and changed hospital operational conditions to identify approaches to reduce the incidence of pathogen transmission in general, and multidrug resistant pathogen transfer in particular.

Materials and Methods

General model

We developed a stochastic IBM that tracks colonization of individual patients with resistant and non-resistant strains of a single bacterial pathogen as the individuals move through a veterinary hospital. For this model, we assumed that the pathogen could be carried asymptomatically in the gastrointestinal tract (colonization) and in some patients cause systemic infections such as wound, bloodstream or urinary tract infections, similar to known veterinary and human nosocomial pathogens such as *E. coli*, *K. pneumoniae*, or *Enterococcus* spp. [14,34,35,36]. Canine patients transit through this network model of the veterinary hospital, with a maximum of P patients in the hospital at any time. During their visits, each patient visits a sequence of transmission points (among T in total), which represent locations within the hospital where colonization can occur (e.g., surgery beds, diagnostic rooms, housing, etc). The patients are attended to by H human healthcare workers, each of whom is assigned to a single patient at any time. In the model, patients may be colonized by the pathogen by either contact with a contaminated transmission point or a contaminated health care worker. The model also incorporates the bacterial loads of colonized and infected patients, as well as the effects of antibiotic treatment of the infections. Specific components of the model discussed below include: 1) the temporal resolution and scope of the model, 2) intake of patients, 3) movement and care of patients in the hospital, 4) colonization and contamination, and 5) treatment.

Temporal Resolution and Scope. The model tracks colonization of patients by the pathogen over a long time horizon (months to years), with model dynamics resolved across several time scales. In particular, the intake of patients into the hospital and treatment with antibiotics is captured at a daily scale. Further, the day is subdivided into several multi-hour shifts (e.g., 3 shifts of eight hours each), after which health-care workers are replaced and treatment efforts re-initiated. Finally, colonization of patients and contamination of healthcare workers and transmission points is modeled at a fine resolution (time step, typically 1–15 minutes). A smaller time step size allows use of an exponential distribution to select values for various duration parameters in the model. We will refer to these different time resolutions in describing different aspects of the model.

Intake of Patients. New patients are taken into the hospital on a daily basis. The number of new patients is modeled as a Poisson random variable with a mean PD, with patients taken in up to the capacity of the hospital. Each patient taken into the hospital is in one of Q classes (labeled 1, ... , Q), which reflect their treatment needs (e.g. surgery, routine visit for a checkup, special diagnostics). Each of these classes would either require hospitalization or not. Specifically, each patient is modeled as being in class q ε 1, ... , Q with probability p_q, independently of the other patients. The duration that each hospitalized patient in a class q remains in the hospital (or the time of visit of the patient) is modeled as an independent exponential random variable, with mean v_q. This duration is specified according to the stochastic model at the time of intake. Each incoming patient may be pre-colonized with resistant, non-resistant, or both strains at small probabilities, independently of the other patients. As soon as the patient is admitted to the hospital a healthcare worker is assigned to that patient.

Patient Movement and Care. Each patient is modeled as following a route through the hospital, i.e. transitioning through a sequence of transmission points during its time at the hospital. Specifically, the routes followed by the patients in each of the Q classes are governed by distinct stochastic-sequence models: for instance, a regular-checkup patient may only transition among the hospital lobby, exam room, and diagnostics facility, while a surgery patient visits a larger number of transmission points (e.g., housing, operating rooms, etc). The route sequence can have both complex pre-determined transitions (to account for restricted movement during certain times of day) or simpler randomized transitions. As each patient follows its route, the patient remains at each transmission point for a stochastically-determined time-duration. Specifically, the patient remains in the transmission point for an exponentially-distributed time with average stay duration of TAV_t depending on the transmission point t, or until the patient's hospital-visit duration is exceeded. Once the healthcare worker's assignment to the patient is completed, he/she is immediately re-assigned to any unassigned patient with equal probability (or is re-assigned as soon as a patient becomes available); the health-care worker continues to transition among patients in this fashion. The healthcare worker remains with each patient for an exponentially distributed duration with mean duration given by AV, unless the assigned patient leaves the hospital.

Colonization, Infection and Contamination. Each patient is in one of four colonization states at each time-step during its visit to the hospital: uncolonized (U), colonized with a non-resistant strain of pathogen (NR), colonized with a resistant strain of pathogen (R) or colonized with both resistant and non-resistant

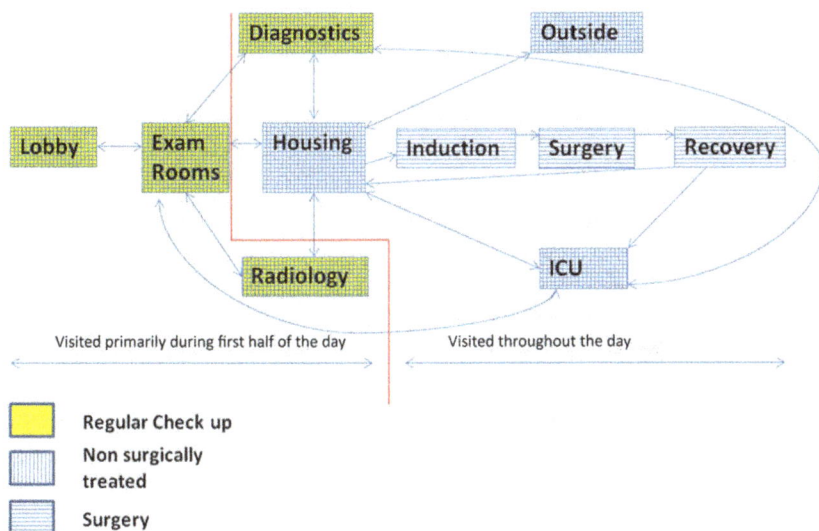

Figure 1. Patient movement inside the hospital. Patients seen for regular exams (yellow) are limited to the lobby, diagnostics and radiology. Patients seen for non-surgical problems (vertical lines) may be housed in wards or in the ICU and are taken outside for walks. Patients coming to WSU VTH for surgery (horizontal lines) have additional movements to the induction, surgery and recovery rooms.

strains of pathogen (NR+R). For each colonized patient, the model also captures the patient's bacterial loads for the non-resistant and resistant strains, and determines infection status. A subset of colonized patients become infected with the colonizing strain; in the model each colonized patient develops an infection with probability *PI*. Similarly, each transmission point and each health care worker may be classified into four contamination categories: uncontaminated, contaminated with the non-resistant strain, contaminated with the resistant strain, or contaminated with both strains. Broadly, patients may become colonized due to contact with either contaminated healthcare workers or contaminated transmission points. Further, colonized patients may contaminate both healthcare workers and transmission points, and there may also be direct cross-contamination between health-care-workers and transmission points.

Within this system of movement, a patient can be colonized with an initial arbitrary bacterial load due to a contaminated healthcare worker and/or transmission point per visit with a probability of *PC* with two provisos. First, the probability of contamination of the transmission point and/or the healthcare worker per patient visit, with the strain from a colonized patient, is directly proportional to the patients' bacterial load and inversely proportional to the surface area of the transmission point. Healthcare worker and transmission point can also cross-contaminate with a probability of *PC*. Contaminated healthcare workers are disinfected and contaminated transmission points are decontaminated with a probability *DE* after time intervals that are exponentially distributed with an average decontamination time *AC*. Secondly, the bacterial load of the colonized patient increases in absence of antibiotic therapy and is updated at the end of every shift. The simultaneous evolution of resistant and non-resistant bacterial loads is derived from a model previously described as equation 2 by Webb *et al.* [37] which simulates transfer of resistance plasmids from plasmid-bearing to non-plasmid bearing bacteria.

Treatment. The probability that a colonized patient becomes infected (i.e., symptomatic of disease) is *PI* and the probability that an infection is detected at the end of shift is *DR* (detection rate). Patients detected with an infection are given a primary antibiotic

treatment immediately, which initiates a decrease in the load of non-resistant strains every shift. After antibiotic susceptibility information is available, the treatment is suitably modified to reduce any resistant strain load carried by the patient as well. When the bacterial load of colonized patients goes below an arbitrary recovery threshold, they become "uncolonized."

Model for the Washington State University Veterinary Teaching Hospital (WSU-VTH)

We modelled the transmission of antibiotic resistant enteric bacteria among canine patients at the WSU-VTH. Data for parameterization of the model was drawn in part from hospital infection control surveillance activities. This surveillance involved collection of individual rectal swab samples from canine patients in three small animal services (intensive care, surgery and neurology) between September, 2009 and April, 2013. Data including antibiotic treatments, which services the animal visited, and the number of days in the hospital were recorded at the time of sample collection. Fecal swabs were plated directly onto MacConkey agar supplemented with ampicillin (16 ug/ml) and nalidixic acid (32 ug/ml) to select for Gram-negative bacteria that were resistant to both of these antibiotics. Any growth was noted and isolated colonies were submitted to the Washington State Animal Disease Diagnostic Laboratory (WADDL) for bacterial species identification. The average number of different categories of patients visiting each day and their duration of stay was calculated using this surveillance data and computerized hospital medical records. Each new patient was classified into one of the three categories: (i) surgery including elective, non-elective and emergency surgery; (ii) non-surgical disease including infectious disease, inflammatory disease, metabolic and other chronic diseases; or (iii) regular check-up involving routine visits for physical exams and vaccinations.

Based on the category assigned in the model, the patients will have different average lengths of stay (surgery and non-surgical disease, 5 days; regular check-up, 0.5 day) and follow different routes in the hospital (Fig. 1). We considered ten areas in the hospital that canine patients may visit during their hospital stay as potential transmission points. These included the lobby, the exam rooms, the diagnostics room (diagnosis of patients is done here and

Table 1. List of parameters and their baseline values.

Parameter name	Base level value in our model	Description
PD	24.372 per day***	Mean number of patients visiting the hospital daily
H	25*	Number of healthcare workers at any time
P	100*	Maximum number of patients in the hospital
T	10	Transmission points considered
Q	3	Routes considered
TAV_1	30 min*	Average time spent in the lobby at a time
TAV_2	120 min*	Average time spent in the exam room at a time
TAV_3	300 min*	Average time spent in the Diagnostics at a time
TAV_4	30 min*	Average visit time at Radiology
TAV_5	600 min*	Average visit time at Housing
TAV_6	600 min*	Average visit time at ICU
TAV_7	30 min*	Average visit time outside
TAV_8	120 min*	Average visit time at Induction room
TAV_9	60 min*	Average visit time at Surgery
TAV_{10}	120 min*	Average visit time at Recovery
AV	60 min**	Average time of healthcare worker visit
AC	60 min**	Average time before disinfection/decontamination of HCW/TP
PC	0.06**	Probability of colonization of patient given contact
$V_{1,2}$	5 days***	Average length of stay of surgery and non-surgical treatment patients
V_3	½ day*	Average length of stay of regular check-up patients
DE	0.9*	Probability of disinfection/decontamination of HCW/TP at the end of contamination period
PI	0.3*	Probability that a colonized patient becomes infected
DR	0.8*	Probability that an infection is detected at the end of shift
p_1	0.211***	Fraction of patients seen at WSU VTH that go to surgery
p_2	0.022***	Fraction of patients coming to WSU VTH for non-surgical or disease treatment
p_3	0.767***	Fraction of patients coming for routine exams at WSU VTH

*values for the WSU VTH were based on information from the hospital staff.
**values used by D'Agata et. al, 2007 [26], in the IBM for human patients.
***values estimated in this study using the hospital records and surveillance data.
HCW- healthcare worker, TP- transmission point.

in rare cases patients stay overnight), radiology, the housing wards (a large area with kennels for hospitalization), the outside dog-walking area, the ICU, the induction room (patients are prepared for surgery here), the surgery rooms, and the recovery room (patients have a transition stay here after surgery before being moved back to housing or ICU). At this hospital most elective surgeries are performed during the morning hours and for the most part patient movement during the night is limited to housing, ICU and diagnostics areas, therefore those movement constraints are included in the model.

Table 2. Variations in model parameters.

Parameter	Variations			
Average length of stay	3 days	6 days	9 days	12 days
Average disinfection/decontamination time for HCW and TP	30 min	60 min	120 min	240min
Number of HCW	15	30	45	60
Probability of colonization of patients given contact with contaminated HCW/TP	0.02	0.04	0.06	0.08
Probability that HCW/TP get disinfected/decontaminated after average contamination period	0.9	0.8	0.7	0.6
Fraction of infected patients detected and given antibiotics	0.9	0.8	0.7	0.6
Starting day of corrected antibiotic therapy	day 1	day 2	day 3	day 4

HCW- healthcare worker, TP- transmission point.

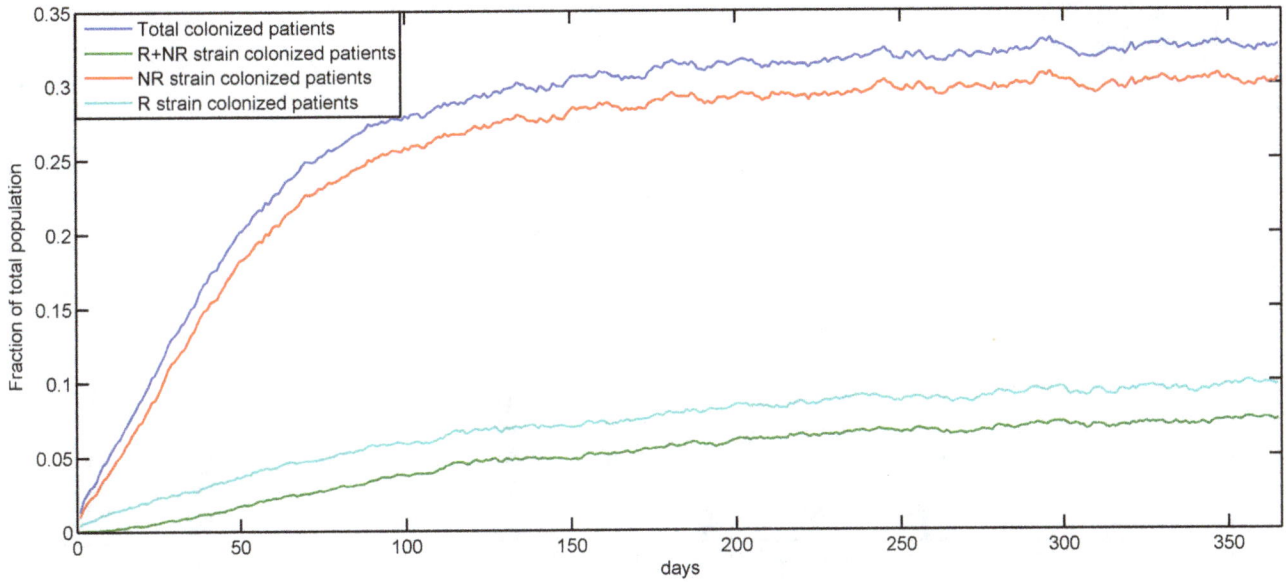

Figure 2. Distribution of strain types and colonization or infection status in the patient population. The fraction of patients in the hospital colonized, colonized with a resistant strain (R), colonized with a non-resistant strain (NR) and colonized with both resistant and non-resistant strains (R+NR), at the end of each day, averaged over 500 simulations.

We assumed that 10% of the daily new arrivals are colonized with a non-resistant strain and an additional 3% are colonized with the resistant strain at the time of entry into the hospital. The number of patients visiting daily averages 24.32. Baseline parameters for average time spent at each transmission point, average number of healthcare workers present in the hospital at any given time, and the maximum hospitalized patient load were based on information from hospital staff. The time required by WADDL to report antibiotic resistance profiles for hospitalized patients was most often 2 days (range, 1–8 days), and this was used

as the time before treatment modification in the model. Baseline parameter values are given in Table 1.

Simulations

Model code was developed using MATLAB vR2012a (Mathworks, Natick, Massachusetts). Simulations begin with an empty hospital and continue over a period of one year. Five hundred simulations using baseline parameter values discussed above (Table 1) were run initially and the results were averaged. To use the model to help indicate relative effectiveness of some control measures, such as changing the duration of hospitalization,

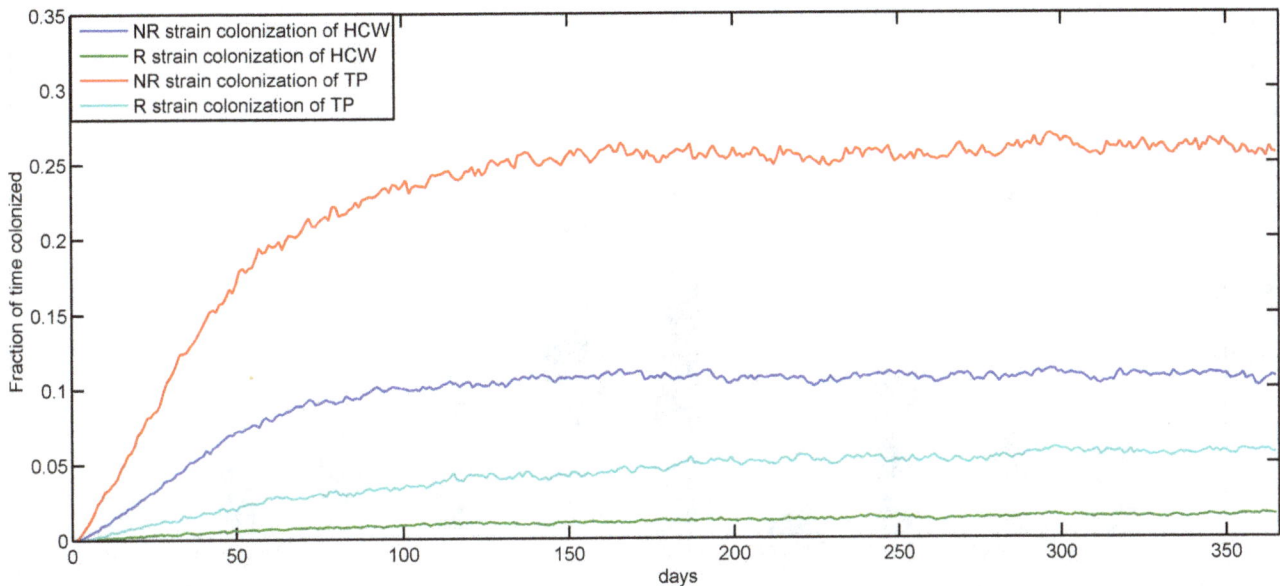

Figure 3. Contamination durations of healthcare workers and transmission points. The fraction of time healthcare workers (HCW) and transmission points (TP) remain contaminated with non-resistant (N) and resistant (R) strains each day averaged over 500 simulations.

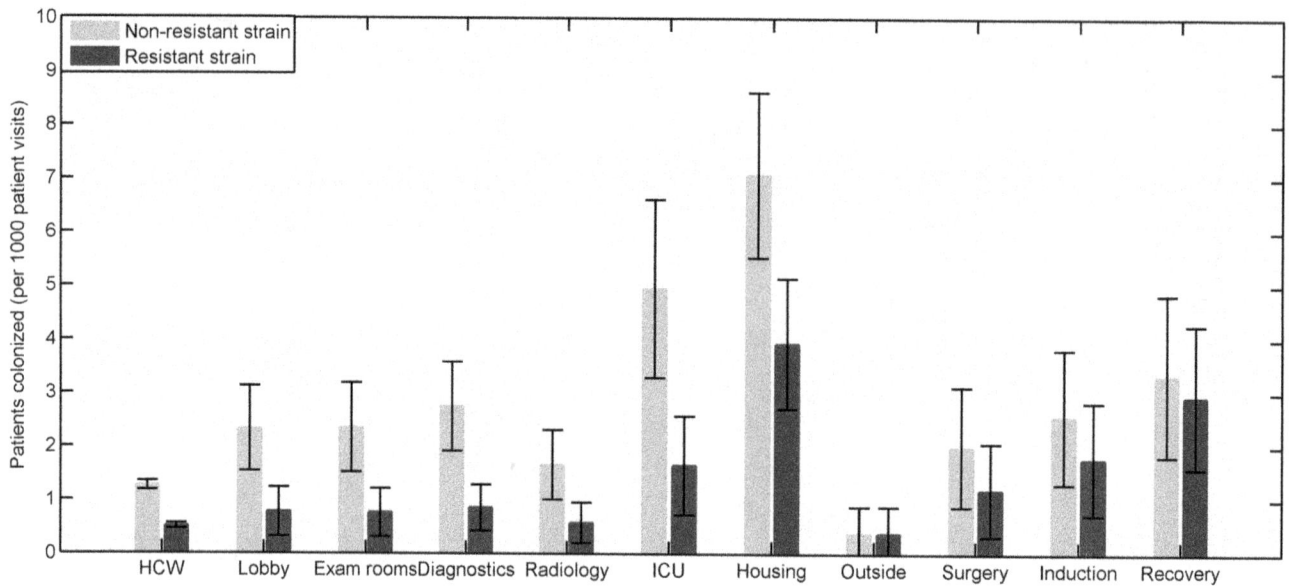

Figure 4. Proportion of visiting patients colonized. The average proportion of patients in contact with the healthcare workers (HCW) and the various transmission points that become colonized with non-resistant (N) and resistant (R) strains over the length of a year averaged over 500 simulations. Bars represent standard deviation across the yearly averages of 500 simulations.

increasing the hospital staff, increasing the frequency of surface decontamination etc., we further ran 600 simulations of our model with different combinations of a range of parameter values (Table 2). For this work parameter values were randomized after every two simulations resulting in 280 unique combinations of parameter values out of a total of 16,384 possible combinations.

Environmental Survey

To compare the model results with the actual contamination prevalence inside the hospital, we conducted environmental sampling at four locations (exam rooms, the diagnostics room,

ICU and the housing wards) in the hospital to estimate the fraction of time these areas were contaminated with *Enterococcus* spp or antibiotic resistant coliforms. Five samples were taken from each area at two hour intervals (midnight, 2am, 4am and so on) for 12 sampling sessions over three weeks. Samples were collected using standard 10 inch^2 sponges (Nasco, Fort Atkinson, Wisconsin) soaked in 30 ml LB broth (Hardy Diagnostics, Santa Maria, California). LB broth (30 ml) was added to each sample sponge and samples were enriched by incubating overnight at 37°C. After incubation 1 ml of each enriched sample was spread on mEnterococcus agar (Neogen Corporation, Lansing, Michigan)

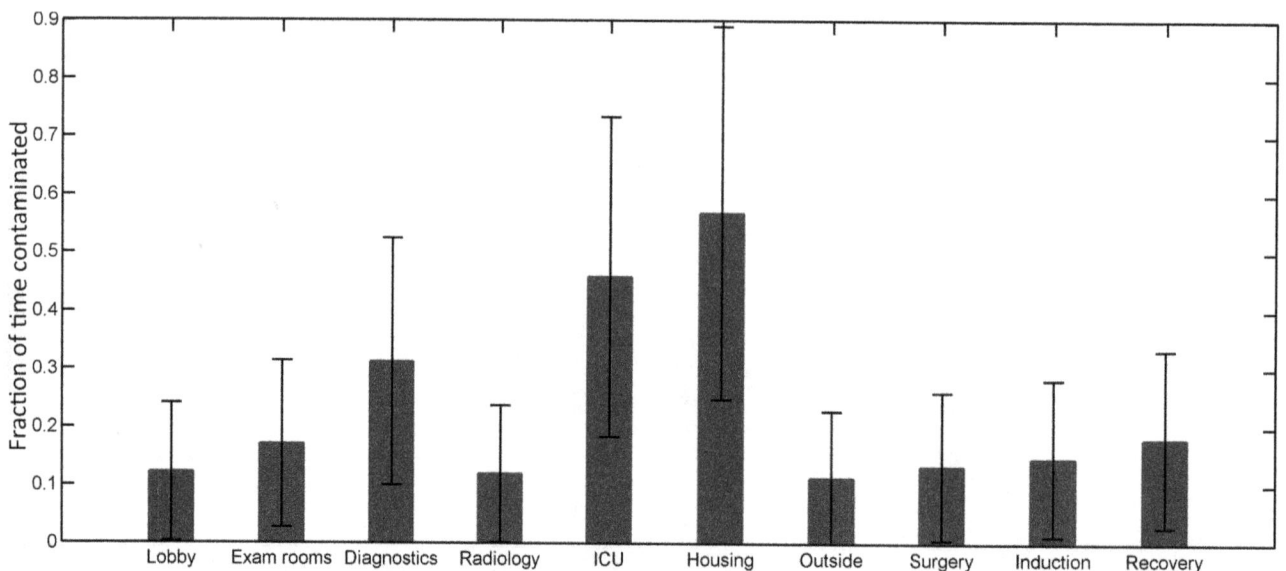

Figure 5. The yearly average of fraction of time that the transmission points remain contaminated. The yearly average of fraction of time each transmission point remains contaminated, averaged further over 500 simulations. Bars represent standard deviation across the yearly averages of 500 simulations.

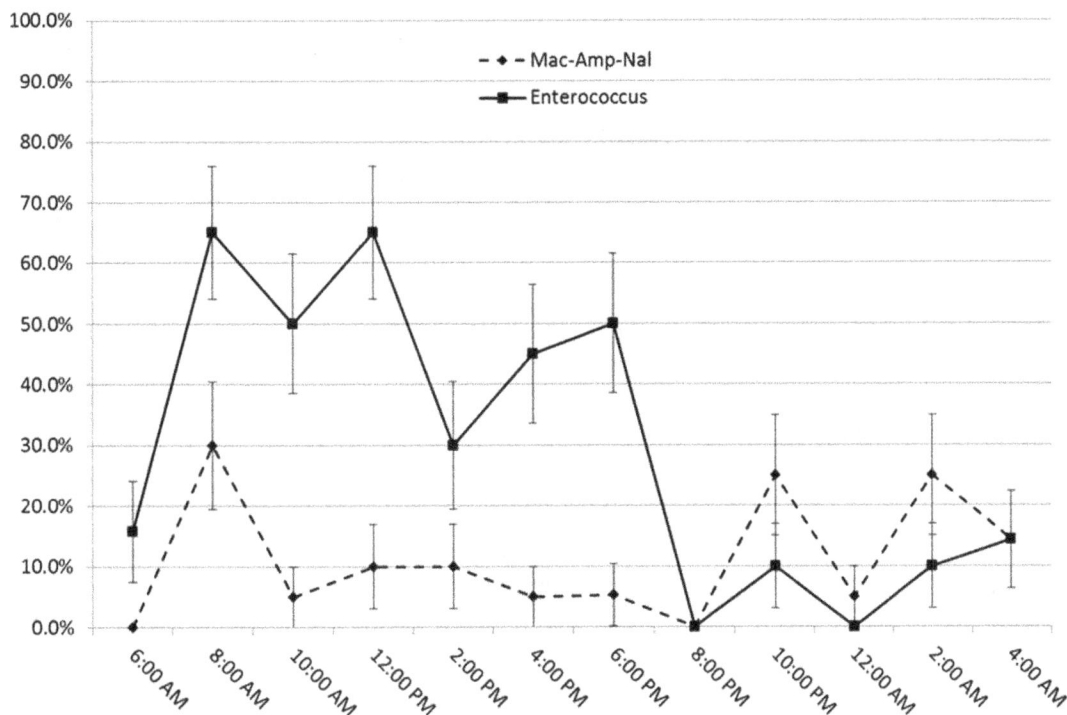

Figure 6. Percentage contamination with *Enterococci* or ampicillin-nalidixic acid-resistant coliforms of four transmission points by time of day. The average combined contamination prevalence of the four places sampled during the validation survey: the exam rooms, the diagnostics, ICU and the housing wards, at different times the sampling was done. Each data point is the average percentage contamination in 20 samples (5 samples per location) for each time. Bars represent the standard error over these 20 samples.

plates and incubated for 48 hrs, at the end of which presence or absence of colonies was recorded. Positive samples on mEnterococcus agar were confirmed to be *Enterococcus* sp. using the PYR-salt tolerance tests [38]. Each enriched sample (1 ml) was also spread onto MacConkey agar (Becton, Dickinson and company, Sparks, Maryland) supplemented with ampicillin (16 µg/ml) and nalidixic acid (32 µg/ml) to select for Gram-negative bacteria that were resistant to both antibiotics (Amp-Nal) and incubated overnight. Average percentage contamination of each area over a 24 hour period and average percentage contamination for all four areas at the time of sampling was calculated.

Statistical Analysis

Following simulations with different parameter sets the mean fraction of patients in the hospital that were colonized with a resistant strain and/or a non-resistant strain was evaluated using multivariate linear regression analysis. Pair-wise comparisons of individual parameters were used to determine the trend of increase or decrease in the mean fraction of patients in the hospital found to be colonized with a resistant and/or non-resistant strain due to an increase or decrease in the parameter value, in effect a sensitivity analysis to determine effects of parameters. Unpaired t-tests were used to compare the percent of times each transmission point remained contaminated according to the model and according to the environmental survey. Results from the environmental survey were also subjected to two-way ANOVA to identify associations between the level of contamination and the transmission points sampled. All statistical analyses were done in SAS analytics software (SAS Inst., Cary, North Carolina)

Results

Results from 500 simulations using baseline parameters

We start the simulation for a year with a clean and empty hospital and as inpatients accumulate, the mean population of patients inside the hospital at any time reaches a stable level. At the baseline values for all parameters, the fraction of the hospital patient population colonized with any strain stabilizes at approximately 32%. Approximately 30% of the patients are colonized with the non-resistant strain, 7% are colonized with the resistant strain, and 5% are colonized with both strains (Fig. 2).

Though the average time interval between decontamination of transmission points and disinfection of healthcare workers is assumed to be the same (60 min), the transmission points are contaminated with both resistant and non-resistant strains for longer durations overall ($P<0.0001$, unpaired t-test) throughout the year (Fig. 3).

Patient visits in the housing wards and the ICU area lead to colonization of the largest proportions of patients by the non-resistant strain. This proportion is significantly higher for housing than for all other transmission points except the ICU. The proportion of patients colonized by the resistant strain is highest for patients visiting the housing area or the recovery room. This proportion is significantly higher for housing, the ICU and diagnostics than for the surgery, exam rooms, lobby, radiology, and outside dog-walking areas (Fig. 4). The average fraction of time these places remain contaminated is also significantly higher amongst all the transmission points considered in the model, with diagnostics remaining contaminated for 31.2% (SD: 21.2%) of the time, ICU for 45.8% (SD: 27.4%) of the time and the housing wards for 56.9% (SD: 33.1%) of the time (Fig. 5).

Table 3. Environmental survey results.

Location[a]	Enterococcus spp.				Amp-Nal Coliforms			
	Day[b]	Night[b]	P[c]	Total[d]	Day[b]	Night[b]	P[c]	Total[e]
Diagnostics Room	60.0	10.0	<0.0001	35.0	13.3	10.0	>0.99	11.6
Exam rooms	43.3	10.0	0.007	26.7	3.3	10.0	0.61	6.7
ICU	50.0	10.0	0.008	30.0	16.7	3.3	0.19	10.0
Housing wards	50.0	3.3	<0.0001	26.7	10.3	23.3	0.30	16.9

[a]Each location was visited a total of 12 times with 5 samples collected at each visit for a total of 30 samples during the day and 30 during the night.
[b]Day includes the hours between 8 AM and 8 PM. Night includes the hours between 8:00 PM and 8:00 AM. Samples were collected at 2-hour intervals.
[c]Fisher exact P-value for the difference in proportion between day and night.
[d]P-value for difference between four mean proportions = 0.71.
[e]P-value for difference between four mean proportions = 0.44.

To determine the accuracy of our model predictions for the relative fractions of time that transmission points were contaminated, an environmental survey was conducted. Each of the four sampled locations (diagnostics room, exam rooms, ICU and housing wards) were frequently contaminated with *Enterococcus* spp: 27 to 35% of samples were positive. With respect to Amp-Nal coliforms, the diagnostics room, exam rooms, the ICU and the housing wards samples had 11.6, 6.7, 10.0 and 16.9 percent positive samples, respectively. The overall sample prevalence of *Enterococcus* spp. and Amp-Nal coliforms was not significantly different between locations (*Enterococcus* spp. contamination: $P=0.71$ and coliform contamination: $P=0.44$), although there were more positive samples for both types of bacteria in the housing wards, the ICU and the diagnostics room than in the exam rooms (Table 3). The prevalence of *Enterococcus*-positive samples was significantly higher in the daytime hours for each location but this day-night difference was not significant for Amp-Nal coliforms (Table 3 and Fig. 6).

Effects of Varying Parameters of the Model

Regression analysis of the mean fraction of patients colonized with a resistant strain produced a statistically significant fit ($P<0.001$) with an $R^2=0.957$. The Type III sums of squares indicated that the average length of stay parameter explained the bulk of the variance in the model with probability of colonization given contact, average time to disinfection of healthcare workers and decontamination of transmission points, and number of healthcare workers in the hospital also being significant in descending order of importance. The starting day of effective antibiotic therapy, efficiency of disinfection of healthcare workers and decontamination of transmission points, and infection detection rate were not significant (Table 4).

Regression analysis of the mean fraction of patients colonized with a non-resistant strain also produced a statistically significant fit ($P<0.001$) with an $R^2=0.965$. The average length of stay parameter again explained most of the variance in the model with probability of colonization given contact, average time of disinfection of healthcare worker and decontamination of transmission point, and number of healthcare workers in the hospital also significant in descending order of importance. The rate of infection detection was also a significant contributor to the mean fraction of the patient population that was colonized with a non-resistant stain (Table 5).

Least square means analysis was used to make pairwise comparisons between the average fractions of the population colonized with the resistant strain and/or non-resistant strain for a range of parameter values. There was a significant increase in the mean fraction of the patient population colonized with increasing length of stay ($P<0.0001$ in all cases) and a consistent decrease in the fraction of population colonized with the non-resistant strain with increases in the detection rate ($P<0.0001$ in all cases). There was a significant increase in the mean fraction of the patient population colonized with increasing duration of TP or HCW contamination ($P<0.0001$ in all cases). Analysis of maximum likelihood parameter estimates for the interaction between increasing the mean time of disinfection/decontamination with a change in transmission point showed that the lobby, exam rooms and diagnostic area have significantly greater increases in proportions of visiting patients that are colonized with resistant and/or non-resistant strains as compared to the housing wards and ICU. Increasing the probability of colonization of a patient given contact (analogous to a hand hygiene lapse) caused a significant increase in the mean fraction of the patient population colonized with ($P<0.0001$ in all cases). There was a significant

Table 4. Type III statistical test results for analysing the significance of various parameters on the mean fraction of the patient population carrying the resistant strain of the potential pathogen.

Source	Type III SS	Mean Square	F Value	Pr>F
Length of stay[a]	8.0319	2.6773	1283.02	<.0001
Detection rate[b]	0.01614	0.00538	2.58	0.054
Decontamination efficiency[c]	0.01143	0.00381	1.83	0.1425
Decontamination time[d]	1.23757	0.41252	197.69	<.0001
Colonization probability[e]	2.0568	0.6856	328.55	<.0001
Starting day of AB therapy[f]	0.00698	0.00233	1.11	0.3434
Number of HCW[g]	0.21583	0.07194	34.48	<.0001

[a]Average length of stay of hospitalized patients.
[b]Rate at which infections are detected.
[c]Efficiency of disinfection/decontamination of healthcare worker and transmission points.
[d]Average time before disinfection/decontamination of contaminated healthcare worker and transmission point.
[e]Probability of colonization of patient given contact with contaminated healthcare workers and transmission points.
[f]Number of days after the initial antibiotic therapy that the effective antibiotic therapy starts.
[g]Number of healthcare workers inside the hospital at any given time.

increase in the mean fraction of patient population colonized given an increasing number of healthcare workers from 15 to 30, but increasing beyond this level did not alter the outcome ($P>0.05$) (Table S1, Table S2).

Discussion

Model simulations done at baseline parameter values indicate that specific transmission points in the hospital such as the ICU, the housing wards and the recovery room, have more influence on transmission of colonization, including transmission of resistant strains, than other locations in the hospital. In the model, the housing and the ICU areas are associated with more transmissions due to the relatively long stays of hospitalized patients in these places [39], particularly at night. The proportions of time that housing wards were contaminated with Amp-Nal resistant coliforms during the environmental survey support this speculation (23.3% at night as compared to 10.3% during the day). However, for *Enterococcus* spp. the reverse was true (Fig. 6). Among the

transmission points exclusive for surgery patients, the recovery room had as much impact on non-resistant strain colonization of patients as the diagnostics room and a greater impact in the case of resistant strain colonization. This may be due to the fact that surgery-related transmission points are visited by patients that stay for longer durations in the hospital as compared to most of the patients visiting the diagnostics area. In the model, this allows for increased bacterial loads among surgery patients, leading to a larger probability of contamination of healthcare workers and the transmission points they visit and eventually increased chances of uncolonized visiting patients getting colonized. In general, the transmission points are contaminated for longer durations as compared to healthcare workers (Fig. 3) and cause colonization of more patients visiting them (Fig. 4). This is mainly because they are assumed to have multiple patient and healthcare worker visits in the model. But in terms of the absolute number of patients colonized, the effect of transmission points and healthcare workers

Table 5. Type III statistical test results for analysing the significance of various parameters on the mean fraction of the patient population carrying the non-resistant strain of the potential pathogen.

Source	Type III SS	Mean Square	F Value	Pr>F
Length of stay[a]	5.81725	1.93908	1483.7	<.0001
Detection rate[b]	0.23787	0.07929	60.67	<.0001
Decontamination efficiency[c]	0.00156	0.00052	0.4	0.7554
Decontamination time[d]	1.1509	0.38363	293.54	<.0001
Colonization probability[e]	1.58922	0.52974	405.33	<.0001
Starting day of AB therapy[f]	0.00474	0.00158	1.21	0.3072
Number of HCW[g]	0.14332	0.04777	36.55	<.0001

[a]Average length of stay of hospitalized patients.
[b]Rate at which infections are detected.
[c]Efficiency of disinfection/decontamination of healthcare worker and transmission points.
[d]Average time before disinfection/decontamination of contaminated healthcare worker and transmission point.
[e]Probability of colonization of patient given contact with contaminated healthcare workers and transmission points.
[f]Number of days after the initial antibiotic therapy that the effective antibiotic therapy starts.
[g]Number of healthcare workers inside the hospital at any given time.

are comparable due to relatively more frequent patient contacts by healthcare workers as compared to transmission points (Table 1).

Results from the simulations done with randomized parameter values and subsequent regression analyses suggest that the model is consistent with previous reports that the incidence of both resistant and non-resistant strain colonization increases with increasing length of stay in the hospital [14,15,33]. As long as the number of patients already hospitalized is below the maximum capacity for the hospital, longer patient stays contribute to a higher number of hospitalized patients, leading to more interactions between patients, healthcare workers and transmission points. Each individual patient also has a greater possibility of getting colonized during a longer stay in the hospital. Veterinary personnel and veterinary hospital environments are reportedly major risk factors in acquisition of antibiotic resistant pathogens by hospitalized dogs [15,40,41]. Consequently, reducing the probability of colonization of a patient given contact with a contaminated healthcare worker or transmission point reduces the percent of patients carrying resistant and/or non-resistant strains. The probability of colonization given contact can be reduced by increasing healthcare worker hand hygiene compliance and by improved cleaning and disinfection of hospital outerwear such as scrubs and white coats [42]. A decrease in the frequency of disinfection/decontamination of the healthcare workers and the transmission points resulted in a general increase in the number and incidence of nosocomial colonization in our model. This effect was most pronounced in the lobby, exam room and diagnostics areas suggesting that those places require more frequent cleaning, possibly because of higher traffic load during the daytime, as compared to the ICU and housing. This idea is supported by the findings of our environmental survey in which prevalence of contamination with Enterococci was higher during the day than during the night. In contrast, Amp-Nal coliform sample prevalence was not different between the day and nighttime hours. The reason for this difference is unknown. Coliforms are less persistent on surfaces in general [43], and therefore the sampling scheme here may not have fully captured their spatial-temporal distribution.

Increasing the number of healthcare workers might lead to safer interactions between patients and healthcare workers because caregivers would have fewer opportunities to cross-contaminate patients, but in our model it also increases the number of interactions between transmission points and healthcare workers leading to more contamination of transmission points and hence no significant change in the mean proportion of patients colonized. If the number of healthcare workers is very low as compared to the average patient population at any time, there is a significant decrease in the percent of patients that are colonized. This presumably occurs due to overall fewer interactions between patients and healthcare workers during their stay. Decreasing the number of healthcare workers is not pragmatic as it would increase the workload on individual healthcare workers and may lead to deterioration of care.

It is well documented that antimicrobial use is associated with antibiotic resistance [6,14,33,44], but our model indicates that giving an early effective antibiotic therapy has no significant impact on either reducing or increasing the incidence of antibiotic resistance. This might be a result of the relatively short average length of stay of the patients and shorter time available for antibiotic therapy completion.

The bacterial species considered in this model are enteric bacterial pathogens like Enterococcus spp., E. coli and K. pneumoniae. All three of these fecal organisms can spread to patients due to surface to body contact, followed by oral ingestion. Enterococcus spp. generally survive longer in the environment than gram-negative

bacteria do which may explain their near ubiquitous presence in our environmental survey. But their presence provides an indication of fecal contamination and inadequate cleaning and disinfection [39]. Gram-negative bacteria provide evidence for more recent fecal contamination [43]. The proportion of time of contamination with Amp-Nal coliforms during the environmental survey better reflected the predictions of the model, although no significant differences were found between the different places sampled. The model does fail to explain the higher level of Enterococcus spp. contamination during daytime than during nighttime hours. A possible explanation for the difference between Enterococci and Amp-Nal resistant coliforms is that the coliforms were specifically selected for resistance to antibiotics which may have co-selected for resistance to disinfectants. Thus after evening disinfection and during low traffic hours the Enterococci were less likely to be reintroduced by patient traffic. The model also indicates that places with shorter visits and higher patient traffic of patients (e.g., the exam room and the lobby) require more frequent disinfection/decontamination.

This model provides a significant contribution to the field of hospital modeling because it accounts for individual patient movements through the hospital rather than assuming a strictly compartmental structure of patient movements. The primary purpose of this effort was to generate a conceptual framework for predicting changes in antimicrobial resistant bacterial transmission in response to changes in the chosen parameters. The determination of baseline parameter values was limited because of a lack of empirical data; for example the true probability of initial colonization and infection given a previous colonization is not known. Nonetheless the relative effect of changing a parameter, for example changing the average length of hospital stay, is unlikely to be biased by the choice of a baseline. While intensive sampling for more empirically based parameterization would strengthen the model, such sampling was beyond the scope of the current effort. This will be included in future work to refine and expand on this model. Regardless of specific parameter values, the sensitivity analysis provides information about which variables will have the most impact and therefore where interventions should be targeted.

In summary, this model suggests that reducing the average length of stay of patients and more frequent disinfection of healthcare workers and decontamination of transmission points are the most important control measures to minimize nosocomial transmission and frequency of colonization or infection with resistant strains inside the hospital. Extensions of this model, such as considering multiple patient and pathogen species, variable healthcare worker population and using empirical data as a basis for the transmission probability estimates used here may give further insight into the risk factors associated with the spread of antibiotic resistance in veterinary hospitals with availability of extensive hospital data.

Supporting Information

Table S1 Results of least square means comparisons between the average fractions of the population colonized with the resistant strain for different parameter values.

Table S2 Results of least square means comparisons between the average fractions of the population colonized with the non-resistant strain for different parameter values.

Acknowledgments

We would like to thank Russell McClanahan and Lisa Jones for help in environmental sampling in the hospital and Dr. Harmon Rogers and the entire staff of VTH-WSU for their views on the dynamics of infection and cooperation in getting the surveillance data. We are also thankful to the Paul G. Allen School for Global Animal Health for supporting the project.

Author Contributions

Conceived and designed the experiments: NS SR MD. Performed the experiments: NS SR. Analyzed the data: NS SR DC MD. Contributed reagents/materials/analysis tools: MD. Wrote the paper: NS SR DC TB MD.

References

1. Frieden DT (2013) Antibiotic Resistance Threats in the United States, 2013. Centers for Disease Control and Prevention, U.S. Department of Health and Human Services.
2. van den Bogaard AE, Stobberingh EE (1999) Contamination of animal feed by multiresistant enterococci. Lancet 354: 163–164.
3. Howard DH, Scott RD, Packard R, Jones D (2003) The Global Impact of Drug Resistance. Clinical Infectious Diseases 36: S4–S10.
4. Guardabassi L, Schwarz S, Lloyd DH (2004) Pet animals as reservoirs of antimicrobial-resistant bacteria. J Antimicrob Chemother 54: 321–332.
5. Murphy C, Reid-Smith RJ, Prescott JF, Bonnett BN, Poppe C, et al. (2009) Occurrence of antimicrobial resistant bacteria in healthy dogs and cats presented to private veterinary hospitals in southern Ontario: A preliminary study. Can Vet J 50: 1047–1053.
6. Lloyd DH (2007) Reservoirs of Antimicrobial Resistance in Pet Animals. Clinical Infectious Diseases 45: S148–S152.
7. Song SJ, Lauber C, Costello EK, Lozupone CA, Humphrey G, et al. (2013) Cohabiting family members share microbiota with one another and with their dogs. Elife 2: e00458.
8. Burke JP (2003) Infection Control — A Problem for Patient Safety. New England Journal of Medicine 348: 651–656.
9. Johnson JA (2002) Nosocomial infections. Vet Clin North Am Small Anim Pract 32: 1101–1126.
10. Morley PS, Apley MD, Besser TE, Burney DP, Fedorka-Cray PJ, et al. (2005) Antimicrobial drug use in veterinary medicine. J Vet Intern Med 19: 617–629.
11. Weinstein RA, Gaynes R, Edwards JR, System NNIS (2005) Overview of Nosocomial Infections Caused by Gram-Negative Bacilli. Clinical Infectious Diseases 41: 848–854.
12. Vatopoulos AC, Kalapothaki V, Legakis NJ (1996) Risk factors for nosocomial infections caused by gram-negative bacilli. The Hellenic Antibiotic Resistance Study Group. J Hosp Infect 34: 11–22.
13. Prescott JF, Hanna WJB, Reid-Smith R, Drost K (2002) Antimicrobial drug use and resistance in dogs. Canadian Veterinary Journal-Revue Veterinaire Canadienne 43: 107–116.
14. Gibson JS, Morton JM, Cobbold RN, Filippich LJ, Trott DJ (2011) Risk factors for dogs becoming rectal carriers of multidrug-resistant Escherichia coli during hospitalization. Epidemiol Infect 139: 1511–1521.
15. Hamilton E, Kruger JM, Schall W, Beal M, Manning SD, et al. (2013) Acquisition and persistence of antimicrobial-resistant bacteria isolated from dogs and cats admitted to a veterinary teaching hospital. J Am Vet Med Assoc 243: 990–1000.
16. Ahmed MO, Williams NJ, Clegg PD, van Velkinburgh JC, Baptiste KE, et al. (2012) Analysis of risk factors associated with antibiotic-resistant Escherichia coli. Microb Drug Resist 18: 161–168.
17. Abraham S, Wong HS, Turnidge J, Johnson JR, Trott DJ (2014) Carbapenemase-producing bacteria in companion animals: a public health concern on the horizon. J Antimicrob Chemother.
18. Opatowski L, Guillemot D, Boelle PY, Temime L (2011) Contribution of mathematical modeling to the fight against bacterial antibiotic resistance. Curr Opin Infect Dis 24: 279–287.
19. Sebille V, Chevret S, Valleron AJ (1997) Modeling the spread of resistant nosocomial pathogens in an intensive-care unit. Infect Control Hosp Epidemiol 18: 84–92.
20. D'Agata EM, Webb GF, Horn MA, Moellering RC, Jr., Ruan S (2009) Modeling the invasion of community-acquired methicillin-resistant Staphylococcus aureus into hospitals. Clin Infect Dis 48: 274–284.
21. Webb GF, Horn MA, D'Agata EM, Moellering RC, Ruan S (2009) Competition of hospital-acquired and community-acquired methicillin-resistant Staphylococcus aureus strains in hospitals. J Biol Dyn 48: 271.
22. Lipsitch M, Bergstrom CT, Levin BR (2000) The epidemiology of antibiotic resistance in hospitals: paradoxes and prescriptions. Proc Natl Acad Sci U S A 97: 1938–1943.
23. McBryde ES, Pettitt AN, McElwain DL (2007) A stochastic mathematical model of methicillin resistant Staphylococcus aureus transmission in an intensive care unit: predicting the impact of interventions. J Theor Biol 245: 470–481.
24. Kouyos RD, zur Wiesch PA, Bonhoeffer S (2011) On Being the Right Size: The Impact of Population Size and Stochastic Effects on the Evolution of Drug Resistance in Hospitals and the Community. Plos Pathogens 7.
25. Raboud J, Saskin R, Simor A, Loeb M, Green K, et al. (2005) Modeling transmission of methicillin-resistant Staphylococcus aureus among patients admitted to a hospital. Infect Control Hosp Epidemiol 26: 607–615.
26. D'Agata EM, Magal P, Olivier D, Ruan S, Webb GF (2007) Modeling antibiotic resistance in hospitals: the impact of minimizing treatment duration. J Theor Biol 249: 487–499.
27. D'Agata EM, Dupont-Rouzeyrol M, Magal P, Olivier D, Ruan S (2008) The impact of different antibiotic regimens on the emergence of antimicrobial-resistant bacteria. PLoS One 3: e4036.
28. Grundmann H, Hori S, Winter B, Tami A, Austin DJ (2002) Risk factors for the transmission of methicillin-resistant Staphylococcus aureus in an adult intensive care unit: fitting a model to the data. J Infect Dis 185: 481–488.
29. D'Agata EM, Horn MA, Ruan S, Webb GF, Wares JR (2012) Efficacy of infection control interventions in reducing the spread of multidrug-resistant organisms in the hospital setting. PLoS One 7: e30170.
30. Levin BR, Rozen DE (2006) Non-inherited antibiotic resistance. Nat Rev Microbiol 4: 556–562.
31. Bootsma MC, van der Horst MA, Guryeva T, ter Kuile BH, Diekmann O (2012) Modeling non-inherited antibiotic resistance. Bull Math Biol 74: 1691–1705.
32. Boerlin P (2004) Molecular epidemiology of antimicrobial resistance in veterinary medicine: where do we go? Anim Health Res Rev 5: 95–102.
33. Ogeer-Gyles J, Mathews KA, Sears W, Prescott JF, Weese JS, et al. (2006) Development of antimicrobial drug resistance in rectal Escherichia coli isolates from dogs hospitalized in an intensive care unit. J Am Vet Med Assoc 229: 694–699.
34. Stolle I, Prenger-Berninghoff E, Stamm I, Scheufen S, Hassdenteufel E, et al. (2013) Emergence of OXA-48 carbapenemase-producing Escherichia coli and Klebsiella pneumoniae in dogs. J Antimicrob Chemother 68: 2802–2808.
35. Ghosh A, Kukanich K, Brown CE, Zurek L (2012) Resident Cats in Small Animal Veterinary Hospitals Carry Multi-Drug Resistant Enterococci and are Likely Involved in Cross-Contamination of the Hospital Environment. Front Microbiol 3: 62.
36. Orsini JA, Snooks-Parsons C, Stine L, Haddock M, Ramberg CF, et al. (2005) Vancomycin for the treatment of methicillin-resistant staphylococcal and enterococcal infections in 15 horses. Can J Vet Res 69: 278–286.
37. Webb GF, D'Agata EM, Magal P, Ruan S (2005) A model of antibiotic-resistant bacterial epidemics in hospitals. Proc Natl Acad Sci U S A 102: 13343–13348.
38. Murray PR, Baron EJ, American Society for Microbiology. (2003) Manual of clinical microbiology. Washington, D.C.: ASM Press.
39. Arias CA, Murray BE (2012) The rise of the Enterococcus: beyond vancomycin resistance. Nat Rev Microbiol 10: 266–278.
40. Heller J, Kelly L, Reid SW, Mellor DJ (2010) Qualitative risk assessment of the acquisition of Meticillin-resistant staphylococcus aureus in pet dogs. Risk Anal 30: 458–472.
41. KuKanich KS, Ghosh A, Skarbek JV, Lothamer KM, Zurek L (2012) Surveillance of bacterial contamination in small animal veterinary hospitals with special focus on antimicrobial resistance and virulence traits of enterococci. J Am Vet Med Assoc 240: 437–445.
42. Banu A, Anand M, Nagi N (2012) White coats as a vehicle for bacterial dissemination. J Clin Diagn Res 6: 1381–1384.
43. Gastmeier P, Schwab F, Barwolff S, Ruden H, Grundmann H (2006) Correlation between the genetic diversity of nosocomial pathogens and their survival time in intensive care units. J Hosp Infect 62: 181–186.
44. Heuer OE, Jensen VF, Hammerum AM (2005) Antimicrobial drug consumption in companion animals. Emerg Infect Dis 11: 344–345.

17

Identification of Myeloid Derived Suppressor Cells in Dogs with Naturally Occurring Cancer

Michelle R. Goulart[1], G. Elizabeth Pluhar[1], John R. Ohlfest[2,3]*

1 Department of Veterinary Clinical Sciences, University of Minnesota, Saint Paul, Minnesota, United States of America, 2 Department of Pediatrics, University of Minnesota, Minneapolis, Minnesota, United States of America, 3 Department of Neurosurgery, University of Minnesota, Minneapolis, Minnesota, United States of America

Abstract

Dogs with naturally occurring cancer represent an important large animal model for drug development and testing novel immunotherapies. However, poorly defined immunophenotypes of canine leukocytes have limited the study of tumor immunology in dogs. The accumulation of myeloid derived suppressor cells (MDSCs) is known to be a key mechanism of immune suppression in tumor-bearing mice and in human patients. We sought to identify MDSCs in the blood of dogs with cancer. Peripheral blood mononuclear cells (PBMCs) from dogs with advanced or early stage cancer and from age-matched healthy controls were analyzed by flow cytometry and microscopy. Suppressive function was tested in T cell proliferation and cytokine elaboration assays. Semi-quantitative RT-PCR was used to identify potential mechanisms responsible for immunosuppression. PBMCs from dogs with advanced or metastatic cancer exhibited a significantly higher percentage of CD11b$^+$CD14$^-$MHCII$^-$ cells compared to dogs diagnosed with early stage non-metastatic tumors and healthy dogs. These CD11b$^+$ CD14$^-$MHCII$^-$ cells constitute a subpopulation of activated granulocytes that co-purify with PBMCs, display polymorphonuclear granulocyte morphology, and demonstrate a potent ability to suppress proliferation and IFN-γ production in T cells from normal and tumor-bearing donors. Furthermore, these cells expressed hallmark suppressive factors of human MDSC including ARG1, iNOS2, TGF-β and IL-10. In summary our data demonstrate that MDSCs accumulate in the blood of dogs with advanced cancer and can be measured using this three-marker immunophenotype, thereby enabling prospective studies that can monitor MDSC burden.

Editor: Sophia N. Karagiannis, King's College London, United Kingdom

Funding: This work was supported by grants to Dr. Ohlfest from the National Institutes of Health (NIH R21-NS055738), and the American Cancer Society (RSG-09-189-01-LIB). The funders had no role in study design, data collection and analysis, decision to publish, or preparation of the manuscript.

Competing Interests: The authors have declared that no competing interests exist.

* E-mail: Ohlfe001@umn.edu

Introduction

Cancer is the leading cause of death in adult dogs in the United States, Australia, Japan and Europe and is considered the major health care concern of pet owners. Approximately four million dogs are diagnosed with cancer each year in the United States [1]. Naturally occurring malignances in dogs share many features with human cancers including similar tumor biology, genetics, incidence rates, histological appearance, and response to conventional treatments (reviewed in [2]). Tumors in dogs progress relatively faster than the same disease in humans, allowing questions related to treatment efficacy (progression and survival) to be addressed more rapidly in dogs. An important advantage of the dog model is the ability to test experimental therapeutics at human scale doses in the setting of minimal residual disease, which is difficult to do in a meaningful way in small rodents that have relatively rapid tumor growth kinetics. In addition, because the standard of care for most canine tumors is poorly established, there is much more flexibility in study design compared to human clinical trials. Collectively these features make the dog an outstanding platform for translational medicine.

Pet dogs with cancer are rapidly becoming an important tool used in drug development. One of the best examples of this is the recent parallel development of SU11654, a multi-targeted tyrosine kinase inhibitor, and sunitinib malate (SU11248). Both drugs are potent inhibitors of PDGFR, VEGFR, KIT, and FLT3. Studies in dogs with various solid tumors revealed that plasma concentration of SU11654, the mutational status of KIT, and the inhibition of KIT phosphorylation were strongly predictive of clinical efficacy. Optimal dosing parameters and toxicity were established in dogs as well. These pioneering studies greatly facilitated the further development of this entire class of drugs, most notably the approval of sunitinib malate by the U.S. Food and Drug Administration for the treatment of renal cell carcinoma (RCC) and gastrointestinal stromal cell tumors, which often contain similar KIT mutations [3]. It was later recognized that sunitinib markedly depletes MDSCs and restores T cell function in human RCC patients [4], an observation that could not have been made in dogs at the time because of limited canine reagents and poorly defined markers for canine leukocytes. We, and others, are testing novel immune-based therapies in dogs with various malignancies, but immune monitoring in these studies has been confounded by the same problem. To put the field in perspective, a surface immunophenotype for canine natural killer cells has not been defined, the MHC alleles are poorly understood, and many of the markers used rely on cross-reactive antibodies whereby specificity must be tested empirically. It is crucial that new reagents are developed and that the immunophenotypes of all major canine leukocytes subsets are determined. Laying this basic foundation will allow unique insights to be made as new small molecule drugs and immunotherapies are tested in dogs as a prelude to human trials.

The accumulation of MDSCs in tumor-bearing mice and humans with cancer is known to be a key mechanism of tumor escape from immune surveillance [5,6,7]. MDSCs comprise a phenotypically heterogeneous population of myeloid cells in early stages of differentiation that expand in cancer and many other pathological conditions, and have a potent ability to suppress T cell function, especially T cell proliferation and effector cytokine production [6,8]. MDSCs may be divided into monocytic and granulocytic subtypes. One source of controversy in this field is that MDSC heterogeneity has made comparisons between cancer patients and murine tumor models challenging (see reference [9] for excellent perspective). The molecular mechanisms by which MDSCs inhibit T cell function are under investigation. Studies have implicated up-regulation of arginase 1 (ARG1), inducible nitric oxide synthase (iNOS2) and reactive oxygen species (ROS) as important factors for MDSC-mediated immune suppression [8,10,11]. ARG1 can profoundly impair T cell function at the tumor site by L-arginine depletion, triggering the amino acid starvation response and apoptosis in lymphocytes [7]. Another mechanism of immune suppression is chemokine nitration, which blunts effector T cell infiltration into the tumor site [12]. Furthermore, MDSC expansion is associated with downregulation of L-Selectin on $CD4^+$ and $CD8^+$ T cells [13]. This reduces T cell trafficking to secondary lymphoid organs where tumor-reactive T cells can be primed [13]. Due to the ability of MDSCs to downregulate the immune response against tumors in mice and in humans, we hypothesized that these cells would also play an important role in tumor-induced immune suppression in dogs with cancer. Hence, the objective of this study was to identify surface markers that characterize the existence of MDSCs in dogs.

Materials and Methods

Study Population and sample collection

The description of all dogs in this study is summarized in **Tables 1** and **2**, with further detail provided in **Tables S1** and **S2**.

Table S3 is a summary of samples assayed in each figure. Clinical data were obtained from medical records. Control dogs were determined to be healthy based on physical examination, owner observations and complete blood count exams. For dogs with cancer, the diagnosis and tumor staging were based on complete physical examinations, histopathology of tumor biopsy specimens, blood work and specialized imaging tests, such as CT scans, ultrasound or radiographs, to assess tumor location and size, as well as the presence of metastatic disease. Dogs with large, necrotic or multiple masses, lytic or severe bone destruction (with osteosarcoma) or presence of metastasis, were placed into the advanced stage/metastatic group. Animals presenting with small masses or no metastatic nodules were placed into the early stage non-metastatic group. **Tables S1** and **S2** also list specifics about any treatment that dogs with cancer had received prior to or at the time of blood collection for this study.

Blood samples from both cancer and healthy control dogs were obtained specifically for this study. Samples were collected in heparinized tubes by the Oncology and Community Practice Services of the Veterinary Medical Center at the University of Minnesota according to Institutional Animal Care and Use Committee guidelines. The samples were drawn after the owners signed the client consent form. The Institutional Animal Care and Use Committee (IACUC) reviewed and approved the study entitled as "Flow Cytometric Immunophenotyping of Peripheral

Table 1. Characteristics of dogs with cancer in the study.

Age (yrs) - Mean (Range)	9 (2–14)
Gender	
Male/Neutered	22
Male/Intact	2
Female/Spayed	21
Processed Samples	
Fresh	21
Frozen	24
Breed	
Labrador Retriever	12
Mixed Breed	5
Golden Retriever	3
Greyhound	2
Boxer	2
Border Collie	2
Beagle	2
Scottish Terrier	1
Bull Mastiff	1
Rottweiler	1
Dalmatian	1
Great Dane	1
Bernese Mountain Dog	1
German Wirehaired Pointer	1
German Shepherd Dog	1
West Highland White Terrier	1
Gordon Setter	1
Weimaraner	1
Rhodesian Ridgeback	1
Rat Terrier	1
Newfoundland	1
Miniature Poodle	1
Chow Chow	1
English Springer Spaniel	1
Total	45

Blood Cells in Dogs" via designated member review under the code number 0912A75493. Unless explicitly stated otherwise, the cells being analyzed for this manuscript co-purified with peripheral blood mononuclear cells (PBMCs) of dogs with cancer or age-matched healthy controls that were isolated using Ficoll (Sigma) gradient centrifugation as follows. Heparinized peripheral blood was diluted 1:3 with sterile PBS (Invitrogen) and layered over Ficoll-Histopaque (Sigma). Samples were centrifuged at 400-× g for 30 min. The PBMCs collected at the interface were transferred to a fresh tube, washed twice with PBS, and resuspended with freezing solution consisting of 90% fetal bovine serum (Invitrogen) 10% Dimethyl sulfoxide (DMSO) (Sigma) and then frozen at −80°C. Lastly, PBMCs were thawed for 2 minutes in a 37°C water bath before staining and analysis. For analysis of fresh samples, PBMCs were isolated as above, resuspended in FACS buffer, stained with antibodies and immediately analyzed by flow cytometry or FACS as indicated.

Table 2. Characteristics of healthy dogs in the study.

Age (yrs) - Mean (Range)	8 (2–13)
Gender	
Male/Neutered	7
Male/Intact	1
Female/Intact	2
Female/Spayed	8
Processed Samples	
Fresh	6
Frozen	12
Breed	
Labrador Retriever	4
Golden Retriever	2
English Setter	1
Shih Tzu	2
Mixed Breed	2
German Shepherd dog	1
German Wirehaired Pointer	1
Red Tick Hound	1
Poodle	1
Cocker Spaniel	1
Catahoula Hound mix	1
Greyhound	1
Total	18

Flow Cytometric Analysis

PBMC samples were isolated from fresh blood or thawed and resuspended in FACS buffer. Nonspecific antibody binding was blocked by pretreatment of cells with 10 μg/mL canine gamma-globulin (Jackson Immunoresearch) for 20 min at room temperature. Cells were first labeled using indirect staining with 0.1 μg of unconjugated mouse anti-dog CD11b antibody (clone CA16.3E10, AbD Serotec) or IgG1 isotype control (AbD Serotec) and 0.5 μg of PE-conjugated goat F(ab')2 anti-mouse IgG (Abcam) secondary antibody at 4°C for 30 min in a dark room. Following indirect staining, cells were washed twice and stained with 0.3 μg of FITC-conjugated rat anti-dog MHCII (clone YKIX334.2, AbD Serotec) and 0.15 μg of the cross-reactive, Alexa fluor 647-conjugated mouse anti-human CD14 antibody (clone TÜK4, AbD Serotec) or isotypes controls at 4°C for 30 min in a dark room according to manufacturer's protocol. Antibody-labeled cells were washed twice and re-suspended in FACS buffer. Cells were incubated for 10 minutes at room temperature in the dark with 7-amino-actinomycin D (7AAD, final concentration of 1 μg/mL; Calbiochem) and then analyzed on a Becton Dickinson Canto three-laser flow cytometer. Data were further analyzed with FlowJo software (Tree Star). Analysis gates were set based on the 7AAD negative population. The percentage of MDSCs was calculated based on the percentage of CD11b$^+$CD14$^-$MHCII$^-$ cells within the overall live PBMC population. In one experiment (**Figure S1**), anti-mouse PE-conjugated CD11b (clone M1/70 eBioscience) and anti-mouse APC-conjugated Gr-1 (clone RB6-8C5 eBioscience) antibodies were also used to verify cross-reactivity with dog cells.

Isolation of MDSCs, PMNs and T cells

For functional assays, RT-PCR and cell morphology analysis, fresh blood samples from a tumor-bearing dog were used for isolation of CD11b$^+$CD14$^-$MHCII$^-$ or CD11b$^+$CD14$^+$MHCII$^-$ cells, as indicated, using a BD FACSAria cell sorter. For T cell isolation, PBMCs were isolated as previously described from fresh blood samples of healthy dogs and stained with 0.3 μg of FITC-conjugated mouse anti-dog CD3 (clone CA17.2A12, AbD Serotec), 0.15 μg of Pacific blue-conjugated mouse anti-dog CD4 (clone YKIX302.9, AbD Serotec) and 0.15 μg of Alexa700-conjugated mouse anti-dog CD8 (clone YCATE55.9, AbD Serotec) antibodies. Polymorphonuclear leukocytes (PMN) were purified from the cell pellet of a Ficoll gradient from healthy dog blood samples, after removal of the PBMCs (at the top of gradient) and erythrocytes by RBC lysis buffer (eBioscience).

Ex Vivo Proliferation

Analysis of MDSC inhibitory activity on T cell proliferation was measured by ^{3}H-thymidine incorporation into DNA. Briefly, PBMCs from the indicated dogs were seeded into U-bottom 96-well plates (5×10^4 cells/well) in medium consisting of RPMI 1640 containing L-arginine (150 μM) (Invitrogen) supplemented with penicillin/streptomycin (Invitrogen) and 10% heat-inactivated fetal bovine serum (Invitrogen) at 37°C, in a 5% CO_2 incubator. CD11b$^+$CD14$^-$MHCII$^-$ or CD11b$^+$ CD14$^+$ MHCII$^-$ cells from a dog with cancer were sorted and added to cancer (autologous) or healthy responder PBMCs as indicated. Concanavalin A (5 μg/ml) (Sigma) and recombinant human IL-2 (10 IU/ml) (R&D systems) were used to stimulate T cell proliferation. Non-stimulated PBMCs were used as negative control. PBMCs or PMNs were co-cultured with healthy PBMCs to control for the effect of simply adding additional cells to the suppression assay as indicated. Plates were cultured for 72 h, then pulsed with 1 μCi of ^{3}H-thymidine (Amersham Pharmacia Biotech) for 18 hrs at 37°C. Cells were harvested onto glass fiber filters (Perkin Elmer), washed, dried, and counted. Proliferative responses were measured by ^{3}H-thymidine incorporation into the DNA using a Matrix 96 Direct Beta Counter (Packard). All experiments were performed in triplicate.

IFN-γ Analyses

FACS-isolated CD11b$^+$CD14$^-$MHCII$^-$ cells from a cancer dog were co-cultured with PBMCs isolated from a healthy dog using the same method as the proliferation assay. After 72 hrs of incubation the cell culture supernatants were collected and measured using a Quantikine canine IFN-γ ELISA kit according to the manufacture's instructions (R&D systems). Samples were assayed colorimetrically, in triplicate, using a Microplate Reader Synergy2 (Biotek) and analyzed with Microplate Data Collection and Analysis Software Gen5 (Biotek).

Cytospin

FACS-isolated CD11b$^+$CD14$^-$MHCII$^-$ cells were stained using a modified Giemsa stain (Diff-quick, Astral Diagnostics Inc) for cell morphology evaluation and observed using a DME microscope (Leica) at 63× power magnification. Pictures were acquired with an EC3 camera (Leica).

RNA extraction and RT-PCR

RNA was extracted from FACS-isolated CD11b$^+$CD14$^-$MHCII$^-$ cells or healthy dog PMNs, using an RNAeasy plus Mini kit (QIAGEN) according to the manufacturer's protocol.

RNA concentrations were evaluated using a ND (100) spectrophotometer (Nanodrop). To detect expression of ARG1 and iNOS2 enzymes, gene-specific primers were designed based on the canine ARG1 and iNOS2 sequence; primer sequences for housekeeping gene were designed from canine β-actin gene using Primer3Plus (http://www.bioinformatics.nl/cgi-bin/primer3plus/primer3plus.cgi). For detection of cytokines IL-10 and TGF-β, primer sequences of IL-10 and TGF-β were obtained from published sources [14]. The BLAST algorithm (http://blast.ncbi.nlm.nih.gov/Blast.cgi) was used to ensure primer specificity to the target gene. First strand cDNA synthesis was done using a QuantiTect Reverse Transcription kit (QIAGEN). The two-step PCR reaction was carried out in a 12.5-μl volume containing 2× SYBR green master mix (Quanta Biosciences), 0.675U GoTaq Polymerase, 2 nM MgCl$_2$ (Promega), 0.2 mM dNTPs (Stratagene), 0.2 μM of each primer pair and 50 ng of cDNA template. Reaction conditions consisted of initial denaturation at 94°C for 2 min, then cycles of denaturation at 94°C for 30 s, annealing at 60°C for 45 s, elongation at 72°C for 45 s and final elongation at 72°C for 5 min in a DNA Engine Thermal Cycler (Bio-rad). The optimum annealing temperature for each primer pair was established prior to the study (see primer sequences in **Table S4**). PCR products were run on 2% agarose gels containing 0.5 μl/ml ethidium bromide and imaged under 590 nm ultraviolet light on a Eagle Eye II image station (Stratagene). Negative control reactions were performed using RNA that was not subjected to reverse transcription PCR.

Statistical Analysis

The differences between two groups were analyzed using unpaired, two-tailed Student's t test. All tests were performed with Prism 4 software (Graph Pad Software, Inc). P values <0.05 were considered to be statistically significant.

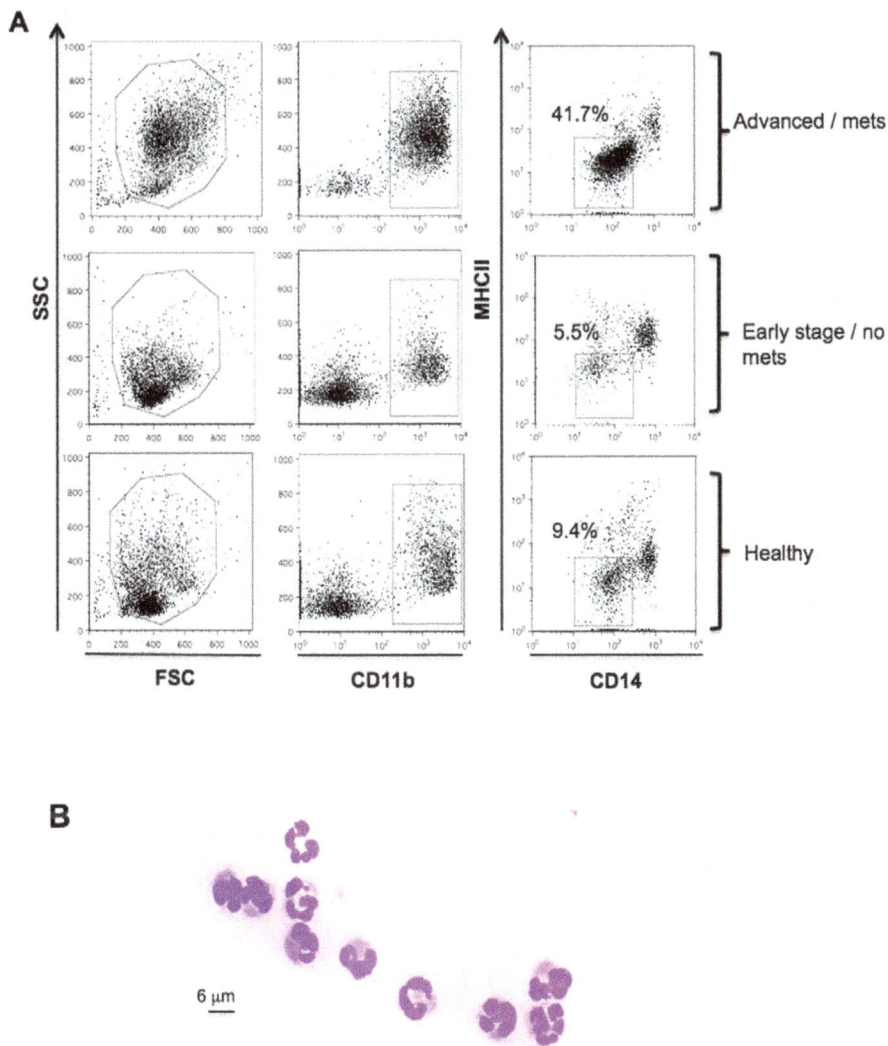

Figure 1. Immunophenotyping gating strategy and morphological analysis for MDSC identification in peripheral blood of dogs. PBMCs from healthy dogs and dogs with cancer were stained for the myeloid marker CD11b, monocytic marker CD14 and MHC II. (A) Representative flow cytometric analysis of forward and side scatter and gated CD11b+CD14−MHCII− cells from dogs with advanced or metastatic tumors compared to dogs with early stage non-metastatic tumors and healthy control dogs. Plots are representative of dog with advanced metastatic hemangiosarcoma (top), early stage bladder transitional cell carcinoma (middle) and a healthy dog. (B) FACS sorted CD11b+CD14−MHCII− cells were stained with diff-quick for cell morphology evaluation. A representative example of polymorphonuclear granulocyte morphology of CD11b+CD14−MHCII− cells is shown at 63× magnification.

Results

Dogs with advanced cancer have elevated levels of granulocytic CD11b$^+$CD14$^-$MHCII$^-$ cells that co-purify with PBMCs

Peripheral blood samples from 45 dogs diagnosed with cancer and 18 healthy control dogs were collected (**Tables 1** and **2**). All dogs with cancer underwent clinical staging of their disease by performing complete physical examinations, blood work, imaging to assess tumor location and size and metastases, and histopathological diagnosis made from diagnostic aspirate or biopsy of the tumor. Among the 45 dogs diagnosed with cancer, 30 dogs were classified as having advanced or metastatic disease and 15 dogs were classified as early stage/non-metastatic or low grade disease based on clinical staging. Each group was further subdivided according to histological diagnosis into sarcomas, carcinomas or mast cell tumors (detailed in **Tables S1** and **S2**). The percentages of putative MDSCs in dogs with cancer and healthy dogs were evaluated by flow cytometry. PBMCs from dogs with advanced or metastatic cancer showed a marked increase in the CD11b$^+$CD14$^-$MHCII$^-$ fraction of cells, which accounted for the majority of the cells in the live cell gate, compared to dogs diagnosed with early stage non-metastatic tumors or healthy dog controls (**Fig. 1A**). This subset of cells exhibited a polymorphonuclear granulocytic morphology at heterogeneous stages of development (**Fig. 1B**), which resembles a granulocytic subset of MDSCs identified in mice [15] and humans [16].

Dogs with advanced or metastatic cancer had a significantly greater fraction of putative MDSCs (36.04±2.542, mean ± SEM) compared to dogs with early stage non metastatic tumors (9.40±0.953, mean ± SEM) and healthy control dogs (10.24±1.412, mean ± SEM) (**Fig. 2A**). Moreover, this elevation in the CD11b$^+$CD14$^-$MHCII$^-$ fraction did not appear to be restricted to a specific tumor type. The differences were statistically significant in dogs with sarcomas, carcinomas, and mast cell tumors compared with healthy controls (**Fig. 2B**). Conversely, the percentage of CD11b$^+$MHCII$^-$ cells that did express CD14 was not significantly different among any group. Therefore, the frequency of CD11b$^+$CD14$^-$MHCII$^-$ cells that co-purify PBMCs correlates with tumor burden. This finding is in agreement with previously published data regarding MDSC levels and tumor burden in mice and humans [17,18].

CD11b$^+$CD14$^-$MHCII$^-$ cells are functionally defined as MDSCs

To test whether the CD11b$^+$CD14$^-$MHCII$^-$ subset was able to inhibit T cell function, we conducted a series of co-culture experiments. Purified CD11b$^+$CD14$^-$MHCII$^-$ cells from three different subtypes of cancer were co-cultured with autologous or healthy responder PBMCs. In all cases, CD11b$^+$CD14$^-$MHCII$^-$ cells exhibited a potent ability to suppress proliferative responses in a dose-dependent manner. Representative examples of proliferative suppression are shown using samples from a dog with tonsillar squamous cell carcinoma (**Fig. 3A**) and prostatic adenocarcinoma (**Fig. 3B**). In order to determine if suppression was an artifact of using responders from tumor-bearing dogs, we assayed for proliferative suppression using normal responders. The addition of CD11b$^+$CD14$^-$MHCII$^-$ cells, but not normal PMNs, impaired the proliferation of PBMCs from healthy dogs (**Fig. 3C**). Moreover, the amount of IFN-γ secretion was assessed in the conditioned medium from these co-cultures, revealing that CD11b$^+$CD14$^-$MHCII$^-$ cells, but not normal PMNs, suppressed the secretion of IFN-γ (**Fig. 3D**).

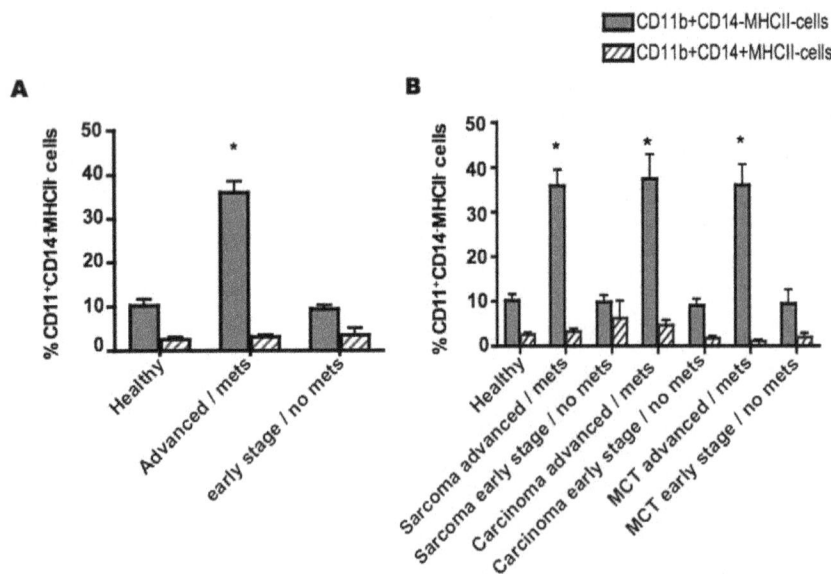

Figure 2. Percentages of circulating CD11b$^+$CD14$^-$MHCII$^-$ cells in dogs with correlates with clinical tumor stage. (A) Analysis of average CD11$^+$CD14$^-$MHCII$^-$ population frequency in dogs with advanced stage or metastatic tumors (n = 30) compared with early stage non-metastatic tumors (n = 15) and control dogs (n = 18). There was a significantly higher percentage of CD11b$^+$CD14$^-$MHCII$^-$ cells in dogs with advanced cancer versus early stage non-metastatic tumors and healthy dogs (36.04% vs. 9.40% and 10.24%, respectively. B) Average CD11b$^+$CD14$^-$MHCII$^-$ population frequency in the major cancer subtypes: advanced stage or metastatic sarcomas (n = 18), early stage non-metastatic sarcomas (n = 6), advanced stage or metastatic carcinomas (n = 7) early stage non-metastatic carcinomas (n = 7), advanced stage or metastatic mast cell tumors (n = 5) and early stage non-metastatic mast cell tumors (n = 2) compared with control dogs (n = 18). Significantly elevated percentages were detected in all advanced tumors subtypes relative to early stage tumors and healthy dogs. Percentages of CD11b$^+$CD14$^+$MHCII$^-$ cells were not significant between groups (* indicates P<0.001). Mean ± SEM are shown.

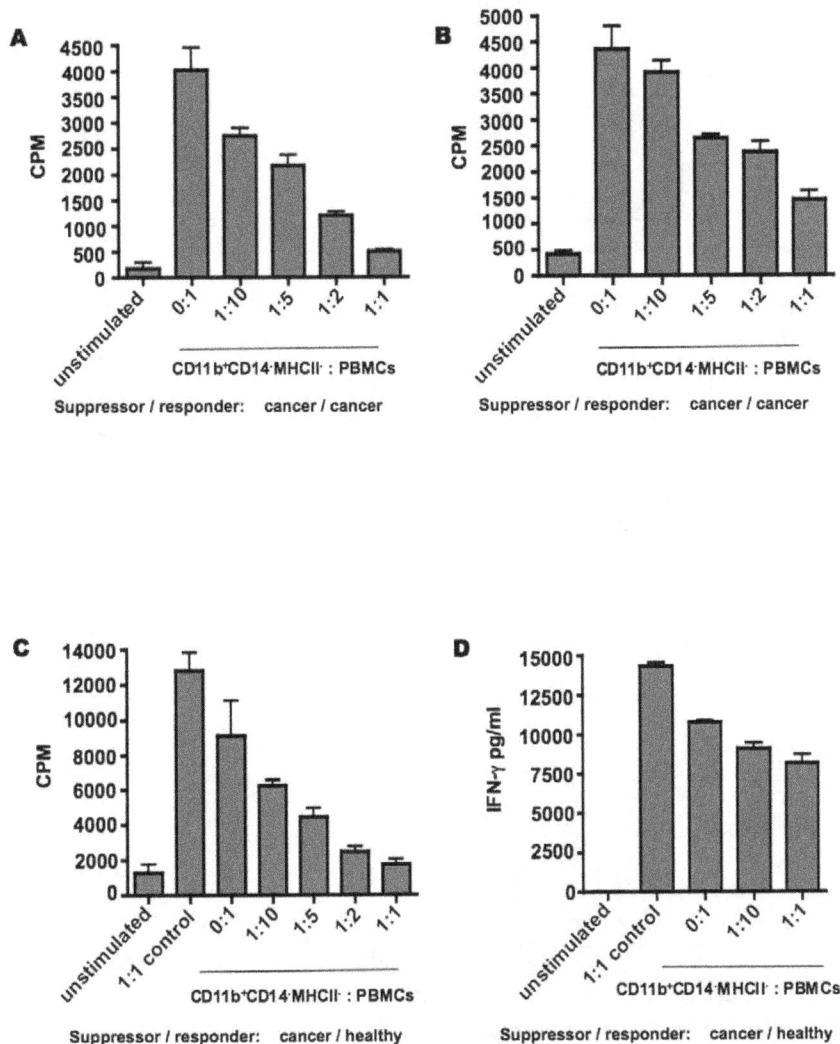

Figure 3. CD11b⁺CD14⁻MHCII⁻ cells suppress T cell proliferation and cytokine elaboration. CD11b⁺CD14⁻MHCII⁻ cells were sorted from peripheral blood sample of dogs with cancer and then co-cultured with autologous PBMCs (A, B) or healthy dog PBMCs (C) in the presence of mitogen for 72 hs. Representative examples from a total of eight dogs are shown. The graphs represent proliferative responses after addition of CD11b⁺CD14⁻MHCII⁻ isolated from a single dog with squamous cell carcinoma (3A), prostatic adenocarcinoma (3B) and osteosarcoma (3C). Non-stimulated PBMCs were used as negative control and PBMCs stimulated in absence of CD11b⁺CD14⁻MHCII⁻ cells were used as positive control for proliferation. PBMCs were also co-incubated with PMNs, to control for presence of additional cells (3C, 3D). Proliferative responses were measured by ³H-thymidine incorporation. CPM, counts per minute. Amount of IFN-γ secretion in the co-culture was determined using canine specific IFN-γ ELISA assay (3D). All experiments were performed in triplicate. Mean ± SEM are shown.

MDSCs suppress both CD4⁺ and CD8⁺ T cells

To further interrogate the direct effect on T lymphocytes, purified CD11b⁺CD14⁻MHCII⁻ cells from a dog with osteosarcoma were co-cultured with purified CD4⁺ and CD8⁺ T cells from a healthy dog for 72 h. Non-stimulated cells and CD4⁺ and CD8⁺ cells co-incubated with healthy PBMCs were used as controls. As expected, CD11b⁺CD14⁻MHCII⁻ cells inhibited the proliferation of CD8⁺ (**Fig. 4A**) and CD4⁺ T cells (**Fig. 4B**) while PBMCs from a normal dog did not. Taken together, these data demonstrate that CD11b⁺CD14⁻MHCII⁻ cells are indeed functionally defined as canine MDSCs.

CD11b⁺CD14⁻MHCII⁻ cells express hallmark MDSC-derived immunosuppressive factors

It has been shown that MDSCs can inhibit T cell function by the production of soluble factors such as arginase-1, reactive

oxygen species, nitric oxide and TGF-β (8–10). In order to assess whether CD11b⁺CD14⁻MHCII⁻ cells from dogs with cancer could possibly utilize these mechanisms to mediate T cell suppression, we evaluated the expression of ARG1 and iNOS2, as well as the immunosuppressive cytokines TGF-β and IL-10, within this cell population and from PMNs isolated from peripheral blood of healthy dogs. PCR analysis of RNA extracted from FACS isolated CD11b⁺CD14⁻MHCII⁻cells confirmed the expression of ARG-1, iNOS2 enzymes and immunosuppressive cytokines TGF-β and IL-10 mRNA (**Fig. 5A**). In contrast, normal dog PMNs did not express ARG1, although iNOS, TGF-β and IL-10 mRNA were detectable (**Fig. 5B**). Because mRNA for ARG-1, iNOS2, TGF- β and IL-10 were all found, we conclude that these factors could play a role in the inhibition of T cell proliferation and effector function. However, since PMNs isolated from healthy dogs did not express detectable ARG-1 mRNA or impair T cell function, suggesting that ARG-1 may be a tumor-

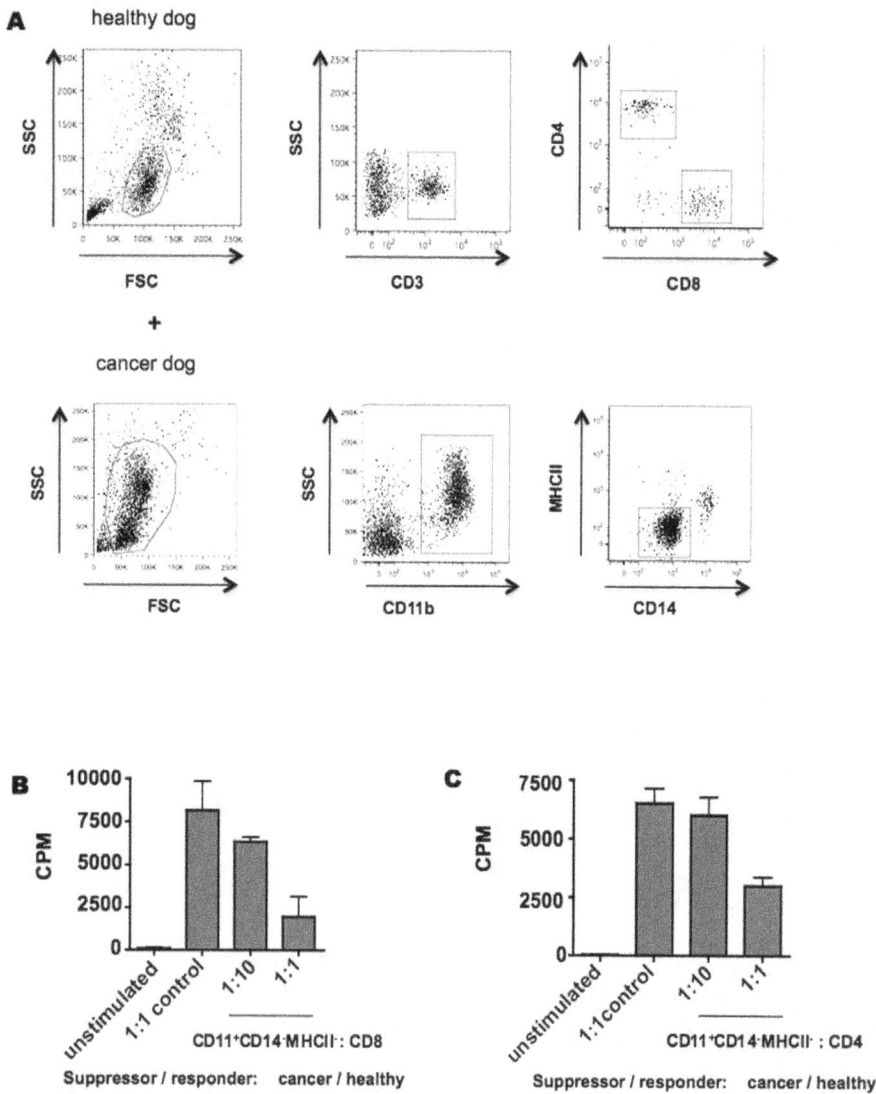

Figure 4. CD11b⁺CD14⁻MHCII⁻ cells suppress T cell proliferation. Facs sorted CD11b⁺CD14⁻MHCII⁻ cells isolated from a dog with osteosarcoma or healthy PBMCs were co-incubated with mitogen-stimulated CD4⁺ and CD8⁺ T cells isolated from a healthy dog for 72 hs. No stimulated cells were used as negative control. Proliferative responses were measured by ³H-thymidine incorporation from experiments performed in triplicate. CPM, counts per minute. Mean ± SEM are shown.

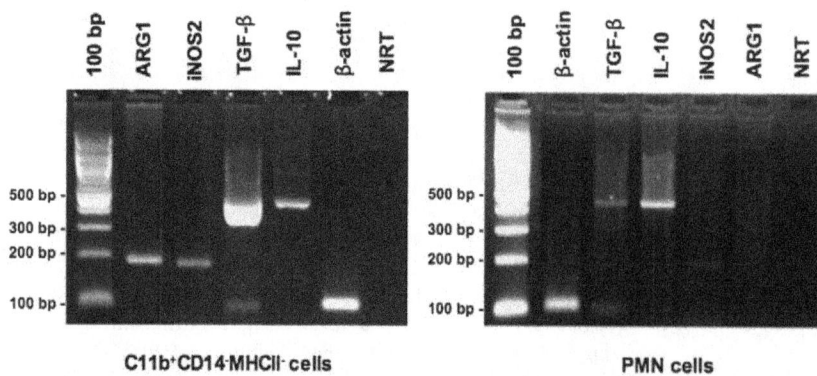

Figure 5. CD11b⁺CD14⁻MHCII⁻ cells express MDSC-derived immunosuppressive factors. RT-PCR analysis of FACS purified CD11b⁺CD14⁻MHCII⁻ cells detected expression of ARG1 and iNOS2, as well TGF-β and IL-10 immunosuppressive cytokines. ARG-1 expression was not detected in normal PMNs. CD11b⁺CD14⁻MHCII⁻ cells were isolated from the peripheral blood of a dog with osteosarcoma and PMNs were isolated from a healthy dog. NRT, RNA template in the absence of reverse transcriptase. Results are representative three experiments.

induced mechanism that MDSCs could employ for T cell suppression. This finding was not unexpected and has been previously documented in human MDSC studies [19].

Discussion

The field of comparative oncology shows great promise to advance the development of novel therapeutics for pet dogs and human patients alike. However, the paucity of reagents and poorly defined immunophenotype of canine leukocytes has restrained our ability to understand tumor immunology in dogs with naturally occurring cancer. Our data demonstrates the existence of MDSCs in the peripheral blood of dogs, which are elevated in all types of advanced or metastatic cancer analyzed compared to early stage non-metastatic cancer and healthy controls. With this basic foundation of knowledge in place, it will now be possible to prospectively monitor MDSC burden in dogs treated with experimental drugs and immunotherapy. The CD11b+CD14− MHCII− cell population that we defined as MDSC co-purified with PBMCs, had polymorphonuclear granulocytic morphology, suppressed T cell proliferation and effector function, expressed hallmark suppressive factors of human MDSC, and positively correlated with tumor burden. Proliferation assays revealed relatively weak proliferation in PBMCs from tumor-bearing dogs (**Fig. 3A,B**) compared to normal responders (**Fig. 3C**) in the absence of exogenous MDSC. This likely reflects elevated levels of endogenous (not experimentally added) MDSCs and regulatory T cells in the PBMCs from dogs with cancer. Furthermore, it is crucial to note that a second subset of MDSC that is more monocytic in nature is widely appreciated in murine and human tumor immunology. We found no evidence for selective expansion of a CD14+ monocyte-like cell in the blood of dogs with cancer. However, CD11b+MHCII− cells that were purified from dogs with advanced cancer that were also CD14+ potently inhibited T cell proliferation (**Figure S2**), revealing that although monocytic MDSC are not a dominant population in dogs with cancer, they are indeed present. This finding of preferential expansion of granulocytic MDSC is not surprising and is in agreement with similar studies carried out in murine tumor models [**15**]. Overall, our data are consistent with a global state of immune suppression in dogs with advanced cancer that is likely attributable to several mechanisms.

The practical deliverable of this study is a simple three marker surface immunophenotype that can be used to prospectively monitor MDSC burden in dogs. We have performed pilot studies to look for additional markers. Specific preliminary results that are worth noting are as follows. We have been unable to demonstrate successful staining using anti-human CD66b antibodies. CD66b is an activation marker expressed on some human MDSC [19]. The most widely used marker for MDSC in the mouse is Gr-1, and an antibody against mouse Gr-1 cross-reacts nicely with canine cells, as does anti-mouse CD11b (**Figure S1**). Further studies will be required to determine if canine cells that are identified by anti-mouse Gr-1 and CD11b antibodies are indeed MDSCs.

One potential limitation of this study that many of the samples we analyzed were frozen, the thawed before analysis, which could have influenced cell viability. However, freeze-thaw did not significantly affect cell viability of either granulocytic or monocytic MDSC (**Figure S3**). We consider this a positive finding because canine MDSCs could be frozen from multiple time points in future prospective studies, then thawed and analyzed simultaneously to limit batch to batch variability. A second limitation is that the RT-PCR analysis of immunosuppressive molecules was qualitative, was performed on a small number of dogs (**Table S3**), and was

not a direct comparison to matched healthy cells. We were not able to obtain adequate viable CD11b+CD14−MHCII− cells from healthy dogs by FACS to directly compare to the same population from dogs with cancer due to their low frequency and apparently high rate of cell death following FACS. For this reason, normal PMNs isolated by gradient centrifugation were used for comparison in our studies. Quantitative mechanistic studies should be conducted to dissect which of the candidate molecules studied herein mediate T cell suppression. Additionally, some of the dogs had received treatment for their cancer. This is relevant because MDSC levels in human cancer patients have been shown to be influenced by prior therapy. It is also known that tumor burden and inflammation significantly affect circulating MDSC levels. Studies in mice have shown that accumulation and suppressive activity of MDSCs are regulated by the inflammatory milieu [20]. Thus treatment, such as surgical excision of the tumor, chemotherapy, and nonsteroidal anti-inflammatory drug (NSAID) administration, can alter the levels of these cells in the peripheral blood. Evaluation of the medical records of dogs in our study revealed that many dogs received some therapy prior to blood sample collection, which could have affected the levels of MDSCs in these samples (see **Tables S1** and **2S**). However, **Figure S4** demonstrates that treatment of dogs with advanced cancer did not significantly alter MDSC burden relative to dogs that had not been previously treated. Therefore, our study provides evidence that expanded MDSCs are likely a robust, general feature of cancer in canines despite genetic heterogeneity and a range of previous treatments (or lack of previous treatment).

In summary, we have identified a granulocytic subset of cells with immunosuppressive function that are elevated in dogs with advanced cancer that can be characterized as MDSCs. Canine MDSCs may be a potential target for therapeutic interventions in dogs with cancer. Furthermore, the study of MDSCs in dogs treated with experimental therapies should reveal unique insights into what might be expected in human patients. This cross-species comparison provides an attractive opportunity to move the field of translational medicine forward.

Supporting Information

Figure S1 Mouse anti-CD11b and Gr-1 antibodies cross-react with canine samples. Fresh PBMCs from healthy dog and cancer patients were isolated by Ficoll, stained with anti-mouse CD11b and anti-mouse Gr-1 antibodies.

Figure S2 CD11b+CD14+MHCII− cells demonstrate ability to suppressive T cell proliferation. (A) CD11b+CD14+MHCII− cells were sorted from peripheral blood sample of an osteosarcoma dog (B) and co-cultured with healthy dog PBMCs in the presence of mitogen for 72 hs. Non-stimulated PBMCs were used as negative control and PBMCs co-cultured with healthy PMNs were used to control for the effect of adding cells to the assay. Proliferative responses were measured by ³H-thymidine incorporation. CPM, counts per minute. The experiment was performed in triplicate. Mean ± SEM are shown.

Figure S3 Frequency of MDSCs measured was not significantly altered by cryopreservation. MDSC percentages in fresh and frozen samples were assessed for comparison. Mean ±SEM are shown.

Figure S4 No significant effect of pretreatment on MDSC burden. Analysis of the average CD11b+CD14−

MHCII$^-$ population frequency in treated (n = 17) or untreated dogs with advanced stage or metastatic tumors (n = 13) compared to control dogs (n = 18). There was a significantly higher percentage of CD11b$^+$CD14$^-$MHCII$^-$ cells in dogs with advanced cancer treated or untreated compared to healthy dogs (32.69±3.24%, 40.42±3.86% vs. 10.24±1.412%, respectively). N.S., not statistically significant (there was no significant difference between samples that had been treated compared to those from untreated samples). Mean ± SEM are shown (* indicates P<0.0001).

Table S1 Summary data for dogs with advanced stage or metastatic tumors.

Table S2 Summary data for dogs with early stage non-metastatic tumors.

Table S3 Table of cancer patient samples and the experiment in which the PBMCs were used.

Table S4 Primer sequences for genes evaluated by semi-quantitative PCR.

Acknowledgments

We thank Dr. Jaime Modiano for his thoughtful perspective and helpful discussions regarding this manuscript.

Author Contributions

Conceived and designed the experiments: JRO. Performed the experiments: MRG. Analyzed the data: MRG JRO GEP. Wrote the paper: MRG JRO GEP.

References

1. Khanna C, Lindblad-Toh K, Vail D, London C, Bergman P, et al. (2006) The dog as a cancer model. Nat Biotechnol 24: 1065–1066.
2. Paoloni M, Khanna C (2008) Translation of new cancer treatments from pet dogs to humans. Nat Rev Cancer 8: 147–156.
3. Khanna C, Gordon I (2009) Catching cancer by the tail: new perspectives on the use of kinase inhibitors. Clin Cancer Res 15: 3645–3647.
4. Ko JS, Zea AH, Rini BI, Ireland JL, Elson P, et al. (2009) Sunitinib mediates reversal of myeloid-derived suppressor cell accumulation in renal cell carcinoma patients. Clin Cancer Res 15: 2148–2157.
5. Diaz-Montero CM, Salem ML, Nishimura MI, Garrett-Mayer E, Cole DJ, et al. (2009) Increased circulating myeloid-derived suppressor cells correlate with clinical cancer stage, metastatic tumor burden, and doxorubicin-cyclophosphamide chemotherapy. Cancer Immunol Immunother 58: 49–59.
6. Nagaraj S, Schrum AG, Cho HI, Celis E, Gabrilovich DI (2010) Mechanism of T cell tolerance induced by myeloid-derived suppressor cells. J Immunol 184: 3106–3116.
7. Ostrand-Rosenberg S, Sinha P (2009) Myeloid-derived suppressor cells: linking inflammation and cancer. J Immunol 182: 4499–4506.
8. Rodriguez PC, Ochoa AC (2008) Arginine regulation by myeloid derived suppressor cells and tolerance in cancer: mechanisms and therapeutic perspectives. Immunol Rev 222: 180–191.
9. Youn JI, Gabrilovich DI (2010) The biology of myeloid-derived suppressor cells: the blessing and the curse of morphological and functional heterogeneity. Eur J Immunol 40: 2969–2975.
10. Gabrilovich DI, Nagaraj S (2009) Myeloid-derived suppressor cells as regulators of the immune system. Nat Rev Immunol 9: 162–174.
11. Serafini P, Borrello I, Bronte V (2006) Myeloid suppressor cells in cancer: recruitment, phenotype, properties, and mechanisms of immune suppression. Semin Cancer Biol 16: 53–65.
12. Molon B, Ugel S, Del Pozzo F, Soldani C, Zilio S, et al. (2011) Chemokine nitration prevents intratumoral infiltration of antigen-specific T cells. J Exp Med 208: 1949–1962.
13. Hanson EM, Clements VK, Sinha P, Ilkovitch D, Ostrand-Rosenberg S (2009) Myeloid-derived suppressor cells down-regulate L-selectin expression on CD4+ and CD8+ T cells. J Immunol 183: 937–944.
14. Biller BJ, Elmslie RE, Burnett RC, Avery AC, Dow SW (2007) Use of FoxP3 expression to identify regulatory T cells in healthy dogs and dogs with cancer. Vet Immunol Immunopathol 116: 69–78.
15. Youn JI, Nagaraj S, Collazo M, Gabrilovich DI (2008) Subsets of myeloid-derived suppressor cells in tumor-bearing mice. J Immunol 181: 5791–5802.
16. Schmielau J, Finn OJ (2001) Activated granulocytes and granulocyte-derived hydrogen peroxide are the underlying mechanism of suppression of t-cell function in advanced cancer patients. Cancer Res 61: 4756–4760.
17. Bronte V, Apolloni E, Cabrelle A, Ronca R, Serafini P, et al. (2000) Identification of a CD11b(+)/Gr-1(+)/CD31(+) myeloid progenitor capable of activating or suppressing CD8(+) T cells. Blood 96: 3838–3846.
18. Almand B, Clark JI, Nikitina E, van Beynen J, English NR, et al. (2001) Increased production of immature myeloid cells in cancer patients: a mechanism of immunosuppression in cancer. J Immunol 166: 678–689.
19. Rodriguez PC, Ernstoff MS, Hernandez C, Atkins M, Zabaleta J, et al. (2009) Arginase I-producing myeloid-derived suppressor cells in renal cell carcinoma are a subpopulation of activated granulocytes. Cancer Res 69: 1553–1560.
20. Bunt SK, Yang L, Sinha P, Clements VK, Leips J, et al. (2007) Reduced inflammation in the tumor microenvironment delays the accumulation of myeloid-derived suppressor cells and limits tumor progression. Cancer Res 67: 10019–10026.

18

Mathematical Model of Plasmid-Mediated Resistance to Ceftiofur in Commensal Enteric *Escherichia coli* of Cattle

Victoriya V. Volkova[1]*, Cristina Lanzas[2], Zhao Lu[1], Yrjö Tapio Gröhn[1]

1 Department of Population Medicine and Diagnostic Sciences, College of Veterinary Medicine, Cornell University, Ithaca, New York, United States of America, **2** Department of Biomedical and Diagnostic Sciences, College of Veterinary Medicine, The University of Tennessee, Knoxville, Tennessee, United States of America

Abstract

Antimicrobial use in food animals may contribute to antimicrobial resistance in bacteria of animals and humans. Commensal bacteria of animal intestine may serve as a reservoir of resistance-genes. To understand the dynamics of plasmid-mediated resistance to cephalosporin ceftiofur in enteric commensals of cattle, we developed a deterministic mathematical model of the dynamics of ceftiofur-sensitive and resistant commensal enteric *Escherichia coli* (*E. coli*) in the absence of and during parenteral therapy with ceftiofur. The most common treatment scenarios including those using a sustained-release drug formulation were simulated; the model outputs were in agreement with the available experimental data. The model indicated that a low but stable fraction of resistant enteric *E. coli* could persist in the absence of immediate ceftiofur pressure, being sustained by horizontal and vertical transfers of plasmids carrying resistance-genes, and ingestion of resistant *E. coli*. During parenteral therapy with ceftiofur, resistant enteric *E. coli* expanded in absolute number and relative frequency. This expansion was most influenced by parameters of antimicrobial action of ceftiofur against *E. coli*. After treatment (>5 weeks from start of therapy) the fraction of ceftiofur-resistant cells among enteric *E. coli*, similar to that in the absence of treatment, was most influenced by the parameters of ecology of enteric *E. coli*, such as the frequency of transfer of plasmids carrying resistance-genes, the rate of replacement of enteric *E. coli* by ingested *E. coli*, and the frequency of ceftiofur resistance in the latter.

Editor: Michael George Roberts, Massey University, New Zealand

Funding: This work was funded by the National Institute of Food and Agriculture of the United States Department of Agriculture (grant # 2010-51110-21083). The funders had no role in study design, analysis, decision to publish, or preparation of the manuscript.

Competing Interests: The authors have declared that no competing interests exist.

* E-mail: vv87@cornell.edu

Introduction

The emergence and spread of antimicrobial resistance (AMR) is progressively demarcating the epochal success of antimicrobial therapies of bacterial infections. Some classes of antimicrobials are used in both human and veterinary medicines; among antibiotics these are β-lactams, including cephalosporins, as well as aminoglycosides, macrolides, tetracyclines, sulphonamides, and in some countries fluoroquinolones [1]. Humans may be exposed to AMR-bacteria from food animals via occupational exposure or contaminated food products. In the 1990s in the USA, a domestically-acquired infection of a boy with ceftriaxone-resistant *Salmonella* was traced to cattle carrying ceftiofur-resistant *Salmonella* after the boy's father had treated the diarrheic calves [2]. Human food-borne infections with AMR-bacteria are clinically challenging [1,3]. Furthermore, ingested strains can become a part of the human enteric microflora [4], and transmit AMR-genetic determinants to other human bacteria [5]. For cephalosporins, the principal mechanism via which resistance disseminates is horizontal transfer of AMR-genes encoded on conjugative plasmids [6,7,8]. The AMR-strains occasionally demonstrate a higher transmissibility via the food chain, *e.g.*, an AMR-strain of *Escherichia coli* (*E. coli*) on pig carcasses has survived processing and chilling better than the parental antimicrobial-sensitive strain [9]. Cattle meat products can be contaminated by animals' feces, and so the enteric microflora [10]. Therefore, minimizing the frequency of AMR in cattle enteric bacteria *en masse* can aid in decreasing human exposure to AMR-strains.

Within animal hosts, enteric commensals may also transmit AMR-genetic determinants to pathogens, *e.g.*, *E. coli* can transmit plasmidic AMR-genes to *Salmonella* [11,12]. However, the *in-vivo* frequency of such transfer is unknown, and may be limited by the number of plasmids shared [12], differences in plasmid developments between bacterial species [11], or restrictions on plasmid establishment in the heterologous recipients [13]. The frequency of plasmid transfer from *E. coli* to *Salmonella* is much lower compared to promiscuous plasmid sharing between *E. coli* cells [12]. However, occasionally AMR-strains themselves exhibit a higher virulence for [14], or a greater ability to colonize animal hosts [15,16]. This necessitates the use of even newer drugs to combat animal infections [1].

A complete cessation of antimicrobial therapies in food animals is impractical [1], and, in the absence of alternatives, unethical [17]. The real challenge is to implement therapies that minimize emergence and spread of AMR [17,18]. Also, farm animals present a model system where the potential of candidate policies for reduction of antimicrobial usage can be evaluated at the population level, with further relevance to policies in humans [19].

The containment of resistance to 3rd generation cephalosporins is categorized by the World Health Organization as critically important. Ceftiofur is the only drug in this class licensed to treat food animals in the USA. Ceftiofur's chemical structure is close to that of ceftriaxone, which is used to treat bacterial meningitis and salmonellosis in humans. Ceftiofur is administered parenterally to individual cattle to treat interdigital necrobacillosis, pneumonia or metritis, and to groups of beef calves for metaphylaxis of bovine respiratory disease (BRD). The drug can also be applied intramammary to treat mastitis or as a dry-off therapy.

Resistance to ceftiofur in enteric bacteria of cattle in the USA is mediated predominantly by plasmid-encoded gene *blaCMY-2* [12,20], which codes for a cephamycinase [21,22,23]. The gene has been reported in *Salmonella* and *E. coli* isolates from feces of food animals and meat products in retail [24], and in *Salmonella* isolates responsible for human illness [25,26]. The resistant *E. coli* have been isolated from feces of beef and dairy cattle, sewage and ground beef [24,27]. Between bacteria, both inter-generational and horizontal transfers of plasmidic *blaCMY-2* occur. In the enteric environment, the horizontal plasmid transfer is the main mechanism of AMR-gene spread within and between bacterial species, both Gram-positive and Gram-negative [13]. *E. coli* can constitute up to 86% of the fecal Gram-negative bacteria in dairy cattle [28], and act as a donor of plasmidic AMR-genes [13]. Recent field studies demonstrate that a fraction of enteric *E. coli* carry plasmidic *blaCMY-2* even in cattle not known to be treated with ceftiofur [27,29,30]. Enteric *E. coli* are primarily commensal and are genetically diverse [10,31]; among them, *E. coli* carrying *blaCMY-2* are not strongly clonal at either serotype or PFGE levels [6,12]. The "background" resistant fraction can have mixed origins. Ecological origins may include adaptation of bacteria to co-exist with fungi that are natural producers of β-lactams, and subsequent transfer of chromosomal AmpC locus from *Citrobacter freundii* to other *Enterobacteriaceae* as a plasmidic gene [21,32]. Also, exposure to resistant *E. coli* can occur on the farm when post-weaned calves are colonized with ruminant-specific microflora (Tom Besser, personal communication). Similarly, ceftiofur-resistant *E. coli* in broilers is associated with its presence at the hatchery and on the farm [33].

During parenteral treatment with ceftiofur, a decline in the numbers of enteric *E. coli* is reported in healthy 3-4 mos old calves [27], healthy adult cattle [34], and lactating dairy cattle treated for metritis or interdigital necrobacillosis [35] (Table S1). Studies employing genetic methods to examine the effects on entire enteric bacterial populations have arrived at similar conclusions [36]. This strongly suggests that parenteral treatment of cattle with ceftiofur results in exposure of their enteric bacteria to antimicrobially-active drug metabolites, with the dose and duration sufficient for prominent effects on the enteric bacteria.

The objectives of this modeling study were to analyze, first, whether the reported fractions of *blaCMY-2*-carrying commensal enteric *E. coli* in cattle could be maintained in the absence of immediate ceftiofur pressure; and, second, how the dynamics of the resistant and sensitive enteric *E. coli* changed during parenteral ceftiofur treatment depending on the treatment protocol.

Materials and Methods

Dynamics of Ceftiofur-sensitive and Resistant Commensal Enteric *E. coli* in the Absence of Immediate Ceftiofur Pressure

Ecology of commensal enteric *E. coli*. A flow-chart of the model is given in Figure 1. Due to unfavorable conditions for *E. coli* growth in the upper parts of the cattle gastrointestinal tract, only *E. coli* in the large intestine was considered (referred to as "commensal enteric *E. coli*"). These may exist in a planktonic "free-living" mode of growth, or by being incorporated into intestinal biofilms [37]. The biofilm-trapped latter likely constitute a small fraction of the total, hence enteric *E. coli* were considered to be free-living. Population growth of *E. coli*, as a facultative anaerobe, slows in anaerobic conditions [38]; the maximum net growth rate (in exponential growth phase) in numbers of enteric *E. coli*, r, was parameterized accordingly. *E. coli* growth in the enteric environment is likely further restricted by intra-specific competition, inter-specific competition with other microflora, and feces substrate composition [39]. A logistic model of bacterial growth was used to reflect the intra-specific competition. The upper limit for total *E. coli* per g of feces, N_{max}, was parameterized from the reported numbers of viable *E. coli* in cattle feces (Table 1), and so bore the expected effects of the inter-specific competition.

E. coli is capable of replicating outside animal hosts; commensal *E. coli* circulate between cattle hosts and their environment [40]. In beef cattle reared at either pasture or feedlot, ~60% of fecal *E. coli* are genetically related to those in animals' oral cavities [31]. From *in vivo* experiments in post-weaned calves [27], an estimated ~20-30% of fecal coliforms are *E. coli* strains fed to the animals on the day of measure or the preceding day. The in-flow of ingested bacteria and the out-flow of bacteria with feces likely ensures a regular partial replacement of *E. coli* "free-living" in the large intestine. To reflect this, the rates of hourly fractional in-flow and outflow of enteric *E. coli* were taken to be equal, both γ. A fraction υ of the ingested bacteria was assumed to carry plasmids with *blaCMY-2*. In-flowing bacteria would mix homogeneously with those already in the intestine.

Plasmid transfer and fitness cost of plasmid-mediated resistance. Various conjugative plasmids of *E. coli* can carry *blaCMY-2* [12]. There is no evidence of enhanced plasmid transfer in enteric *E. coli* during parenteral ceftiofur therapy [27]. The maximum number of cells to which a donor *E. coli* can transfer a plasmid per unit time is inherently restricted by biology of conjugation; the transconjugant (recipient cell) undergoes a 40-80 minutes maturation before becoming a proficient donor [41]. Therefore, the transfer was modeled as a contagious process [65,66] with frequency-dependent transmission. β was the transmission term for *blaCMY-2*-carrying plasmids from resistant donor to sensitive cells, N_r - number of resistant cells, N_s - number of sensitive cells, and N - total number of *E. coli* cells. Then, "force of transfer" per a sensitive cell per unit time was $\beta*N_r/N$, and the total transfer was $\beta*N_r*N_s/N$.

The growth rate of a bacterial strain is considered to represent its evolutionary fitness [38]. Having *blaCMY-2*-carrying plasmids is associated with either a fitness cost, *i.e.*, reduced growth [42], or a fitness gain, *i.e.*, enhanced growth [43]; or no change in growth [44]. The fitness cost appears more often, and was modeled as a fractional reduction, α, in net growth rate, r [45].

The fate of AMR-bacterial strains in the absence of antimicrobial pressure is unclear. In some laboratory experiments, a gradual loss of AMR-gene-carrying plasmids during cell divisions after thousands of bacterial generations (several months) is reported [42]; others, however, report maintenance of the plasmid profile, in particular by *E. coli* [44]. The AMR-strains can acquire compensatory mutations to restore fitness without losing resistance, *e.g.*, a better growth performance of *E. coli* with chromosomal-encoded resistance to streptomycin [46], or plasmid-encoded resistance to tetracycline [43]. Notably, these processes occur over extended time horizons. The period of parenteral treatment of cattle with ceftiofur is at most 7 days, followed by at most a 13-day pre-slaughter withdrawal period. Hence the possibility of loss of plasmidic *blaCMY-2* by enteric *E. coli* was not considered in this analysis.

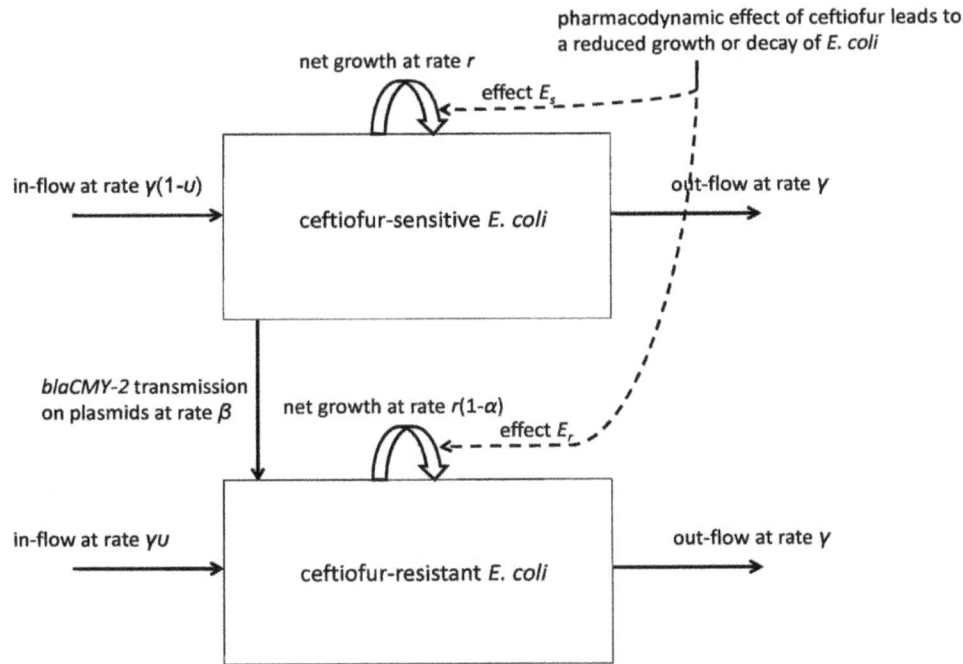

Figure 1. Flow-chart of the model of the dynamics of ceftiofur-sensitive and resistant commensal *E. coli* in the cattle large intestine.
Bacterial growth is density-dependent with fractional net growth rate r; fitness cost for cells with *blaCMY-2*-carrying plasmids manifests as a reduction α in r. Resistant cells transfer *blaCMY-2* to the progeny during cell division. Horizontally, *blaCMY-2* is transferred to the sensitive cells at rate β; the transmission is frequency-dependent with the total of $\beta * N_r * N_s / N$. There is fractional in-flow and out-flow of *E. coli* at rate γ; fraction υ of in-flowing *E. coli* are ceftiofur-resistant. Antimicrobial action of ceftiofur metabolites, depending on their concentration, results in either reduced growth or decay in number of *E. coli*.

Dynamics of Ceftiofur-sensitive and Resistant Commensal Enteric *E. coli* During Parenteral Ceftiofur Treatment

Pharmacokinetics and biodegradation of ceftiofur metabolites. Ceftiofur in cattle is metabolized shortly post injection (p.i.) [47]. Major ceftiofur metabolites retain the β-lactam

Model for dynamics without treatment.

The ordinary differential Equations [1] and [2] described the changes in N_s and N_r, respectively, over time in the absence of immediate ceftiofur pressure:

$$\frac{dN_S}{dt} = \underbrace{r\left(1 - \frac{N}{N_{max}}\right)N_S}_{\text{growth}}$$
$$\underbrace{-\frac{\beta N_r N_S}{N}}_{\substack{\text{plasmid}\\\text{transfer}}} + \underbrace{(1-\upsilon)\gamma N}_{\text{in-flow}} - \underbrace{\gamma N_S}_{\text{out-flow}} \quad (1)$$

$$\frac{dN_r}{dt} = \underbrace{r(1-\alpha)(1-\frac{N}{N_{max}})N_r}_{\text{growth}}$$
$$+ \underbrace{\frac{\beta N_r N_S}{N}}_{\substack{\text{plasmid}\\\text{transfer}}} + \underbrace{\upsilon\gamma N}_{\text{in-flow}} - \underbrace{\gamma N_r}_{\text{out-flow}} \quad (2)$$

ring [48]; their antimicrobial activity against *E. coli* is close to that of ceftiofur [49,50]. The total of ceftiofur and its active metabolites is termed the concentration of ceftiofur equivalents (CE) [51]. The pharmacokinetics of ceftiofur in cattle following an intramuscular (IM) or a subcutaneous (SC) injection in cattle are similar in terms of CE-pattern in the plasma [52]. The pharmacokinetics of formulations containing ceftiofur sodium and ceftiofur hydrochloride salts are similar in terms of CE-pattern in the plasma of pigs [53]; this is considered to hold for cattle [48].

In humans, ceftriaxone (its structure is close to that of ceftiofur) is excreted via both renal and hepatic pathways [54]. There is no evidence of a correlation between ceftriaxone concentrations in bile (bile metabolite is structurally similar to ceftriaxone) and in plasma [54], or of ceftriaxone intestinal absorption and enterohepatic circulation [55]. The rate of ceftriaxone biliary excretion in humans positively correlates with the rate of bile acid secretion [56]; experimental data in rats suggest a common mechanism for hepatic transport of ceftriaxone and bile acids [57]. There is inter-individual variability in achieved ceftriaxone concentrations in bile [54,56,58], and in feces [54] of humans.

In cattle, ceftiofur administered parenterally is also excreted via both urine (~65%) and, through bile, feces (~35%) [47]. There are no published data on the pattern or inter-individual variability of the biliary excretion. We assumed that in cattle, as in humans, there was no enterohepatic ceftiofur circulation, and CE-concentration in the intestine was independent of that in systematic distribution. Of (radio-labeled) ceftiofur dose injected IM, 29% is detected in cattle feces in 8 hours, and 37% in 12 hours p.i. [51]. The exact structure of intestinal metabolites is unknown; although it is likely that they enter the large intestine having an intact β-lactam ring. However, most of the (radio-labeled) amounts in feces lack antimicrobial activity [48,59]. This

Table 1. Parameter definitions and values.

Parameter	Definition, units	Value	Reference
Bacteria			
r	Specific growth rate, h^{-1}	0.17	estimated from [39]
γ	Fractional in-flow/out flow, h^{-1}	0.01	estimated from [27]
N_{max}	Max *E. coli*, log CFU/*g* of feces		
	6-mos beef (220 kg)	5.5	[31]
	6-mos dairy (180 kg)	6.5	[27]
	adult dairy (600 kg)	4.3	[90]
	post-partum/lactating dairy (600 kg)	4.3	–
AMR			
pAMR	Fraction of ceftiofur-resistant enteric *E. coli* at start of treatment		
	6-mos beef (220 kg)	0.018	[80]
	6-mos dairy (180 kg)	0.050	[78]
	adult dairy (600 kg)	0.007	[79]
	post-partum/lactating dairy (600 kg)	0.018	–
β	Plasmid transmission term, h^{-1}	0.004	[27,42]
a	Resistance fitness cost as fraction of r	0.05	[42]
υ	Resistant *E. coli* fraction in in-flow (pAMR*0.6 based on [31])		
	6-mos beef (220 kg)	0.0110	
	6-mos dairy (180 kg)	0.0310	
	adult dairy (600 kg)	0.0042	
	post-partum/lactating dairy (600 kg)	0.0110	
Biliary ceftiofur metabolites			
p	Bile-excreted fraction of injected dose	0.37	[47,51]
$T\delta$	Passage time to large intestine, h	6	–
V	Volume of large intestine, L		
	6-mos beef or dairy	5	–
	adult cattle	20	–
λ	Biodegradation decay constant, h^{-1}	0.2	estimated from [48,60]
H	Hill coefficient in E_{max} model	1.5	estimated using [68]
MICs	MIC for sensitive *E. coli*, μg/mL	1	–
MICr	MIC for resistant *E. coli*, μg/mL	8	–

is attributed to enteric bacteria biodegrading metabolites within and outside the intestinal environment [60], because of variable timing of metabolite degradation in normal *vs.* sterilized cattle feces [60]. In normal cattle feces fortified with 100 μg/g of CE, under aerobic conditions it takes ~8 hours for these to entirely degrade to antimicrobially inactive compounds [48,60]. The dynamics of decline in CE-concentration appears to be an exponential decay [48,60]. The exact enteric species producing β-lactamases involved are unknown [48]; different species may be involved, as plasmid-mediated β-lactamases are widely produced by Gram-negative bacteria [61].

Let D denote ceftiofur dose in one injection. Fraction p of D was excreted in bile, and the volume of the animal's large intestine was V.

First consider a therapy with repeated injections of a non-sustained-release ceftiofur formulation (Table S1, scenarios R1-R3). D was, and p and V were taken to be equal for every injection n_j, which occurred at time Tj since start of treatment, $t = 0$. As the pattern of ceftiofur biliary excretion is unknown, two possibilities

were explored. Under pattern 1, amount $D*p$ was excreted at 1 hour p.i. After a passage time $T\delta$, biliary metabolites entered the large intestine. At entry, for a given n_j, CE-concentration per g of feces (assuming weight-to-volume ratio of feces of 1) was $D*p/V$, then decayed exponentially due to the biodegradation at rate λ. Total CE-concentration per g of feces in large intestine, C (CE μg/g), at time t was:

$$C(t) = \sum_{j=1}^{n} c^j(t) \qquad (3)$$

$$c^j(t) = \begin{cases} 0; & t < Tj + 1 + T\delta \\ \frac{Dp}{V} exp(-\lambda(t - (Tj + 1 + T\delta))); & t \geq Tj + 1 + T\delta \end{cases} \qquad (4)$$

where $Tj = 24(n_j - 1)$; $j =$ injection number: 1, ..., n, $n = 5$

Under pattern 2, $m = 6$ equal fractions of $D*p$ were excreted hourly at hour 1 to 6 p.i. (similarly to uniform patterns of ceftriaxone biliary excretion in rabbits [62], and of bile flow in

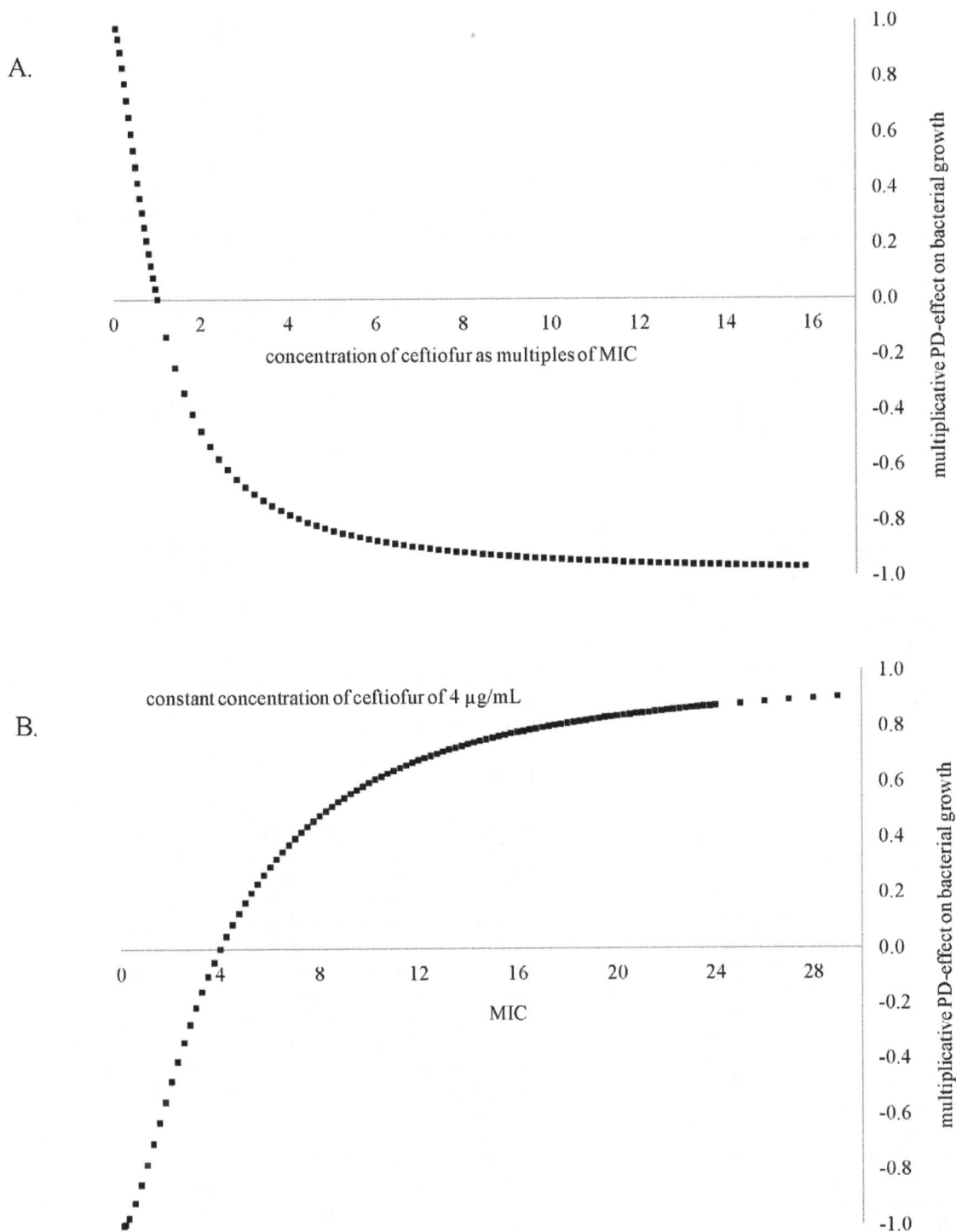

Figure 2. Pharmacodynamic model. A. Multiplicative pharmacodynamic effect on *E. coli* net growth with a constant minimum inhibitory concentration (MIC = 1 µg/mL) and changing ceftiofur concentration expressed as multiples of MIC; Hill coefficient = 1.5. B: Multiplicative pharmacodynamic effect on *E. coli* net growth with changing MIC and a constant ceftiofur concentration; Hill coefficient = 1.5.

cattle [63]). k was excretion fraction number. The choice of hours 1 to 6 p.i. was based on the working hypothesis that $T\delta = 6$ hours, thus the entire amount $D*p$ would reach the large intestine by 12 hours p.i (as in experimental observations [51]). Initial CE µg/g feces was $D*p/6*V$. The concentration C (CE µg/g), at time t was as in Equation [3]; c^j for a given n_j was:

$$c^j(t) = \sum_{k=1}^{m} c^k(t) \qquad (5)$$

$$c^k(t) = \begin{cases} 0; & t < Tj + T\delta + k \\ \dfrac{Dp}{6V}exp(-\lambda(t-(Tj+T\delta+k))); & t \geq Tj + T\delta + k \end{cases} \quad (6)$$

where $Tj = 24(n_j - 1)$, j = injection number: 1, ..., n, $n = 5$ and $k = 1, ... m$, $m = 6$.

Now consider a SC injection of a sustained-release ceftiofur formulation (Table S1, scenarios SB1-SB3 and SD1). According to the data published by the drug manufacturer, plasma CE-concentration peaks at hours 1 to 2 p.i., then declines but remains above the therapeutic threshold (0.2 μg/mL) for ~10 days [64,65]. Due to the quality of these data, data for 60 time points over 10 days p.i. were extracted to detail the plasma pattern. We assumed that the plasma pattern paralleled the pattern of drug release, and that entire drug dose, D, was released within 10 days p.i. At each time point i, amount d_i of ceftiofur (so that $\sum_{i=1}^{n=60} d_i = D$; what fraction of D was d_i was determined by the drug release pattern) was released at the site of injection. Fraction p of d_i was excreted in bile 1 hour later. The passage of metabolites to the large intestine, and decay in their concentration due to the biodegradation were modeled similarly to the above.

Pharmacodynamic effect. Antimicrobial action of β-lactams results in the death of growing, preparing to divide bacteria (both the dividing cell and its "daughter" cell are killed); unaffected growing cells replicate (survive and produce "daughter" cells) [66]. What fraction of growing cells is killed vs. is replicating at a given time, and so what is net growth or decline of the bacterial population, depends on the concentration of β-lactams [67,68]. The changes in net growth of ceftiofur-sensitive and resistant enteric E. coli depending on CE-concentration were modeled using a fractional inhibitory E_{max} pharmacodynamic (PD) model, where E_{max} term specifies the maximum possible PD-effect [69,70]. The 50% PD-effect was with stationary concentration of CE, at which half of the growing cells were replicating, and half were killed (no net change in number of bacteria) [71]. In the case of β-lactams, for a given drug and microbe, the stationary concentration is close to a commonly measured minimum inhibitory concentration (MIC) [71]. Therefore, in this PD-model at a CE-concentration <MIC, net population growth was positive (as more growing cells were able to replicate than were killed). At a CE-concentration >MIC, the population declined. The maximum decline was when all growing cells were killed; the population declined at the rate of attempted growth. This was specified by setting $E_{max} = 2$ (giving -1 as the multiplier for growth rate at a sufficiently high CE-concentration). If CE-concentration rose further, the PD-effect saturated, as no more cells could be killed than those growing to divide. The PD-model behavior is illustrated in Figure 2. The total kill depended on how long CE-concentration was at or above that producing maximum effect. The model therefore depicted time-dependent PD of cephalosporins [68,72,73], with a point of maximum effect (at a drug concentration of low multiples of MIC) after which further concentration rise does not enhance the rate of killing [68,72,74]. The model also accounted for that for antimicrobial resistance via enzymatic deactivation that can be surmounted by a higher drug dose, the change in antimicrobial activity against resistant bacteria should be reflected as an increase in the drug concentration producing the 50% PD-effect [75].

Denoting MIC_s for ceftiofur-sensitive and MIC_r for resistant E. coli, E_s in Equation [7] and E_r in Equation [8] described fractional changes in net growth of ceftiofur-sensitive and resistant E. coli, respectively, at CE-concentration C:

$$E_s = 1 - \frac{E_{max}C^H}{MIC_s{}^H + C^H} \quad (7)$$

$$E_r = 1 - \frac{E_{max}C^H}{MIC_r{}^H + C^H} \quad (8)$$

where $E_{max} = 2$, and H is Hill coefficient.

Postantibiotic effect, the period post exposure to antibiotic after which surviving bacteria begin to multiply normally, in Gram-negative bacilli after the majority of β-lactams is from none to brief [68,76,77], and so was not considered.

Model for dynamics during treatment. The ordinary differential Equations [9] and [10] described the changes in N_s and N_r, respectively, over time of parenteral ceftiofur treatment:

$$\frac{dN_S}{dt} = r\left(1 - \frac{N}{N_{max}}\right)E_sN_S - \frac{\beta N_r N_S}{N} + (1-v)\gamma N - \gamma N_S \quad (9)$$

$$\frac{dN_r}{dt} = r(1-\alpha)\left(1 - \frac{N}{N_{max}}\right)E_r N_r + \frac{\beta N_r N_S}{N} + v\gamma N - \gamma N_r \quad (10)$$

Post treatment, when ceftiofur metabolites had been eliminated from the large intestine ($C = 0$, $E_s = 1$, $E_r = 1$), the dynamics reverted to Equations [1] and [2].

Parameterization

Table 1 details the parameters and their values. The maximum number of E. coli per g of feces in large intestine, N_{max}, was based on reported numbers of viable fecal E. coli (colony-forming units, CFU, of E. coli or fecal coliforms were considered as a measurement of viable E. coli). Starting values of N_s and N_r were calculated using N (set at 90% of N_{max}), and pAMR - fraction of ceftiofur-resistant E. coli at start of treatment. pAMR estimates were adopted from tests of E. coli sensitivity at start of or without connection to ceftiofur treatments. The available estimates varied depending on cattle age and purpose: 6% of ceftriaxone-resistant E. coli for breakpoint ≥16 μg/mL in 2-6 mos post-weaned dairy calves (estimated from [78]); 7.4% of ceftiofur-resistant E. coli for breakpoint ≥16 μg/mL in dairy cattle [28]; 0.7% of ceftazidime-resistant coliforms for breakpoint ≥8 μg/mL across samples from 39 dairy herds [79]; and 1.8% of ceftazidime-resistant E. coli for breakpoint ≥8 μg/mL in feedlot steers [80].

E. coli doubling time in the large intestine was assumed to be 4 hours [39]; hence hourly net growth rate in the exponential phase of population growth (in bacteriological terms, the specific growth rate), r, was 0.17. The fitness cost of resistance (fractional decrease in r) was parameterized from in vitro competition assays between E. coli strains carrying plasmids with blaCMY-2 and those that do not; a crude average of experimental data $\alpha = 0.05$ was used [42].

Rates of horizontal transfer of individual plasmids with blaCMY-2 in vitro vary from 10^{-8} to 10^{-3} [42,81]. In vivo in post-weaned calves fed a donor and a recipient E. coli strains, the overall rate of generation of blaCMY-2-transconjugates in fecal E. coli is 8^{-5} to 2^{-3} [27].

The rates of hourly fractional in-flow and out-flow of E. coli "free-living" in the large intestine, $\gamma = 0.01$ (to the daily total of

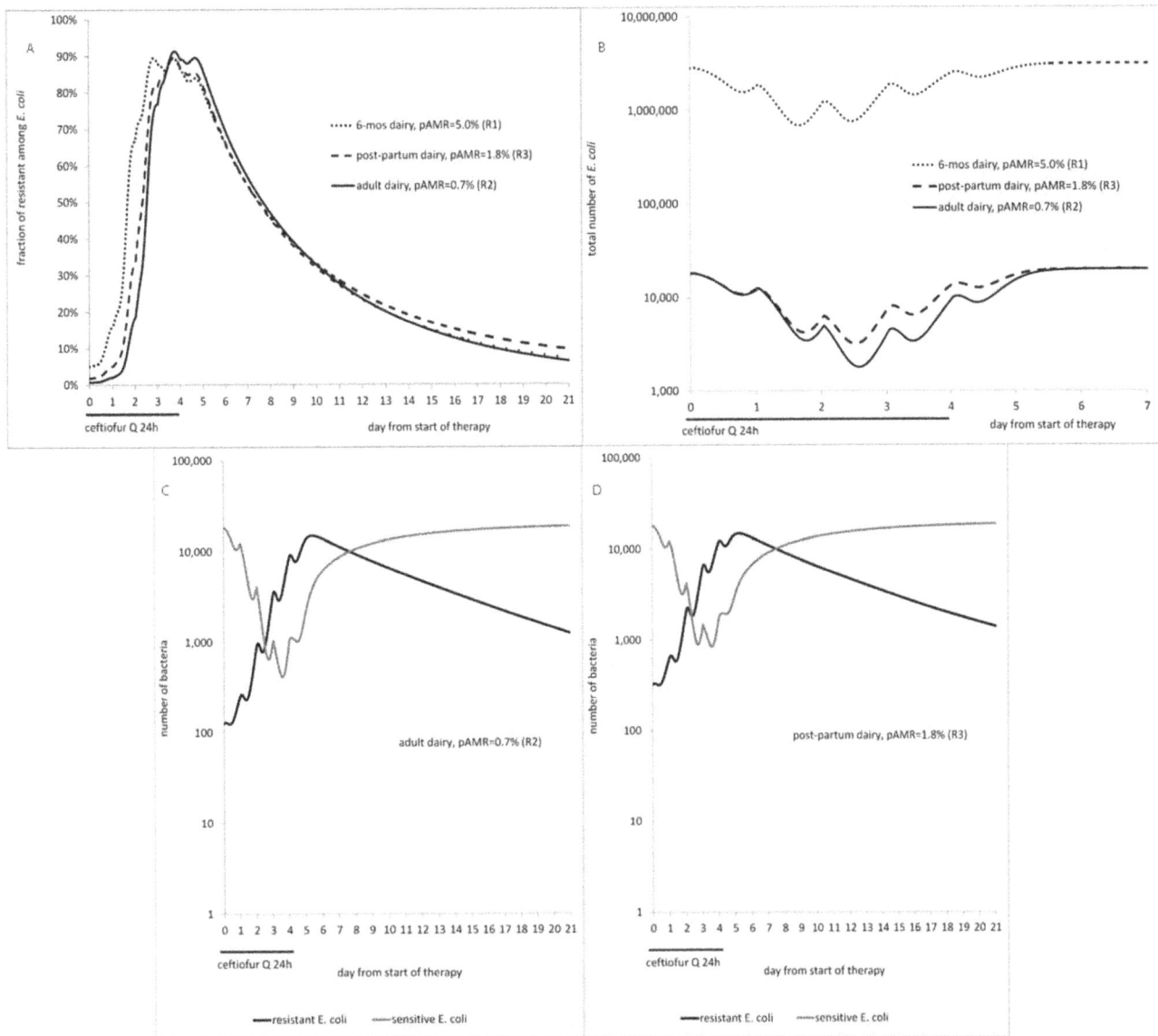

Figure 3. Effect of therapy with repeated ceftiofur administration on enteric *E. coli* in the deterministic case considered ($r = 0.17$, $\alpha = 0.05$, $\beta = 4^{-3}$, $\gamma = 0.01$; all h^{-1}). A: Fraction of ceftiofur-resistant among *E. coli*. B: Total number of *E. coli*. C: Dynamics of ceftiofur-sensitive and resistant *E. coli* in an adult dairy. D: Dynamics of ceftiofur-sensitive and resistant *E. coli* in a post-partum dairy. pAMR = frequency of resistance at start of therapy.

0.24), were estimated from an *in vivo* study in post-weaned dairy calves [27]. The fraction of ceftiofur-resistant cells in in-flow was set at 0.6*pAMR, based on 60% genetic similarity of *E. coli* in oral cavities and in feces of beef cattle reared at either pasture or feedlot [31].

Of parenteral ceftiofur dose, D, fraction $p = 0.37$ was excreted in bile within 6 hours p.i. (under excretion pattern 1 or 2) [51]; metabolites reached the large intestine in $T\delta = 6$ hours post excretion. Volume of the large intestine was 20L in an adult cattle, and 5L in a 6-mos calf. The rate of exponential decay in CE-concentration in the large intestine was twice lower compared to feces under aerobic conditions [48,60].

As there are no published data from a time-kill experiment for *E. coli* and ceftiofur, the PD-model was applied to reproduce the data from *in vitro* time-kill experiments for *E. coli* and β-lactam ticarcillin [68], and performed well; H of 1.5 performed optimally for both concentrations below and above MIC. Under aerobic

conditions, ceftiofur and its major metabolites are highly active against veterinary isolates of *E. coli*, with $MIC_{50} = 0.25$ μg/mL and $MIC_{90} = 0.50$ μg/mL [50]. Decrease in activity under anaerobic conditions appears to be limited ("one 2-fold dilution" *in vitro*), but the data are scarce. For the PD-model, $MIC_s = 1$ μg/mL and $MIC_r = 8$ μg/mL were used.

Sensitivity of methods based on bacteriological culture to detect a strain of *E. coli* in bovine feces is generally restricted to when >100 CFU/g is present [82]. We processed model outputs, N_s and N_r, to separate scenarios when ceftiofur-resistant *E. coli* likely would not be detected by culturing the feces.

Model Solving, and Uncertainty and Global Parameter Sensitivity Analysis

Solutions of the ordinary differential equations were approximated numerically using the fourth-order Runge–Kutta method

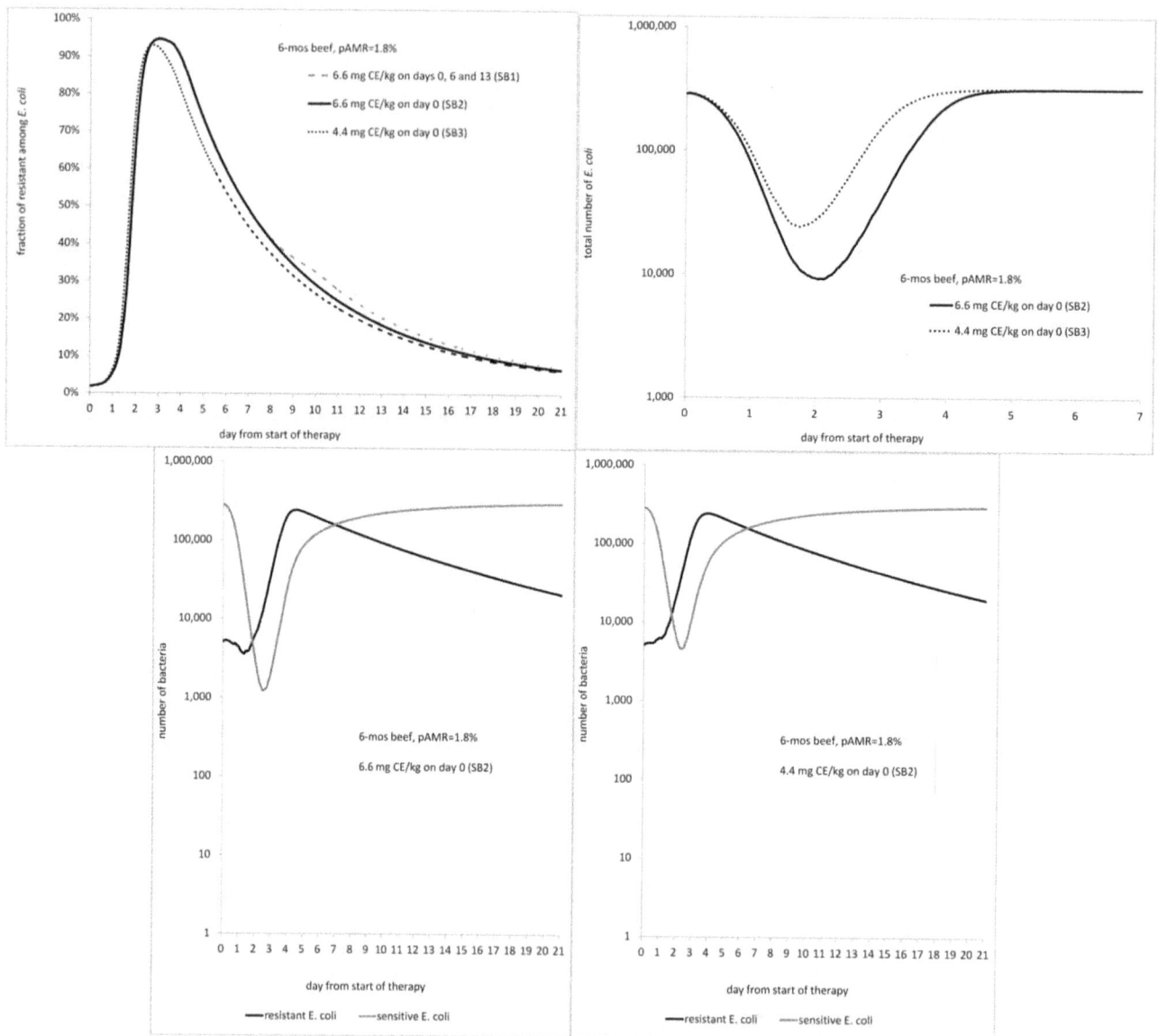

Figure 4. Effect of therapy using a sustained-release ceftiofur formulation on enteric *E. coli* in the deterministic case considered ($r=0.17$, $\alpha=0.05$, $\beta=4^{-3}$, $\gamma=0.01$; all h^{-1}). A: Fraction of ceftiofur-resistant among *E. coli*. B: Total number of *E. coli*. Dynamics of ceftiofur-sensitive and resistant *E. coli* in a 6-mos beef treated with C: 6.6 mg CE/kg dosage, and D: 4.4 mg CE/kg dosage. pAMR = frequency of resistance at start of therapy.

implemented in Vensim® PLE Plus software (Ventana Systems, Inc.; Harvard, MA, USA). In the deterministic analysis, first, for each treatment scenario (Table S1), the model without treatment (Equations [1] and [2]) was solved varying parameter values to reproduce the reported pAMR (Table 1). Then concentration C, and PD-effects E_s and E_r were calculated. These were introduced into the model (Equations [9] and [10]) and the equations were solved. The models were solved starting with total *E. coli*, N, at 90% of N_{max}.

The analysis of uncertainty and global parameter sensitivity of the model outputs was conducted for the treatment scenarios R2 and SB2 (Table S1). Given the dynamics of ceftiofur metabolites in the large intestine during therapy (section *Pharmacokinetics and biodegradation of ceftiofur metabolites* above), the sensitivity analysis was targeted at how the model outputs correlated with changes in the parameters of ecology of enteric *E. coli* (r, α, β, γ and υ), and of

pharmacodynamics of the metabolites against *E. coli* (MIC_s, MIC_r and H). A uniform distribution (U) was assumed for all, because of the lack of knowledge of distributions of individual parameters. The minimum and maximum values were specified based on the literature review (all rates h^{-1}): $r \sim U(0.05, 0.5)$, $\alpha \sim U(-0.2, 0.2)$, $\beta \sim U(10^{-5}, 0.01)$, $\gamma \sim U(10^{-3}, 0.02)$, $\upsilon \sim U(10^{-5}, 0.10)$, $MIC_s \sim U(0.2, 1.9)$, $MIC_r \sim U(2, 16)$, and $H \sim U(0.5, 4)$. For each of the two treatment scenarios, 500 Monte Carlo simulations were performed with Latin Hypercube sampling of each parameter space at each time point over 90 days from start of therapy for the model with treatment, and for 180 days for the model without treatment. This was implemented in Vensim® PLE Plus software. The uncertainty in model outputs was explored graphically. The sensitivity of model outputs to changes in values of each parameter was evaluated with the Spearman correlation coefficient (ρ) [83]. Whether ρ was significantly different from zero was tested with a

A.

B.

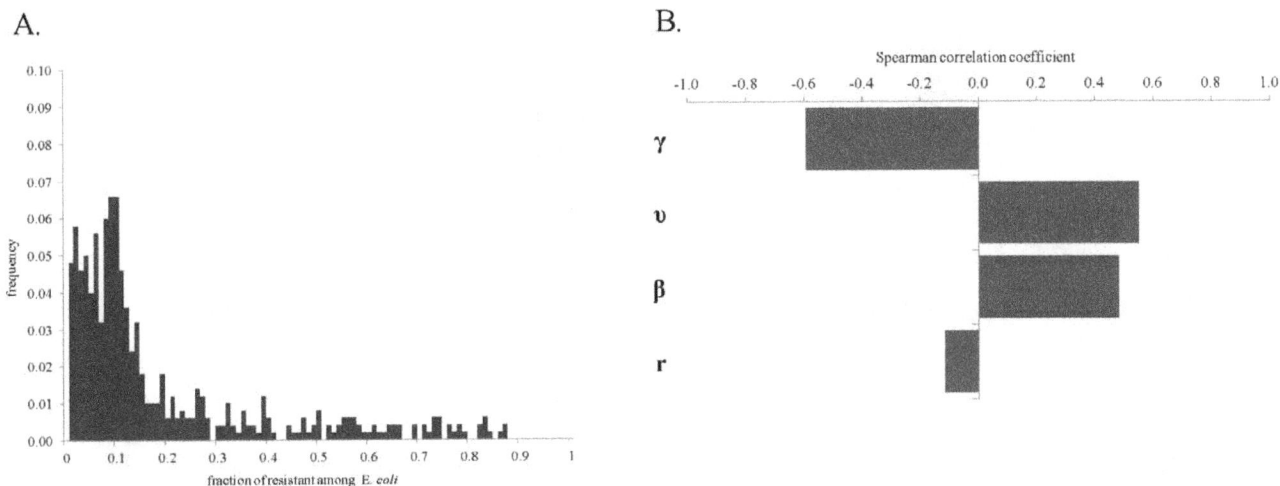

Figure 5. Fraction of ceftiofur-resistant among enteric *E. coli* in long-term absence of ceftiofur pressure. A: Uncertainty: frequency histogram for 500 model simulations with randomly varying parameters of bacterial ecology. B: Sensitivity: significant linear correlations (*p*-value ≤0.05) between ranked-transformed values of the parameters of bacterial ecology and the fraction of resistance.

Student's *t*-test, with the test statistics, denoting the number of simulations as *w*, calculated as $T = |\rho| \sqrt{\dfrac{w-2}{1-\rho^2}}$ and assumed to follow a *t*-distribution with (w-2) degrees of freedom. If the test's *p*-value was ≤0.05, the correlation was considered as significant.

Results

Deterministic Analysis

Maintenance of ceftiofur resistance in commensal enteric *E. coli* in the absence of immediate ceftiofur pressure. In the model without treatment (Equations [1–2]), for every scenario (Table S1) the reported pAMR could be reproduced with $r = 0.17$, $\alpha = 0.05$, $\beta = 4^{-3}$, $\gamma = 0.01$, and $\upsilon = 0.6*$pAMR. (These parameter values were used for the deterministic analysis of treatment

scenarios: Table 1). N_{max} corresponded to the scenario, and had no influence on the dynamics observed. pAMR was most sensitive to β and υ (or, if υ was kept constant, to γ). $\beta > 0.01$ (somewhat unrealistic, see the discussion below) allowed reproducing the reported pAMR if there was no ceftiofur resistance among ingested *E. coli*, $\upsilon = 0$. In all the scenarios, the resulting N_r was over 100; hence, culture-based methods would likely detect the presence of resistance.

Effects of parenteral ceftiofur therapy on commensal enteric *E. coli*: repeated ceftiofur administration. Models with both hypothesized biliary excretion patterns produced outputs resembling experimental data (Table S1); thus, biliary excretion of ceftiofur likely occurs within the first several hours p.i. Further results and discussion refer to the model with excretion pattern 2 (uniform excretion hourly at hour 1 to 6 p.i.).

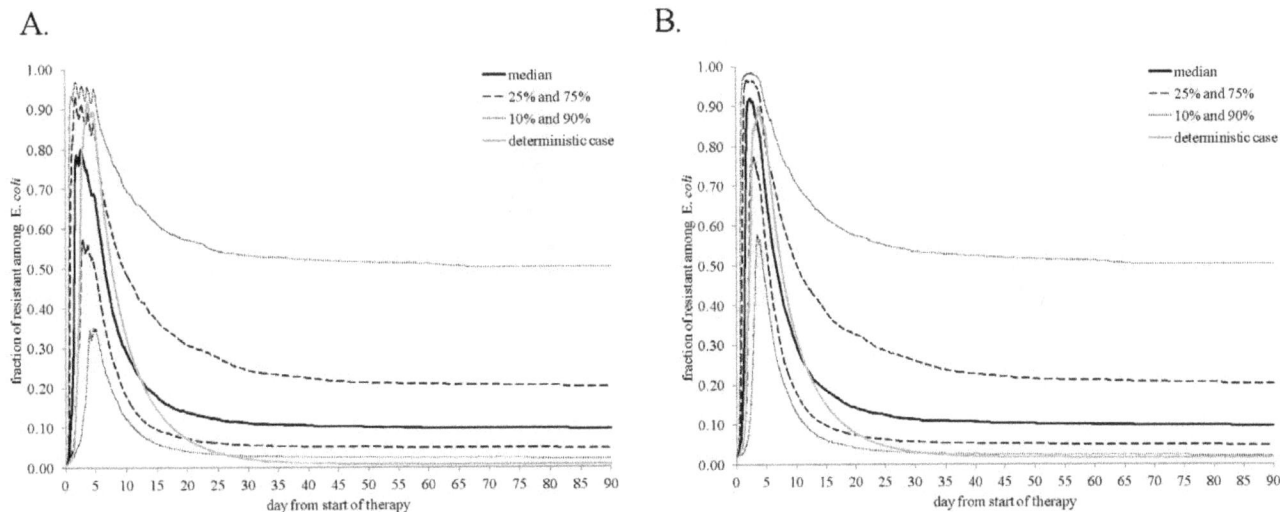

A.

B.

Figure 6. Uncertainty in the fraction of ceftiofur-resistant among enteric *E. coli* during 90 days from start of therapy. Statistics are for 500 model simulations at each time point randomly varying parameters of bacterial ecology and pharmacodynamics. A: A 5-day repeated ceftiofur administration to an adult dairy (frequency of resistance at start of therapy 0.7%). B: An injection of a sustained-release ceftiofur formulation to a 6-mos beef (frequency of resistance at start of therapy 1.8%).

A.

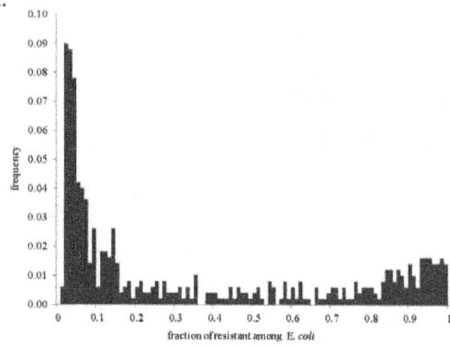

B.

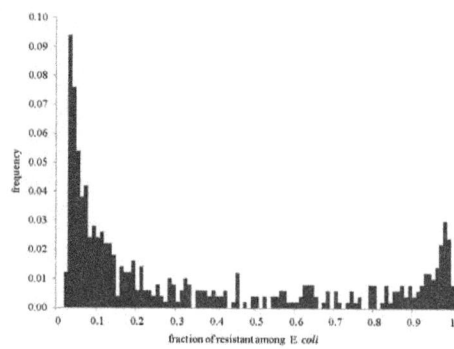

Day 1

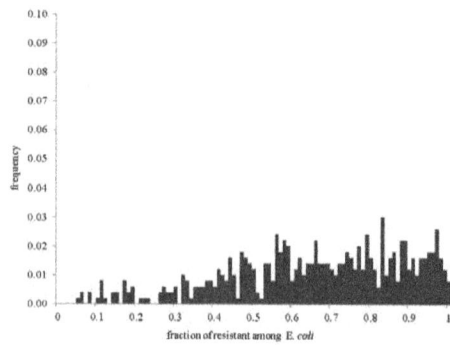

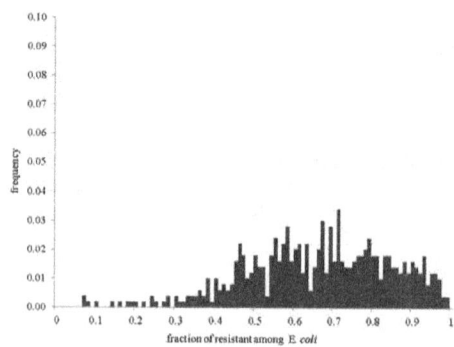

Day 5

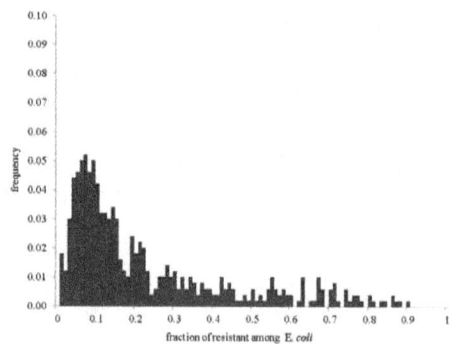

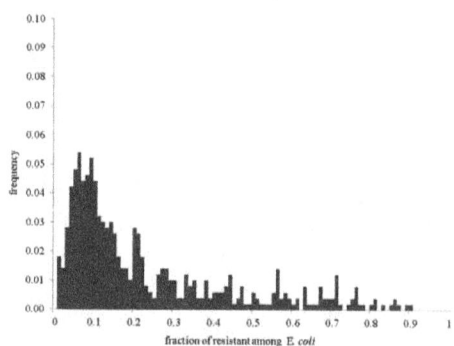

Day 21

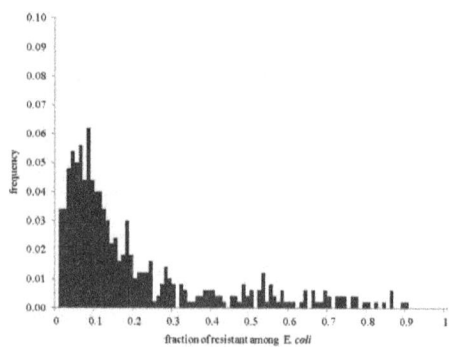

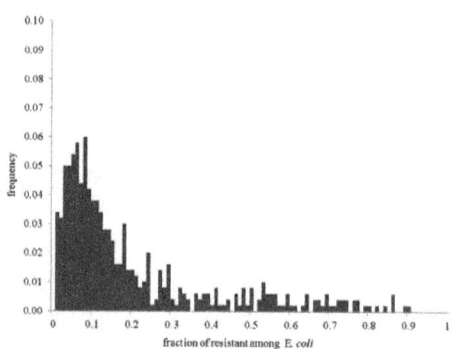

Day 35

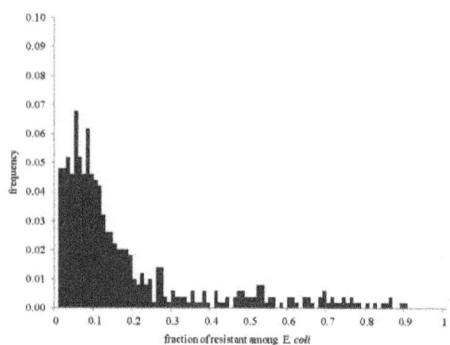

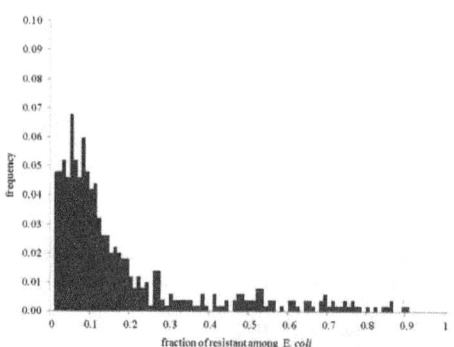

Day 90

Figure 7. Frequency histograms for the fraction of ceftiofur-resistant among enteric *E. coli* on days 1, 5, 21, 35 and 90 from start of therapy. Histograms are of 500 model simulations at each time point randomly varying parameters of bacterial ecology and pharmacodynamics. A: A 5-day repeated ceftiofur administration to an adult dairy (frequency of resistance at start of therapy 0.7%). B: An injection of a sustained-release ceftiofur formulation to a 6-mos beef (frequency of resistance at start of therapy 1.8%).

For all the treatment scenarios, the model (Equations [9–10]) outputs showed a decrease in counts of total and of ceftiofur-sensitive enteric *E. coli*, and a rise in the fraction of resistant among *E. coli* during therapy, similar to experimental observations (Fig. 3 *cf.* Table S1, scenarios R1-R3). For a 5-day therapy in an adult dairy, the model showed a decrease in total count from day 1, to a minimum on day 3, remaining decreased until day 4, and then returning to pre-treatment level on day 7 (Fig. 3B). The timing was close to the results for an on-farm 5-day ceftiofur therapy reporting fecal *E. coli* decreasing from day 1, to a minimum on day 6 (the samples were not collected every day), returning to pre-treatment level by day 9 (Table S1, R2). The maximum drop differed between the model, ~1.05 log CFU/g, and the on-farm study, estimated ~4.0 log CFU/g. However, the count change in the model corresponded to a 91% reduction in number of *E. coli*. Also, there may have been inter-individual variability in the count and its dynamics in the cattle treated on-farm, but only average numbers were reported. For a 5-day therapy in a 6-mos dairy, the model output of a 0.66 log CFU/g drop in total *E. coli* resembled well the field data of 0.5-1 log CFU/g drop in culturable fecal bacteria in individual 2-6 mos calves [78] (Fig. 3B *cf.* Table S1, R1). In both these scenarios, the total *E. coli* count dropped starting from day 1 of therapy.

As total *E. coli* was composed of both ceftiofur-sensitive and resistant cells, propagation of the latter offset the decline in total count, but this took time. *E.g*, in an adult dairy the total *E. coli* count was lowest on day 3 of therapy, dropping by 1.05 log CFU/g (Fig. 3B); but the count of ceftiofur-sensitive cells was lowest on day 4, dropping by 1.68 log CFU/g (Fig. 3C). These corresponded to a 91% and 98% reduction in number of bacteria, respectively. The fraction of resistant among *E. coli* peaked on day 4 (Fig. 3A). At this point, resistant cells filled most of the "carrying capacity", sensitive cells grew less and were less exposed to antimicrobial action (hence no further reduction in sensitive counts). Similarly, in a 6-mos calf the number of sensitive *E. coli* dropped to its minimum and the fraction of resistant *E. coli* rose to its maximum (Fig. 3A) the next day after the maximum drop in total *E. coli* (Fig. 3B).

In cattle of a given age treated under a given protocol, the lower was the initial frequency of resistance, pAMR, the larger was the decline in total count of *E. coli* (Fig. 3B, R2 *vs.* R3) and of sensitive *E. coli* (Fig. 3C *vs.* 3D) during therapy. However, the maximum fraction of resistant among *E. coli* during therapy did not seem to depend on pAMR in the range explored, peaking to 90-91% in either an adult (pAMR = 0.7%), post-partum (pAMR = 1.8%), or 6-mos (pAMR = 5.0%) dairy (Fig. 3A). Yet it took longer for the fraction to completely return to pre-treatment level if this already had been elevated, *e.g.*, ~16 weeks in a 6-mos (pAMR = 5.0%) *cf.* ~10 weeks in an adult (pAMR = 0.7%) dairy.

Scenarios R1-R3 were repeated with ceftiofur dosage 1.1 mg CE/kg (with biliary excretion pattern 1). In an adult dairy, including post-partum, there was a slightly lesser peak in number and relative fraction of resistant *E. coli*, and a day later in therapy compared to using 2.2 mg CE/kg. There was however a difference in a 6-mos dairy; the drop in total *E. coli* was 26% with 1.1 mg *vs.* 64% with 2.2 mg dosage, and the fraction of resistant cells rose to 27% *vs.* 80%, returning to pre-treatment level in 104 *vs.* 110 days, respectively.

Effects of parenteral ceftiofur therapy on commensal enteric *E. coli*: sustained-release ceftiofur formulation. For a 6-mos beef administered a sustained-release ceftiofur formulation, lowering the dosage to 4.4 from 6.6 mg CE/kg (Table S1, SB3 *vs.* SB2), resulted in a smaller drop in total *E. coli*, 1.11 *vs.*1.54 log CFU/g, occurring a day earlier, day 2 *vs.* day 3, of therapy (Fig. 4B). The count of sensitive *E. coli* dropped by 1.83 log CFU/g with 4.4 mg *vs.* by 2.4 log CFU/g with 6.6 mg (98.5% *vs.* 99.6% reduction in number of sensitive bacteria), in either case being the lowest on day 3 (Fig. 4D *vs.* 4C). Quantitatively, the decrease in total *E. coli* matched field data; the timing was not contrasted because in the field study available for comparison with the scenarios SB1-SB3, the fecal samples were only obtained on days 0, 2, 6, 9, 13, 16, 20, and 28 of therapy [84]. The fraction of resistant *E. coli*, however, still rose to its highest of 93% on day 3 with 4.4 mg, *cf.* 95% on day 4 with 6.6 mg (Fig. 4A). The fraction reported by the field study varied from 40% to 90% [84]. In both scenarios SB2 and SB3, it took 111-112 days for the fraction of resistant *E. coli* to completely return to pre-treatment level.

With 6.6 mg CE/kg dosage, whether this was administered once on day 0, or 3 times on days 0, 6 and 13 (Table S1, SB1 *vs.* SB2) had a very limited effect on the dynamics observed (Fig. 4A). This is because the fraction of resistant *E. coli* was still high, and the number of sensitive *E. coli* depressed, following the 1st dose at the time the 2nd dose was given; similarly for doses 2 and 3. This agreed with field observations [84].

For an adult dairy (SD1), the model outputs were similar to a single administration of sustained-release ceftiofur formulation in 4.4 mg CE/kg dosage to a 6-mos beef (SB3).

Sensitivity of model outputs to variability in parameter values. In the absence of immediate ceftiofur pressure, the maintenance of a fraction of ceftiofur-resistant cells among commensal enteric *E. coli* depended on the rate of in-flow and out-flow of *E. coli*, the prevalence of ceftiofur resistance in the in-flow, and the rate of transfer of *blaCMY-2*-carrying plasmids between *E. coli* within the intestine, and, to a lesser extent, on the rate of bacterial growth (Fig. 5B). Certain, although infrequent, combinations of the parameters produced a largely elevated frequency of resistance (Fig. 5A).

There were similar tendencies in the dynamics of ceftiofur-resistant enteric *E. coli* under the scenarios of a 5-day treatment of an adult dairy with a non-sustained release ceftiofur formulation in 2.2 mg CE/kg dosage (R2), and a single injection of a sustained-release ceftiofur formulation to a 6-mos beef in 6.6 mg CE/kg dosage (SB2) (Fig. 6). However, the median (over 500 model simulations) peak fraction of resistant among enteric *E. coli* was in the upper 70% range in the former *vs.* over 90% in the latter scenario (Fig. 6A *vs.*6B). There was a substantial uncertainty in the fraction of resistant *E. coli*, as during so after treatment, with the explored parameter ranges (Figs. 6 and 7). The largest uncertainty was observed on days 1 and 5 from start of therapy (Fig. 7). At those time points the variability in both the ecology of enteric *E. coli*, and in antimicrobial action of enteric ceftiofur metabolites against *E. coli* contributed to the outcome. On day 1 (Fig. 8), a higher fraction of resistance strongly correlated with a higher rate of bacterial growth, and a lower MIC$_s$, which would correspond to a larger kill of growing sensitive *E. coli*, hence a larger niche for

A.

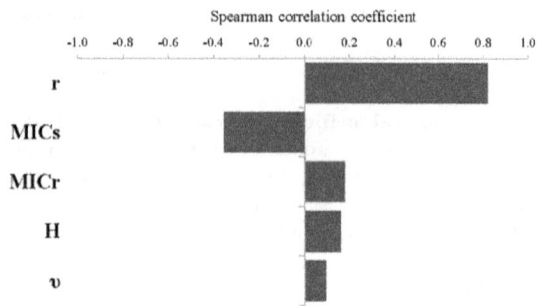

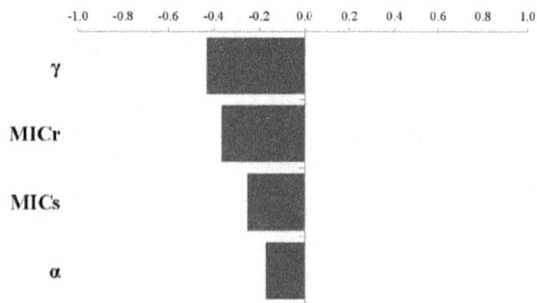

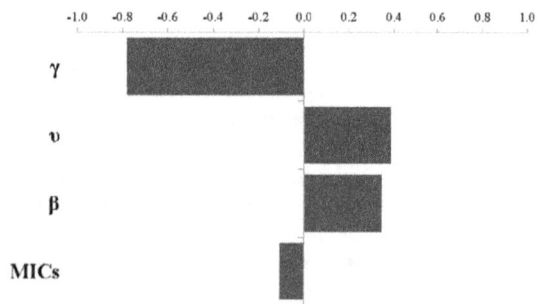

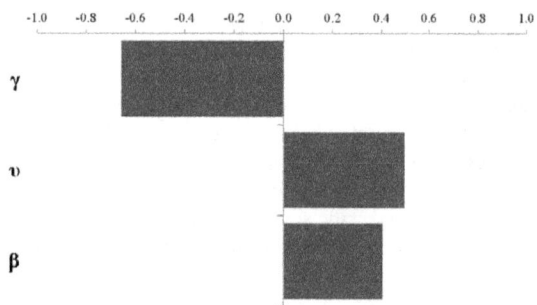

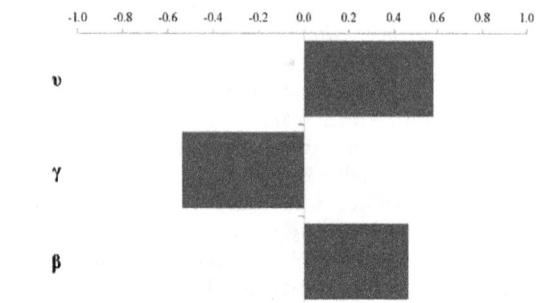

B.

Day 1

Day 5

Day 21

Day 35

Day 90

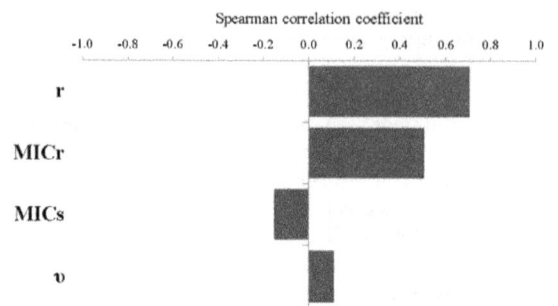

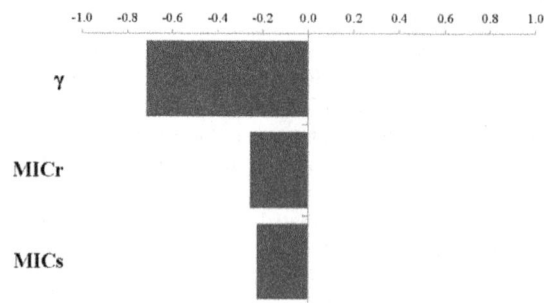

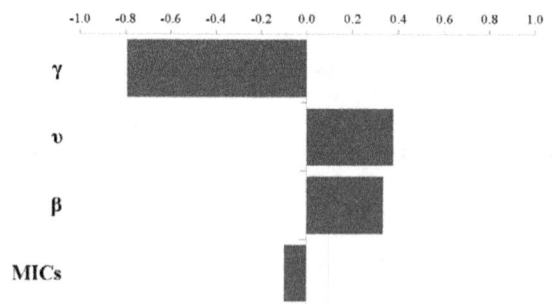

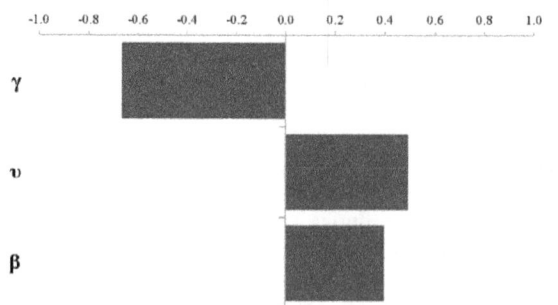

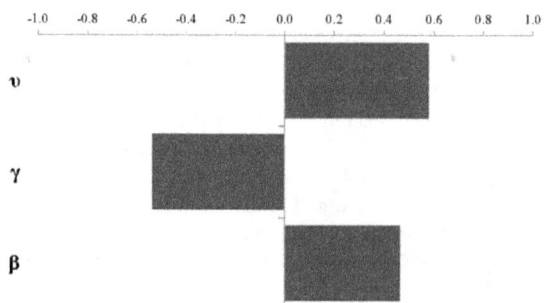

Figure 8. Significant linear correlations (p-value ≤ 0.05) between ranked-transformed values of the parameters of bacterial ecology and pharmacodynamics and the frequency of ceftiofur-resistant among enteric *E. coli* on days 1, 5, 21, 35 and 90 from start of therapy. A: A 5-day repeated ceftiofur administration to an adult dairy (frequency of resistance at start of therapy 0.7%). B: An injection of a sustained-release ceftiofur formulation to a 6-mos beef (frequency of resistance at start of therapy 1.8%).

expansion of the resistant cells, in turn ensured by the higher growth potential. A higher fraction of resistance also correlated with a higher MIC_r, *i.e.*, a larger expansion of resistant *E. coli* if these were less sensitive at the start of therapy. The importance of individual parameters changed by day 5 when the fraction of resistance, after reaching its maximum, was still correlated with the pharmacodynamical parameters, but also became influenced again by the rate of fractional replacement of enteric *E. coli* (Fig. 8). By day 35, the fraction of resistance tended to settle at lower than 20%, further clustering toward lower values by day 90 (Fig. 7). This outcome depended on the same parameters that were most important for resistance maintenance in the absence of treatment: the rate of horizontal transfer of *blaCMY-2*, the rate of in-flow and out-flow of enteric *E. coli*, and the prevalence of ceftiofur-resistance in the in-flow (Fig. 8, Days 35 and 90 *vs.* Fig. 5B).

Discussion

This modeling study suggested that ceftiofur-resistant commensal enteric *E. coli* in cattle could persist between treatments. A low but stable fraction of resistance can be maintained even if the number of resistant *E. coli* grows slower than that of the sensitive ones, when the rate of *blaCMY-2* transfer in enteric *E. coli* is sufficiently high or a sufficient fraction of ingested *E. coli* is ceftiofur-resistant. The latter could occur if the conditions on the farm allow for a close circulation of commensal *E. coli* between cattle and their environment.

The values reported by field studies of the fraction of ceftiofur-resistant cells among fecal *E. coli* in the absence of immediate ceftiofur pressure were reproduced in the deterministic analysis with a transfer rate for *blaCMY-2*-carrying plasmids of 4^{-3}. For individual plasmids, *in vitro* transfer rates are up to 2^{-3} [42]. *In vivo* in post-weaned calves fed a donor and a recipient strain, a rate of *blaCMY-2*-transconjugant generation in fecal *E. coli* of 2^{-3} has been reported [27]. Several plasmids may be present in enteric *E. coli*, and the *blaCMY-2*-transfer rate *in vivo* may be the cumulative of those for individual plasmids. Generally, conjugation frequency may depend on the physiological status of donor cells, phase of growth of donor population [85], and physical conditions [13,86,87]. As the enteric environment is *E. coli*'s ecological niche, the cells are likely in normal physiological condition; this, coupling with nutrient availability for population growth, absence of light and favorable temperatures, may allow for the bacterial conjugation, and so plasmid transfer rate, to be at the high end of the biological maximum [87,88].

Ceftiofur-resistant *E. coli* in this study were defined as cells having a plasmid with *blaCMY-2*. A possibility of variability in the degree of resistance conferred by presence of more than one copy of the gene, or by presence of another mechanism of resistance, and how this may be reflected in MIC-values, was not considered; neither are such data available in experimental literature. This complicated interpretation of the correlations of MIC_r with the fraction of resistant among *E. coli* during therapy (Fig. 8).

The increase in absolute number of *E. coli* cells carrying *blaCMY-2* per g of feces during parenteral ceftiofur therapy could lead to a higher frequency of horizontal transfer of this plasmidic gene to the other enteric bacteria, including potential zoonotic pathogens. However, this would require not only the donor but also the recipient populations to be present in sufficient numbers [89]. The numbers of ceftiofur-sensitive cells among the other bacteria may be diminishing during therapy, similar to the numbers of ceftiofur-sensitive *E. coli*. Hence, the net effect on the frequency of *blaCMY-2*-transmission from *E. coli* to the other bacteria would depend on the degree of sensitivity of the latter to antimicrobial action of enteric ceftiofur metabolites. Importantly, the only origin and spread of AMR considered here for ceftiofur and *E. coli* were the *a-priori* presence of plasmidic *blaCMY-2*, and its vertical and horizontal transfers, respectively. Other mechanisms, *e.g.* resistance mediated by chromosomal genes or that due to plasmid-mediated extended-spectrum beta-lactamases, may need to be considered to understand AMR dynamics across the species. Therefore, based on the current model, we could not infer what effect ceftiofur therapy might have on inter-species spread of *blaCMY-2*. Furthermore, evaluating the potential for spread of AMR-determinants requires accounting for not only the within-host dynamics addressed here, but also how the resistant bacteria spread among the hosts, and between the hosts and their environment.

This study highlighted that results of ceftiofur treatment trials would be more informative for modeling if the data reported would include the dynamical change in fraction of the resistant fecal bacteria, and description of variability among individual cattle. Frequent sampling during treatment would help with detailing the length of time available for expansion of resistant bacteria; continuing sampling post treatment would help with understanding the mechanisms involved in resistance maintenance. On the epidemiological side, important knowledge gaps are details of *E. coli* cycling between cattle and their environment, including the degree of replacement of enteric *E. coli*, the prevalence of ceftiofur resistance in *E. coli* ingested by cattle, and the rates of horizontal *blaCMY-2*-transfer *in vivo*. Absence of publicly accessible data on the concentration and antimicrobial activity of ceftiofur metabolites in cattle intestine during parenteral therapy hinders more detailed research into the selective pressure experienced by enteric bacteria. On the pharmacological side, time-kill experiments (as opposed to experiments establishing MIC-values) mimicking intestinal conditions are needed to describe the pharmacodynamics of ceftiofur metabolites against enteric bacteria.

To conclude, first, the results showed that reported low fractions of ceftiofur-resistant commensal enteric *E. coli* in cattle could be maintained without immediate ceftiofur pressure. Second, during parenteral ceftiofur therapy there likely are antibiotically-active drug metabolites in the large intestine, circumventing a slash in the number of ceftiofur-sensitive enteric *E. coli*. These conclusions are strongly supported by the concordance of the model outputs with experimental data. Hence, there is a window during therapy when ceftiofur-resistant *E. coli* could expand in absolute number and relative frequency; the degree of expansion depends on the parameters of antimicrobial action of the metabolites against *E. coli*, as well as on the rates of enteric *E. coli* growth and replacement. However, whether the post-treatment fraction of resistance would remain elevated in the long-term depends on a present combination of the parameters of bacterial ecology, the same parameters that are important for maintenance of resistance in the absence of ceftiofur pressure. Namely, these are the rate of horizontal transfer of plasmids with *blaCMY-2* between enteric *E. coli*, which may be determined by which plasmids are present, and the frequency of resistance in *E. coli* ingested by cattle, which may be determined by the extent of *E. coli* circulation between cattle and their environment.

Supporting Information

Table S1 Modeled scenarios of treatment of cattle with ceftiofur, and experimental data considered for comparison.

Acknowledgments

We are grateful to Craig Altier of Cornell University and Thomas Besser of Washington State University for generous sharing of their expertise in

biology of ceftiofur resistance; and to Morgan Scott of Kansas University for informative discussions. We thank scholars of the Leadership Program for Veterinary Scholars at Cornell University: summer 2010 scholar Clinton Doering for starting-up literature research on the topic, and summer 2011 scholar Sarah Wood for interactive discussions.

Author Contributions

Conceived and designed the experiments: CL YTG. Wrote the paper: VVV. Partook in model development: VVV CL ZL YTG. Supported VVV in model implementation: ZL. Worked on model parameterization, collated the treatment scenarios, and solved the models: VVV. Helped edit the manuscript: CL ZL YTG. Read and approved the final version of the manuscript: VVV CL ZL YTG.

References

1. McDermott PF, Zhao S, Wagner DD, Simjee S, Walker RD, et al. (2002) The food safety perspective of antibiotic resistance. Animal Biotechnology 13: 71–84.
2. Fey PD, Safranek TJ, Rupp ME, Dunne EF, Ribot E, et al. (2000) Ceftriaxone-resistant salmonella infection acquired by a child from cattle. N Engl J Med 342: 1242–1249.
3. Cohen ML, Tauxe RV (1986) Drug-resistant Salmonella in the United States: an epidemiologic perspective. Science 234: 964–969.
4. Linton AH, Howe K, Bennett PM, Richmond MH, Whiteside EJ (1977) The colonization of the human gut by antibiotic resistant Escherichia coli from chickens. J Appl Bacteriol 43: 465–469.
5. Salyers AA, Gupta A, Wang Y (2004) Human intestinal bacteria as reservoirs for antibiotic resistance genes. Trends Microbiol 12: 412–416.
6. Winokur PL, Vonstein DL, Hoffman LJ, Uhlenhopp EK, Doern GV (2001) Evidence for transfer of CMY-2 AmpC beta-lactamase plasmids between Escherichia coli and Salmonella isolates from food animals and humans. Antimicrob Agents Chemother 45: 2716–2722.
7. Boerlin P, Reid-Smith RJ (2008) Antimicrobial resistance: its emergence and transmission. Anim Health Res Rev 9: 115–126.
8. McCuddin Z, Carlson SA, Rasmussen MA, Franklin SK (2006) Klebsiella to Salmonella gene transfer within rumen protozoa: Implications for antibiotic resistance and rumen defaunation. Veterinary Microbiology 114: 275–284.
9. Delsol AA, Halfhide DE, Bagnall MC, Randall LP, Enne VI, et al. (2010) Persistence of a wild type Escherichia coli and its multiple antibiotic-resistant (MAR) derivatives in the abattoir and on chilled pig carcasses. International Journal of Food Microbiology 140: 249–253.
10. Aslam M, Nattress F, Greer G, Yost C, Gill C, et al. (2003) Origin of contamination and genetic diversity of Escherichia coli in beef cattle. Appl Environ Microbiol 69: 2794–2799.
11. Call DR, Kang MS, Daniels J, Besser TE (2006) Assessing genetic diversity in plasmids from Escherichia coli and Salmonella enterica using a mixed-plasmid microarray. J Appl Microbiol 100: 15–28.
12. Daniels JB, Call DR, Besser TE (2007) Molecular epidemiology of blaCMY-2 plasmids carried by Salmonella enterica and Escherichia coli isolates from cattle in the Pacific Northwest. Appl Environ Microbiol 73: 8005–8011.
13. Licht TR, Wilcks A (2006) Conjugative gene transfer in the gastrointestinal environment. Adv Appl Microbiol 58: 77–95.
14. Ravel J, Fricke WF, McDermott PF, Mammel MK, Zhao SH, et al. (2009) Antimicrobial Resistance-Conferring Plasmids with Similarity to Virulence Plasmids from Avian Pathogenic Escherichia coli Strains in Salmonella enterica Serovar Kentucky Isolates from Poultry. Applied and Environmental Microbiology 75: 5963–5971.
15. Khachatryan AR, Hancock DD, Besser TE, Call DR (2004) Role of calf-adapted Escherichia coli in maintenance of antimicrobial drug resistance in dairy calves. Appl Environ Microbiol 70: 752–757.
16. Khachatryan AR, Hancock DD, Besser TE, Call DR (2006) Antimicrobial drug resistance genes do not convey a secondary fitness advantage to calf-adapted Escherichia coli. Appl Environ Microbiol 72: 443–448.
17. Apley MD, Brown SA, Fedorka-Cray PJ, Ferenc S, House JK, et al. (1998) Role of veterinary therapeutics in bacterial resistance development: animal and public health perspectives. Journal of the American Veterinary Medical Association 212: 1209–1213.
18. Morley PS, Apley MD, Besser TE, Burney DP, Fedorka-Cray PJ, et al. (2005) Antimicrobial drug use in veterinary medicine. Journal of Veterinary Internal Medicine 19: 617–629.
19. Lanzas C, Ayscue P, Ivanek R, Grohn YT (2010) Model or meal? Farm animal populations as models for infectious diseases of humans. Nature Reviews Microbiology 8: 139–148.
20. Bauernfeind A, Stemplinger I, Jungwirth R, Ernst S, Casellas JM (1996) Sequences of beta-lactamase genes encoding CTX-M-1 (MEN-1) and CTX-M-2 and relationship of their amino acid sequences with those of other beta-lactamases. Antimicrob Agents Chemother 40: 509–513.
21. Barlow M, Hall BG (2002) Origin and evolution of the AmpC beta-lactamases of Citrobacter freundii. Antimicrob Agents Chemother 46: 1190–1198.
22. Bush K, Jacoby GA, Medeiros AA (1995) A functional classification scheme for beta-lactamases and its correlation with molecular structure. Antimicrob Agents Chemother 39: 1211–1233.
23. Bauernfeind A, Stemplinger I, Jungwirth R, Giamarellou H (1996) Characterization of the plasmidic beta-lactamase CMY-2, which is responsible for cephamycin resistance. Antimicrob Agents Chemother 40: 221–224.
24. Heider LC, Hoet AE, Wittum TE, Khaitsa ML, Love BC, et al. (2009) Genetic and phenotypic characterization of the bla(CMY) gene from Escherichia coli and Salmonella enterica isolated from food-producing animals, humans, the environment, and retail meat. Foodborne Pathogens and Disease 6: 1235–1240.
25. Dunne EF, Fey PD, Kludt P, Reporter R, Mostashari F, et al. (2000) Emergence of domestically acquired ceftriaxone-resistant Salmonella infections associated with AmpC beta-lactamase. JAMA 284: 3151–3156.
26. Dutil L, Irwin R, Finley R, Ng LK, Avery B, et al. (2010) Ceftiofur resistance in Salmonella enterica serovar Heidelberg from chicken meat and humans, Canada. Emerging Infectious Diseases 16: 48–54.
27. Daniels JB, Call DR, Hancock D, Sischo WM, Baker K, et al. (2009) Role of ceftiofur in selection and dissemination of blaCMY-2-mediated cephalosporin resistance in Salmonella enterica and commensal Escherichia coli isolates from cattle. Appl Environ Microbiol 75: 3648–3655.
28. Sawant AA, Hegde NV, Straley BA, Donaldson SC, Love BC, et al. (2007) Antimicrobial-resistant enteric bacteria from dairy cattle. Appl Environ Microbiol 73: 156–163.
29. Tragesser LA, Wittum TE, Funk JA, Winokur PL, Rajala-Schultz PJ (2006) Association between ceftiofur use and isolation of Escherichia coli with reduced susceptibility to ceftriaxone from fecal samples of dairy cows. American Journal of Veterinary Research 67: 1696–1700.
30. Morley PS, Dargatz DA, Hyatt DR, Dewell GA, Patterson JG, et al. (2011) Effects of restricted antimicrobial exposure on antimicrobial resistance in fecal Escherichia coli from feedlot cattle. Foodborne Pathogens and Disease 8: 87–98.
31. Aslam M, Greer GG, Nattress FM, Gill CO, McMullen LM (2004) Genetic diversity of Escherichia coli recovered from the oral cavity of beef cattle and their relatedness to faecal E. coli. Lett Appl Microbiol 39: 523–527.
32. Philippon A, Arlet G, Jacoby GA (2002) Plasmid-determined AmpC-type beta-lactamases. Antimicrob Agents Chemother 46: 1–11.
33. Persoons D, Haesebrouck F, Smet A, Herman L, Heyndrickx M, et al. (2011) Risk factors for ceftiofur resistance in Escherichia coli from Belgian broilers. Epidemiol Infect 139: 765–771.
34. Singer RS, Patterson SK, Wallace RL (2008) Effects of therapeutic ceftiofur administration to dairy cattle on Escherichia coli dynamics in the intestinal tract. Appl Environ Microbiol 74: 6956–6962.
35. Mann S, Siler JD, Jordan D, Warnick LD (2011) Antimicrobial susceptibility of fecal Escherichia coli isolates in dairy cows following systemic treatment with ceftiofur or penicillin. Foodborne Pathogens and Disease.
36. Alali WQ, Scott HM, Norby B, Gebreyes W, Loneragan GH (2009) Quantification of the bla(CMY-2) in feces from beef feedlot cattle administered three different doses of ceftiofur in a longitudinal controlled field trial. Foodborne Pathogens and Disease 6: 917–924.
37. Ketyi I (1994) Effectiveness of antibiotics on the autochthonous Escherichia coli of mice in the intestinal biofilm versus its planktonic phase. Acta Microbiol Immunol Hung 41: 189–195.
38. Durso LM, Smith D, Hutkins RW (2004) Measurements of fitness and competition in commensal Escherichia coli and E. coli O157:H7 strains. Appl Environ Microbiol 70: 6466–6472.
39. Freter R, Brickner H, Botney M, Cleven D, Aranki A (1983) Mechanisms That Control Bacterial-Populations in Continuous-Flow Culture Models of Mouse Large Intestinal Flora. Infection and Immunity 39: 676–685.

40. Ayscue P, Lanzas C, Ivanek R, Grohn YT (2009) Modeling On-Farm Escherichia coli O157:H7 Population Dynamics. Foodborne Pathogens and Disease 6: 461–470.

41. Andrup L, Andersen K (1999) A comparison of the kinetics of plasmid transfer in the conjugation systems encoded by the F plasmid from Escherichia coli and plasmid pCF10 from Enterococcus faecalis. Microbiology-Uk 145: 2001–2009.

42. Subbiah M, Top EM, Shah DH, Call DR (2011) Selection Pressure Required for Long-Term Persistence of blaCMY-2-Positive IncA/C Plasmids. Appl Environ Microbiol 77: 4486–4493.

43. Lenski RE, Simpson SC, Nguyen TT (1994) Genetic analysis of a plasmid-encoded, host genotype-specific enhancement of bacterial fitness. J Bacteriol 176: 3140–3147.

44. Poole TL, Brichta-Harhay DM, Callaway TR, Beier RC, Bischoff KM, et al. (2011) Persistence of resistance plasmids carried by beta-hemolytic Escherichia coli when maintained in a continuous-flow fermentation system without antimicrobial selection pressure. Foodborne Pathogens and Disease 8: 535–540.

45. Bergstrom CT, Lipsitch M, Levin BR (2000) Natural selection, infectious transfer and the existence conditions for bacterial plasmids. Genetics 155: 1505–1519.

46. Schrag SJ, Perrot V, Levin BR (1997) Adaptation to the fitness costs of antibiotic resistance in Escherichia coli. Proc Biol Sci 264: 1287–1291.

47. Jaglan PS, Kubicek MF, Arnold TS, Cox BL, Robins RH, et al. (1989) Metabolism of ceftiofur - nature of urinary and plasma metabolites in rats and cattle. Journal of Agricultural and Food Chemistry 37: 1112–1118.

48. Hornish RE, Kotarski SF (2002) Cephalosporins in veterinary medicine - ceftiofur use in food animals. Curr Top Med Chem 2: 717–731.

49. Ritter L, Kirby G, Cerniglia C (1996) Toxicological evaluation of certain veterinary drug residues in food. (857) Ceftiofur WHO Food Additives Series 36.

50. Salmon SA, Watts JL, Yancey RJ (1996) In vitro activity of ceftiofur and its primary metabolite, desfuroylceftiofur, against organisms of veterinary importance. Journal of Veterinary Diagnostic Investigation 8: 332–336.

51. Beconi-Barker MG, Roof RD, Vidmar TJ, Hornish RE, Smith EB, et al. (1996) Ceftiofur sodium: Absorption, distribution, metabolism, and excretion in target animals and its determination by high-performance liquid chromatography. Veterinary Drug Residues 636: 70–84.

52. Brown SA, Chester ST, Speedy AK, Hubbard VL, Callahan JK, et al. (2000) Comparison of plasma pharmacokinetics and bioequivalence of ceftiofur sodium in cattle after a single intramuscular or subcutaneous injection. Journal of Veterinary Pharmacology and Therapeutics 23: 273–280.

53. Brown SA, Hanson BJ, Mignot A, Millerioux L, Hamlow PJ, et al. (1999) Comparison of plasma pharmacokinetics and bioavailability of ceftiofur sodium and ceftiofur hydrochloride in pigs after a single intramuscular injection. J Vet Pharmacol Ther 22: 35–40.

54. Arvidsson A, Alvan G, Angelin B, Borga O, Nord CE (1982) Ceftriaxone - Renal and Biliary-Excretion and Effect on the Colon Microflora. Journal of Antimicrobial Chemotherapy 10: 207–215.

55. Bakken JS, Cavalieri SJ, Gangeness D (1990) Influence of plasma exchange pheresis on plasma elimination of ceftriaxone. Antimicrob Agents Chemother 34: 1276–1277.

56. Arvidsson A, Leijd B, Nord CE, Angelin B (1988) Interindividual Variability in Biliary-Excretion of Ceftriaxone - Effects on Biliary Lipid-Metabolism and on Intestinal Microflora. European Journal of Clinical Investigation 18: 261–266.

57. Xia Y, Lambert KJ, Schteingart CD, Gu JJ, Hofmann AF (1990) Concentrative biliary secretion of ceftriaxone. Inhibition of lipid secretion and precipitation of calcium ceftriaxone in bile. Gastroenterology 99: 454–465.

58. Hoffmann-La Roche Limited (2010) Prepared June 16, 1987. 9 RevisedFebruary, ed. 2010. Product monograph: Rocephin (sterile ceftriaxone sodium). 46 pp.

59. United States Food and Drug Administration (1990) Environmental Assessment of Excenel Sterile Suspension (Ceftiofur Hydrochloride). 46 pp.

60. Gilbertson TJ, Hornish RE, Jaglan PS, Koshy KT, Nappier JL, et al. (1990) Environmental Fate of Ceftiofur Sodium, a Cephalosporin Antibiotic - Role of Animal Excreta in Its Decomposition. Journal of Agricultural and Food Chemistry 38: 890–894.

61. Livermore DM (1991) Mechanisms of resistance to beta-lactam antibiotics. Scand J Infect Dis Suppl 78: 7–16.

62. Merle-Melet M, Seta N, Farinotti R, Carbon C (1989) Reduction in biliary excretion of ceftriaxone by diclofenac in rabbits. Antimicrob Agents Chemother 33: 1506–1510.

63. Symonds HW, Mather DL, Hall ED (1982) Surgical procedure for modifying the duodenum in cattle to measure bile flow and the diurnal variation in biliary manganese, iron, copper and zinc excretion. Res Vet Sci 32: 6–11.

64. Pfizer Animal Health website. Graph of plasma concentrations of ceftiofur equivalents following a single injection of a sustained-release ceftiofur formulation in lactating dairy: Available: http://www.excede.com/Excede.aspx?country = US&drug = XT&species = DA&sec = 310. Accessed 1 Oct 2011.

65. Pfizer Animal Health website. Graph of plasma concentrations of ceftiofur equivalents following a single injection of a sustained-release ceftiofur

66. Tipper DJ (1985) Mode of action of beta-lactam antibiotics. Pharmacol Ther 27: 1–35.

67. Mattie H, van Dokkum AM, Brus-Weijer L, Krul AM, van Strijen E (1990) Antibacterial activity of four cephalosporins in an experimental infection in relation to in vitro effect and pharmacokinetics. J Infect Dis 162: 717–722.

68. Craig WA, Ebert SC (1990) Killing and regrowth of bacteria in vitro: a review. Scand J Infect Dis Suppl 74: 63–70.

69. Mouton JW, Dudley MN, Cars O, Derendorf H, Drusano GL (2005) Standardization of pharmacokinetic/pharmacodynamic (PK/PD) terminology for anti-infective drugs: an update. J Antimicrob Chemother 55: 601–607.

70. Goutelle S, Maurin M, Rougier F, Barbaut X, Bourguignon L, et al. (2008) The Hill equation: a review of its capabilities in pharmacological modelling. Fundam Clin Pharmacol 22: 633–648.

71. Mouton JW, Vinks AA (2005) Pharmacokinetic/pharmacodynamic modelling of antibacterials in vitro and in vivo using bacterial growth and kill kinetics: the minimum inhibitory concentration versus stationary concentration. Clin Pharmacokinet 44: 201–210.

72. Drusano GL (2004) Antimicrobial pharmacodynamics: critical interactions of 'bug and drug'. Nat Rev Microbiol 2: 289–300.

73. Drusano GL (1991) Human Pharmacodynamics of Beta-Lactams, Aminoglycosides and Their Combination. Scandinavian Journal of Infectious Diseases. pp 235–248.

74. Hanberger H (1992) Pharmacodynamic effects of antibiotics. Studies on bacterial morphology, initial killing, postantibiotic effect and effective regrowth time. Scand J Infect Dis Suppl 81: 1–52.

75. Czock D, Keller F (2007) Mechanism-based pharmacokinetic–pharmacodynamic modeling of antimicrobial drug effects. J Pharmacokinet Biopharm 34: 727–751.

76. Ambrose PG, Bhavnani SM, Rubino CM, Louie A, Gumbo T, et al. (2007) Pharmacokinetics-pharmacodynamics of antimicrobial therapy: it's not just for mice anymore. Clinical Infectious Diseases 44: 79–86.

77. Vogelman B, Gudmundsson S, Turnidge J, Leggett J, Craig WA (1988) Invivo Postantibiotic Effect in a Thigh Infection in Neutropenic Mice. Journal of Infectious Diseases 157: 287–298.

78. Jiang X, Yang H, Dettman B, Doyle MP (2006) Analysis of fecal microbial flora for antibiotic resistance in ceftiofur-treated calves. Foodborne Pathogens and Disease 3: 355–365.

79. Daniels JB, Call DR, Hancock D, Sischo WM, Baker K, et al. (2009) Role of Ceftiofur in Selection and Dissemination of bla(CMY-2)-Mediated Cephalosporin Resistance in Salmonella enterica and Commensal Escherichia coli Isolates from Cattle. Applied and Environmental Microbiology 75: 3648–3655.

80. Alexander TW, Yanke LJ, Topp E, Olson ME, Read RR, et al. (2008) Effect of subtherapeutic administration of antibiotics on the prevalence of antibiotic-resistant Escherichia coli bacteria in feedlot cattle. Applied and Environmental Microbiology 74: 4405–4416.

81. Fricke WF, Welch TJ, McDermott PF, Mammel MK, LeClerc JE, et al. (2009) Comparative genomics of the IncA/C multidrug resistance plasmid family. J Bacteriol 191: 4750–4757.

82. LeJeune JT, Hancock DD, Besser TE (2006) Sensitivity of Escherichia coli O157 detection in bovine feces assessed by broth enrichment followed by immunomagnetic separation and direct plating methodologies. Journal of Clinical Microbiology 44: 872–875.

83. Marino S, Hogue IB, Ray CJ, Kirschner DE (2008) A methodology for performing global uncertainty and sensitivity analysis in systems biology. Journal of Theoretical Biology 254: 178–196.

84. Lowrance TC, Loneragan GH, Kunze DJ, Platt TM, Ives SE, et al. (2007) Changes in antimicrobial susceptibility in a population of Escherichia coli isolated from feedlot cattle administered ceftiofur crystalline-free acid. American Journal of Veterinary Research 68: 501–507.

85. Muela A, Pocino M, Arana I, Justo JI, Iriberri J, et al. (1994) Effect of growth phase and parental cell survival in river water on plasmid transfer between Escherichia coli strains. Appl Environ Microbiol 60: 4273–4278.

86. Fernandez-Astorga A, Muela A, Cisterna R, Iriberri J, Barcina I (1992) Biotic and abiotic factors affecting plasmid transfer in Escherichia coli strains. Appl Environ Microbiol 58: 392–398.

87. Arana II, Justo JI, Muela A, Pocino M, Iriberri J, et al. (1997) Influence of a Survival Process in a Freshwater System upon Plasmid Transfer Between Escherichia coli Strains. Microb Ecol 33: 41–49.

88. Arana I, Pocino M, Muela A, Fernandez-Astorga A, Barcina I (1997) Detection and enumeration of viable but non-culturable transconjugants of Escherichia coli during the survival of recipient cells in river water. J Appl Microbiol 83: 340–346.

89. Stecher B, Denzler R, Maier L, Bernet F, Sanders MJ, et al. (2012) Gut inflammation can boost horizontal gene transfer between pathogenic and commensal Enterobacteriaceae. Proc Natl Acad Sci U S A 109: 1269–1274.

90. Sorum H, Sunde M (2001) Resistance to antibiotics in the normal flora of animals. Vet Res 32: 227–241.

19

Irradiated Male Tsetse from a 40-Year-Old Colony Are Still Competitive in a Riparian Forest in Burkina Faso

Adama Sow[1,2,3], Issa Sidibé[1,2], Zakaria Bengaly[1], Augustin Z. Bancé[1], Germain J. Sawadogo[3], Philippe Solano[1,4], Marc J. B. Vreysen[5], Renaud Lancelot[6], Jeremy Bouyer[6,7]*

1 Centre International de Recherche-Développement sur l'Elevage en Zone subhumide (CIRDES), Bobo-Dioulasso, Burkina Faso, 2 Pan-African Tsetse and Trypanosomosis Eradication Campaign (PATTEC), Projet de Création de Zones Libérées Durablement de Tsé-tsé et de Trypanosomoses (PCZLD), Bobo-Dioulasso, Burkina Faso, 3 Ecole Inter-Etats des Sciences et Médecine Vétérinaires (EISMV), Dakar-Fann, Sénégal, 4 Institut de Recherche pour le Développement (IRD), UMR 177 IRD-CIRAD INTERTRYP, Montpellier, France, 5 Insect Pest Control Laboratory, Joint FAO/IAEA Programme of Nuclear Techniques in Food and Agriculture, Vienna, Austria, 6 Institut Sénégalais de Recherches Agricoles, Laboratoire National d'Elevage et de Recherches Vétérinaires, Hann, Dakar, Sénégal, 7 UMR Contrôles des Maladies Animales et Emergentes, Centre de Coopération Internationale en Recherche Agronomique pour le Développement (CIRAD), Campus International de Baillarguet, Montpellier, France

Abstract

Background: Tsetse flies are the cyclical vectors of African trypanosomosis that constitute a major constraint to development in Africa. Their control is an important component of the integrated management of these diseases, and among the techniques available, the sterile insect technique (SIT) is the sole that is efficient at low densities. The government of Burkina Faso has embarked on a tsetse eradication programme in the framework of the PATTEC, where SIT is an important component. The project plans to use flies from a *Glossina palpalis gambiensis* colony that has been maintained for about 40 years at the Centre International de Recherche-Développement sur l'Elevage en zone Subhumide (CIRDES). It was thus necessary to test the competitiveness of the sterile males originating from this colony.

Methodology/Principal Findings: During the period January–February 2010, 16,000 sterile male *G. p. gambiensis* were released along a tributary of the Mouhoun river. The study revealed that with a mean sterile to wild male ratio of 1.16 (s.d. 0.38), the abortion rate of the wild female flies was significantly higher than before ($p = 0.026$) and after ($p = 0.019$) the release period. The estimated competitiveness of the sterile males (Fried index) was 0.07 (s.d. 0.02), indicating that a sterile to wild male ratio of 14.4 would be necessary to obtain nearly complete induced sterility in the female population. The aggregation patterns of sterile and wild male flies were similar. The survival rate of the released sterile male flies was similar to that observed in 1983–1985 for the same colony.

Conclusions/Significance: We conclude that gamma sterilised male *G. p. gambiensis* derived from the CIRDES colony have a competitiveness that is comparable to their competitiveness obtained 35 years ago and can still be used for an area-wide integrated pest management campaign with a sterile insect component in Burkina Faso.

Editor: Basil Brooke, National Institute for Communicable Diseases/NHLS, South Africa

Funding: This work was carried out with the financial support of Institute of Tropical Medicine Anvers and Pan African Tsetse and Trypanosomosis Eradication-Projet de Création de Zones Libérées Durablement de Tsé-tsé et de Trypanosomoses, Burkina Faso. The funders had no role in study design, data collection and analysis, decision to publish, or preparation of the manuscript.

Competing Interests: The authors have declared that no competing interests exist.

* E-mail: bouyer@cirad.fr

Introduction

African animal trypanosomosis (AAT) constitutes a major constraint to livestock production in sub-Saharan Africa. The disease is enzootic in an area covering ca. 10 million km^2 and threatens nearly 50 million cattle [1]. The disease causes many direct losses due to lower production, mortality and treatment costs, as well as indirect losses such as the opportunity of genetic improvement, and intensification of livestock production [2]. Direct losses and cost of AAT control is estimated to range between USD 600 and 1200 million year^{-1} for sub-Saharan Africa [3].

Tsetse flies are the sole cyclical vectors of trypanosomes, the causative agents of AAT. The maintenance of non-trypanotolerant cattle in tsetse-infested areas is often only feasible through continuous prophylactic and curative treatment with trypanocidal drugs and as a result, more than 35 million doses are being administered annually [4]. Chemoresistance against these drugs is however, becoming more and more widespread [4,5] making tsetse control the only way to sustainably manage AAT. According to Budd [6], the eradication of trypanosomosis would increase agricultural production in Africa with a value of USD 4.5 billion/year. In addition, tsetse are the vectors of human sleeping sickness, a major neglected disease [7].

Most control tactics against tsetse flies are effective and allow quick reduction of their abundance. The use of insecticide impregnated targets and the application of insecticide pour-ons on cattle reduced tsetse populations in Burkina Faso and in some East African countries drastically [8–11] and this was usually followed by a reduction of the AAT incidence [8,12,13]. However, these control methods generally do not eradicate the tsetse population because their efficiency is density dependent [14]. Other vector control methods, such as the Sequential Aerosol Technique (SAT), are not tsetse density dependent and can be used to manage tsetse populations in open savannah areas such as *Glossina morsitans centralis* in the Okavango Delta of Botswana [15]. The SAT relies on a high percentage of adult mortality (>99%) during each spraying cycle, which can rarely be attained in the humid or sub-humid areas of West Africa, in view of the dense gallery forests. Finally, the SIT has "negative" density dependent properties, i.e. its efficiency is inversely proportional to the density of the target population because of an increase of the ratio of sterile to wild males at each generation [16]. Therefore, the combination of the SIT (effective at low population densities) with other control techniques that are effective at high population densities is an optimal strategy to achieve eradication of riverine tsetse fly populations in West Africa [17,18]. However, to warrant a sustainable impact, these tsetse control tactics must be applied area-wide, i.e directed against an entire tsetse population within a delimited area, especially if eradication is the strategy of choice. For example in West-Africa, riverine tsetse species occur in large distribution belts, with established gene flows between the various river basins [19,20]: their eradication would thus require a sequential approach, including the implementation of barriers between eradication blocks.

Knipling conceived the idea of using sterile insects to manipulate the reproduction rate of a natural insect population in 1937, but it was not until the 1950's that a method was found to sterilize insects and the idea could be given a practical follow-up [21–23]. It was for the first time applied in 1954 to eradicate the New World screwworm fly *Cochliomyia hominivorax* (Coquerel) from the Island of Curaçao, Netherlands Antilles [24]. This successful trial was followed by the eradication of the pest from the southern USA, Mexico, Central America (1950–2000) [25,26], and from Libya in 1990–1991 [27]. Since then, the SIT as part of area-wide integrated pest management (AW-IPM) approaches, has been successfully used to suppress or eradicate several lepidopteran and dipteran pests, including fruit and tsetse flies [16,28]. It was tested for the first time against *Glossina morsitans morsitans* in Tanzania [29] in the 1970's where sterile males released at a 1.12:1 ratio managed to maintain the population suppressed for 15 months at a 80–95% reduction level obtained after an initial application of insecticides by air. Thereafter, the release of sterile males was successfully integrated with the deployment of insecticide impregnated targets to eradicate *Glossina palpalis gambiensis* Vanderplank, *Glossina tachinoides* Westwood, and *Glossina morsitans submorsitans* Newstead from an agro pastoral zone of Sidéradougou in Burkina Faso (3,000 km^2, 1983–1985) and *Glossina palpalis palpalis* Rob. Desv. from a pastoral area in Nigeria (1,500 km^2, 1982–1985) [18,30,31]. Although initially successful, these campaigns in Burkina Faso and Nigeria were not sustainable as the approach was not area-wide (i.e. it did not target the entire tsetse population in a circumscribed geographical area [32]) and the local beneficiary communities and authorities failed to create or maintain adequate buffer areas to prevent re-invasion of the cleared areas [33]. The AW-IPM approach was introduced into the area of tsetse control on the Island of Unguja, Zanzibar, where a population of *Glossina austeni* Newstead was eradicated using the SIT combined with pour-on treatment of cattle and insecticide impregnated targets/screens [34]. The success of this area-wide campaign was a strong argument for the Pan African Tsetse and Trypanosomosis Eradication Campaign (PATTEC), to promote the use of SIT for the eradication of tsetse populations from selected areas in Africa after pre-release reduction of tsetse populations with 90–99% using other effective techniques. In Burkina Faso, more than 20,000 insecticide impregnated targets were deployed along the Mouhoun River and its tributaries to drastically reduce tsetse densities in the PATTEC intervention area. Cypermethrin-based pour-on treatment was applied on cattle in the buffer areas, located at the borders of the study area along 10 km of the Mouhoun River and its tributaries [35]. In addition the eastern branch of the Mouhoun River was treated with the SAT using deltamethrin as active ingredient in collaboration with the PATTEC Ghana office. As a result of this suppression campaign (2009–2010), the populations of *G. p. gambiensis* and *G. tachinoides*, the sole cyclical vectors of trypanosomosis in the area [36,37], were reduced by 95% in the PATTEC Burkina Faso intervention area [35].

In addition to the mass-rearing of male flies to be sterilized by ionizing irradiation, the SIT can only be successful if these sterile males (i) can locate the wild virgin females and successfully transfer their sterile sperm, and (ii) disperse and aggregate in a similar pattern as their wild counterparts [38]. The Centre International de Recherche-Développement sur l'Elevage en zone Subhumide (CIRDES), Bobo Dioulasso, Burkina Faso has been maintaining a *G. p. gambiensis* colony since 1972, with introduction of wild pupae from time to time. The colony however, has, since the eradication campaign in Sidéradougou in the early 1980's not been used for any operational releases [30]. It is intended to use the sterile flies from this colony for AW-IPM programmes in Burkina Faso and Senegal and it was therefore deemed necessary to re-confirm its field competitiveness [39].

In this study, field releases of sterilized male *G. p. gambiensis* were carried out in riverine gallery forest habitat in Burkina Faso to study their survival, dispersal and aggregation pattern, as well as their mating frequencies with wild female tsetse flies.

Materials and Methods

Study area

The study area was situated close to the village of Kadomba (11°53′ North; 3°97′ West), 70 km north of Bobo-Dioulasso (fig. 1) and contained guinean riverine forest [40] along the Leyessa River (a tributary of the Mouhoun River) which has its origin in the protected forest of Maro. Previous entomological surveys showed that almost all caught tsetse were *G. p. gambiensis*, with an average apparent density of 10 flies per trap per day [41]. Laboratory-reared *G. p. gambiensis* were released over 3 km along the river (fig. 1) in geo-referenced release sites. One km upstream of the release area, a 1-km barrier was established with 20 biconical traps impregnated with deltamethrin (800 mg/m^2) and deployed every ~50 meters during the whole study. Other studies had revealed that the tsetse population of the study area was genetically differentiated (and thus partially isolated) from that of the Mouhoun River [42].

Tsetse sterile males

Laboratory-reared tsetse flies used for this study were produced at the CIRDES in Bobo Dioulasso, Burkina Faso. Newly emerged adult male flies were irradiated in a Cs^{137} GAAA ® irradiator with a dose of 110 Gy (dose rate of 4.49 Gy/min), routinely used at CIRDES since the Sideradougou eradication campaign [43]. Irradiated males were marked with acrylic paint on the thorax using different colours to differentiate between series of released insects. Before release, flies were offered twice a blood meal containing isometamidium chloride (Trypamidium® MERIAL SAS, Lyon, France batch nDG/20058) at a concentration of 10 mg/L to prevent the development of trypanosomes in the released flies [44,45]. Batches of 50 4-day-old male flies were

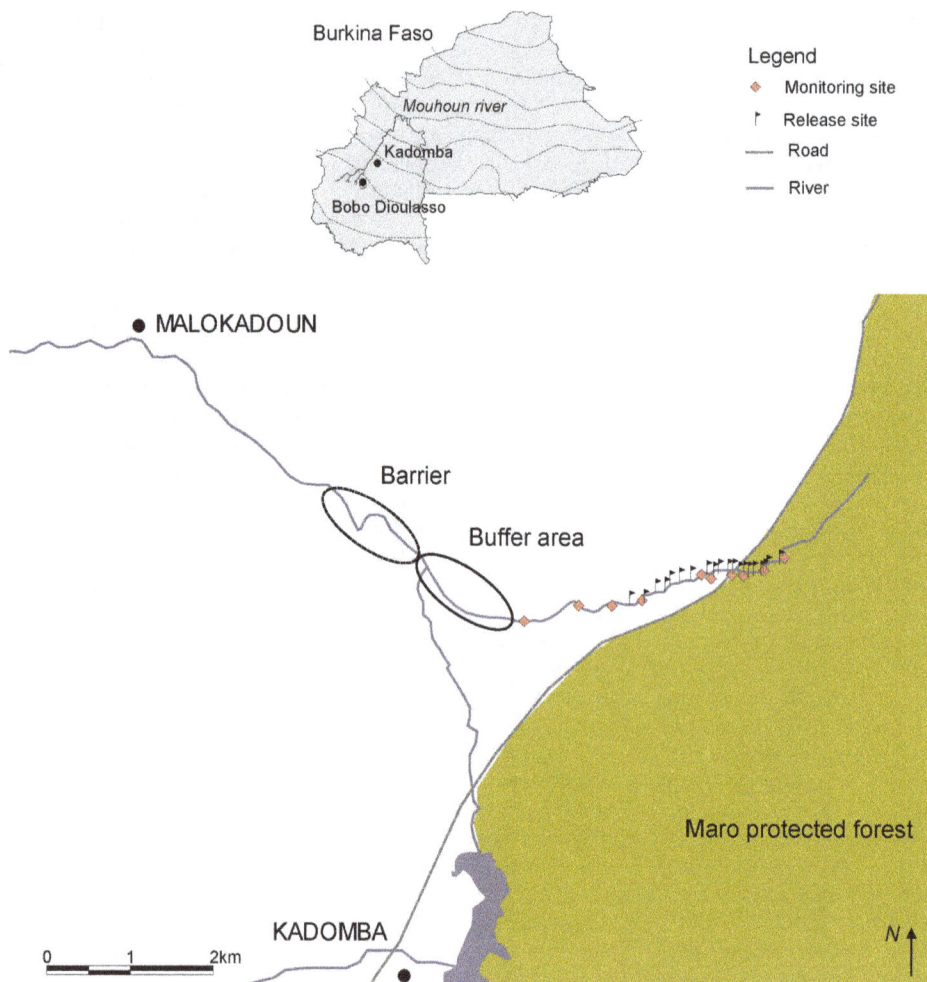

Figure 1. Location of the study area in Burkina Faso. The release and monitoring sites along the Leyessa River are displayed. The 1-km barrier was established with 20 biconical traps impregnated with deltamethrin (see M&M for details).

transferred to Roubaud cages (4.5×13×8 cm) that were covered with a net of mesh 1×1 mm. Cages were then put in a humidified container and transported to the release sites.

Preliminary entomological data collection

Before initiating the field releases, two entomological sampling efforts were carried out during 5 consecutive days, at 10-day intervals. Tsetse flies were sampled with 20 biconical traps [46] deployed at 150 m intervals along the river. All trapping sites were georeferenced. Caught female flies that were still alive were dissected. The same person assessed the percentage of pregnant females and the spermathecal fill during these preliminary sampling periods and during intervention period.

Release of sterile males

Seven releases were carried out at weekly intervals in January–February 2010. A thousand sterile males were released during each of the first 2 releases, and the number of males released was increased to 2,000 and 4,000 sterile males for the 3 following releases and the last two releases, respectively. A total of 16,000 sterile males were thus released over the 7-week interval, to obtain a ratio of irradiated to wild males upon 1:1. Releases were made along the river between 4h30 and 6h30 p.m. at equal proportions in 10 different sites interspaced at approximately 300 m. During

the releases, dead flies and non-flyers were recorded after opening the Roubaud cages.

Sterility levels of irradiated male *G. p. gambiensis*

Twenty newly emerged virgin *G. p. gambiensis* females from the CIRDES colony were mated with 10 newly emerged irradiated males and maintained under normal insectary conditions (both males and females were 4 days old). Produced pupae were regularly collected, weighed and stored. Females were dissected after 4 weeks to assess spermathecal fill and their reproductive status. The results were compared to those of a control group of 2000 females the main colony, maintained in the same conditions.

Dissection of sampled wild female *G. p. gambiensis*

All trapped live female flies were dissected for ovarian ageing to determine the physiological age of the population [47]. Proportions of nulliparous, young (less than 4 ovulations) and old (4 ovulations or more) parous females were determined [48]. Pregnant females were classified as having a larva or a developing egg *in utero*, and non-pregnant females as having an empty uterus. The rate of sterility (natural abortion and induced sterility) was determined taking into consideration the status of the uterus and the follicle next in ovulation sequence: i.e, those females that had recently aborted an egg in embryonic arrest or still had the degenerated egg *in utero*.

The competitiveness of the irradiated males was assessed using the Fried index [49] by comparing the abortion rates obtained during the entomological surveys carried out before, during and after the releases of sterile males. After dissection, spermathecae were placed in a droplet of normal saline solution and were observed under the microscope at $40\times$ magnitude. Spermathecal fill was scored as empty (0) quarter-full (0.25), half-full (0.5), three quarter-full (0.75) and full (1.0) [50,51].

Dispersal and population dynamics of the irradiated males

Trapping surveys were implemented weekly after each sterile male release session using 10 biconical traps set along the release area during 2 to 5 days to assess the relative abundance of wild and irradiated males. The colour of the acrylic spot on the thorax indicated the date of release, and thus the age of the trapped flies. The ratio of irradiated to wild male flies in the samples was also calculated.

Recapture of released irradiated males provided an estimate of the number of alive, marked flies for the different series of releases. After the last release, entomological monitoring was continued every week, up to one month after the last release.

Statistical analyses

Mortality rate and survival of the released male flies were estimated using the temporal relative abundance data, assuming a constant daily mortality rate within each released batch. The linear evolution of the captures of the sterile males released on 06/02/10 is presented in fig. 2: this is illustrative of what was observed with other batches. The daily survival rate was thus estimated as the exponential of the slope of the natural logarithm (ln) of total captures for each batch against time.

To assess similarities or differences in the spatial pattern of apparent densities of wild and sterile male flies using trap records, the existence of a spatial trend in log(wild male counts) was tested [38]. This trend was subtracted from log-counts before assessing the independence of trap locations and wild male fly abundance. This was achieved with a Monte Carlo test for marked point processes [52]: the point process being the set of trap locations, and the marks being the wild male fly counts. Secondly, we used

a X^2 test to assess the spatial heterogeneity in wild male fly abundance, and correlation tests to assess the independence of wild males and females, and sterile males.

To plot the data, we transformed fly counts into standardized contributions. For each fly category i (wild male or female, sterile male) and trap j ($j = 1,...$ J), each observed trap count n_{ij} was divided by the total observed count N_i for this fly category to give the observed relative contribution of each trap $o_{ij} = n_{ij}/N_i$. The expected relative contribution of trap j under the assumption of homogeneous spatial distribution ($e_{ij} = 1/J$) was then subtracted to o_{ij} and the result was divided by e_{ij}, thus providing the standardized contribution $c_{ij} = (o_{ij} - e_{ij})/e_{ij} = J n_{ij}/N_i - 1$.

The proportion of flies having aborted and the spermathecal fill were compared using X^2 tests. A Pearson's correlation test was used to assess the correlation between the ratio of sterile to wild male flies and the abortion rate of wild females, and between the mortality of the sterile males and the number of flies released.

Ethical statement

All necessary permits were obtained by « Projet de Création de zones libérées durablement de la mouche Tsé-Tsé et de la Trypanosomose » (national project of the Ministry of Animal Resources, N° SAP PZ1-AAO-009), particularly that of the Ministry of Environment of Burkina Faso, which is in charge of the follow up of the environmental impact of this project, for conducting the described field studies as a part of the feasibility study of tsetse eradication in the first block (Mouhoun river loop).

Results

Baseline situation

During the two pre-release entomological sampling events, 1950 wild *G. p. gambiensis* were caught giving a relative abundance of 12.2 tsetse flies/trap/day. The sample contained 53.4% female flies of which 166 were dissected. Of these dissected females, 25.9% were nulliparous, 36.1% young and 38% old parous flies. The natural abortion rate was 3.3%, an additional 4.9% of the female flies had an empty uterus (post larviposition) while 39.8% of the female flies contained an egg and 52% a larva.

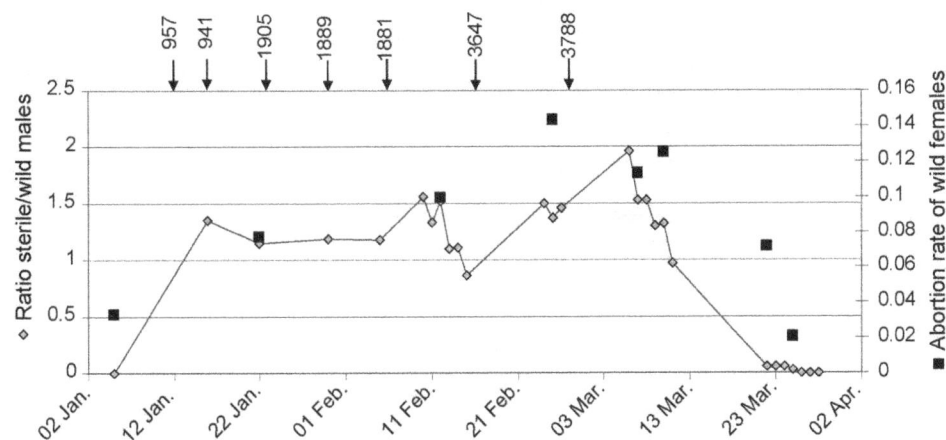

Figure 2. Impact of sterile males releases on wild female abortion rates. Temporal pattern of the ratio of sterile to wild males and the abortion rates of wild females during the study period (Jan.–Apr. 2010) are displayed. The number and dates of sterile flies released are represented by the black arrows at the top.

Sterile male fly losses during transport

Of the 16,000 irradiated males shipped to the release points, 15,008 (93.8%) were actually released (Table 1), i.e. mortality rate of the male flies at the release sites was 1.9% due to handling, marking, transport or irradiation, and 4.3% were non-flyers and either too weak to take off or had non-functional wings due to acrylic painting.

Population dynamics of the irradiated males

During the monitoring of the dispersal of the irradiated males, 1,068 wild females, 1,048 wild males and 1,142 released males (i.e. 7.6% of the released flies) were trapped. The mean daily mortality rate of the released sterile males was 14.9±4.0%, corresponding to a mean lifespan of 4.6±1.3 days (fig. 3 and table 1). There was no significant correlation between the mortality rate and the number of released flies (p=0.15). The population of irradiated flies decreased quickly and, one month after the last release no more marked flies were trapped during 3 consecutive days of trap deployment (fig. 2).

Mating of virgin females with irradiated males

In the laboratory, 48.9% of the colony G. p. gambiensis females that had mated with 110 Gy irradiated males had an empty uterus due to abortion, and 6.7% and 44.4% of the female flies had a larva and a degenerating egg in utero respectively. The abortion rate was thus higher (p<0.001) than in the control group, where only 1.1%±0.7% of the females aborted. The weight of pupae collected from the different experimental batches was significantly lower (p<0.001) than that of pupae produced by the untreated control group i.e. a mean weight of 20.7±2.3 mg vs. 26.8±0.3 mg. Moreover, no adult flies emerged from these pupae. The abortion rate and the spermathecal fill did not vary significantly from one experimental group to another (F=0.40; df=6; p=0.75). However, less than one third of females mated with the irradiated males had full spermathecae (31.1%) while 20% had empty spermathecae, which was significantly lower than the mean spermathecal fill of the wild females dissected during the pre-release entomological sampling (χ^2 = 5.90; p=0.015).

Competitiveness of irradiated males as compared to wild males

From the second week of sterile male fly releases, the rate of induced sterility increased from 3.3% to 7.7% (s.e. 7.7%) reaching 14% at the end of the releases (fig. 2). It dropped again to 2.1% (s.e. 1.5%) one month after the last release. During the release period, the abortion rate was significantly higher than the natural abortion rate before (n = 338, X2 = 4.932, p = 0.026) and after

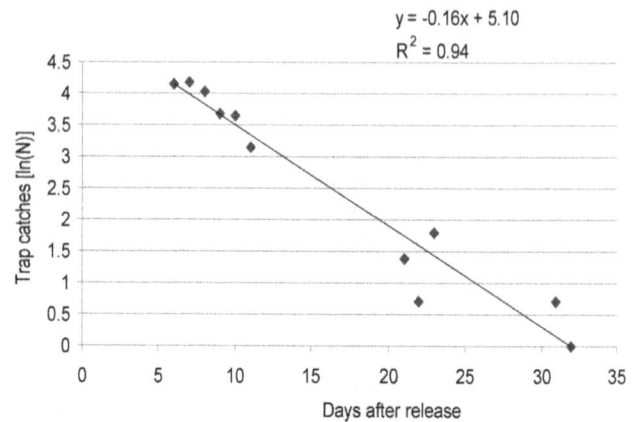

$$y = -0.16x + 5.10$$
$$R^2 = 0.94$$

Figure 3. Dynamics of the number of sterile males recaptured. The data correspond to the batch released on 06/02/2010 in Kadomba.

(n = 311, X2 = 5.548, p = 0.019) the release period. There was no significant difference between the natural abortion rates recorded before and after the releases (n = 219, X2 = 0.012, p = 0.914).

During the entire experiment, the ratio of irradiated to wild males fluctuated between 1 and 2 (fig. 2), and was on average 1.16 (s.d. 0.38). There was a strong positive correlation (r = 0.95, p<0.001) between the ratio of sterile to wild males and the abortion rate measured during the same week. The competitiveness of the sterile males (Fried index) was 0.07 (s.d. 0.02), corresponding to a sterile to wild male ratio of 14.4 required to obtain 100% induced sterility in female flies.

Spermathecal fill

During the preliminary fly sampling there was no significant difference between spermathecal fill of the 3 age groups, i.e. teneral/nulliparous, young and old parous wild flies (F = 0.13; df = 2; p = 0.88). During the release period, no significant difference was observed between the spermathecal fill of the various age groups (F = 2.05; df = 2; p = 0.130). More than 50% of the flies had spermathecae completely filled with sperm and less than 5% had empty spermathecae. Average spermathecal fill of the wild female flies before and after the releases was similar (p = 0.149).

Spatial distribution of the sterile males

Significant spatial trends were observed in the count data: a non-linear (quadratic-like) trend ($p<10^{-4}$) was observed for longitude

Table 1. Characteristics of the batches of irradiated male G. p. gambiensis released in Kadomba.

Date	Colour	Released flies	Flyers (%)	Daily mortality rate (%)	Mean lifespan (days)	Recapture rate (%)
12 Jan	White*	1,000	95.7	10.0	6.60	3.6
16 Jan	Red	1,000	94.1	11.9	5.45	5.6
23 Jan	Yellow	2,000	95.3	16.8	3.76	4.7
30 Jan	Green	2,000	94.4	16.1	3.95	5.0
6 Feb	White*	2,000	94.0	14.7	4.34	15.0
16 Feb	Light red	4,000	91.2	12.5	5.19	4.4
26 Feb	Brillant green	4,000	94.7	22.0	2.79	9.4
Total		16,000	93.8±1.5	14.9±4.0	4.6±1.3	7.2±0.1

*The difference between the released males of these two groups was done by the wing fray interpretation.

with a maximum close to the eastern region of the study area, and a linear trend ($p < 10^{-4}$) was observed in latitude, with a maximum in the northern region of the study area.

Similar trends were observed for wild female and sterile male flies, with significant and very similar p values. These spatial trends were removed from the data sets for further analyses. The point marked process analysis showed that wild male fly counts were independent from trap locations (Monte Carlo test, $p > 0.05$), i.e., no interaction was detected between trap locations and fly counts.

Although sterile male flies were released rather homogeneously along the river (fig. 1, mean distance between release sites = 102 m, s.d. = 49 m) their spatial distribution of recapture was highly heterogeneous, as evidenced by trapping counts with spatial trend removed ($X^2 = 34$, df = 9, $p = 10^{-4}$). The distributions of male and female wild fly catches were also heterogeneous ($X^2 = 133$, df = 9, $p < 10^{-4}$; $X^2 = 25$, df = 9, $p = 0.003$). The joint distribution of these de-trended counts is shown in Figure 4. The spatial distribution of sterile and wild male fly catches was similar ($p = 0.94$).

Discussion

The use of sterile insects as part of AW-IPM can only be successful if the male flies released are of the highest biological quality. They should have adequate survival, intermingle with the wild insect population and be capable of transferring their sterile sperm to virgin females preferably in the same frequency as their natural male counterparts. The competitiveness of sterile insects becomes the more questionable when they have been colonised for multiple generations, as is the case with the G. p. gambiensis colony maintained at the CIRDES in Burkina Faso. Recently, it was demonstrated that this strain was still competitive with two field strains originating from Mali and Senegal in experimental conditions [53]. The results of these experimental releases clearly indicate that the competitiveness and behaviour of irradiated male

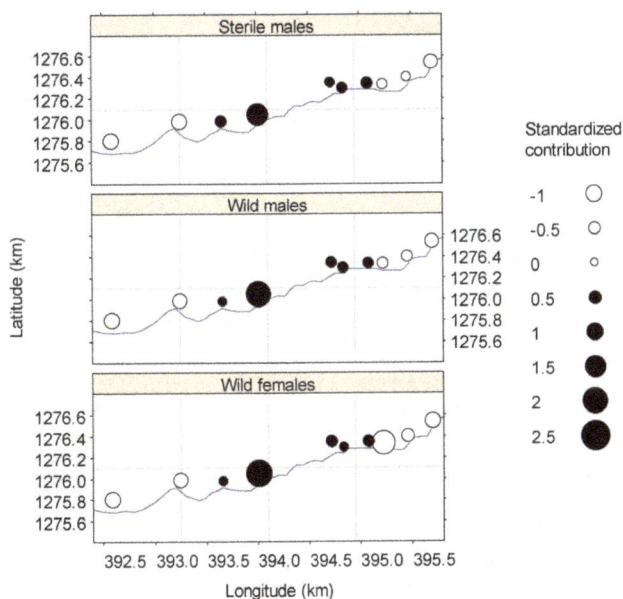

Figure 4. Aggregation patterns of wild and sterile *Glossina palpalis gambiensis*. The figure displays the spatial distribution (standardized abundance) of wild and sterile tsetse sampled with 10 biconical traps along the Leyessa River. See text for explanations on standardized abundance. Longitude and latitude are expressed according to the coordinate reference system UTM 30N, Clarke 1880 ellipsoid.

G. p. gambiensis derived from the CIRDES colony under field conditions was comparable with data obtained 30 years ago.

The percentage of flies actually released (94%) as a proportion of total flies transported, was satisfactory and similar to that obtained by Clair et al. (1976) in Burkina Faso [54]. Mortality rates before release and the proportion of non-flying alive flies in our experiment were very close to their observations, indicating adequate handling, irradiation, transport, and release procedures. Although the average daily mortality rate after release can be considered as high i.e. 14.9% and corresponding to a mean lifespan of 4.6 days, these data are in line with results obtained from January to March 1984 during the Sidéradougou eradication campaign using flies derived from the same colony [30,31]. A re-analysis of the raw data available during this period (Bouyer J., unpublished) revealed a daily mortality of 13.6%, s.d. 6%. However, during the rainy season of the same year (August–October 1984) a much lower daily mortality rate of 9% (s.d. 3%) was observed. The high mortality rates in our experiment could therefore be attributed to the hot dry season in the area when temperatures were high and the stress on the sterile flies considerable. It would be useful to expand this study and assess performance of the sterile males during the rainy season. The mean lifespan obtained during our study is also close to the one obtained with irradiated males of G. tachinoides released around N'Djamena (Chad) in 1973 (4.8 days) [55]. Generally, the longevity of irradiated male tsetse flies is reduced as compared with wild flies due to (i) successive anaesthesia using cold temperatures, (ii) handling in the insectary for sorting and marking, and (iii) irradiation using ionizing radiation that inflicts somatic cell damage [56]. Former studies in the laboratory showed that mean longevity was considerably reduced in irradiated G. tachinoides, G. fuscipes fuscipes Newstead, and G. brevipalpis [57]. These shorter lifespans must be compensated for by regular (twice weekly) releases during an eradication campaign to maintain critical sterile to wild male overflooding ratios [58]. In the case of tsetse, the shorter lifespan presents however an advantage as it reduces the risk of sterile males transmitting the trypanosomoses [44,45].

The spatial analysis showed that the observed heterogeneous fly distribution among traps was not related to differences in trap efficiency, but to a fly aggregation in preferred sites (and fly emigration from other sites) as was observed on Unguja Island (Zanzibar) during the eradication campaign of G. austeni [38]. Barclay [59] has shown the importance of insect aggregation in pest control, especially when using the SIT or any other genetic control method. The weaker correlation between wild males and females, and absence of correlation between sterile males and wild females might be related to different, sex-specific preferences in fly habitat, as observed on Unguja Island [38]. In addition, the present data confirm that tsetse fly dispersal cannot be solely considered as a homogeneous diffusion process, as often assumed [60,61]. It also confirms that mass-reared and gamma-sterilized male tsetse flies were able to respond to environmental cues and to aggregate in the preferred sites of the wild males, even after being colonised for about 40 years. Their aggregation behaviour was therefore similar to that of wild males, confirming that sterile male flies derived from the CIRDES colony are still very good candidates for genetic control.

The competitiveness of irradiated males was assessed through the comparison of the abortion rate and spermathecal fill before, during and after the releases of irradiated males, and the analysis of their spatial distribution, as compared with their wild counterparts. During the collection of initial baseline data, the observed natural abortion rate of 3.3% was close to the rate of natural abortion noted in *G. austeni* [34]. Under adverse climatic conditions, the abortion rate in female tsetse can reach 9%, as observed in *G. m. morsitans* in Zambia [62]. However, there was no climatic accident during the study, but instead a progressive increase of the mean temperature from 27.6°c to 32.6°c and of the mean relative hygrometry from 16.6% to 35.8% (data not shown), whereas the abortion rate dropped again after the release period. The low spermathecal fill observed in laboratory cage conditions in comparison to the wild females is probably related to the use of 4 day-old males, which are not as competitive as older males. During 11 weeks of monitoring, the ratio of irradiated/wild males was on average 1.16 (s.d. 0.38). These results confirmed that 110 Gy-irradiated, previously fed male *G. p. gambiensis* disperse well and have a significant impact on the reproduction of wild females. Obviously, such a low release rate would neither allow a significant induction of sterility in the wild female population or/and a significant reduction of the wild tsetse population in the release area. In our experiment, the wild *G. p. gambiensis* population was deliberately not suppressed before release of sterile male flies because we needed an adequate number of wild female flies for dissection to assess the impact of sterile males on their sterility. The data of the experiment clearly indicated that irradiated male *G. p. gambiensis* reared at CIRDES are still compatible with the wild females and competitive with the wild males in the Mouhoun River basin. This is probably due to the slow reproductive cycle of tsetse (one offspring every 10 days resulting in a mean number of

only 4.7 pupae by female in the insectarium of CIRDES), which imposes relatively low selection pressures on flies maintained in a colony. This makes it necessary to keep a large colony to produce the sterile males, as it was done in CIRDES (between 50 000 and 100 000 females during the last 20 years), thus allowing to maintain the genetic diversity.

Within the framework of the eradication project in Burkina Faso, it will however be necessary to overflood the wild male population with a higher ratio (>14.4). That is why pre-release suppression by other effective techniques (target, pour on treatment of cattle, SAT and ground fogging) will be implemented in the Mouhoun River basin before using the SIT as was done in the 1980's in the Sidéradougou area [30,31].

Acknowledgments

Special thanks are due to the National Coordinator of PATTEC Burkina and the director general of CIRDES, Prof. Abdoulaye Gouro, for provision of excellent working conditions, and to Sanogo Lassina and Bila Cene for their assistance during the field studies.

Author Contributions

Conceived and designed the experiments: AS JB. Performed the experiments: AS AZB. Analyzed the data: AS MJBV RL JB. Contributed reagents/materials/analysis tools: IS ZB AZB GJS PS. Wrote the paper: AS PS MJBV RL JB.

References

1. Kristjanson PM, Swallow BM, Rawlands GJ, Kruska RL, Leeuw PN (1999) Measuring the cost of African Animal Trypanosomiasis, the potential benefits of control and returns to research. Agr syst 59: 79–98.
2. Shaw APM (2004) Economics of African trypanosomosis. In: Maudlin I, Holmes PH, Miles MA, eds. The trypanosomosis. Wallingford: CABI Publishing. pp 369–402.
3. Swallow BM (1999) Impacts of Trypanosomiasis on African Agriculture. Rome: FAO. 46 p.
4. Geerts S, Holmes PH, Diall O, Eisler MC (2001) African bovine trypanosomiasis: the problem of drug resistance. Trends Parasitol 17: 25–28.
5. Delespaux V, Geysen D, Van Den Bossche P, Geerts S (2008) Molecular tools for the rapid detection of drug resistance in animal trypanosomes. Trends Parasitol 24: 236–242.
6. Budd L (1999) DFID-funded tsetse and trypanosome research and development since 1980. Volume 2: Economic Analysis, Livestock Production Programme. Chatham Maritime: NRInternational. 123 p.
7. Simarro PP, Cecchi G, Paone M, Franco JR, Diarra A, et al. (2010) The Atlas of human African trypanosomiasis: a contribution to global mapping of neglected tropical diseases. Int J Health Geogr 9: e57.
8. Bauer B, Amsler-Delafosse S, Kaboré I, Kamuanga M (1999) Improvement of cattle productivity through rapid alleviation of African Trypanosomosis by integrated disease management practices in the Agropastoral zone of Yalé, Burkina Faso. Trop Anim Health Prod 31: 89–102.
9. Bauer B, Amsler-Delafosse S, Clausen P, Kabore I, Petrich-Bauer J (1995) Successful application of deltamethrin pour on to cattle in a campaign against tsetse flies (*Glossina* spp.) in the pastoral zone of Samorogouan, Burkina Faso. Trop Med Parasitol 46: 183–189.
10. Hargrove JW, Torr SJ, Kindness HM (2003) Insecticide-treated cattle against tsetse (Diptera: Glossinidae): what governs success? Bull Entomol Res 93: 203–217.
11. Kagbadouno MS, Camara M, Bouyer J, Courtin F, Morifaso O, et al. (2011) Tsetse control in Loos islands, Guinea. Parasites & Vectors 4: 18.
12. Rowlands GJ, Leak SGA, Mulatu W, Nagda SM, Wilson A, et al. (2000) Use of deltamethrin 'pour-on' insecticide for the control of cattle trypanosomosis in the presence of high tsetse invasion. Med Vet Entomol 15.
13. Bouyer J, Stachurski F, Gouro A, Lancelot R (2009) Control of bovine trypanosomosis by restricted application of insecticides to cattle using footbaths. Vet Parasitol 161: 187–193.
14. Bouyer J, Solano P, Cuisance D, Itard J, Frézil J-L, et al. (2010) Trypanosomosis: Control methods. In: Lefèvre P-C, Blancou J, Chermette R, Uilenberg G, eds. Infectious and parasitic diseases of livestock. Paris: Éditions Lavoisier (Tec & Doc). pp 1936–1943.
15. Kgori PM, Modo S, Torr SJ (2006) The use of aerial spraying to eliminate tsetse from the Okavango Delta of Botswana. Acta Trop 99: 184–199.
16. Dyck VA, Hendrichs J, Robinson AS (2005) Sterile insect technique. Dordrecht: Springer. 787 p.
17. Vloedt van der AMV, Baldry DAT, Politzar H, Kulzer H, Cuisance D (1980) Experimental helicopter applications of decamethrin followed by release of sterile males for the control of riverine vectors of trypanosomiasis in Upper Volta. Insect Sci Applic 1: 105–112.
18. Takken V, Oladunmade MA, Dengwat L, Feldmann HU, Onah JA, et al. (1986) The eradication of Glossina palpalis palpalis (Robineau-Desvoidy) (Diptera: Glossinidae) using traps, insecticide-impregnated targets and the sterile insect technique in central Nigeria. Bull Entomol Res 76: 275–286.
19. Bouyer J, Ravel S, Guerrini L, Dujardin JP, Sidibé I, et al. (2010) Population structure of *Glossina palpalis gambiensis* (Diptera: Glossinidae) between river basins in Burkina-Faso: consequences for area-wide integrated pest management. Inf Gen Evol 10: 321–328.
20. Koné N, Bouyer J, Ravel S, Vreysen MJB, Domagni KT, et al. (2011) Contrasting Population Structures of Two Vectors of African Trypanosomoses in Burkina Faso: Consequences for Control. PLoS Negl Trop Dis 5: e1217.
21. Knipling EF (1955) Possibilities of insect population control through the use of sexually sterile males. J Econ Entomol 48: 443–448.
22. Klassen W (2003) Edward F. Knipling: Titan and driving force in ecologically selective area-wide pest management. J Am Mosq Control Assoc 19: 94–103.
23. Knipling EF (1959) Sterile-Male Method of Population Control: Successful with some insects, the method may also be effective when applied to other noxious animals. Science 9: 902–904.
24. Baumhover AH, Graham AJ, Bitter BA, Hopkins DE, New WD, et al. (1955) Screwworm control through release of sterile flies. J Econ Entomol 48: 462–466.
25. Vargas-Terán M (1991) The New World Screwworm in Mexico and Central America. World Anim Rev Special Issue October. pp 28–35.
26. Novy JE (1991) Screwworm control and eradication in the southern United States of America. World Anim Rev. pp 18–27.
27. Vargas-Terán M, Hursey BS, Cunningham EP (1994) Eradication of the screwworm from Libya using the sterile insect technique. Parasitol Today 10: 119–122.
28. Dagnachew S, Sangwan AK, Abebe G (2005) Epidemiology of Bovine Trypanosomosis in the Abay (Blue Nile) Basin Areas of Northwest Ethiopia. Rev Elev Méd vét Pays trop 58: 151–157.
29. Williamson DL, Baumgartner HM, Mtuya AG, Warner PV, Tarimo SA, et al. (1983) Integration of insect sterility and insecticides for control of Glossina morsitans morsitans (Diptera: Glossinidae) in Tanzania: I. Production of tsetse flies for release. Bull Entomol Res 73: 267–273.
30. Cuisance D, Politzar H, Merot P, Tamboura I (1984) Les lâchers de mâles irradiés dans la campagne de lutte intégrée contre les glossines dans la zone pastorale de Sidéradougou, Burkina Faso. Rev Elev Méd vét Pays trop 37: 449–468.
31. Politzar H, Cuisance D (1984) An integrated campaign against riverine tsetse flies *Glossina palpalis gambiensis* and *Glossina tachinoides* by trapping and the release of sterile males. Insect Sci Applic 5: 439–442.

32. Vreysen M, Robinson AS, Hendrichs J (2007) Area-Wide Control of Insect Pests, From research to field implementation. Dordrecht: Springer. 789 p.

33. Sow A, Sidibé I, Bengaly Z, Bouyer J, Bauer B, et al. (2010) Fifty years of research and fight against tsetse flies and animal trypanosomosis in Burkina Faso. An overview. Bull Anim Hlth Prod 58: 95–118.

34. Vreysen MJB, Saleh KM, Ali MY, Abdulla AM, Zhu Z-R, et al. (2000) *Glossina austeni* (Diptera: Glossinidae) Eradicated on the Island of Unguja, Zanzibar, Using the Sterile Insect Technique. J Econ Entomol 93: 123–135.

35. Pan-African Tsetse, Trypanosomosis Eradication Campaign (PATTEC)/Projet de Création de Zones Libérées Durablement de Tsé-tsé et de Trypanosomoses (PCZLD) (2010) Bobo-Dioulasso, Burkina Faso. 47 p.

36. Bouyer J, Guerrini L, Desquesnes M, de la Rocque S, Cuisance D (2006) Mapping African Animal Trypanosomosis risk from the sky. Vet Res 37: 633–645.

37. Van den Bossche P, de La Rocque S, Hendrickx G, Bouyer J (2010) A changing environment and the epidemiology of tsetse-transmitted livestock trypanosomiasis. Trends Parasitol 26(5): 236–243.

38. Vreysen MJB, Saleh KM, Lancelot R, Bouyer J (2011) Factory tsetse flies must behave like wild flies: a prerequisite for the sterile insect technique. PLoS Negl Trop Dis 5(2): e907.

39. Bouyer J, Seck MT, Sall B, Guerrini L, Vreysen MJB (2010) Stratified entomological sampling in preparation of an area-wide integrated pest management programme: the example of *Glossina palpalis gambiensis* in the Niayes of Senegal. J Med Entomol 47(4): 543–552.

40. Bouyer J, Guerrini L, César J, de la Rocque S, Cuisance D (2005) A phytosociological analysis of the distribution of riverine tsetse flies in Burkina Faso. Med Vet Entomol 19: 372–378.

41. Koné N, N'Goran EK, Sidibé I, Kombassere AW, Bouyer J (2011) Spatiotemporal distribution of tsetse (Diptera: Glossinidae) and other biting flies (Diptera: Tabanidae and Stomoxinae) in the Mouhoun River Basin, Burkina Faso. Med Vet Entomol 25: 156–168.

42. Esnault O (2007) Etude de la structuration de deux sous-populations de Glossina palpalis gambiensis Vanderplank sur la Leyessa, un affluent du Mouhoun au Burkina Faso. Bobo: CIRDES. 37 p.

43. Taze Y, Cuisance D, Politzar H, Clair M, Sellin E, et al. (1977) Essais de détermination de la dose optimale d'irradiation des mâles de *Glossina palpalis gambiensis* (Vanderplank, 1949) en vue de la lutte biologique par lâchers de mâles stériles dans la région de Bobo-Dioulasso (Haute Volta). Rev Elev Méd vét Pays trop 30: 269–279.

44. Van den Bossche P, Akoda K, Djagmah B, Marcotty T, De Deken R, et al. (2006) Effect of Isometamidium Chloride Treatment on Susceptibility of Tsetse Flies (Diptera: Glossinidae) to Trypanosome Infections. J Med Entomol 43: 564–567.

45. Bouyer J (2008) Does isomethamidium chloride treatment protect tsetse flies from trypanosome infections during SIT campaigns? Med Vet Entomol 22: 140–144.

46. Challier A, Laveissière C (1973) Un nouveau piège pour la capture des glossines (*Glossina:* Diptera, Muscidae): description et essais sur le terrain. Cah ORSTOM, sér Ent Méd et Parasitol 10: 251–262.

47. Challier A (1965) Amélioration de la méthode de détermination de l'âge physiologique des glossines. Bull Soc Path Ex 58: 250–259.

48. Laveissière C, Grébaut P, Herder S, Penchenier L (2000) Les glossines vectrices de la Trypanosomiase humaine africaine; IRD, editor. Yaoundé: IRD and OCEAC. 246 p.

49. Fried M (1971) Determination of Sterile-Insect Competitiveness. J Econ Entomol 64: 869–872.

50. Pollock JN (1982) Training Manual for Tsetse Control Personnel. Vol. 1: Tsetse biology, systematics and distribution, techniques. Rome: FAO. 243 p.

51. Abila PP, Kiendrebeogo M, Mutika GN, Parker AG, Robinson AS (2003) The effect of age on the mating competitiveness of male *Glossina fuscipes fuscipes* and *G. palpalis palpalis*. J Insect Sci: 3: 13.

52. Schlather M, Ribeiro PJ, Diggle PJ (2004) Detecting dependence between marks and locations of marked point processes. J Roy Stat Soc Ser B (Stat Method) 66: 79–93.

53. Mutika GN, Kabore I, Seck MT, Sall B, Bouyer J, et al. (2012) Mating performance of *Glossina palpalis gambiensis* strains from Burkina Faso, Mali and Senegal. Entomol Exp Appl in press.

54. Clair M, Politzar H, Cuisance D, Lafaye A (1976) Observations sur un essai préliminaire de lâchers de mâles stériles de *Glossina palpalis gambiensis* (Haute-Volta). Rev Elev Méd vét Pays trop 29: 341–351.

55. Cuisance D, Itard J (1973) Comportement de mâles stériles de Glossina tachinoides West. lâchés dans les conditions naturelles – environs de Fort-Lamy (Tchad). II. Longévité et dispersion. Rev Elev Méd vét Pays trop 26: 169–186.

56. Vreysen MJB (2001) Principles of area-wide integrated tsetse fly control using the Sterile Insect Technique. Med Trop 61: 397–411.

57. Vreysen MJB, Van der Vloedt AMV, Barnor H (1996) Comparative gamma radiation sensitivity of *G. tachinoides* Westw., *G. f. fuscipes* Newst., and *G. brevipalpis* Newst. Int J Radiat Biol 69: 67–74.

58. Hendrichs J, Vreysen MJB, Enkerlin WR, Cayol JP (2005) Strategic Options in Using Sterile Insects for Area-Wide Integrated Pest Management. In: Dyck VA, Hendrichs J, Robinson AS, eds. Sterile insect technique. Dordrecht: Springer. pp 563–600.

59. Barclay HJ (1992) Modelling the effects of population aggregation on the efficiency of insect pest control. Res Pop Ecol 34: 131–141.

60. Bouyer J, Balenghien T, Ravel S, Vial L, Sidibé I, et al. (2009) Population sizes and dispersal pattern of tsetse flies: rolling on the river? Mol Ecol 18: 2787–2797.

61. Hargrove JW (2000) A theoretical study of the invasion of cleared areas by tsetse flies (Diptera: Glossinidae). Bull Entomol Res 90: 201–209.

62. Challier A (1982) The ecology of tsetse (*Glossina* spp.)(Diptera, Glossinidae): a review. Insect Sci Applic 3: 97–143.

20

Multiple Loci Are Associated with Dilated Cardiomyopathy in Irish Wolfhounds

Ute Philipp[1]*, **Andrea Vollmar**[2], **Jens Häggström**[3], **Anne Thomas**[4], **Ottmar Distl**[1]

1 Institute for Animal Breeding and Genetics, University of Veterinary Medicine Hannover, Hannover, Germany, 2 Veterinary Clinic for Small Animals, Wissen, Germany, 3 Department of Clinical Sciences, Faculty of Veterinary Medicine and Animal Science, Swedish University of Agricultural Sciences, Uppsala, Sweden, 4 ANTAGENE, Animal Genetics Laboratory, Limonest, France

Abstract

Dilated cardiomyopathy (DCM) is a highly prevalent and often lethal disease in Irish wolfhounds. Complex segregation analysis indicated different loci involved in pathogenesis. Linear fixed and mixed models were used for the genome-wide association study. Using 106 DCM cases and 84 controls we identified one SNP significantly associated with DCM on CFA37 and five SNPs suggestively associated with DCM on CFA1, 10, 15, 21 and 17. On CFA37 *MOGAT1* and *ACSL3* two enzymes of the lipid metabolism were located near the identified SNP.

Editor: Rongling Wu, Pennsylvania State University, United States of America

Funding: This work was funded thanks to grants from Deutsche Forschungsgemeinschaft (PH188_1/1) and European Commission (LUPA-GA.201270. The funders had no role in study design, data collection and analysis, decision to publish, or preparation of the manuscript.

Competing Interests: AT is the Head of Research and Development at Antagene.

* E-mail: ute.philipp@tiho-hannover.de

Introduction

Dilated cardiomyopathy (DCM) is a myocardial disorder which affects dogs as well as humans. The disease is characterized by systolic dysfunction caused by an impaired myocardial contractility and progressive dilation of the left or both ventricles. Affected dogs often develop signs of congestive heart failure (CHF) during the progession of the disease or die from sudden cardiac death. A familial background for DCM has been suggested in several dog breeds and in people [1–3].

In humans, DCM is a genetically heterogenic disease [4,5]. Rare variants of genes encoding predominantly sarcomeric, cytoskeletal or nuclear proteins have been shown to account for monogenic familial forms of DCM [6]. Until now, mutations in more than 30 genes have been associated with DCM [7]. There is, however, also some evidence that common genetic variants might play a role for causing DCM in humans [8].

Several human candidate genes have been ruled out as causative in Doberman Pinschers, Irish wolfhounds and Newfoundland dogs [9–18].

Recently, using mainly a linkage, candidate gene or genome-wide association analyses evidence was found for genomic loci being associated with cardiac diseases in dogs. In Boxer dogs from US, a mutation in the striatin gene was found associated with arrhythmogenic right ventricular cardiomyopathy (ARVC) but could not explain all cases of ARVC [19]. In Portuguese waterdogs, for a genomic region spanning 3.9 Mb on dog chromosome 8 linkage has been demonstrated for a juvenile form of DCM [20].

A mutation in the *ACTN2* gene has been associated with DCM in some, but not all, affected Doberman Pinschers [21]. In addition, it has been shown that a locus on canine chromosome (CFA) 5 was associated with DCM in Doberman Pinschers

explaining about 50 percent of DCM cases in dogs from Germany and the United Kingdom [22].

In Irish wolfhounds, the incidence of DCM reaches approximately 20 percent [23] which leads to the highest cause-specific mortality rate for cardiac disease in the breed compared to all other breeds [24]. The mean age of onset has been estimated at 4.52 ± 2.0 years and female dogs are less frequently affected and develop the disease at an older age than males [23–25]. This suggests a protective effect in female Irish wolfhounds. A major gene model with sex-specific allele effects was the most plausible explanation for the inheritance of DCM in Irish wolfhounds whereas a monogenic mode of inheritance of DCM had been rejected using complex segregation analysis [26]. Echocardiographic reference values have been established for Irish wolfhounds, facilitating the diagnosis of DCM in this breed [27,28]. The objective of this study was to identify loci associated with DCM in Irish wolfhounds. Therefore, we conducted a genome-wide association study (GWAS) to identify susceptibility loci for DCM in Irish wolfhounds.

Results

Mapping Genomic Regions

A genome-wide association study was performed for 106 Irish wolfhound-DCM-cases and 84 Irish wolfhound-DCM-controls using the canine Illumina high density (HD) beadchip (Illumina, San Diego, CA, USA). The 190 Irish wolfhound samples (Table S1) were collected in Central Europe (including samples from Germany, The Netherlands and Belgium), France and Sweden (including samples from Denmark and Norway). Using general linear model analysis (GLM) with sex, inbreeding coefficient and the first three principal components as covariates a significant association with DCM was identified on dog chromosome 37 (Figure 1, Table 1). The corresponding quantile-quantile (Q-Q) plot illustrates the level of potential p-value inflation (Figure S1). The error probability threshold was 9.72×10^{-6} for DCM using Bonferroni correction at a p-value of 0.05 for 5142 independent tests. The assumption of 5142 independent tests was based on pairwise correlation coefficients among alleles for all SNPs used in GWAS and threshold for $r^2 < 0.2$. In order to provide moderate evidence of association a threshold of 1×10^{-4} was used [29,30]. Applying this less stringent threshold resulted in five additional SNPs associated with DCM on CFA1, 10, 15, 17 and 21 (Figure 1, Table 1).

Mixed model analysis (MLM) including sex, inbreeding coefficient and the first three principal components as covariates confirmed the GLM analysis (Figure S2). The SNP highest associated with DCM on CFA37 was identical in both analyses. Due to fact that we included dogs of several countries the possible impact of population stratification on the GWAS result was evaluated for the first three principal components in scatter plots (Figure S3). The results indicated that stratification probably did not impair the association results.

In order to quantify the impact of the single SNPs on occurrence of DCM the odds ratios (OR) were estimated. The ORs for the single SNPs were between 1.31 for BICF2P5199741 on CFA21 and 3.62 for BICF2P801304 on CFA10.

The highest associated SNP BICF2G630134189 on CFA37 is located about 40 kb distal to *MOGAT1* and 80 kb proximal to *ACSL3*. The SNPs on CFA10, 15 and 21 are located in the genes *ARGHAP8*, *FSTL5* and *PDE3B*, respectively (Table 1) while the other two SNPs moderately associated with DCM are located in intergenic regions (Figure S4, S5, S6, S7, S8, S9).

To identify haplotypes associated with DCM linkage disequilibrium and haplotype block analysis was performed. Haplotype blocks containing the SNPs associated with DCM were identified for five chromosomes (Table S2). On CFA21, no significantly associated hapotype block (p-value <0.05) was observed. The size of the associated haplotype blocks varied from 78 kb on CFA15 to 794 kb on CFA17. On CFA17, the genes *SPAG17* and *TBX15* are

within the associated haplotype block. On CFA37, the associated haplotype block of 294 kb contains the genes *MOGAT1* and *ACSL3*.

Discussion

The genome-wide association study in Irish wolfhounds demonstrated the potential involvement of six loci in DCM. We identified one SNP significantly associated with DCM on CFA37 and five SNPs with evidence of association with DCM on CFA1, 10, 15, 17 and 21. The same SNPs were consistently mapped using GLM and MLM analyses. Our results suggest that DCM in Irish wolfhounds is not inherited as a simple Mendelian trait. This finding is in agreement with a previous complex segregation analysis which found an autosomal dominant major gene model with sex-specific allelic effects as the best suited inheritance model for DCM in Irish Wolfhounds [26]. An oligogenic inheritance of DCM might be explained by the fact that dogs from several breeds including Great Danes, Scottish deerhounds, Barsoi and Tibet mastiffs were crossed with few remaining Irish wolfhounds to conserve this breed, which at the time, was close to extinction. This admixture may have lead to many gene variants contributing to development of DCM in Irish wolfhound population. This is in contrast to dog breeds with pure bred founders which are classified as closed populations and might harbour only a limited number of disease causing alleles.

For association study we included Irish wolfhounds originated from several European countries. Nonetheless, dog breeds are composed of related individuals across national boundaries. Therefore, it is important to take population structure and relatedness into account in models avoiding false positive associations. For this purpose we used a compressed linear model approach that has been proven useful in controlling for these effects in GWAS [31]. Concomitantly, this way reduced power for any mutation whose effects confounded with population structure. So, we may have missed contributory loci.

For eliminating potential associations due to population structure or relatedness we fitted the first three principal

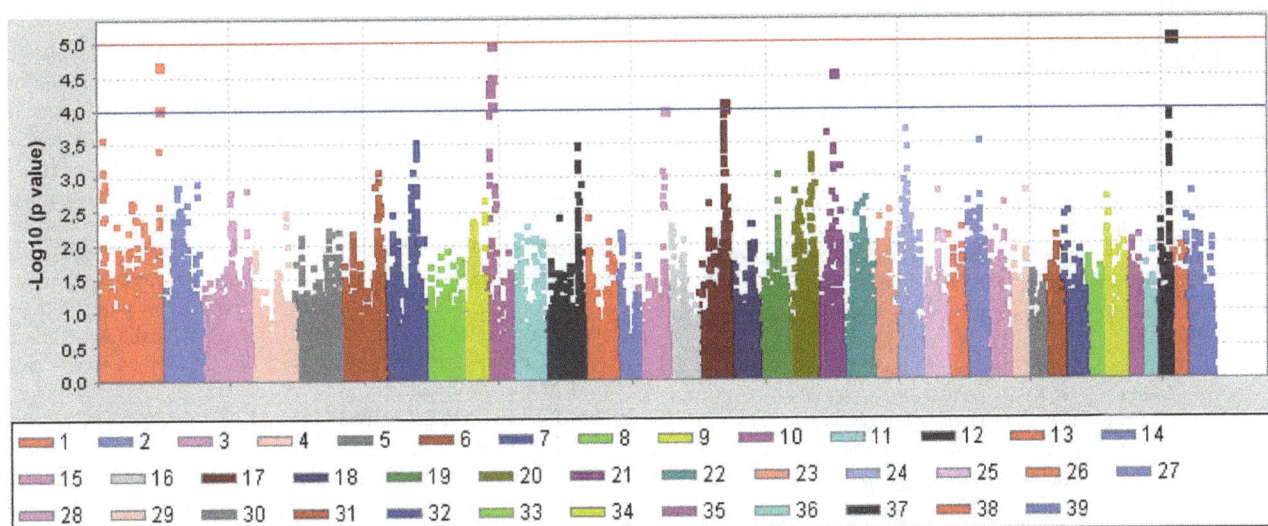

Figure 1. Manhattan plot of the genome-wide association study for dilated cardiomyopathy in Irish wolfhounds from Europe using a general linear model analysis. The genome-wide p-values (–log10 p-values) for the SNP effect are plotted against marker position on each chromosome. X-axis indicates marker number. Chromosomes are differentiated by colours. Colours are given below the plot. Red line indicates threshold value of probability for significant association with DCM. Blue line indicates threshold value of probability for suggestive association with DCM.

Table 1. Summary of results for the genome-wide association study using a mixed model analysis for dilated cardiomyopathy in European Irish wolfhounds.

Locus CFA	Position (bp)	SNP	Gene	Major allele	Minor allele	MAF all	MAF AFF	MAF UNAFF	OR	OR-L	OR-U	-log10P GLM	-log10P MLM
1	123,630,555	BICF2P937484	–	C	T	0.12	0.08	0.18	2.48	1.32	4.67	4.72	3.70
10	24,159,608	BICF2P801304	*ARHGAP8*	A	C	0.06	0.03	0.11	3.62	1.46	9.01	4.51	3.56
15	61,260,406	BICF2S23319191	*FSTL5*	C	A	0.26	0.22	0.32	1.63	1.03	2.59	4.02	3.64
17	58,604,566	BICF2S23232515	–	C	T	0.48	0.52	0.41	1.56	1.03	2.36	4.12	3.59
21	40,670,543	BICF2P5199741	*PDE3B*	G	A	0.29	0.32	0.26	1.31	1.20	2.06	4.57	4.08
37	31,801,266	BICF2G630134189	–	G	A	0.43	0.37	0.51	1.73	1.14	2.61	5.10*	4.14

Identified loci on dog chromosome (CFA), position in base pair (bp), SNP identification and localization, gene name (Gene) for intragenic SNPs, major and minor allele, the minor allele frequency (MAF) in all dogs, affected and unaffected dogs (MAF all, aff, unaff) odds ratios (OR) with lower and upper 95% confidence limits (-L, -U), −log10 p-value of a general linear model (GLM) and mixed model analysis (MMA) is given.

components derived from a pruned SNP set as covariates capturing false positive association due to population structure. Scatter plots for the first three principal components indicated only minor stratification due to sampling from the different European countries. Correction for multiple testing was done using 5142 SNPs which were considered as independent due to their correlation coefficients ($r^2 < 0.2$). Using another less stringent threshold for moderate associations compensated for reduced power applying the compressed approach.

We identified one region significantly associated with DCM and five putative loci. Interestingly, we did not map DCM to regions harbouring known genes causing DCM in human. This fact might be explained that in human monogenic familial DCM cases were investigated. Here, causative mutations are rare in the population but have a strong effect on the phenotype. In Irish wolfhounds, DCM has a high incidence. Therefore, we looked for more common variants with smaller phenotypic effects. Our findings are supported by GWAS on ARCV in Boxers [19] and on DCM in Doberman Pinschers [22]. In the Boxer dog, the *striatin* gene seems to be causative for many ARVC cases in the United States. But the associated mutation explained not all cases and there are also unaffected dogs carrying the disease related mutation. Therefore, other still unknown genes are involved in developing ARCV. For DCM in Doberman Pinschers, one QTL on CFA5 was mapped. However, the best associated SNP identified about 50 percent of DCM cases in this breed. Further genomic regions were not mapped which supports the hypothesis that other loci with smaller effects contribute to the Doberman Pinscher DCM. Incidentally, it is worth to mention that the genomic region observed in Doberman Pinschers is not identical with any region mapped in Irish wolfhounds.

In Irish wolfhounds, the SNPs contributed in different degrees to the occurrence of DCM in Irish wolfhounds which could be shown by their odds ratios. Indeed, these loci were not able to explain all DCM cases in our cohort either due to incomplete linkage disequilibrium with the causative mutations or due to missing loci involved in DCM. There might be rare risk alleles or alleles with small effects which did not lead to significant peaks due to the limited numbers of diagnosed dogs. Due to inbreeding and to a genetic bottleneck by breed foundation, Irish wolfhounds share the longest linkage disequilibrium blocks observed in dog populations [32]. This fact facilitated identification of DCM associated regions but also impedes refinement of detected regions.

SNP BICF2G630134189 on CFA37 (g.31801266G>A) is the only marker which showed significant association with DCM in our study. It is located between *MOGAT1* and *ACSL3* two enzymes of the lipid synthesis. In rats, increased mRNA expression of *ACSL3* was observed in the progression of diabetic cardiomyopathy in the myocardium [33]. It was not shown if the elevated expression of *ACSL3* is cause or the result of the cardiomyopathy.

On CFA10, 15 and 21 the SNPs associated with DCM are located within genes. On CFA10, *ARHGAP8* (BICF2P801304, g.24159608A>C) is an interesting positional candidate gene. It is a member of the RhoA activating protein family which have been shown to regulate many aspects of intracellular actin dynamics. Actins are components of thin filaments of (cardiac) muscle cells and constituents of the cytoskeleton. Based on OR, BICF2P801304 on CFA10 might have the strongest effect on pathogenesis of DCM in Irish wolfhounds. However, the frequency of the minor allele of 0.06 in the Irish wolfhound population indicates only minor involvement in pathogenesis of DCM in Irish wolfhound population.

The positional candidate gene *FSTL5* (BICF2S23319191, g.61260406A>C) on CFA15 is proposed to be a prognostic marker for medullablastoma [34]. The gene is conserved in human, chimpanzee, dog, rat, chicken and zebrafish but a functional pathway has not been identified. On CFA21, *PDE3B* (BICF2P5199741, g.40670543G>A) is a cGMP inhibited phosphodiesterase. There is evidence that *PDE3B* is involved in regulation of lipolysis, lipogenesis, and insulin secretion [35]. For *ARGHAP*, *FSTL5* and *PDE3B* functional pathways need to be elucidated more detailed. Currently, we cannot evaluate if these genes might be involved in pathophysiology of cardiomyocytes or if one of proximate genes may have any impact on developing DCM in Irish wolfhounds.

On CFA1, SNP BICF2P937484 (g.123630555C>T) is associated with DCM suggesting that the nearest gene *TSHZ3* located 270 kb upstream may play a role in DCM in Irish wolfhounds. The gene is a zincfinger transcription factor which has been associated with respiratory rhythm and breathing control [36]. But, the gene may impact regulation in other pathways. On CFA17, four positional candidate genes GDAP2, WDR3, SPAG17 and TBX15 are located near SNP BICF2S23232515 (g.58604566C>T). These genes have not been connected to cardiovascular diseases. However, *HMGCS2*, 1.1 Mb away from SNP BICF2S23232515 encodes a mitochondrial enzyme of the metabolic pathway providing lipid derived energy for brain, heart and kidney in times of carbohydrate deprivation [37].

In total, we identified four positional candidate genes involved in lipid metabolism (*MOGAT1* and *ASCL3* on CFA37, *PDE3B* on CFA21 and *HMGCS2* on CFA 17). Until now, no causative mutation for DCM in genes of lipid metabolism has been reported. However, it is known that cardiac cells use mainly fatty acids as fuel. Between 60 to 90 percent of myocardial energy is supplied by them. There seem to be two pathways for lipid up-take either for VLDL-derived fatty acids or for chylomicron-derived fatty acids [38]. Generally, the uptake of fatty acids occurs either as lipoproteins or as free fatty acid associated with albumin. The key enzyme for breaking down the first ones is lipoprotein lipase (LPL). It was shown that over- or under-expression of *LPL* leads to deficient hearts in mice. Increased lipid up-take led to dilated cardiomyopathy [39]. Therefore, disturbances within pathways connected to or involved in lipid metabolism might play a role in developing DCM in Irish wolfhounds.

In summary, we identified one SNP significantly associated with DCM and five loci suggestively associated with DCM in Irish wolfhounds. The most interesting locus is located on CFA37. The risk allele is a common variant which might impair a big part of Irish wolfhound population.

Materials and Methods

Ethics Statement

All animal work has been conducted according to the national and international guidelines for animal welfare. The dogs in this study were included with consent of their owners. Data were collected during the routine veterinary cardiologic examination for DCM, diagnostic procedures which had to be carried out anyway. All blood-sampling of dogs was done in veterinary clinics for small animals by trained staff.

Animals

In total, 190 samples from Germany, The Netherlands, Belgium, France and Sweden (the Swedish cohort includes dogs from several Scandinavian countries) were used for analysis (Table S1). There were 21 samples from France (19 cases and two controls) and five Scandinavian samples (one case and four controls). Mean age of diagnosis of all cases was 4.9 years. Dogs in the control cohort had to be DCM unaffected and 7 years old at diagnosis (mean age 7.7 years).

Diagnosis of DCM

DCM affected dogs had to be diagnosed by veterinary cardiology specialists. The mean age of diagnosis was 4.9 years for all dogs. The diagnosis of DCM was based on the results of echocardiographic examinations. For diagnosing DCM in Irish wolfhounds echocardiographic criteria were left ventricular internal dimension at end-diameter systolic wider than 41 mm and wider than 61.2 mm at end-diastole, fractional shortening below 25%, and end-systolic volume indices greater than 41 ml/m^2. Right ventricular dilatation was diagnosed when right ventricular internal dimensions, measured during end-diastole, were wider than 36.0 mm. Left or right atrial enlargement was present when the two-dimensional systolic internal diameter of the atrium measured parallel to the AV-valve, was wider than 56 mm [27]. Dogs in the control cohort had to be DCM unaffected and at least 7 years old at diagnosis (mean age 7.7 years).

DNA Extraction

Genomic DNA was extracted from EDTA blood samples through a standard ethanol fractionation with concentrated sodiumchloride (6 M NaCl) and sodium dodecyl sulphate (10% SDS). Alternative, genomic DNA was extracted from buccal samples preserved in ethanol using the NucleoSpin 96 Tissue DNA Kit (NucleoSpin 96 Tissue DNA kit, Macherey Nagel, Hoerdt, France) according to the manufacturer's instructions. Concentration of extracted DNA was determined using the Nanodrop ND-1000 (Peqlab Biotechnology, Erlangen, Germany). DNA concentration of samples for SNP chip analysis was adjusted to 70–120 ng/µl.

Statistical Analysis

For genome-wide association analyses, DNA samples were genotyped on the canine high density bead chip (Illumina, San Diego, CA, USA) containing a total of 172,942 SNPs. Quality criteria were minor allele frequencies (MAF) >0.05, genotyping rate per SNP>0.90 and HWE test (p<0.00001). After filtering for quality criteria, 83,621 SNPs remained for analysis. The mean genotyping rate per individual was 0.995.

We performed a mixed model analysis (MMA) and a general linear model (GLM) analysis procedure using TASSEL version 3.088 [40]. The advantage of MMA or GLM over a simplistic approach without considering any other effects in modeling association can be seen in removing disturbing effects caused by data structure, different levels of relationships among animals and inbreeding. The model included the respective SNP genotypes, sex and inbreeding coefficients and the first three principal components as fixed effects and the genomic relationship matrix for the random genetic effect of the animal. For multiple testing we used a SNP set consisting of 5142 markers due to LD between SNPs, respectively. For representing linkage disequilibrium blocks we considered a window of 20 SNPs and shifted the window 5 SNPs forward in each step. One of a pair of SNPs was removed if the LD is greater than 0.2. The threshold of multiple tests was 9.72×10^{-6} at 0.05 of single test threshold. To obtain moderate evidence of association we used a less stringent threshold of 1×10^{-4}.

For visualization and plotting of whole genome association, haplotype block analysis and haplotype association tests and results Haploview analysis was employed [41].

For allele frequencies of the SNPs, allele odds ratios, their corresponding CHI square and probability values the proc allele procedure of SAS, version 9.3 was carried out.

Supporting Information

Figure S1 Q-Q plot of general linear model using inbreeding coefficients, sex and the first three principal components as fixed effects. The plot compares expected versus observed –log10 p-value for all 83,621 included in GWAS with the grey line corresponding to the null hypothesis of no association.

Figure S2 Manhattan plot of genome-wide association study for dilated cardiomyopathy in Irish wolfhounds from Europe using a mixed model analysis. X-axis indicates marker number. The genome-wide p-values (–log10 p-values) for the SNP effect are plotted against marker position on each chromosome. Chromosomes are differentiated by colours. Colours are given below the plot. Blue line indicates threshold value of probability for moderate association with DCM.

Figure S3 Scatter plots of the first three principal components. A: Principal component PC1 versus PC2 **B**: Principal component PC1 versus PC3 Turquoise triangels: Samples from Continental Europe (Germany, The Netherlands and Belgium) Blue diamonds: Scandinavian samples (Denmark, Norway and Sweden) Pink squares: samples from France

Figure S4 Genome-wide association study in 190 European Irish Wolfhounds showed significant association for dilated cardiomyopathy on CFA1. (A) SNPs and their corresponding −log10 p-values in a 1 Mb interval on dog chromosome 1 are shown (**B**). Gene annotation of the highest associated chromosomal region is shown (**C**). Gene annotation is based on dog genome assembly build 2.1. Some genes are still annotated as loc and numbers.

Figure S5 Genome-wide association study in 190 European Irish Wolfhounds showed significant association for dilated cardiomyopathy on CFA10. (A) SNPs and their corresponding −log10 p-values in a 0.5 Mb interval on dog chromosome 10 are shown (**B**). Gene annotation of the highest associated chromosomal region is shown (**C**). Gene annotation is based on dog genome assembly build 2.1. Some genes are still annotated as loc and numbers.

Figure S6 Genome-wide association study in 190 Irish Wolfhounds from Europe showed significant association for dilated cardiomyopathy on CFA15. (A) SNPs and their corresponding −log10 p-values in a 1 Mb interval on dog chromosome 15 are shown (**B**). Gene annotation of the highest associated chromosomal region is shown (**C**). Gene annotation is based on dog genome assembly build 2.1. Some genes are still annotated as loc and numbers.

Figure S7 Genome-wide association study in 190 Irish Wolfhounds from Europe showed significant association for dilated cardiomyopathy on CFA17. (A) Several SNPs in a 2 Mb interval on dog chromosome 17 were suggestively associated (**B**). Gene annotation of the highest associated chromosomal region is shown (**C**). Gene annotation is based on dog genome assembly build 2.1. Some genes are still annotated as loc and numbers.

Figure S8 Genome-wide association study in 190 European Irish Wolfhounds showed significant association for dilated cardiomyopathy on CFA21. (A) SNPs and their corresponding −log10 p-values in a 2 Mb interval on dog chromosome 21 are shown (**B**). Gene annotation of the highest associated chromosomal region is shown (**C**). Gene annotation is based on dog genome assembly build 2.1. Some genes are still annotated as loc and numbers.

Figure S9 Genome-wide association study in 190 Irish Wolfhounds from Europe showed significant association for dilated cardiomyopathy on CFA37. (A) SNPs and their corresponding −log10 p-values in a 3 Mb interval on dog chromosome 37 are shown (**B**). Gene annotation of the highest associated chromosomal region is shown (**C**). Gene annotation is based on dog genome assembly build 2.1. Some genes are still annotated as loc and numbers.

Table S1 Irish wolfhounds used for the genome-wide association study. Distribution by diagnosis of dilative cardiomyopathy (DCM), sex, country of sampling and age at diagnosis or at last examination in years (AGE) is given.

Table S2 Haplotype blocks associated to DCM in Irish wolfhounds. Dog chromosome (CFA), haplotype block (bold letters are highest associated SNPs in GLM), bold, size of haplotype block in kb, frequency of haplotype block in all 190 Irish wolfhounds from Europe, frequency of haplotype block in affected and control dogs, CHI square value and corresponding p-value is given.

Acknowledgments

We thank all breeders and dog owners for donating EDTA-blood samples of their dogs and the RALIE club in France.

Author Contributions

Conceived and designed the experiments: UP AV OD. Performed the experiments: UP AT AV. Analyzed the data: UP JH AT AV OD. Contributed reagents/materials/analysis tools: UP JH AT AV OD. Wrote the paper: UP OD.

References

1. Mestroni L, Rocco C, Gregori D, Sinagra G, Di Lenarda, et al. (1999) Familial dilated cardiomyopathy: evidence for genetic and phenotypic heterogeneity. Heart Muscle Disease Study Group. J Am Coll Cardiol 34: 181–190.
2. Meurs KM (1998) Insights into the hereditability of canine cardiomyopathy. Vet Clin North Am Small Anim Pract 28: 1449–1457.
3. Meurs KM, Miller MW, Wright NA (2001) Clinical features of dilated cardiomyopathy in Great Danes and results of a pedigree analysis: 17 cases (1999–2000). J Am Vet Med Assoc 218: 729–732.
4. Amara ME, Villard E, Komajda M (2005). Review: genetics of familial dilated cardiomyopathy. Ann Cardiol Angeiol 54: 151–156.
5. Hershberger RE, Cowan J, Morales A, Siegfried JD (2009) Progress with genetic cardiomyopathies: screening, counseling, and testing in dilated, hypertrophic, and arrhythmogenic right ventricular dysplasia/cardiomyopathy. Circ Heart Fail 2: 253–261.
6. Morimoto S (2008) Sarcomeric proteins and inherited cardiomyopathies. Cardiovasc Res 1: 659–666.
7. Stark K, Esslinger UB, Reinhard W, Petrov G, Winkler T, et al. (2011) Genetic association study identifies HSPB7 as a risk gene for idiopathic dilated cardiomyopathy. PLoS Genet 6 (10) e1001167.
8. Rampersaud E, Kinnamon DD, Hamilton K, Khuri S, Hershberger RE, et al. (2010) Common susceptibility variants examined for association with dilated cardiomyopathy. Ann Hum Genet 74: 110–116.
9. Stabej P, Leegwater PA, Imholz S, Versteeg SA, Zijlstra C, et al. (2005) The canine sarcoglycan delta gene: BAC clone contig assembly, chromosome assignment and interrogation as a candidate gene for dilated cardiomyopathy in Dobermann dogs. Cytogenet Genome Res 111: 140–146.
10. Stabej P, Leegwater PA, Stokhof AA, Domanjko-Petric A, van Oost BA (2005) Evaluation of the phospholamban gene in purebred large-breed dogs with dilated cardiomyopathy. Am J Vet Res 66: 432–436.
11. Stabej P, Imholz S, Versteeg SA, Zijlstra C, Stokhof AA, et al. (2004) Characterization of the canine desmin (DES) gene and evaluation as a candidate gene for dilated cardiomyopathy in the Dobermann. Gene 340: 241–249.
12. Schatzberg S, Olby N, Steingold S, Keene B, Atkins C, et al. (1999) A polymerase chain reaction screening strategy for the promoter of the canine dystrophin gene Am J Vet Res 60: 1040–1046.
13. Meurs KM, Magnon AL, Spier AW, Miller MW, Lehmkuhl LB, et al. (2001) Evaluation of the cardiac actin gene in Doberman Pinschers with dilated cardiomyopathy Am J Vet Res 62: 33–36.
14. Meurs KM, Hendrix KP, Norgard MM (2008) Molecular evaluation of five cardiac genes in Doberman Pinschers with dilated cardiomyopathy. Am J Vet Res 69: 1050–1053.
15. Philipp U, Broschk C, Vollmar A, Distl O (2007) Evaluation of tafazzin as candidate for dilated cardiomyopathy in Irish wolfhounds. J Hered 98: 506–509.

16. Philipp U, Vollmar A, Distl O (2008) Evaluation of six candidate genes for dilated cardiomyopathy (DCM) in Irish wolfhounds. Animal Genet 39: 88–89.

17. Philipp U, Vollmar A, Distl O (2008) Evaluation of *TCAP* as candidate gene for dilated cardiomyopathy in Irish wolfhounds. Animal Biotech 19: 231–236.

18. Wiersma AC, Stabej P, Leegwater PA, Van Oost BA, Ollier WE, et al. (2008) Evaluation of 15 Candidate Genes for Dilated Cardiomyopathy in the Newfoundland Dog. J Hered 99: 73–80.

19. Meurs KM, Mauceli E, Lahmers S, Acland GM, White SN, et al. (2010) Genome-wide association identifies a deletion in the 3' untranslated region of striatin in a canine model of arrhythmogenic right ventricular cardiomyopathy. Hum Genet 128: 315–324.

20. Werner P, Raducha MG, Prociuk U, Sleeper MM, Van Winkle TJ, et al. (2008) A novel locus for dilated cardiomyopathy maps to canine chromosome 8. Genomics 91: 517–521.

21. O'Sullivan ML, O'Grady MR, Pyle WG, Dawson JF (2011) Evaluation of 10 genes encoding cardiac proteins in Doberman Pinschers with dilated cardiomyopathy. Am J Vet Res 72: 932–939.

22. Mausberg TB, Wess G, Simak J, Keller L, Drögemüller M, et al. (2011) A locus on chromosome 5 is associated with dilated cardiomyopathy in Doberman Pinschers. PLoS One 6: e20042.

23. Vollmar A (2000) The prevalence of cardiomyopathy in the Irish wolfhound: a clinical study of 500 dogs. J Am Anim Hosp Assoc 36: 125–32.

24. Egenvall A, Bonnett BN, Häggström J (2006) Heart disease as a cause of death in insured Swedish dogs <10 years of age – data from 1995 to 2002. J Vet Intern Med 20: 894–903.

25. Brownlie SE, Cobb MA (1999) Observations on the development of congestive heart failure in Irish wolfhounds with dilated cardiomyopathy. J Small Anim Pract 40: 371–377.

26. Distl O, Vollmar AC, Broschk C, Hamann H, Fox PR (2007) Complex segregation analysis of dilated cardiomyopathy (DCM) in Irish wolfhounds. Heredity 99: 460–465.

27. Vollmar A (1999) Echocardiographic measurements in the Irish wolfhound, reference values for the breed. J Am Anim Hosp Assoc 35: 271–277.

28. Vollmar A (1999) Use of echocardiography in the diagnosis of dilated cardiomyopathy in Irish wolfhounds. J Am Anim Hosp Assoc 35: 279–283.

29. Teyssèdre S, Dupuis MC, Guérin G, Schibler L, Denoix JM, et al. (2012) Genome-wide association studies for osteochondrosis in French Trotter horses. J Anim Sci 90: 45–53.

30. Wellcome Trust Case Control Consortium (2007) Genome-wide association study of 14,000 cases of seven common diseases and 3,000 shared controls. Nature 447: 661–678.

31. Zhang Z, Ersoz E, Lai CQ, Todhunter RJ, Tiwari HK, et al. (2010) Mixed linear model approach adapted for genome-wide association studies. Nat Genet 42: 355–360.

32. Karlsson EK, Baranowska I, Wade CM, Salmon Hillbertz NH, Zody MC, et al. (2007) Efficient mapping of mendelian traits in dogs through genome-wide association. Nat Genet 39: 1321–1328.

33. Cheng Y, Liu G, Pan Q, Guo S, Yang X (2011) Elevated expression of liver X receptor alpha (LXRα) in myocardium of streptozotocin-induced diabetic rats. Inflammation 34: 698–706.

34. Remke M, Hielscher T, Korshunov A, Northcott PA, Bender S, et al. (2011) FSTL5 is a marker of poor prognosis in non-WNT/non-SHH medulloblastoma J Clin Oncol 29: 3852–3861.

35. Choi YH, Park S, Hockman S, Zmuda-Trzebiatowska E, Svennelid F, et al. (2006) Alterations in regulation of energy homeostasis in cyclic nucleotide phosphodiesterase 3B-null mice. J Clin Invest 116: 3240–3251.

36. Caubit X, Thoby-Brisson M, Voituron N, Filippi P, Bévengut M, et al. (2010) "Teashirt 3 regulates development of neurons involved in both respiratory rhythm and airflow control". J Neurosci 30: 9465–9476.

37. Robinson AM, Williamson DH (1980) Physiological roles of ketone bodies as substrates and signals in mammalian tissues. Physiol Rev 60: 143–87.

38. Bharadwaj KG, Hiyama Y, Hu Y, Huggins LA, Ramakrishnan R, et al. (2010) Chylomicron- and VLDL-derived lipids enter the heart through different pathways: in vivo evidence for receptor- and non-receptor-mediated fatty acid uptake. J Biol Chem 3: 37976–37986.

39. Noh HL, Yamashita H, Goldberg IJ (2006) Cardiac metabolism and mechanics are altered by genetic loss of lipoprotein triglyceride lipolysis.Cardiovasc Drugs Ther 20: 441–444.

40. Bradbury PJ, Zhang Z, Kroon DE, Casstevens TM, Ramdoss Y, et al. (2007) TASSEL: software for association mapping of complex traits in diverse samples. Bioinformatics 19: 2633–2635.

41. Barrett JC, Fry B, Maller J, Daly MJ (2005) Haploview: analysis and visualization of LD and haplotype maps. Bioinformatics: 21: 263–265.

21

Household Risk Factors for Colonization with Multidrug-Resistant *Staphylococcus aureus* Isolates

Meghan F. Davis[1]*, **Amy E. Peterson**[2], **Kathleen G. Julian**[3], **Wallace H. Greene**[3], **Lance B. Price**[4], **Kenrad Nelson**[2], **Cynthia J. Whitener**[3], **Ellen K. Silbergeld**[1]

1 Department of Environmental Health Sciences, Johns Hopkins Bloomberg School of Public Health, Baltimore, Maryland, United States of America, 2 Department of Epidemiology, Johns Hopkins Bloomberg School of Public Health, Baltimore, Maryland, United States of America, 3 Penn State Hershey Medical Center, Hershey, Pennsylvania, United States of America, 4 Division of Pathogen Genomics, The Translational Genomics Research Institute (TGen North), Phoenix, Arizona, United States of America

Abstract

Antimicrobial resistance, particularly in pathogens such as methicillin-resistant *Staphylococcus aureus* (MRSA), limits treatment options and increases healthcare costs. To understand patient risk factors, including household and animal contact, potentially associated with colonization with multidrug-resistant MRSA isolates, we performed a prospective study of case patients colonized with MRSA on admission to a rural tertiary care hospital. Patients were interviewed and antimicrobial resistance patterns were tested among isolates from admitted patients colonized with MRSA in 2009–10. Prevalence of resistance was compared by case-patient risk factors and length-of-stay outcome among 88 MRSA case patients. Results were compared to NHANES 2003–04. Overall prevalence of multidrug resistance (non-susceptibility to ≥four antimicrobial classes) in MRSA nasal isolates was high (73%) and was associated with a 1.5-day increase in subsequent length of stay ($p = 0.008$). History of hospitalization within the past six months, but not antimicrobial use in the same time period, was associated with resistance patterns. Within a subset of working-age case patients without recent history of hospitalization, animal contact was potentially associated with multidrug resistance. History of hospitalization, older age, and small household size were associated with multidrug resistance in NHANES data. In conclusion, recent hospitalization of case patients was predictive of antimicrobial resistance in MRSA isolates, but novel risk factors associated with the household may be emerging in CA-MRSA case patients. Understanding drivers of antimicrobial resistance in MRSA isolates is important to hospital infection control efforts, relevant to patient outcomes and to indicators of the economic burden of antimicrobial resistance.

Editor: Herminia de Lencastre, Rockefeller University, United States of America

Funding: Research was supported by grants from the Johns Hopkins Center for a Livable Future (http://www.jhsph.edu/clf/) and the Heinz Foundation (http://www.heinzfamily.org/aboutus/philanthropies_02.html). AEP and MFD were supported by Johns Hopkins Center for a Livable Future Predoctoral Fellowships. Additionally, MFD was supported by a Sommer Scholarship. The funders had no role in the study design, data collection and analysis, decision to publish, or preparation of the manuscript.

Competing Interests: The authors have declared that no competing interests exist.

* E-mail: mdavis@jhsph.edu

Introduction

Methicillin-resistant *Staphylococcus aureus* (MRSA) is a pandemic antimicrobial-resistant pathogen [1]. In 2004, an estimated 1.5% of the United States population, or approximately 4 million people, were nasally colonized with MRSA [2]. Nasal colonization increases risk for development of clinical infection [3]. Antimicrobial-resistant pathogens, which include MRSA, have human costs in morbidity and mortality, and they have been estimated to have healthcare costs in excess of $4 billion annually in the U.S. [4]. As a result, understanding the epidemiology of multidrug-resistant MRSA case-patients is both clinically and economically relevant to healthcare surveillance and control efforts.

MRSA epidemiology in the United States is shifting rapidly, as strains historically considered community-associated enter hospitals, and hospital strains disseminate into the community [5–8]. However, some authors have suggested that isolate antimicrobial susceptibility may continue to distinguish community-acquired (CA-)MRSA isolates from those acquired in the hospital, and that

isolate resistance to certain antimicrobials (ciprofloxacin, clindamycin, and aminoglycosides) may typify hospital-acquired (HA-)MRSA isolates [9–12]. In addition, new risk factors for acquisition of MRSA may be emerging. Human households [13–15] and animals [16,17] recently have been described as potential community reservoirs for MRSA.

To describe case-patient epidemiology and evaluate novel household and animal risk factors as potential drivers of antimicrobial resistance, we interviewed MRSA positive case patients identified from nasal colonization surveillance at a tertiary care center serving largely rural and suburban communities. MRSA isolates were tested for antimicrobial susceptibility. We also evaluated associations between isolate drug resistance and subsequent length-of-stay (LOS) among case-patients, using LOS as an economic and human cost marker for potential associations between drug resistance and factors related to hospitalization. Risk factor results were compared to data from MRSA-colonized participants in the National Health and Nutrition Examination Survey (NHANES) 2003–04.

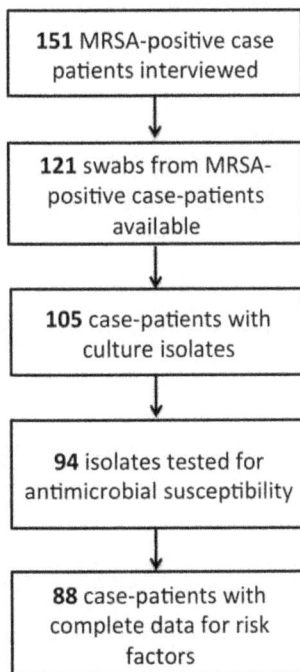

Figure 1. Study design for analysis of risk factors from case-patients interviewed at Penn State Hershey Medical Center.

Methods

Research Design

We enrolled patients over the age of 18 years at Penn State Hershey Medical Center (PSHMC) between August 2009 and March 2010 as previously described [18]. As part of a larger case-control study, MRSA case patients identified on admission via screening nasal swabs were interviewed as a prospective case cohort to characterize MRSA isolates by multi-locus sequence typing (MLST) and antimicrobial susceptibility patterns from a hospital source population that included predominantly rural and suburban communities [18]. This manuscript is limited to analysis of the case-patients from whom a MRSA isolate was available for antimicrobial susceptibility testing and who had complete data for all risk factors.

Survey

Patients were interviewed for self-reported risk factors that included demographic information; hospitalization within the past month, six months, or year prior to admission for themselves and for family members; antimicrobial drug use within the past month, six months or year prior to admission for themselves and for family members; animal contact, including livestock (cows, pigs, and poultry); household pet ownership (dogs and cats only); and number of people living in the household. Subsequent length of stay was determined through record review.

Sample Collection

Swabs of the anterior nares of patients were collected within 48 hours of admission and these swabs were processed at the PSHMC virology laboratory using the BD GeneOhm™ MRSA Assay (Becton Dickinson Diagnostics, San Diego, CA). MRSA-positive swabs by this PCR method were archived and subsequently cultured for viable MRSA isolates using commercial MRSA

Select™ agar plates (Bio-Rad Laboratories, Hercules, CA). Isolates were confirmed as MRSA using a real-time PCR assay by detection of *mecA* and *femA* genes (Pathogene, LLC). Due to potential presence of variant *mecA* genes, MSSA isolates found to be beta-lactam resistant were tested for presence of *mecC* using a newly designed universal primer as previously described [19,20].

Antimicrobial Susceptibility Testing

MRSA and MSSA isolates were tested for antimicrobial susceptibility using disc diffusion methods [21,22], including erythromycin-induced resistance to clindamycin (D-test), following CLSI guidelines [23] to nine antimicrobials: chloramphenicol, quinupristin/dalfopristin (Synercid), tetracycline, gentamicin, amikacin, trimethoprim/sulfamethoxazole, clindamycin, ciprofloxacin, and erythromycin. Multi-drug resistance (MDR4) was defined as beta-lactam resistance by *mecA* gene presence plus nonsusceptibility (inducible, intermediate or high-level resistance) to three additional classes of antimicrobial drugs by disc diffusion methods, based on a definition reported by SENTRY [24]. An additional category of high multidrug resistance (MDR5) was included to evaluate whether risk factors differed for isolates more difficult to treat, and this was defined as beta-lactam resistance (*mecA* gene presence, all isolates by definition) plus high-level (complete) resistance to four additional classes of antimicrobial drugs (*i.e.*, resistance to ≥ five antimicrobials). For MDR5 and for individual antimicrobial drug evaluation, risk factors were compared to high-level (complete) resistance only, including intermediate with susceptible isolates in models, because high-level resistance may be associated with a higher probability of acquired resistance [25], as opposed to resistance based on other mechanisms, *e.g.* via multiple mutations in cell wall biosynthesis. For clindamycin, inducible resistance was included with high-level resistance phenotypes [26].

All isolates were screened for vancomycin resistance by real-time PCR assay for the *vanA* gene (Pathogene, LLC) and disc diffusion testing. Because of previous findings of hVISA isolates in this patient population [27], 33 of the isolates were selected for further vancomycin susceptibility testing on the basis of their susceptibility profiles (*e.g.* quinupristin/dalfopristin non-susceptibility or MDR4). These isolates were screened using a standard VA E-test and also a GRD E-test (vancomycin and teicoplanin) for potential hGISA phenotype as previously described [27]. Isolates with positive GRD E-tests [28] were tested using a population analysis as previously described [27]. Briefly, 10^7 and 10^6 inoculations were placed on agar plates containing 1, 2, 4, 7, and 8 ug/ml vancomycin. Growth at the level of 4 ug/ml with a 10^6 inoculation was considered indicative of hGISA positivity. Results were validated against quality control strains ATCC 29213, ATCC Mu3 (hGISA) and ATCC Mu50 (GISA).

Statistical Analysis

We estimated unadjusted and adjusted associations for antimicrobial resistance by risk factor using prevalence ratios (PRs). We calculated PRs using Poisson models with robust estimation of standard errors as described previously [29,30] using Stata 11 (College Station, TX). P-values ≤0.05 were considered statistically significant, and p-values ≤0.10 were considered to approach statistical significance.

A priori, covariates included self-reported age, gender, race, history of hospitalization, prior use of antimicrobials, exposure to animals, and household size. Categorical dummy variables for hospitalization or antimicrobial use within one month compared to within six months were created, assigning 0 if patients self-reported no hospital contact or antimicrobial use within six

---

Table 1. Prevalences of antimicrobial resistance by risk factor among 88 MRSA isolates from Penn State Hershey Medical Center admitted patients, August 2009 to February 2010.

	Multidrug Resistance (MDR4)	High Multidrug Resistance (MDR5)	Ciprofloxacin Resistant (CIPR)	Clindamycin Resistant (CLIR)	Amikacin Resistant (AMKR)
	4+ classes of non-susceptibility	*5+ classes of high-level resistance*	*high-level resistance*	*high-level resistance*	*high-level resistance*
Overall, N (%)	64 (73%)	20 (23%)	72 (82%)	51 (58%)	21 (24%)
Gender					
Female, *n* = 35	25 (71%)	11 (31%)	29 (83%)	20 (57%)	10 (29%)
Male (*ref*), *n* = 53	39 (74%)	9 (17'%)	43 (81%)	31 (58%)	11 (21%)
Age					
65 years or older, *n* = 38	30 (80%)	10 (26%)	35 (92%)	26 (68%)	7 (19%)
Under 65 (*ref*), *n* = 50	34 (68%)	10 (20%)	37 (74%)	25 (50%)	14 (28%)
Hospitalization					
Within 1 month, *n* = 24	20 (83%)	9 (38%)	22 (92%)	17 (71%)	8 (33%)
1–6 mo, *n* = 18	17 (94%)	5 (28%)	17 (94%)	13 (72%)	2 (11%)
Over 6 mo (*ref*), *n* = 46	27 (59%)	6 (13%)	33 (72%)	21 (46%)	11 (24%)
Antimicrobial use					
Within 1 month, *n* = 36	31 (86%)	11 (31%)	33 (92%)	24 (67%)	10 (28%)
1–6 mo, *n* = 24	18 (75%)	4 (17%)	20 (83%)	13 (54%)	6 (25%)
Over 6 mo (*ref*), *n* = 28	15 (54%)	5 (18%)	19 (68%)	14 (50%)	5 (18%)
Livestock Exposure					
Direct contact, *n* = 12[‡]	7 (58%)	1 (8%)	8 (67%)	7 (58%)	3 (25%)
No direct contact (*ref*), *n* = 76	57 (75%)	19 (25%)	64 (84%)	44 (58%)	18 (24%)
Household pets					
Have pets, *n* = 49[‡‡]	39 (80%)	12 (24%)	40 (82%)	30 (61%)	12 (24%)
Don't have pets (*ref*), *n* = 39	25 (64%)	8 (21%)	32 (82%)	21 (54%)	9 (23%)
Household Size*					
Over 2, *n* = 32	24 (75%)	8 (25%)	23 (72%)	18 (56%)	9 (28%)
2 or fewer (*ref*), *n* = 56	40 (71%)	12 (21%)	49 (88%)	33 (59%)	12 (21%)

N (%) shown are for the resistant population compared to the susceptible population. Intermediates are included with resistant isolates for the SENTRY MDR definition, but are included with the susceptible population for the remainder of the categories. Race was not included due to small numbers of non-white participants (N = 6).
[‡]Six case patients reported living on a farm; six reported farm occupation; two reported chicken contact, six reported cow contact; and one reported pig contact (categories non-exclusive).
[‡‡]34 dogs and 22 cats.
*Household size includes index patient.

months, assigning 1 if patients self-reported hospitalization or antimicrobial use within six months prior to admission, and 2 if patients self-reported hospitalization or antimicrobial use within a month of admission. The six-month cut-off and definitions for HA- versus CA-MRSA assignment were selected based on prior work in this study population [18]. Self-reported contact with dogs and cats was colinear with self-reported household pet ownership; hence these variables were aggregated. Due to small numbers, livestock contact was aggregated from individual reporting of pig, poultry, or cow contact. Age, household size, and animal exposure variables were dichotomized. Because of the small numbers with non-white race (*n* = 6), this risk factor was not examined further.

Linear regression models were run with log-transformed length of stay (LOS) as an outcome, evaluating potential association with antimicrobial resistance patterns. Beta coefficients from log-transformed models were exponentiated to return a point estimate, in days, for average LOS increase in patients colonized with MDR isolates.

The Penn State Hershey Medical Center and Johns Hopkins Bloomberg School of Public Health Institutional Review Boards reviewed and approved this study. Patients provided written informed consent to participate in the study.

NHANES Analysis

To provide a descriptive comparison between this geographically-limited study of hospital inpatients and data from a wider U.S. population, statistical analysis was run on a subset of all MRSA-colonized participants in NHANES 2003–04, which represented the most recent national data available to the public on MRSA colonization [31]. Risk factor data available in NHANES 2003–04 included gender, age, self-reported history hospitalization within the past year, and household size [31]. Antimicrobial use data was available only for the prior one month; this variable was not included in analysis due to the inconsistent time frame with the hospitalization variable. Data on animal contact or pet ownership was not available. Methods for

Table 2. Unadjusted and adjusted prevalence ratios for antimicrobial resistance by risk factor among 88 MRSA isolates from Penn State Hershey Medical Center admitted patients, August 2009 to February 2010.

	Multidrug Resistance (MDR4) 4+ classes of non-susceptibility			High Multidrug Resistance (MDR5) 5+ classes of high-level resistance			Ciprofloxacin Resistant (CIPR) high-level resistance			Clindamycin Resistant (CLIR) high-level resistance			Amikacin Resistant (AMKR) high-level resistance		
	PR	95% CI	p-value	PR	95% CI	p-value	PR	95% CI	p-value	PR	95% CI	p-value	PR	95% CI	p-value
Gender (male is ref)															
Unadjusted	0.97	0.74-1.27	0.83	1.85	0.85-4.02	0.12	1.02	0.84-1.25	0.84	0.98	0.68-1.41	0.90	1.38	0.65-2.90	0.40
Adjusted	0.96	0.73-1.26	0.78	1.70	0.79-3.64	0.18	1.00	0.82-1.21	0.97	0.91	0.63-1.31	0.61	1.58	0.74-3.38	0.24
Age (under 65 is ref)															
Unadjusted	1.16	0.90-1.49	0.25	1.32	0.61-2.85	0.49	**1.24**	**1.03-1.50**	**0.02**	*1.37*	*0.96-1.95*	*0.08*	0.66	0.29-1.48	0.31
Adjusted	1.23	0.93-1.61	0.15	1.12	0.51-2.47	0.78	**1.24**	**1.02-1.51**	**0.03**	*1.42*	*0.98-2.06*	*0.07*	0.58	0.26-1.27	0.17
Hospitalization (>6 mo is ref)															
Within 1 month, unadjusted	**1.42**	**1.05-1.92**	**0.02**	**2.88**	**1.15-7.16**	**0.02**	**1.28**	**1.03-1.59**	**0.03**	**1.55**	**1.03-2.34**	**0.04**	1.39	0.65-3.01	0.40
Within 1 month, adjusted	*1.14*	*0.79-1.65*	*0.49*	**3.15**	**1.16-8.57**	**0.03**	1.12	0.88-1.44	0.36	1.42	0.82-2.45	0.22	1.28	0.45-3.62	0.64
1-6 months, unadjusted	**1.61**	**1.23-2.10**	**0.001**	2.13	0.74-6.15	0.16	**1.32**	**1.06-1.63**	**0.01**	**1.58**	**1.03-2.43**	**0.04**	0.46	0.11-1.91	0.29
1-6 months, adjusted	**1.46**	**1.09-1.96**	**0.01**	*2.38*	*0.85-6.67*	*0.10*	**1.28**	**1.02-1.62**	**0.04**	**1.72**	**1.06-2.79**	**0.03**	*0.31*	*0.08-1.19*	*0.09*
Antimicrobial use (>6 mo is ref)															
Within 1 month, unadjusted	**1.61**	**1.11-2.33**	**0.01**	1.71	0.67-4.38	0.26	**1.35**	**1.03-1.78**	**0.03**	1.33	0.86-2.07	0.20	1.56	0.60-4.06	0.37
Within 1 month, adjusted	*1.42*	*0.93-2.15*	*0.10*	0.84	0.29-2.46	0.75	*1.31*	*0.98-1.75*	*0.06*	1.10	0.61-1.97	0.75	1.51	0.46-4.99	0.50
1-6 months, unadjusted	1.40	0.92-2.13	0.11	0.93	0.28-3.11	0.91	1.23	0.90-1.68	0.20	1.08	0.64-1.83	0.77	1.40	0.48-4.04	0.53
1-6 months, adjusted	1.16	0.74-1.82	0.51	0.57	0.18-1.84	0.35	1.15	0.83-1.59	0.42	0.81	0.45-1.45	0.47	1.74	0.57-5.34	0.33
Livestock Exposure (no contact is ref)															
Bivarite	0.78	0.47-1.28	0.32	0.33	0.04-2.29	0.26	0.79	0.52-1.20	0.27	1.01	0.60-1.69	0.98	1.06	0.36-3.07	0.92
Adjusted	0.79	0.53-1.17	0.24	0.31	0.04-2.39	0.26	0.81	0.57-1.15	0.24	1.03	0.63-1.67	0.92	0.93	0.31-2.79	0.89
Household pets (no pets is ref)															
Unadjusted	1.24	0.94-1.64	0.12	1.19	0.54-2.64	0.66	0.99	0.82-1.21	0.96	1.14	0.79-1.64	0.49	1.06	0.50-2.27	0.88
Adjusted	1.23	0.93-1.61	0.14	1.12	0.49-2.55	0.79	1.03	0.84-1.24	0.80	1.07	0.73-1.57	0.71	0.83	0.37-1.88	0.66
Household Size* (2 or fewer is ref)															
Unadjusted	1.05	0.81-1.36	0.71	1.17	0.53-2.56	0.70	0.82	0.65-1.04	0.11	0.95	0.65-1.39	0.81	1.31	0.62-2.78	0.48
Adjusted	0.93	0.73-1.20	0.59	1.05	0.49-2.27	0.90	**0.79**	**0.63-0.99**	**0.04**	0.94	0.64-1.38	0.51	1.42	0.68-2.96	0.35

Intermediates are included with resistant isolates for the SENTRY MDR definition, but are included with the susceptible population for the remainder of the categories. Unadjusted and adjusted results are limited to the 88 individuals for whom complete data on all potential covariates is available. Adjusted models control for gender, age, history of hospitalization, history of antimicrobial use, livestock exposure, household pets, and household size. Prevalence ratios (PRs) shown are estimated from poisson regression models (categorical models used for hospitalization and antibiotic use). Significant associations (two-sided $p<0.05$) are shown in bold. Associations that are non-significant but approach significance (two-sided $p<0.10$) are italicized. Race was not included due to small numbers of non-white participants ($n=6$).
*Household size includes index patient.

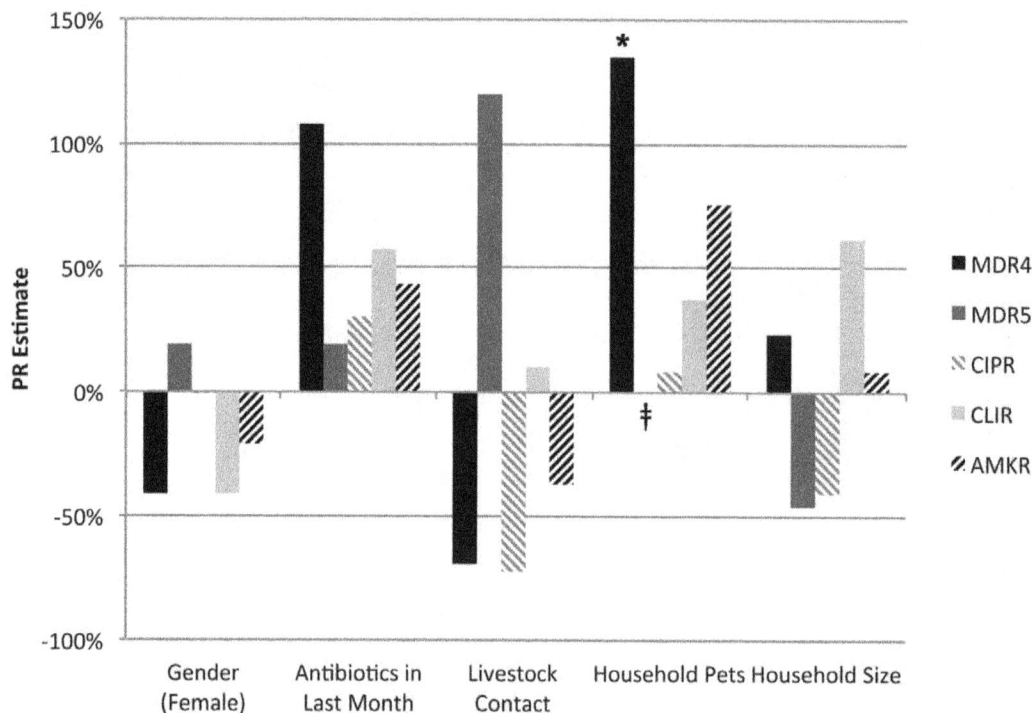

Figure 2. Risks for antimicrobial resistance in CA-MRSA case-patients of working age (18–65), $n = 27$. *$p<0.10$. No estimates were statistically significant at the $p<0.05$ level. ‡ A PR could not be estimated for MDR5 (high multi-drug resistance, 5+ classes of antimicrobial) for household pet presence due to a 0 stratum. Antimicrobial resistance patterns: MDR4: nonsusceptibility to four or more classes of antimicrobial drug; MDR5 ("high multidrug resistance"): high-level (complete) resistance to five or more classes of antimicrobial drug; CIPR: high-level resistance to ciprofloxacin; CLIR: high-level (complete) resistance to clindamycin, including inducible resistance; AMKR: high-level (complete) resistance to amikacin.

antimicrobial susceptibility testing in NHANES previously have been described [32]. Identical analysis was run on the NHANES data and the PSHMC datasets for descriptive comparison. Trends also were evaluated for *S. aureus* nasal colonization and identified risk factors in NHANES. Survey weighting was not used for NHANES models limited to MRSA-positive individuals due to the small sample size.

Results

Case-patient Selection

Figure 1 presents the selection process for case-patient inclusion in these analyses. Analysis was restricted to 88 individuals for whom data was complete for risk factors and from whom isolates were available for antimicrobial susceptibility testing. Epidemiologic comparison of the 63 case patients not included in this analysis demonstrated that these patients did not differ significantly in demographic characteristics, rates of prior hospitalization, or self-reported antimicrobial use as the included 88 case patients.

Prevalence of Antimicrobial Resistance

Overall, the prevalence of inducible and high-level resistance to individual antimicrobial drugs among the 88 isolates was: erythromycin, 90%; ciprofloxacin, 82%; clindamycin, 58%; amikacin, 24%; trimethoprim-sulfamethoxazole, 15%; gentamicin, 10%; tetracycine, 7%; quinupristin/dalfopristin (Synercid), 1%; and chloramphenicol, 1%.

All isolates were negative for *vanA* by real-time PCR and were susceptible on vancomycin disc diffusion testing. Based on

antimicrobial susceptibility profile screening, we selected a subset of 33 isolates to evaluate further. All were classified as vancomycin-susceptible based on a MIC of 2 or less by standard vancomycin E-test analysis. However, 16 (48%) were considered suspect for heterogeneous glycopeptide intermediate resistant *S. aureus* (hGISA) phenotype by vancomycin-teicoplanin (GRD) E-test. One (6%) of these 16 isolates was confirmed as a heterogeneous glycopeptide intermediate resistant *S. aureus* (hGISA) on the basis of population analysis, and details on this case are described below. Due to the low prevalence in this cohort ($n = 1$), vancomycin, quinupristin-dalfopristin, and chloramphenicol resistance were excluded from further analysis.

Case Report

This paper reports on the finding of a methicillin-resistant and heterogeneous glycopeptide-intermediate *S. aureus* (hGISA) isolate, typed as a ST5 (CC5) on the basis of multi-locus sequence testing [33], from a nasally colonized 76-year old Caucasian female case-patient who reported no personal or household member ($n = 1$) history of hospitalization, antimicrobial drug use, or healthcare occupational contact in the past year and who did not currently reside in a nursing home or have home nursing care on the basis of record review. She did have routine outpatient contact for follow up of chronic medical conditions. Her isolate was highly resistant to all nine antimicrobials tested and represented the only strain we identified with high-level resistance to quinupristin-dalfopristin and chloramphenicol. Although CC5 isolates historically have been associated with healthcare acquisition, recent reports have demonstrated that these strains may be establishing circulation patterns in the community [7], and the finding of such a highly-

Table 3. Antimicrobial resistance by risk factor among MRSA isolates comparing data from NHANES 2003–04 and data from Penn State Hershey Medical Center 2009–10.

	NHANES 2003–04						PSHMC 2009–10					
	n=133						n=88					
	Multidrug Resistance (MDR4)			Clindamycin Resistant (CLIR)			Multidrug Resistance (MDR4)			Clindamycin Resistant (CLIR)		
	4+ classes of non-susceptibility			high-level resistance			4+ classes of non-susceptibility			high-level resistance		
Prevalence	73%			63%			73%			58%		
	PR	95% CI	p-value	PR	95% CI	p-value	PR	95% CI	p-value	PR	95% CI	p-value
Gender (male is ref)												
Unadjusted	1.00	0.81–1.23	0.98	1.04	0.80–1.35	0.78	0.97	0.74–1.27	0.83	0.98	0.68–1.41	0.90
Adjusted	0.98	0.81–1.20	0.87	1.01	0.79–1.30	0.91	0.93	0.71–1.22	0.60	0.91	0.64–1.32	0.63
Age (18–65 is ref)												
Over 65, Unadjusted	**1.61**	**1.24–2.09**	**<0.001**	**1.82**	**1.34–2.48**	**<0.001**	1.16	0.90–1.49	0.25	*1.37*	*0.96–1.95*	*0.08*
Over 65, Adjusted	**1.36**	**1.03–1.78**	**0.03**	**1.46**	**1.03–2.04**	**0.03**	1.20	0.93–1.55	0.17	*1.40*	*0.97–2.02*	*0.07*
Under 18, Unadjusted	*1.30*	*0.97–1.75*	*0.08*	1.17	0.80–1.71	0.41	–			–		
Under 18, Adjusted	**1.44**	**1.05–1.97**	**0.02**	1.31	0.89–1.93	0.17	–			–		
Hospitalization (>1 year is ref)												
Within 1 year, unadjusted	**1.30**	**1.08–1.57**	**0.005**	**1.53**	**1.22–1.92**	**<0.001**	1.22	0.90–1.67	0.20	1.13	0.76–1.68	0.54
Within 1 month, adjusted	**1.22**	**1.00–1.48**	**0.05**	**1.36**	**1.07–2.04**	**0.01**	1.23	0.91–1.66	0.19	1.13	0.77–1.67	0.53
Household Size* (under 2 is ref)												
Unadjusted	**0.79**	**0.65–0.96**	**0.02**	**0.68**	**0.53–0.88**	**0.003**	1.05	0.81–1.36	0.71	0.95	0.65–1.39	0.81
Adjusted	0.93	0.73–1.20	0.59	*0.76*	*0.55–1.06*	*0.10*	1.10	0.85–1.41	0.47	1.04	0.70–1.52	0.86

Adjusted models include gender, age, hospitalization, and household size.

drug resistant isolate in a patient with CA-MRSA epidemiology is notable.

Prevalence of Antimicrobial Resistance by Risk Factor

Table 1 presents prevalence for individual resistance patterns and for multidrug resistance (MDR4 and MDR5) according to self-reported variables for gender, age, history of hospitalization and antimicrobial use, animal contact (livestock and household pets separately), and human household size for the 88 case-patients. The rate of multidrug resistance (MDR4) was high overall (73%). Highly multidrug-resistant isolates (MDR5) comprised almost a quarter of isolates. Almost half (48%) of case-patients reported a history of hospitalization within the prior six months, and antimicrobial use in the same period (68%) frequently was found.

Three antimicrobials–clindamycin, ciprofloxacin, and amikacin–were selected to demonstrate trends according to risk factor in part based on the potential utility of these resistance patterns to differentiate isolates as HA-MRSA or CA-MRSA [9–11]. Erythromycin was excluded from analysis due to extremely high resistance prevalence, and others were excluded due to low prevalence, which led to unstable model estimates (zero strata).

Unadjusted and Adjusted Models

Table 2 presents unadjusted and adjusted model estimates of prevalence ratios for each resistance pattern by risk factor. In adjusted models, history of hospitalization was associated with multidrug resistance, clindamycin resistance, and ciprofloxacin resistance, controlling for the effects of other covariates. Such

associations with hospitalization were not present for amikacin resistance; instead, history of hospitalization in the one to six months prior to admission had a prevalence ratio (PR) of 0.31, although this association was not significant ($p = 0.09$). A sensitivity analysis including self-reported information on healthcare occupation reported by the case patient or a household member as recent (≤ 1 mo) hospital contact produced no significant changes in inference, although estimates of association strengthened slightly in all cases.

Estimates of association between resistance patterns and antimicrobial use were weaker, and attenuated to non-significance in adjusted models in all cases. When sensitivity analysis was performed including intermediate with high-level (complete) resistance, antimicrobial use in the previous month was significantly associated with risk for resistance to ciprofloxacin or to multidrug resistance (MDR4), and antimicrobial use remained a significant predictor in adjusted models. In these adjusted models, estimates of association with hospitalization were attenuated and generally non-significant.

Most animal contact or household variables did not show strong trends for association with high-level resistance patterns, except that greater household size was negatively associated with ciprofloxacin resistance (PR 0.79 for household sizes over two, $p = 0.04$). However, 29 (76%) of the older case-patients lived in households with, at most, one other person. No significant trends in multidrug resistance over time (August 2009 to March 2010) were found (results not shown).

We also performed a sensitivity analysis examining inclusion of indirect effects from household members. We created a dummy variable in which we assigned: (2) the patient reported hospitalization and/or antimicrobial use within the past six months, (1) the patient reported that a he or she had not been hospitalized or taken antimicrobial drugs, but a household member had done so in the last six months, or (0) neither patient nor household member reported a history of hospitalization or antimicrobial use in the past six months. Patient history of hospitalization or antimicrobial use was associated with a 1.51 [95% CI: 1.01–2.25] fold higher risk of multidrug resistance (MDR4) in the patient's isolate, and this was statistically significant ($p = 0.05$). Household member risk in the absence of patient risk was not associated with multidrug resistance (PR 0.46 [95% CI: 0.08–2.64], $p = 0.38$), but only four patients reported household member risk in the absence of patient risk.

Associations in CA-MRSA Case-patients

Because of interest in evaluating risks for colonization with multidrug-resistant MRSA among community associated (CA-)MRSA case-patients, we also performed analysis restricted to PSHMC case-patients who had reported no history of hospitalization in the past six months. We stratified this analysis by age due to *a priori* concerns with potential differences in risk factors for community acquisition of MRSA by age, and also based on evidence from the data that age independently was associated with increases in risk for antimicrobial resistance. We evaluated 27 CA-MRSA case-patients of working age (18–65) and 18 CA-MRSA case-patients over the age of 65. Due to statistical properties (strata with zero observations) in the older sub-cohort, few associations could be estimated for case-patients over the age of 65, but estimates that could be made sometimes were associated in the opposite direction from those of working-age CA-MRSA case-patients, supporting our decision to stratify by age. For working-age CA-MRSA case-patients, **Figure 2** presents the predicted PR estimates according to gender, use of antimicrobials in the last month, contact with livestock, household pet contact, and human household size. Household pet contact was associated with a 2.35-fold higher prevalence of multidrug resistance (MDR4), but this association was not significant ($p = 0.09$). Although a PR could not be estimated for associations between MDR5 and household pet contact due to a zero stratum, data from other strata suggested that this was a high-risk category. Estimates of risk with livestock were heavily influenced by a single case patient reporting direct contact with livestock who had an isolate resistant to beta-lactam, erythromycin, ciprofloxacin, clindamycin, and amikacin antimicrobials.

Length of Stay Outcome

Geometric mean length of stay (LOS) was 5.73 days, ranging from 1.25 to over 45 days. On average, among PSHMC case-patients, having a multidrug-resistant isolate (MDR4) on admission was associated with a 1.5-day [95% CI: 1.11–1.97] increase in subsequent length of stay (LOS) in unadjusted models, and this association was statistically significant ($p = 0.008$). LOS estimates were similar for having a clindamycin-resistant or ciprofloxacin-resistant isolate. When history of hospitalization within the prior six months was included in LOS models, the estimate attenuated to a 1.3-day [95% CI: 1.01–1.80] increase ($p = 0.05$) and for having a clindamycin resistant isolate attenuated to a 1.4-day [95% CI: 1.06–1.80] increase ($p = 0.02$); the association between ciprofloxacin resistance and LOS lost significance.

NHANES Analysis

In the 2003–04 NHANES population, prevalence of multidrug resistance (MDR4) was 73%, but prevalence of high multidrug resistance (MDR5) was only 4%, precluding further analysis. Prevalence of clindamycin resistance (inducible or high-level resistance) was 63%. Susceptibility to amikacin and ciprofloxacin were not tested; prevalence of levofloxacin resistance was 46%. Age distribution was: $n = 47$ for under 18, $n = 49$ for 18–65, and $n = 37$ for over 65 years of age. **Table 3** provides results of unadjusted and adjusted models from 133 NHANES MRSA-colonized individuals (2003–04) and 88 PSHMC MRSA-colonized inpatients (2009–10). In both the NHANES 2003–04 and PSHMC 2009–10 populations, older age and history of hospitalization were positively associated with multidrug resistance. In the NHANES 2003–04 population, greater household size was negatively associated with multidrug resistance in MRSA isolates.

Conversely, among the 9004 NHANES participants tested in 2003–04 for any nasal colonization with *S. aureus* (MRSA and MSSA combined), odds were 1.32 fold higher [95% CI: 1.10–1.57] for colonization among participants who lived in larger households ($p = 0.005$). This association remained significant in survey-weighted, adjusted models controlling for gender, age, and hospitalization within the prior year (OR 1.37 [95% CI: 1.15–1.62], $p = 0.001$).

Discussion

In this cohort of MRSA case-patients from primarily rural and suburban Pennsylvania, most isolates were susceptible to quinupristin-dalfopristin (Synercid); chloramphenicol; tetracycline; gentamicin; and trimethoprim/sufamethoxazole. Low rates of resistance to tetracycline and trimethoprim/sulfamethoxazole have been found in clinical MRSA isolates in other studies [34,35]. Overall, most isolates were resistant to erythromycin and ciprofloxacin. Other studies have shown high levels of erythromycin resistance in MRSA isolates [9,35–37] and increasing resistance to fluoroquinolones [9,37], including in NHANES [32]. However, the 82% rate of resistance to ciprofloxacin in this cohort was much higher than rates of 40–45% reported in a North American hospital-based prevalence study in 2001–02 [35] or 50–55% rates reported through NHANES for 2001–2004 [32]. The 58% overall rate of resistance to clindamycin in this study was higher than the 30–35% reported in the 2001–02 North American hospital data [35], but was comparable with national trends of inducible or constitutive resistance in isolates collected between 2001–2004 [32].

In this study, recent hospitalization was associated with patient risk for carrying a multidrug-resistant strain of MRSA, and carriage of such strains was associated with increases in length of stay among case-patients admitted to the hospital for medical reasons unrelated to colonization status. Patients with prior hospital contact were more likely to be colonized with multidrug resistant isolates, and patients with prior hospital contact might have been a biased group with more severe medical conditions. However, inclusion of history of hospitalization in models did not negate the association.

When patients with recent hospital contact were excluded from PSHMC analysis and models were limited to working-age case-patients, potential but non-significant associations with animal contact emerged, particularly with dogs and cats. We did not collect information on antimicrobial use in pets, which might be a source of selective pressure for antimicrobial resistance in households. A prior study by Lin and colleagues described five MRSA isolates in animals from PA, with four of canine origin, from a study of clinical isolates collected during 2006–08 [38]. These isolates were of human HA-MRSA MLST types (primarily CC5) and displayed high levels of antimicrobial non-susceptibility to erythromycin, and additionally to veterinary fluoroquinolones, *e.g.*, enrofloxacin, (clindamycin was not tested) [38]. Clinical veterinary data analyzed by Rankin, Morris and colleagues from the Matthew J. Ryan veterinary hospital in Philadelphia demonstrated 100% resistance to clindamycin, ciprofloxacin, and erythromycin among nine PVL-positive clinical MRSA isolates from tested dogs and cats [39], and high clindamycin (72%), erythromycin (85%) and fluoroquinolone (90%) resistance among all 39 MRSA companion animal isolates submitted for 2003–04 [40]. The epidemic of MRSA in humans has been speculated to drive the parallel epidemic in companion animals, in part because companion animals tend to carry strains of MRSA typically associated with human transmission, and in part because households may be points of transmission between humans and companion animals [41–44]. The pilot data we report here may suggest that companion animals can serve as sources of antimicrobial resistance (potentially by harboring drug-resistant *S. aureus*, veterinary pathogens methicillin-resistant *S. pseudintermedius* and *S. schleiferi*, and other staphylococci [15]), but conclusions are limited by the small sample size and cross-sectional nature of the study. Longitudinal studies are needed to evaluate the potential association between animal contact and antimicrobial resistance in MRSA strains found in humans.

This study evaluated isolates from nasal colonization of newly-admitted hospital inpatients, a group likely to have greater prior exposure to healthcare settings and antimicrobial use than an outpatient population. Due to this potential bias, we also evaluated data from NHANES 2003-04 for similar risk factors. Typically, associations with antimicrobial resistance were in the same direction, although somewhat stronger in the NHANES data, for older age, hospitalization history, and smaller household size risk factors among individuals with MRSA colonization. However, larger household size was a risk factor for *S. aureus* nasal colonization in the U.S. population generally, indicating that household size may play a complicated role in *S. aureus* and MRSA epidemiology. Evaluation of MRSA-colonized individuals demonstrated higher risk for isolate antimicrobial resistance in smaller households, although this association was attenuated when models accounted for gender, age, and history of hospitalization. Comparisons between PSHMC and NHANES data are limited

by differences in methodology and potential temporal trends in MRSA epidemiology between 2003–04 (NHANES) and 2009–10 (PSHMC). Future NHANES surveys of national *S. aureus* colonization should consider including survey questions on pet ownership and animal contact.

In conclusion, carriage of ciprofloxacin-resistant, clindamycin-resistant, MDR4 and MDR5 MRSA was associated with prior history of hospitalization, but not with history of antimicrobial use, in MRSA case-patients colonized at admission to a tertiary care center. Similarly, prior history of hospitalization, older age (over 65), younger age (under 18), and small household size were risk factors for multidrug resistance and resistance to clindamycin in MRSA-colonized individuals who participated in NHANES 2003–04. Colonization with multidrug-resistant isolates was associated with increases in subsequent length-of-stay for patients in the hospital, with economic and clinical implications. Animal contact, particularly with household pets, may be an emerging risk factor for isolate antimicrobial resistance in case-patients lacking recent history of hospitalization, but this potential association should be confirmed with larger studies.

Acknowledgments

The authors are grateful to Dr. Avanthi Doppalapudi, Nancy L. Sperry and Dr. Michael Spitzer from PSHMC, and Dr. Beth Feingold and Grace Awantang from JHSPH for their invaluable assistance in sample collection. The authors would like to thank Drs. Peter Appelbaum and Klaudia Kosowska-Shick for their perspectives on MRSA in this PSHMC cohort; the PSHMC Diagnostic Virology Medical Technologists for their assistance in isolate collection; and Tania Contente, Jordan Buchhagen, Lindsey Watson, and Lauren Buck for their assistance in MLST preparation and analysis. AEP and MFD appreciate the assistance of thesis mentors, particularly Drs. Patti Gravitt, Jackie Agnew, and Bill Moss from JHSPH and Dr. Karen Carroll from JHSOM.

Author Contributions

Conceived and designed the experiments: MFD AEP KGJ KN CJW EKS. Performed the experiments: MFD AEP KGJ WHG LBP CJW. Analyzed the data: MFD AEP KJG CJW EKS. Contributed reagents/materials/ analysis tools: MFD AEP WHG LBP EKS. Wrote the paper: MFD AEP KGJ WHG LBP KN CJW EKS.

References

1. Monecke S, Coombs G, Shore AC, Coleman DC, Akpaka P, et al (2011) A field guide to pandemic, epidemic and sporadic clones of methicillin-resistant *Staphylococcus aureus*. PloS One 6(4): e17936.

2. Gorwitz RJ, Kruszon-Moran D, McAllister SK, Mcquillan G, McDougal LK, et al (2008) Changes in the prevalence of nasal colonization with *Staphylococcus aureus* in the United States, 2001–2004. The Journal of Infectious Diseases 197(9): 1226–1234.

3. Huang SS, Platt R (2003) Risk of methicillin-resistant *Staphylococcus aureus* infection after previous infection or colonization. Clinical Infectious Diseases 36(3): 281–285.

4. American Society for Microbiology (1995) Report of the ASM task force on antibiotic resistance.

5. Freitas EAF, Harris RM, Blake RK, Salgado CD (2010) Prevalence of USA300 strain type of methicillin-resistant *Staphylococcus aureus* among patients with nasal colonization identified with active surveillance. Infection Control and Hospital Epidemiology 31(5): 469–475.

6. Milstone AM, Carroll KC, Ross T, Shangraw KA, Perl TM (2010) Community-associated methicillin-resistant *Staphylococcus aureus* strains in pediatric intensive care unit. Emerging Infectious Diseases 16(4): 647–655.

7. Miller R, Walker AS, Knox K, Wyllie D, Paul J, et al (2010) 'Feral' and 'wild'-type methicillin-resistant *Staphylococcus aureus* in the United Kingdom. Epidemiology and Infection 138(5): 655–665.

8. Alvarez CA, Yomayusa N, Leal AL, Moreno J, Mendez-Alvarez S, et al (2010) Nosocomial infections caused by community-associated methicillin-resistant *Staphylococcus aureus* in Colombia. American Journal of Infection Control 38(4): 315–318.

9. David MZ, Glikman D, Crawford SE, Peng J, King KJ, et al (2008) What is community-associated methicillin-resistant *Staphylococcus aureus*? The Journal of Infectious Diseases 197(9): 1235–1243.

10. Popovich K, Hota B, Rice T, Aroutcheva A, Weinstein RA (2007) Phenotypic prediction rule for community-associated methicillin-resistant *Staphylococcus aureus*. Journal of Clinical Microbiology 45(7): 2293–2295.

11. Popovich KJ, Weinstein RA, Hota B (2008) Are Community-Associated Methicillin-Resistant *Staphylococcus aureus* (MRSA) strains replacing traditional nosocomial MRSA strains? Clinical Infectious Diseases 46(6): 787–794.

12. Millar BC, Loughrey A, Elborn JS, Moore JE (2007) Proposed definitions of community-associated meticillin-resistant *Staphylococcus aureus* (CA-MRSA). Journal of Hospital Infection 67(2): 109–113.

13. Lautenbach E, Tolomeo P, Nachamkin I, Hu B, Zaoutis TE (2010) The impact of household transmission on duration of outpatient colonization with methicillin-resistant *Staphylococcus aureus*. Epidemiology and Infection 138(5): 683–685.

14. Lucet J, Paoletti X, Demontpion C, Degrave M, Vanjak D, et al (2009) Carriage of methicillin-resistant *Staphylococcus aureus* in home care settings: Prevalence, duration, and transmission to household members. Archives of Internal Medicine 169(15): 1372–1378.

15. Davis MF, Iverson SA, Baron P, Vasse A, Silbergeld EK, et al (2012) Household transmission of meticillin-resistant *Staphylococcus aureus* and other staphylococci. The Lancet Infectious Diseases 12(9): 703–716.

16. Smith TC, Moritz ED, Leedom Larson K,R., Ferguson DD (2010) The environment as a factor in methicillin-resistant *Staphylococcus aureus* transmission. Reviews on Environmental Health 25(2): 121–134.

17. Cuny C, Friedrich A, Kozytska S, Layer F, Nubel U, et al (2010) Emergence of methicillin-resistant *Staphylococcus aureus* (MRSA) in different animal species. International Journal of Medical Microbiology 300(2–3): 109–117.

18. Peterson AE, Davis MF, Julian KG, Awantang G, Greene WH, et al (2012) Molecular and phenotypic characteristics of healthcare- and community-associated methicillin-resistant *Staphylococcus aureus* at a rural hospital. PloS One 7(6): e38354.

19. Garcia Alvarez L, Holden M, Lindsay H, Webb CR (2011) Meticillin-resistant *Staphylococcus aureus* with a novel *mecA* homologue in human and bovine populations in the UK and Denmark: a descriptive study. The Lancet Infectious Diseases 11(8): 595–603.

20. Ito T, Hiramatsu K, Tomasz A, de Lencastre H, Perreten V, et al (2012) Guidelines for reporting novel *mecA* gene homologues. Antimicrobial Agents and Chemotherapy 56(10): 4997–4999.

21. Barry AL, Garcia F, Thrupp LD (1970) An improved single-disk method for testing the antibiotic susceptibility of rapidly-growing pathogens. American Journal of Clinical Pathology 53(2): 149–158.

22. Bauer AW, Kirby WM, Sherris JC, Turck M (1966) Antibiotic susceptibility testing by a standardized single disk method. American Journal of Clinical Pathology 45(4): 493–496.

23. Clinical Laboratory Standards Institute (2010) 2009 S. aureus CLSI breakpoint guide.

24. Moet G, Jones R, Biedenbach D, Stilwell M, Fritsche T (2007) Contemporary causes of skin and soft tissue infections in North America, Latin America, and Europe: Report from the SENTRY antimicrobial surveillance program (1998–2004). Diagnostic Microbiology and Infectious Disease 57(1): 7–13.

25. Turnidge J, Kahlmeter G, Kronvall G (2006) Statistical characterisation of bacterial wild-type MIC value distributions and the determination of epidemiological cut-off values. Clinical Microbiology and Infection 12(5): 418–425.

26. Fiebelkorn KR, Crawford SA, McElmeel ML, Jorgensen JH (2003) Practical disk diffusion method for detection of inducible clindamycin resistance in *Staphylococcus aureus* and coagulase-negative staphylococci. Journal of Clinical Microbiology 41(10): 4740–4744.

27. Kosowska-Shick K, Ednie LM, McGhee P, Smith K, Todd CD, et al (2008) Incidence and characteristics of vancomycin nonsusceptible strains of methicillin-resistant *Staphylococcus aureus* at Hershey Medical Center. Antimicrobial Agents and Chemotherapy 52(12): 4510–4513.

28. Appelbaum PC (2007) Reduced glycopeptide susceptibility in methicillin-resistant *Staphylococcus aureus* (MRSA). International Journal of Antimicrobial Agents 30(5): 398–408.

29. Deddens JA, Petersen MR (2008) Approaches for estimating prevalence ratios. Occupational and Environmental Medicine 65(7): 501–506.

30. Barros AJD, Hirakata V (2003) Alternatives for logistic regression in cross-sectional studies: An empirical comparison of models that directly estimate the prevalence ratio. BMC Medical Research Methodology 3(1): 21.

31. Centers for Disease Control and Prevention (2003–2004) National Center for Health Statistics (NCHS). National Health and Nutrition Examination Survey data. Hyattsville, MD: U.S. Department of Health and Human Services, Centers for Disease Control and Prevention.

32. Tenover FC, McAllister S, Fosheim G, McDougal LK, Carey RB, et al (2008) Characterization of *Staphylococcus aureus* isolates from nasal cultures collected from individuals in the United States in 2001 to 2004. Journal of Clinical Microbiology 46(9): 2837–2841.

33. Enright MC, Day NP, Davies CE, Peacock SJ, Spratt BG (2000) Multilocus sequence typing for characterization of methicillin-resistant and methicillin-susceptible clones of *Staphylococcus aureus*. Journal of Clinical Microbiology 38(3): 1008–1015.

34. Bordon J, Master RN, Clark RB, Duvvuri P, Karlowsky JA, et al (2010) Methicillin-resistant *Staphylococcus aureus* resistance to non beta-lactam antimicrobials in the United States from 1996 to 2008. Diagnostic Microbiology and Infectious Disease 67(4): 395–398.

35. Winston LG (2009) Antimicrobial resistance in staphylococci: Mechanisms of resistance and clinical implications. Chapter in: Antimicrobial Drug Resistance.

36. Limbago B, Fosheim GE, Schoonover V, Crane CE, Nadle J, et al (2009) Characterization of methicillin-resistant staphylococcus aureus isolates collected in 2005 and 2006 from patients with invasive disease: A population-based analysis. Journal of Clinical Microbiology 47: 1344–1351.

37. Diep BA, Chambers HF, Graber CJ, Szumowski JD, Miller LG, et al (2008) Emergence of multidrug-resistant, community-associated, methicillin-resistant *Staphylococcus aureus* clone USA300 in men who have sex with men. Annals of Internal Medicine 148: 249–257.

38. Lin Y, Barker E, Kislow J, Kaldhone P, Stemper ME, et al (2011) Evidence of multiple virulence subtypes in nosocomial and community-associated MRSA genotypes in companion animals from the upper midwestern and northeastern United States. Clinical Medicine & Research 9(1): 7–16.

39. Rankin S, Roberts S, O'Shea K, Maloney D, Lorenzo M, et al (2005) Panton Valentine Leukocidin (PVL) toxin positive MRSA strains isolated from companion animals. Veterinary Microbiology 108(1–2): 145–148.

40. Morris DO, Rook KA, Shofer FS, Rankin SC (2006) Screening of *Staphylococcus aureus*, *Staphylococcus intermedius*, and *Staphylococcus schleiferi* isolates obtained from small companion animals for antimicrobial resistance: A retrospective review of 749 isolates (2003–04). Veterinary Dermatology 17(5): 332–337.

41. Weese JS, van Duijkeren E (2010) Methicillin-resistant *Staphylococcus aureus* and *Staphylococcus pseudintermedius* in veterinary medicine. Veterinary Microbiology 140(3–4): 418–429.

42. Loeffler A, Lloyd DH (2010) Companion animals: A reservoir for methicillin-resistant *Staphylococcus aureus* in the community? Epidemiology and Infection 138(5): 595–605.

43. Bramble M, Morris D, Tolomeo P, Lautenbach E (2011) Potential role of pet animals in household transmission of methicillin-resistant *Staphylococcus aureus*: A narrative review. Vector Borne and Zoonotic Diseases 11(6): 617–620.

44. Baptiste KE, Williams K, Willams NJ, Wattret A, Clegg PD, et al (2005) Methicillin-resistant staphylococci in companion animals. Emerging Infectious Diseases 11(12): 1942–1944.

22

Seroepidemiological Survey for *Coxiella burnetii* Antibodies and Associated Risk Factors in Dutch Livestock Veterinarians

René Van den Brom[1]*, Barbara Schimmer[2], Peter M. Schneeberger[3], Wim A. Swart[4], Wim van der Hoek[2], Piet Vellema[1]

1 Department of Small Ruminant Health, Animal Health Service, Deventer, The Netherlands, 2 Centre for Infectious Disease Control, National Institute for Public Health and the Environment, Bilthoven, The Netherlands, 3 Department of Medical Microbiology and Infection Control, Jeroen Bosch Hospital, 's-Hertogenbosch, The Netherlands, 4 Department of Diagnostics, Research and Epidemiology, Animal Health Service, Deventer, The Netherlands

Abstract

Since 2007, Q fever has become a major public health problem in the Netherlands and goats were the most likely source of the human outbreaks in 2007, 2008 and 2009. Little was known about the consequences of these outbreaks for those professional care providers directly involved. The aim of this survey was to estimate the seroprevalence of antibodies against *C. burnetii* among Dutch livestock veterinarians and to determine possible risk factors. Single blood samples from 189 veterinarians, including veterinary students in their final year, were collected at a veterinary conference and a questionnaire was filled in by each participant. The blood samples were screened for IgG antibodies against phase I and phase II antigen of *C. burnetii* using an indirect immunofluorescent assay, and for IgM antibodies using an ELISA. Antibodies against *C. burnetii* were detected in 123 (65.1%) out of 189 veterinarians. Independent risk factors associated with seropositivity were number of hours with animal contact per week, number of years graduated as veterinarian, rural or sub urban living area, being a practicing veterinarian, and occupational contact with swine. Livestock veterinarians should be aware of this risk to acquire an infection with *C. burnetii*. Physicians should consider potential infection with *C. burnetii* when treating occupational risk groups, bearing in mind that the burden of disease among veterinarians remains uncertain. Vaccination of occupational risk groups should be debated.

Editor: Tara C. Smith, University of Iowa, United States of America

Funding: No external funding was received for this survey.

Competing Interests: The authors have declared that no competing interests exists.

* E-mail: r.vd.brom@gddeventer.com

Introduction

Q fever is a zoonotic disease caused by the obligate intracellular bacterium, *Coxiella burnetii*, and ruminants are considered to be the primary source of infection for humans. In cattle, the disease is mainly asymptomatic [1], but in sheep and goats the main symptom is abortion, stillbirth and retention of foetal membranes [2–6]. The bacterium is shed in urine, milk, faeces and birth products of infected animals. The main route of transmission of the bacterium to humans is by aerosols [4,7,8].

Until 2007, about 20 Q fever cases were reported in the Netherlands annually [9]. In that year, Q fever became a major public health problem in the Netherlands with 168, 1000 and 2,357 human cases notified in 2007, 2008 and 2009, respectively [10]. These unprecedented annual outbreaks are largely explained by exposure of the general population living in the surroundings of infected dairy goat farms to airborne contaminated dust particles. Only 5% of the notified Q fever patients in the Netherlands report an occupation in agriculture, transporting or handling animal products, or animal care [11]. However, since its first description in abattoir workers in Australia in 1935 [12], Q fever has been considered primarily an occupational zoonotic disease for abattoir workers, sheep shearers, livestock farmers, and especially veteri-

narians because of their direct contact with potentially infected animals [13–19].

The aim of this survey was to estimate the seroprevalence of antibodies against *C. burnetii* among Dutch livestock veterinarians and to determine possible risk factors.

Materials and Methods

Human Population and Data Collection

In November 2009, professional laboratory assistants collected a single blood sample from Dutch livestock veterinarians and final-year veterinary students attending a veterinary conference.

Each participant filled in a self-administered questionnaire to obtain epidemiological and clinical information. The questionnaire existed of three parts, and took approximately fifteen minutes to complete. The first part focused on demographic data and included age, gender, and residence in urban, sub urban or rural area. The second part consisted of occupation-related questions regarding work location, type of veterinary occupation, years in veterinary practice, contact with livestock and livestock farms, contact with animal related products as straw, hay, soil, birth products and urine and faeces, contact with aborted animals, use of personnel protective equipment, work related wounds and accidental vaccine exposure. The third part consisted of non-occupation related questions regarding possession of animals in the last five years, consumption of raw dairy products, outdoor activities and health conditions, including smoking, tick bites during the last five years and a known history of a clinical Q fever infection, pregnancy and abortion.

This study was approved by the Medical Ethical Committee of the University Medical Centre Utrecht, Utrecht, the Netherlands (reference number 09–322). All participants received a book to express appreciation for their cooperation.

Laboratory Methods

A serum sample from each participant was tested for the presence of IgG antibodies against C. burnetii using a Q fever indirect immunofluorescent assay (IFA; Focus Diagnostics, Cypress, CA), according to the manufacturer's protocol. Sera were screened for phase I and phase II IgG using a cut-off of 1:32. Samples with both IgG phase I and II titres of ≥1:32 were considered to be positive, while solitary IgG phase II samples were scored positive if they had a single titre of ≥1:512.

All samples were also screened for IgM using an ELISA (Focus Diagnostics), according to the manufacturer's protocol, and positive samples were confirmed with IFA. Samples with a titre of ≥1:32, both for IgM phase I and II, were considered to be positive, indicating a possibly recent infection.

Within the group of participants with a past infection, a distinction was made between serological profiles considered not likely to be compatible with a chronic infection, and serological profiles which could indicate a chronic infection. Serum samples from participants with a possibly chronic Q fever infection, having an IgG phase I titre ≥1:1024, were additionally analysed by performing a C. burnetii PCR.

Statistical Data Analysis

All individual laboratory results were merged with the self-administered questionnaires. Statistical analysis was carried out using STATA 11. The Chi square test and the two-sided proportion-test were used to estimate univariate associations between exposures and seropositivity. Analyses were carried out to calculate odds ratio's with 95% confidence intervals. The odds ratio (OR) was defined, in this context as the odds of a given exposure among veterinarians seropositive for C. burnetii divided by the odds of exposure among seronegative veterinarians. Veterinarians who did not completely fill in the questionnaire were excluded for the analysis of that particular question.

For the multivariable logistic regression, initially all variables with (2-sided) p<0.20 and with sufficient numbers (>10) were selected. To avoid multicollinearity, from groups of variables that had a correlation of more than 0.50 with each other, only one, the most plausible biological variable, was left in the multivariable analysis.

Stepwise backward logistic regression was carried out, starting with all data and excluding stepwise each variable that had a p-value of >0.05. All remaining variables were considered to be risk or protective factors.

Results

Descriptive Results

A total of 189 participants, being more than 90% of the attendants, completed the questionnaire and provided a blood sample during the conference. The median age of the participants was 44 years (interquartile range, 34–52 years). Of the participants, 130 (68.8%) were male and 59 (31.2%) were female

(Table 1). One hundred and twelve of the participants worked as a livestock practitioner, 20 were non-practicing, 37 worked as livestock veterinarian at a veterinary institute (Utrecht University (UU) or Animal Health Service (GD)) and 20 were livestock veterinary students in their final year. A total of 108 (57.1%) of the participants had contact with livestock for more than 50% of working hours in their current job.

The overall seroprevalence was 65.1% (n = 189). In livestock veterinarians the seroprevalence was 69.2% (n = 169). The seroprevalence in livestock veterinary students was 30.0% (n = 20). Among the group of 169 livestock veterinarians the seroprevalence was 87.5% in practicing livestock veterinarians (n = 112), 45.0% in non-practicing livestock veterinarians (n = 20) and 27.0% in livestock veterinarians working at a veterinary institute (n = 37). IgG antibody titers against C. burnetii measured for both phase I and II ranged from 1:32 to 1:2048. Seven out of nine participants with a positive IgM ELISA result were confirmed with IFA, suggesting a recent infection. Four of those seven IFA positive study participants were livestock veterinary students. The other three were practicing livestock veterinarians. Seven participants with an IgG phase I titre ≥1:1024, a possible indication of a chronic Q fever infection, were followed up by performing a C. burnetii PCR on a blood sample, and in all cases PCR results were negative. Additionally, participants with an IgG phase I titre ≥1:512 are offered to participate in a follow-up study and are advised to be controlled for risk factors of a chronic Q fever infection.

Univariable Analysis

Participants who were seropositive were likely to be male over the age of 32 years (Table 1). Participants living in rural or suburban areas were significantly more often seropositive than participants living in an urban area. Occupational risk factors in univariable analysis were: graduated as a veterinarian more than two years ago; more than 10 hours of animal contact per week; practicing as livestock veterinarian; and working with cattle, horses, dogs and cats. Participants with frequent contact with animal products, like straw, hay, roughage, raw milk, birth products of ruminants as well as of pets, urine of ruminants, practicing on cattle farms with abortion, and one or more contacts on farms with abortion problems in the last five years, were significantly more often seropositive. Accidental needle injections and cutting incidents were also found to be associated with seropositivity. Non-occupational activities like cycling and shopping were associated with seronegativity. In contrast, gardening and having dogs and (pet) birds were found to be associated with seropositivity. Consumption of dairy products, health conditions like smoking behaviour, and not wearing protective clothes during work were not found to be a significant univariate risk factor. The number of participants primarily working with sheep and goats, with a history of a clinical Q fever infection, or with pregnancy and abortion was too small for statistical analysis.

Multivariable Analysis

Variables with a p-value <0.20 in the univariable analysis were used as input for the multivariable analysis. The number of years as a veterinarian was highly correlated with age and gender; the latter two were left out of the analysis. Working category and contacts with ruminants were very highly correlated to contact with hay/straw, roughage, raw milk, birth products of ruminants and with urine of ruminants; the latter 5 were left out of the analysis.

In this group of livestock veterinarians, risk factors for C. burnetii seropositivity in the multivariable analysis (Table 2) were: number

Table 1. Results of univariable analysis of risk factors for presence of antibodies against *Coxiella burnetii*.

	Participants						
	Seropositive[#]		Seronegative				
	No.	%	No.	%	Odds Ratio	95% confidence interval	P
Gender							
Female	24	40.7	35	59.3	1.0	. .	.
Male	99	76.2	31	23.8	4.7	2.3 9.4	<0.001
Age							
<=32 year	19	40.4	28	59.6	1.0	.	
33–44 year	35	71.4	14	28.6	3.7	1.6 8.6	0.003
45–52 year	37	75.5	12	24.5	4.5	1.9 10.9	0.001
53–65 year	32	72.7	12	27.3	3.9	1.6 9.5	0.002
Living region							
Urban	8	30.8	18	69.2	1.0	. .	.
Sub-urban	21	56.8	16	43.2	3.0	1.0 8.5	0.037
Rural	94	74.6	32	25.4	6.6	2.6 16.7	<0.001
Veterinarian (years)							
Veterinarian (<=2)	13	27.7	34	72.3	1.0		
veterinarian (3–13)	36	70.6	15	29.4	6.3	2.6 15.1	<0.001
veterinarian (14–21)	33	75.0	11	25.0	7.9	3.1 20.0	<0.001
veterinarian (>=22)	40	87.0	6	13.0	17.4	6.00 50.8	<0.001
Animal contact (hours/week)							
<10 hours	9	24.3	28	75.7	1.0		
10–19 hours	25	55.6	20	44.4	3.9	1.5 10.1	0.005
20–29 hours	42	80.8	10	19.2	13.1	4.7 36.2	<0.001
>=30 hours	43	89.6	5	10.4	26.8	8.1 88.2	<0.001
Work category							
Others	23	30.7	52	69.3	1.0		
Practicing	100	87.7	14	12.3	16.2	7.7 34.0	<0.001
Contact with cows							
No	11	31.4	24	68.6	1.0	. .	.
Yes	112	72.7	42	27.3	5.8	2.6 12.9	<0.001
Contact with swine							
No	80	61.5	50	38.5	1.0	.	.
Yes	43	72.9	16	27.1	1.7	0.9 3.3	0.131
Contact with birth products of ruminants							
No	16	33.3	32	66.7	1.0	.	.
Yes	107	75.9	34	24.1	6.3	3.1 12.9	<0.001
Contact with birth products of pets							
No	101	61.2	64	38.8	1.0	. .	.
Yes	22	91.7	2	8.3	7.0	1.5 31.9	0.004
Practice on cow farm with abortion							
No	32	43.8	41	56.2	1.0	. .	.
Yes	91	78.4	25	21.6	4.7	2.4 9.3	<0.001

[#]Sera were screened for phase I and phase II IgG using a cut-off of 1:32. Samples with both IgG phase I and II ≥1:32 were considered to be positive, while solitary IgG phase II samples were scored positive if they had a single titre of ≥1:512 (Focus Diagnostics, Cypress, CA).

of hours with animal contact per week, number of years graduated as veterinarian, living in a rural (OR, 17.9 (95% CI: 3.6–88.1)) or semi urban area (OR, 11.9 (95% CI: 2.1–68.5)), working as practicing livestock veterinarian (OR, 15.8 (95% CI: 2.9–87.2)), and occupational contact with swine (OR, 3.4 (95% CI: 1.1–10.2)).

Discussion

In this cross-sectional study, an overall *C. burnetii* seroprevalence of 65.1% among Dutch livestock veterinarians was found. The number of hours with animal contact per week, the number of

Table 2. Final multivariable model for risk factors associated with presence of antibodies against *Coxiella burnetii* in 189 veterinarians.

Variable	Category	No.	OR	[95% CI]		P
Animal contacts (hours/week)	<10 hours	37	1.0			
	10–19 hours	45	12.0	2.5	57.1	0.002
	20–29 hours	52	1.2	0.2	7.6	0.869
	>=30 hours	48	16.0	1.8	141.8	0.013
Veterinarian (years)	<=2	47	1.0			
	3–13	51	17.5	4.0	77.4	<0.001
	14–21	44	26.5	4.8	145.9	<0.001
	>=22	46	58.1	10.3	328.0	<0.001
Living region	Urban	26	1.0			
	Sub-urban	37	11.9	2.1	68.5	0.005
	Rural	126	17.9	3.6	88.1	<0.001
Work category	Others	75	1.0			
	Practicing	114	15.8	2.9	87.2	0.002
Contact with swine	No	130	1.0			
	Yes	59	3.4	1.1	10.2	0.029

years the participants were graduated and practicing as a veterinarian, were the main independent risk factors in this study. These risk factors suggest a high dose-effect relation for seropositivity in Dutch livestock veterinarians. In 1984, 84% of 222 Dutch livestock veterinarians were seropositive for IgG antibodies against *C. burnetii* [17]. The use of a different laboratory test and cut-offs, differences in study population and different infection rates of livestock over time could be possible explanations for other seroprevalence estimates.

Dutch livestock veterinarians have a high risk of getting *C. burnetii* seropositive because of intensive contact with potentially infected livestock, and the immune system can be boosted frequently because of a high prevalence in Dutch livestock [20,21]. Contact with swine was found to be an independent risk factor, but the group of veterinarians involved was also exposed to cattle. Further, the main geographical areas where pigs are kept in the Netherlands corresponds with the high-incidence areas where the human Q fever epidemic related to dairy goats was situated and where high seroprevalences were found in the rural population. On the other hand, treatment of swine has previously been described as a risk factor for seropositivity for veterinarians [19]. The natural susceptibility of swine to *C. burnetii* was demonstrated during a Q fever epidemic in Uruguay. A seroprevalence of 21.4% was measured in 391 healthy slaughter pigs [22]. No information about Q fever prevalences in swine in the Netherlands is available.

In this survey, 20 veterinary students participated, and the seroprevalence was 30%. In a survey in Spain, a seroprevalence of 11% among veterinary students was found. First course students showed a significant lower seroprevalence. Multiple risk factors were associated with *C. burnetii*: study course, contact with live animals especially ruminants and contact with persons working with animals [18]. A large serological survey (n = 674) was already carried out in the Netherlands in 2006. At that time 18.7% of the

veterinary students were seropositive. Students in their final year with the livestock study direction had a seroprevalence of 37.3%. The main risk factors were a study direction focusing on large animals, advanced year of study, having had a zoonosis during study and having ever lived on a farm with ruminants [23]. To detect possible recent exposure to *C. burnetii*, testing was also performed by ELISA IgM, and it is not remarkable that four out of seven possible recent infections occurred in veterinary livestock students, indicating this group is susceptible for the infection during the practical rotations during their study. The lower prevalence in veterinary students, an indication for recent infection in seven of whom four were students, and the main risk factors we found, are another indication for a high dose-effect relation for seropositivity.

Our study clearly indicates that livestock veterinarians are an occupational risk group. The prevalence found in this study was much higher than described in several international sero-epidemical studies among livestock veterinarians [13–15,18,19,24,25], with the exception of a small survey among 12 veterinarians in southern Italy, which revealed a seroprevalence of 100% [16]. In other studies, contact with livestock is described as an important risk factor for seropositivity [14,19,24], and exposure to goats was the most important risk factor associated with *C. burnetii* infection in Southern Taiwan [14]. Treatment of cattle, swine or wildlife were main risk factors associated with *C. burnetii* seropositivity in US veterinarians [19]. In Slovakia and Nova Scotia, professional orientation and regular contact with farm animals and pets [24], and exposure to sheep placentas [15] were described as important risk factors, respectively. In contrast, in Japan, no significant correlation was found between years of occupational experience and *C. burnetii* seropositivity [13].

The final independent risk factor was living in a rural or sub-urban area. Participants living in these areas were significantly more often seropositive than participants living in an urban area. Rural and sub-urban living areas have been described before as a risk factor [26–30], although urban outbreaks also have been described, but could mostly be related to exposure to animals or animal products [31–33]. In the Netherlands, livestock farms are mainly situated in rural or sub-urban areas. The knowledge that ruminants are the main reservoir for *C. burnetii* [1,34] and the fact that *C. burnetii* can easily be spread by aerosols [4,7,8], presumably explains why living in rural or sub-urban area is a risk factor for seropositivity.

In the univariable analysis, age and gender were risk factors for seropositivity. Nevertheless, both were left out of the multivariable analysis because they were highly correlated with the number of years participants were graduated as veterinarian. The higher incidence in males than in females has been reported in several sero-epidemical studies among veterinarians, but without a clear explanation [15,17–19]. Also a Spanish study among veterinary students revealed that male students in the fifth study year had a significantly higher risk to be seropositive than female students [18]. A higher clinical incidence in males and persons aged between 40–60 years in the Dutch population has been described during the Q fever outbreaks between 2007–2010 [11]. Age above 46 years, was also previously described as a risk factor for seropositivity in veterinarians [19].

To differentiate in the group of practicing veterinarians, all analyses were repeated in the multivariable analysis for the subset of practicing veterinarians only, mainly working with cattle, swine and poultry, or individual housed animals. The analysis on the subset of practicing veterinarians did not result in additional significant results (data are not shown), and was less robust than the multivariable analysis based on the full data set.

In conclusion, Dutch livestock veterinarians are an occupational risk group with increased risk for *C. burnetii* infection presumably because of their direct contact with infected livestock. Dutch livestock veterinarians should be aware of this risk and be extra alert regarding symptoms of Q fever. Most of the infections are not notified, as they remain asymptomatic or result in only mild flu-like symptoms. Serious infections leading to pneumonia or hepatitis may occur. A *C. burnetii* infection can cause serious complications during pregnancy and in those with underlying disease, therefore these groups should be monitored properly. Vaccination of occupational groups at risk is common in Australia [35,36]. In the Netherlands, vaccination has been made available in the first half of 2011, but only for specific risk groups, as those patients with heart valve and vascular disorders. During the community Q fever outbreaks between 2007 and 2009 in the Netherlands, few patients reported occupational exposure [11]. Most veterinarians are not eligible for vaccination because the presence of antibodies is an absolute contraindication for administering the currently available Australian vaccine. However, vaccination could be considered for seronegative veterinary students at the beginning of their study [35]. Routine serological follow-up is useful as well as basic safety rules, like hygiene measures and the use of protection clothes [18,19,24,37], although in this study disregard of protective measures was not found to be an independent risk factor. Occupational exposure to several zoonotic diseases makes basic safety rules useful for protecting the livestock veterinarian.

Acknowledgments

This study was facilitated by the GGL (Dutch society for livestock veterinarians). We would like to thank all participants for their cooperation in this seroepidemical survey. In addition, we would like to thank Diagnostiek Nederland for collecting blood samples and Jeroen Bosch Hospital, and especially Jamie Meekelenkamp for examining the blood samples. Last but not least we would like to thank Lammert Moll, and Gerdien van Schaik of the Animal Health Service (GD) for their help with the data-analysis and their comments on the manuscript, and Roel Coutinho of the National Institute for Public Health and the Environment (RIVM) for his comments on the manuscript.

Author Contributions

Revised the manuscript: BS PV. Read and approved the final manuscript: RV BS PS WS Wvdh PV. Conceived and designed the experiments: RV BS WvdH PV. Performed the experiments: PS. Analyzed the data: WS RV BS. Wrote the paper: RV.

References

1. Arricau-Bouvery N, Rodolakis A (2005) Is Q fever an emerging or re-emerging zoonosis? Vet Res 36: 327–349.
2. Damoser J, Hofer E, Muller M (1993) [Abortions in a lower Austrian sheep facility caused by Coxiella burnetii]. Berl Munch Tierarztl Wochenschr 106: 361–364.
3. Hatchette TF, Hudson RC, Schlech WF, Campbell NA, Hatchette JE, et al. (2001) Goat-associated Q fever: a new disease in Newfoundland. Emerg Infect Dis 7: 413–419.
4. Maurin M, Raoult D (1999) Q fever. Clin Microbiol Rev 12: 518–553.
5. Wouda W, Dercksen DP (2007) [Abortion and stillbirth among dairy goats as a consequence of Coxiella burnetii]. Tijdschr Diergeneeskd 132: 908–911.
6. Zeman DH, Kirkbride CA, Leslie-Steen P, Duimstra JR (1989) Ovine abortion due to Coxiella burnetti infection. J Vet Diagn Invest 1: 178–180.
7. Marrie TJ (1990) Q fever - a review. Can Vet J 31: 555–563.
8. Schimmer B, Dijkstra F, Vellema P, Schneeberger PM, Hackert V, et al. (2009) Sustained intensive transmission of Q fever in the south of the Netherlands, 2009. Euro Surveill 14.
9. Van Steenbergen JE, Morroy G, Groot CA, Ruikes FG, Marcelis JH, et al. (2007) [An outbreak of Q fever in The Netherlands–possible link to goats]. Ned Tijdschr Geneeskd 151: 1998–2003.
10. van der Hoek W, Dijkstra F, Wijers N, Rietveld A, Wijkmans CJ, et al. (2010) [Three years of Q fever in the Netherlands: faster diagnosis]. Ned Tijdschr Geneeskd 154: A1845.
11. Dijkstra F, van der Hoek W, Wijers N, Schimmer B, Rietveld A, et al. (2012) The 2007–2010 Q fever epidemic in The Netherlands: characteristics of notified acute Q fever patients and the association with dairy goat farming. FEMS Immunol Med Microbiol 64: 3–12.
12. Derrick EH (1937) Q fever, new fever entity: clinical features, diagnosis and laboratory investigation. Med J Aus 2: 282–299.
13. Abe T, Yamaki K, Hayakawa T, Fukuda H, Ito Y, et al. (2001) A seroepidemiological study of the risks of Q fever infection in Japanese veterinarians. Eur J Epidemiol 17: 1029–1032.
14. Chang CC, Lin PS, Hou MY, Lin CC, Hung MN, et al. (2010) Identification of risk factors of Coxiella burnetii (Q fever) infection in veterinary-associated populations in southern Taiwan. Zoonoses Public Health 57: e95–101.
15. Marrie TJ, Fraser J (1985) Prevalence of Antibodies to Coxiella burnetii Among Veterinarians and Slaughterhouse Workers in Nova Scotia. Can Vet J 26: 181–184.
16. Monno R, Fumarola L, Trerotoli P, Cavone D, Giannelli G, et al. (2009) Seroprevalence of Q fever, brucellosis and leptospirosis in farmers and agricultural workers in Bari, Southern Italy. Ann Agric Environ Med 16: 205–209.
17. Richardus JH, Donkers A, Dumas AM, Schaap GJ, Akkermans JP, et al. (1987) Q fever in the Netherlands: a sero-epidemiological survey among human population groups from 1968 to 1983. Epidemiol Infect 98: 211–219.
18. Valencia MC, Rodriguez CO, Punet OG, de Blas Giral I (2000) Q fever seroprevalence and associated risk factors among students from the Veterinary School of Zaragoza, Spain. Eur J Epidemiol 16: 469–476.
19. Whitney EA, Massung RF, Candee AJ, Ailes EC, Myers LM, et al. (2009) Seroepidemiologic and occupational risk survey for Coxiella burnetii antibodies among US veterinarians. Clin Infect Dis 48: 550–557.
20. Muskens J, Mars MH, Franken P (2007) [Q fever: an overview]. Tijdschr Diergeneeskd 132: 912–917.
21. Van den Brom R, van Engelen E, Luttikholt S, Moll L, van Maanen K, et al. (2012) Coxiella burnetii in bulk tank milk samples from dairy goat and dairy sheep farms in The Netherlands in 2008. Vet Rec 170: 310.
22. Somma-Moreira RE, Caffarena RM, Somma S, Perez G, Monteiro M (1987) Analysis of Q fever in Uruguay Rev Infect Dis 9: 386–387.
23. De Rooij MM, Schimmer B, Versteeg B, Schneeberger P, Berends BR, et al. (2012) Risk factors of Coxiella burnetii (Q fever) seropositivity in veterinary medicine students. PloS One 7: e32108.
24. Dorko E, Kalinova Z, Weissova T, Pilipcinec E (2008) Seroprevalence of antibodies to Coxiella burnetii among employees of the Veterinary University in Kosice, eastern Slovakia. Ann Agric Environ Med 15: 119–124.
25. Ergonul O, Zeller H, Kilic S, Kutlu S, Kutlu M, et al. (2006) Zoonotic infections among veterinarians in Turkey: Crimean-Congo hemorrhagic fever and beyond. Int J Infect Dis 10: 465–469.
26. Gardon J, Heraud JM, Laventure S, Ladam A, Capot P, et al. (2001) Suburban transmission of Q fever in French Guiana: evidence of a wild reservoir. J Infect Dis 184: 278–284.
27. Karagiannis I, Schimmer B, Van Lier A, Timen A, Schneeberger P, et al. (2009) Investigation of a Q fever outbreak in a rural area of The Netherlands. Epidemiol Infect 137: 1283–1294.
28. Lyytikainen O, Ziese T, Schwartlander B, Matzdorff P, Kuhnhen C, et al. (1998) An outbreak of sheep-associated Q fever in a rural community in Germany. Eur J Epidemiol 14: 193–199.
29. Nebreda T, Contreras E, Jesus Merino F, Dodero E, Campos A (2001) [Outbreak of Q fever and seroprevalence in a rural population from Soria Province]. Enferm Infecc Microbiol Clin 19: 57–60.
30. Stein A, Raoult D (1999) Pigeon pneumonia in provence: a bird-borne Q fever outbreak. Clin Infect Dis 29: 617–620.
31. Langley JM, Marrie TJ, Covert A, Waag DM, Williams JC (1988) Poker players' pneumonia. An urban outbreak of Q fever following exposure to a parturient cat. N Engl J Med 319: 354–356.
32. Oren I, Kraoz Z, Hadani Y, Kassis I, Zaltzman-Bershadsky N, et al. (2005) An outbreak of Q fever in an urban area in Israel. Eur J Clin Microbiol Infect Dis 24: 338–341.
33. Schimmer B, Ter Schegget R, Wegdam M, Zuchner L, de Bruin A, et al. (2010) The use of a geographic information system to identify a dairy goat farm as the most likely source of an urban Q-fever outbreak. BMC Infect Dis 10: 69.
34. Raoult D, Marrie T, Mege J (2005) Natural history and pathophysiology of Q fever. Lancet Infect Dis 5: 219–226.
35. Gidding HF, Wallace C, Lawrence GL, McIntyre PB (2009) Australia's national Q fever vaccination program. Vaccine 27: 2037–2041.
36. Marmion B (2007) Q fever: the long journey to control by vaccination. Med J Aust 186: 164–166.
37. Henning K, Hotzel H, Peters M, Welge P, Popps W, et al. (2009) [Unanticipated outbreak of Q fever during a study using sheep, and its significance for further projects]. Berl Munch Tierarztl Wochenschr 122: 13–19.

23

Isolation and Characterization of Methicillin-Resistant *Staphylococcus aureus* from Pork Farms and Visiting Veterinary Students

Timothy S. Frana[1]*, Aleigh R. Beahm[1], Blake M. Hanson[2], Joann M. Kinyon[1], Lori L. Layman[1], Locke A. Karriker[1], Alejandro Ramirez[1], Tara C. Smith[2]

1 Department of Veterinary Diagnostic and Production Animal Medicine, College of Veterinary Medicine, Iowa State University, Ames, Iowa, United States of America,
2 University of Iowa, Center for Emerging Infectious Diseases, Department of Epidemiology, College of Public Health, Iowa City, Iowa, United States of America

Abstract

In the last decade livestock-associated methicillin-resistant *S. aureus* (LA-MRSA) has become a public health concern in many parts of the world. Sequence type 398 (ST398) has been the most commonly reported type of LA-MRSA. While many studies have focused on long-term exposure experienced by swine workers, this study focuses on short-term exposures experienced by veterinary students conducting diagnostic investigations. The objectives were to assess the rate of MRSA acquisition and longevity of carriage in students exposed to pork farms and characterize the recovered MRSA isolates. Student nasal swabs were collected immediately before and after farm visits. Pig nasal swabs and environmental sponge samples were also collected. MRSA isolates were identified biochemically and molecularly including *spa* typing and antimicrobial susceptibility testing. Thirty (30) veterinary students were enrolled and 40 pork farms were visited. MRSA was detected in 30% of the pork farms and in 22% of the students following an exposure to a MRSA-positive pork farm. All students found to be MRSA-positive initially following farm visit were negative for MRSA within 24 hours post visit. Most common *spa* types recovered were t002 (79%), t034 (16%) and t548 (4%). *Spa* types found in pork farms closely matched those recovered from students with few exceptions. Resistance levels to antimicrobials varied, but resistance was most commonly seen for spectinomycin, tetracyclines and neomycin. Non-ST398 MRSA isolates were more likely to be resistant to florfenicol and neomycin as well as more likely to be multidrug resistant compared to ST398 MRSA isolates. These findings indicate that MRSA can be recovered from persons visiting contaminated farms. However, the duration of carriage was very brief and most likely represents contamination of nasal passages rather than biological colonization. The most common *spa* types found in this study were associated with ST5 and expands the range of livestock-associated MRSA types.

Editor: J. Ross Fitzgerald, University of Edinburgh, United Kingdom

Funding: TCS is partially supported through research funding from The National Institute for Occupational Safety and Health K01OH009793 (http://www.cdc.gov/niosh/). The funders had no role in study design, data collection and analysis, decision to publish, or preparation of the manuscript. No additional external funding was received for this study.

* E-mail: tfrana@iastate.edu

Introduction

Staphylococcus aureus is a common bacterium found on the skin and nasal passages of healthy people. Approximately 25–40% of the population is colonized with *S. aureus*. It is also a common cause of skin and soft tissue infections and sometimes causes severe disease such as pneumonia, bacteremia, meningitis, sepsis, and pericarditis. *S. aureus* bacteria harboring the *mecA* gene are resistant to methicillin and other β-lactam antimicrobials and are referred to as methicillin-resistant *S. aureus* (MRSA). In the United States it is estimated that 1.5% of the population (~4.1 million persons) is colonized with MRSA [1] leading to at least 94,000 invasive infections and over 18,000 deaths annually [2]. Various categories of MRSA based on epidemiologic characteristics are commonly used and include healthcare-associated MRSA (HA-MRSA), community-associated MRSA (CA-MRSA) and livestock-associated MRSA (LA-MRSA). HA-MRSA infections are most commonly found in immunocompromised people who have spent time in hospitals or healthcare centers, while CA-MRSA infections occur among otherwise healthy adults and children in the wider community. Livestock-associated MRSA (LA-MRSA) refers to strains of MRSA in which animals, particularly production animals, serve as the main reservoir of infection to humans.

LA-MRSA emerged as a public health concern in 2005 with reports of a specific multilocus sequence type (ST398) being found in higher than expected numbers in swine workers in France and the Netherlands [3–5]. Since ST398 was found at high levels in both pigs and pig farmers and very low levels in the general population, it was initially referred to as the "swine-associated" MRSA. Several studies attempting to determine the prevalence of ST398 in pigs have been conducted including a large multinational study conducted by the European Food Safety Authority (EFSA) which found the prevalence of MRSA ST398 in swine farms to be 25.5% but varied from 0% to 50.2% among European Union Member States [6]. In Ontario, Canada a study found that 25% of the pigs from 20 farms were colonized with MRSA and that ST398 was the predominant sequence type [7]. A study in the U. S. examined 299 animals from two swine production systems in Iowa and Illinois and 45% were found to carry MRSA. All isolates typed were ST398 [8].

It is apparent that those workers who spend considerable time in production animal farms are more likely to carry MRSA than those who don't. One study in The Netherlands demonstrated a 26% carriage rate among pig farmers [4]. The Canadian and U. S. studies previously mentioned found MRSA is 20% and 45%, respectively, in the swine workers tested. Isolates obtained from swine and their human caretakers are frequently indistinguishable, suggesting transmission between the two animal species [7]. Several studies have indicated that veterinarians working with swine are more likely to carry MRSA, primarily ST398, than non-swine focused colleagues [9–12]. While there are concerns that ST398 may establish itself in people, it appears that human to human spread of ST398 is limited [13,14] and transmissibility within hospitals is less likely than non-ST398 MRSA strains [15,16]. Additionally, colonization in persons exposed to livestock appears to be dependent on intensity of animal contact [17]. Studies indicate that short-term exposure to MRSA-positive pig farms does not lead to long-term colonization [17,18]. Similar studies assessing the risk of short but intense exposure to MRSA-positive pork farms in the U. S. have not been done. Therefore the objectives of this study were to: i) assess the rate of MRSA acquisition and longevity of carriage in uncolonized students exposed to pork farms during the two week course, ii) characterize recovered MRSA isolates by *spa* typing and antimicrobial susceptibility testing to assess the relatedness between pork farms and veterinary student isolates.

Methods

Ethics Statement

The ISU Institutional Review Board (IRB) approved the protocols. Animal samples tested were obtained from samples submitted as part of the diagnostic workup for field case investigations and did not require institutional animal care committee (IACUC) approval. All animals sampled were under a valid veterinary-client-patient relationship (VCPR).

Enrollment

Veterinary students were provided written informed consent and voluntarily enrolled during participation in swine courses at Iowa State University (ISU) from May to November, 2010. Students answered a short questionnaire related to potential risk factors for MRSA such as recent respiratory illness with fever and sore throat, skin or soft tissue infections (SSTI), antibiotic use, hospitalization, visitation to pork production or prior diagnosis of MRSA. Age and gender information was also collected. Students participated in diagnostic investigations at pork farms as would normally occur during the two-week clinical swine medicine fourth year elective course. Diagnostic investigations at pork farms were based on requests to ISU Veterinary Diagnostic and Production Animal Medicine (VDPAM) department by swine veterinarians and producers seeking assistance with animal health-related problems. Students were randomly assigned to an investigation and were generally at the pork farms for 3 to 4 hours. No prior knowledge of MRSA status or MRSA-related disease in pigs or humans at the pork farms was available. The type of farm and approximate age of animals were recorded at the time of visit, but no further farm data was made available for this study.

Sample collection

Student. Students were sampled at the following intervals: 1) the beginning of the course before any visits to pork farms, 2) before entry into a pork farm, 3) immediately after leaving a pork farm, 4) weekends or non-visit weekdays during the course, 5) daily for 4 consecutive days after the end of the clinical swine medicine course. Sample collection was accomplished by using sterile swabs (BBL CultureSwab, Sparks, MD) containing Stuart's medium inserted approximately 2 cm into one naris, rotated against the anterior nasal mucosa and repeated with same swab in second naris. The swabs were transported on ice to the ISU Veterinary Diagnostic Laboratory (VDL) within 6 hours. All samples were submitted using an assigned student study ID and date.

Animal. As part of the routine diagnostic investigation, when nasal samples were collected from manually restrained pigs for other diagnostic purposes, 3–5 of these nasal samples where then also submitted for MRSA testing. All samples were obtained as part of normal diagnostic investigation during student visit using materials and techniques described above for students. Samples were identified using a sample kit ID and date. Pigs were selected from pens with and without illness. Health status of the pig was not included when the sample was forwarded for MRSA testing.

Environmental. The environmental samples were collected from the same farms visited by participating students during the time of the visit. The sampling sites included, but were not limited to, treatment carts, fences and gates. Typically swab samples were collected from 3–5 areas in each farm. Samples were acquired by swabbing an approximate three square inch area with a sterile Speci-Sponge (Nasco, Fort Atkinson, WI) in 5 ml of enrichment broth, placed in Whirlpak bag, and transported on ice to the ISU VDL within 6 hours. Samples were identified using the date and same sample kit ID used for animal samples.

To maintain client confidentiality, each farm was assigned a farm study ID by an individual not involved in the study. A master spreadsheet was created that included the farm ID, sample kit ID, student IDs that visited the farm, sampling date, farm type, and approximate pig age.

Isolation and identification of bacteria

Student and pig nasal swabs were inoculated directly into 2 ml of enrichment broth containing 10 g tryptone/L, 75 g NaCl/L, 10 g mannitol/L and 2.5 g yeast extract/L. Bags containing environmental sponges received an additional 10 ml of enrichment broth. Samples were incubated for 24 h at 35°C, then inoculated onto selective MRSA agar plates (MRSASelect, Bio-Rad, Hercules, CA), which were then incubated for 24–48 hours at 35°C. All plates were examined for MRSA and *Staphylococcus* species. Up to 3 suspect colonies from each sample were further identified by biochemical tests (coagulase, maltose, lactose, trehalose, and Voges-Proskauer). All *S. aueus* isolates were screened for methicillin resistance by disc diffusion (6 µg/ml oxacillin) on Mueller Hinton agar with 2% NaCL. Oxacillin-resistant isolates were tested for the presence of penicillin binding protein 2′ (PBP 2a) using latex agglutination kit (MRSA latex agglutination test, Oxoid Ltd., Hants, UK). At least one *S. aureus* isolate which was also PBP 2a positive from given sample was forwarded for molecular testing.

Molecular testing

Genomic DNA was extracted using the Wizard Genomic DNA preparation kit (Promega, Madison, WI). Polymerase Chain Reaction (PCR) was performed on all isolates. A multiplex PCR assay was used to determine the presence of the *mecA* gene, and the *nuc* gene (present only in *S. aureus*) [19]). Amplification of the

Staphylococcus protein A (*spa*) gene was performed through PCR as previously described [20], using primers validated for use with Ridom-StaphType software [21]. The presence of PVL toxin genes (*lukS*, *lukF*) was determined by an additional PCR [22]. All molecular procedures utilized known positive and negative controls.

Antimicrobial Susceptibility Testing

Isolates were selected for antimicrobial susceptibility testing by broth dilution using minimum inhibitory concentration (MIC) method as described by the Clinical and Laboratory Standards Institute [23] using TREK Veterinary Sensititre equipment (Thermo Fisher Scientific, Cleveland, OH). Isolates were tested for susceptibility to chlortetracycline (CHL), clindamycin (CLI), enrofloxacin (ENR), florfenicol (FLO), gentamicin (GEN), neomycin (NEO), oxytetracycline (OXY), spectinomycin (SPE), sulfadimethoxine (SUL), tiamulin (TIA), tilmicosin, (TIL) and trimethoprim/sulfamethoxazole (TMP/SMZ). Beta-lactam antimicrobials were not considered. Breakpoints used for interpretation of resistance were based on information provided by TREK Diagnostic Systems and were as follows: CHL ($\geq$8 μg/ml), CLI ($\geq$2 μg/ml), ENR ($\geq$1 μg/ml), FLO ($\geq$4 μg/ml), GEN ($\geq$8 μg/ml), NEO ($\geq$8 μg/ml), OXY ($\geq$8 μg/ml), SPE ($\geq$32 μg/ml), TIA ($\geq$32 μg/ml), TIL ($\geq$16 μg/ml), TMP/SMZ ($\geq$2 μg/ml). Multidrug resistance was defined as resistance to $\geq$4 antimicrobials. The reference strain *S. aureus* ATCC 29213 served as a quality control strain in the MIC determinations.

Data Analysis

Descriptive analyses were initially performed. Factor associations were investigated using χ^2 analysis and assessed with Fisher's exact test. Associations were deemed significant at $p<0.05$ level and subsequently odd ratios (OR) determined as appropriate. No allowance was made for multiple comparisons. Statistical analysis of data sets was performed using SAS software, version 9.1 (SAS Institute, Inc., Cary, NC).

Results

Pork farms samples

Forty (40) pork farms of various types and animal age groups were visited during the study period. No farm was visited more than once. MRSA was detected in 30% (12/40) of the pork farms tested by either pig or environmental sampling. Two sites did not have pig samples collected, but were positive for MRSA from the environmental samples. A total of 362 samples were collected from these sites including 194 from pigs and 168 from the environment. Overall MRSA was detected in 17.4% (63/362) of the samples tested including 17.5% (34/194) of the pig samples and 17.3% (29/168) of the environmental samples. In MRSA-positive farms, either animal or environmental samples were positive 60.1% (63/104) of the time. Of these, 69.4% (34/49) of pig samples and 52.7% (29/55) of environmental samples were MRSA-positive. There was no significant differences in MRSA detection between pig and environmental samples ($p=0.08$). Pig and environmental sample results at the farm level matched 97.4% (37/38) of the time. The type of farm and age of animals was recorded for 82.5% (33/40) farms visits. In MRSA-positive farms, pigs less than 10 weeks of age were nearly 6 times (OR 5.95; 95% CI 1.22–28.95) more likely to also be present than not. Pork farm sample testing results are summarized in Table 1.

Student samples

Thirty (30) veterinary students were enrolled in a study. Only one student elected not to participate as she was taking the clinical swine course for a second time. Complete questionnaires were available for 29 students. The mean student age was 26.4 with a range of 24–35. Twenty females and 10 males participated in the study. Seven students reported using antibiotics in the previous 3 months. Also in previous 3 months, 0, 3, 1, 17 students reported hospitalization, respiratory disease with fever, SSTI, and pork farm visit, respectively. One student reported diagnosis of MRSA occurring 7 years prior. All students were negative for MRSA by nasal swab on the initial sampling. Six hundred and four (604) student samples were collected during the study period and MRSA was detected in 8 samples (1.3%, 8/604). Twenty-one (70%, 21/30) students visited MRSA-positive pork farms at least once and 6 students visited MRSA-positive farms on two separate occasions. Therefore, there were 27 student exposure events and MRSA was detected 6 times in separate students (22.2%, 6/27). MRSA was detected in 5 of these 6 students from the first nasal sample following the visit to a MRSA-positive farm. In one student MRSA was not detected until 5 days after a visit to a MRSA-positive farm. MRSA was not detected in any student for more than 24 hours, and no student subsequently became MRSA-positive again during the study period. MRSA was not detected in any student following visits to pork farms which were negative for MRSA. There was no significant association between detection of MRSA and recent respiratory disease with fever ($p=0.53$), recent antimicrobial use ($p=0.29$), SSTI ($p=0.29$), or recent swine farm visit ($p=0.15$). Additionally MRSA detection was not associated with gender ($p=1.00$) or multiple exposures to MRSA-positive farms ($p=0.62$). Age range in the exposed group was 24–35 years old. However, all except one student were between 24 and 28 years old. Therefore, age was not analyzed for risk. No students reported symptoms compatible with staphylococcal infections during the study period.

Molecular testing

One hundred and six isolates from 69 separate samples were positive for both *mecA* and *nuc* genes and negative for PVL genes. All 106 MRSA isolates were *spa*-typed and results are shown in Table 2. In summary, six *spa* types were found including: t002 (78.3%; n=83), t034 (14.2%; n=15), t548 (4.7%; n=5), t10065 (0.9%, n=1), t126 (0.9%; n=1), and t1107 (0.9%; n=1). The *spa* types found in pork farms from either pig or environmental samples included: t002, t034, t548 and t10065. The *spa* types found in students included: t002, t034, t548, t1107, and t126. The sequence types (MLST) that have been associated with these *spa* types includes: ST398 (t034, t10065) [24,25], ST5 (t002, t548, t1107) [21,25,26], and ST72 (t126) [21].

Pig and environmental *spa* types matched in all MRSA-positive farms with two exceptions. In one site, t034 was recovered from pig samples and one environmental sample. However, a second environmental sample from the same site was positive for MRSA with *spa* type t10065, which appears be a derivative of t034. In another site, t548 was recovered from all pig samples and t002 recovered from all environment samples. Both of these *spa* types (t548, t002) are associated with ST5 [25]. The *spa* type recovered from students and the pork farms closely matched those recovered from students with two exceptions; i) three *spa* types (t1107, t002, t548) were recovered from a student within 24 hours following exposure to a MRSA-positive farm where only t002 and t548 was detected. However, t1107 is also considered to be associated with ST5. ii) *spa* type t126, ST72-associated, was isolated from a student 5 days following exposure to a MRSA-positive farm with only *spa*

Table 1. Overview of the characteristics for the pork farms visited in this study.

Facility Type	Age Range/Group	Pigs <10 weeks of age present	Number in study	Number with MRSA
Finisher	10–27 weeks	No	20	4
Farrow to finish	All age groups	Yes	3	0
Farrow to feeder	Birth – 10 weeks and Adults	Yes	5	5
Nursery	3–10 weeks	Yes	1	1
Sow Farm	Birth – 3 weeks and Adults	Yes	3	1
Gilt Developer	3–8 months	No	1	0
Unknown	NA*	NA*	7	1
Total			40	12

*NA = Not available.

type t002 detected. This isolate may represent exposure to a MRSA source not associated with pork farms. The combined results from pork farms and veterinary students are shown in Table 3.

Antimicrobial Susceptibility

Antimicrobial susceptibility panel testing (AST) was performed on 67 MRSA isolates from separate samples. Sources of MRSA isolates for AST included: pigs (n = 31), environment (n = 28) and students (n = 8). The spa types for AST included: t002 (n = 51), t034 (n = 12) and t548 (n = 4). Resistant levels to antimicrobials for all isolates included: CHL (n = 58, 86.6%), CLI (n = 31, 46.3%), ENR (n = 11, 16.4%), FLO (n = 26, 38.8%), GEN (n = 15, 22.4%), NEO (n = 49, 73.1%), OXY (n = 58, 86.6%), SPE (n = 67, 100%), SUL (n = 2, 3.0%), TIA (n = 15, 22.4%), TIL (n = 23, 34.3%), TMP-SMZ (n = 0, 0.0%) Percentage of all isolates that were resistant to a given antimicrobial is shown in Figure 1. Significant differences in level of resistance by source were seen only with enrofloxacin ($p = 0.024$) and florfenicol ($p = 0.0006$). The student isolates were more resistant than farm isolates for both anti-microbials. Significant differences in level of antimicrobial resistance among spa types were seen for: FLO ($p = 0.0002$), NEO ($p = <0.0001$), and TIL ($p = 0.01$) as shown in Figure 2. When related spa types (t002, t548) were combined, significant differences compared to t034 were found for only FLO ($p = 0.002$) and NEO ($p = <0.0001$) (Figure 3). In the case of NEO, if resistance was found the odds that the isolate was either t002 or t548 was very high (OR = 75.4, 95% CI = 8.4–677.6). There was 23 different resistant profiles in the isolates tested. The most common resistant phenotypes are shown in Table 4. Sixty -four (95.5%, 64/67)

isolates were resistant to 3 or more antimicrobials. One isolate was resistant to 10 antimicrobials (t002; CHL-CLI-FLO-GEN-NEO-OXY-SPE-SUL-TIA-TIL). Combined resistance to tetracyclines (CHL, OXY), neomycin, and spectinomycin was seen in 67.2% (45/67) of the isolates overall but only in 8.3% (1/12) of the ST398 isolates. The proportion of multidrug-resistant isolates (≥4 antimicrobials) was higher in non-ST398 MRSA (94.5%, 52/55) versus ST398 (58.3%, 7/12) isolates ($p = 0.0005$).

Discussion

MRSA transmission to students

In this study we investigated the transmission dynamics associated with MRSA found in pork farms. We found that following short-term exposure (3–4 hr) to MRSA-positive pork farms, MRSA could be detected in students approximately 22% of the time. However, MRSA was not detected in any students for more than one day post-farm visit and did not reappear later on in the study. This suggests that the strains of MRSA from the pork farms did not become established in the students. These findings are consistent with other studies investigating LA-MRSA that have shown that short-term exposure to production animal farms does not lead to colonization [18,27] or that carriage rapidly decreases when exposure is removed [17]. Studies have investigated the prevalence of MRSA in occupationally exposed people such as veterinarians with varying results. Some studies have used convenience sampling conducted at meetings or conferences and found detectable MRSA in swine veterinarians at levels such as 3% [28], 3.9% [11], and 12.5% [29]. A cross-sectional study found the prevalence of MRSA in livestock veterinarians to be

Table 2. Summary of the spa types and motifs from MRSA isolates found in this study overall and by source of isolation.

Spa type	Associated MLST	Motif	Overall	Pigs	Environment	Students
t002	ST5	26-23-17-34-17-20-17-12-17-16	83/106 (78.3%)	42/56 (75.0%)	31/37 (83.8%)	10/13 (76.9%)
t034	ST398	08-16-02-25-02-25-34-24-25	15/106 (14.2%)	10/56 (17.9%)	5/37 (13.5%)	-
t548	ST5	26-23-17-34-17-20-17-12-16	5/106 (4.7%)	4/56 (7.1%)	-	1/13 (7.7%)
t10065	ST398	02-16-12-25-02-25-34-24-25	1/106 (0.9%)	-	1/37 (2.7%)	-
t126	ST72	07-23-12-21-17-12-12-17	1/106 (0.9%)	-	-	1/13 (7.7%)
t1107	ST5	26-17-20-17-12-16	1/106 (0.9%)	-	-	1/13 (7.7%)

Table 3. Combined results of environmental, pig, and veterinary student testing from MRSA-positive pork production sites.

Type of Facility	Pig Results[a]	Pig *spa* types	Environmental Results[a]	Environmental *spa* types	Student Results[b]	Student *spa* types
Finisher	NA		2/3	t002	0/1	
Finisher	NA		3/3	t002	0/1	
Sow Farm	4/5	t002	1/5	t002	3/3	t002; t126[c]
Nursery	1/5	t034	2/5	t034	0/3	
Finisher	5/5	t034	2/5	t034; t10065	0/3	
Finisher	2/5	t034	2/5	t034	0/2	
Farrow to Feeder	4/4	t002	2/4	t002	0/1	
Farrow to Feeder	5/5	t002	3/5	t002	1/3	t002
Farrow to Feeder	0/5		1/5	t002	0/3	
Farrow to Feeder	3/5	t002	2/5	t002	0/2	
Farrow to Feeder	5/5	t002	4/5	t002	1/3	t002
Unknown	5/5	t548	5/5	t002	1/2	t002; t548; t1107[d]
Total	**34/49**		**29/55**		**6/27**	

[a]Number of MRSA-positive samples/number of samples collected. [b]Number of MRSA-positive students/number of students exposed. [c]*Spa* type t126 was isolated from a student 5 days following exposure to MRSA-positive site. [d]Three *spa* types (t002, t548, t1107) from same student.

1.4% and 9.5% in Denmark and Belgium, respectively [30], while an epidemiological study in Germany found 23% of meat inspectors, laboratory personnel, and veterinarians tested were positive for MRSA ST398 [12]. Differences in prevalence can be expected based on geographic location, frequency of exposure, time since exposure, veterinary practices and study design. However, the level of MRSA detection in students enrolled in this study is rather consistent with other veterinarian prevalence

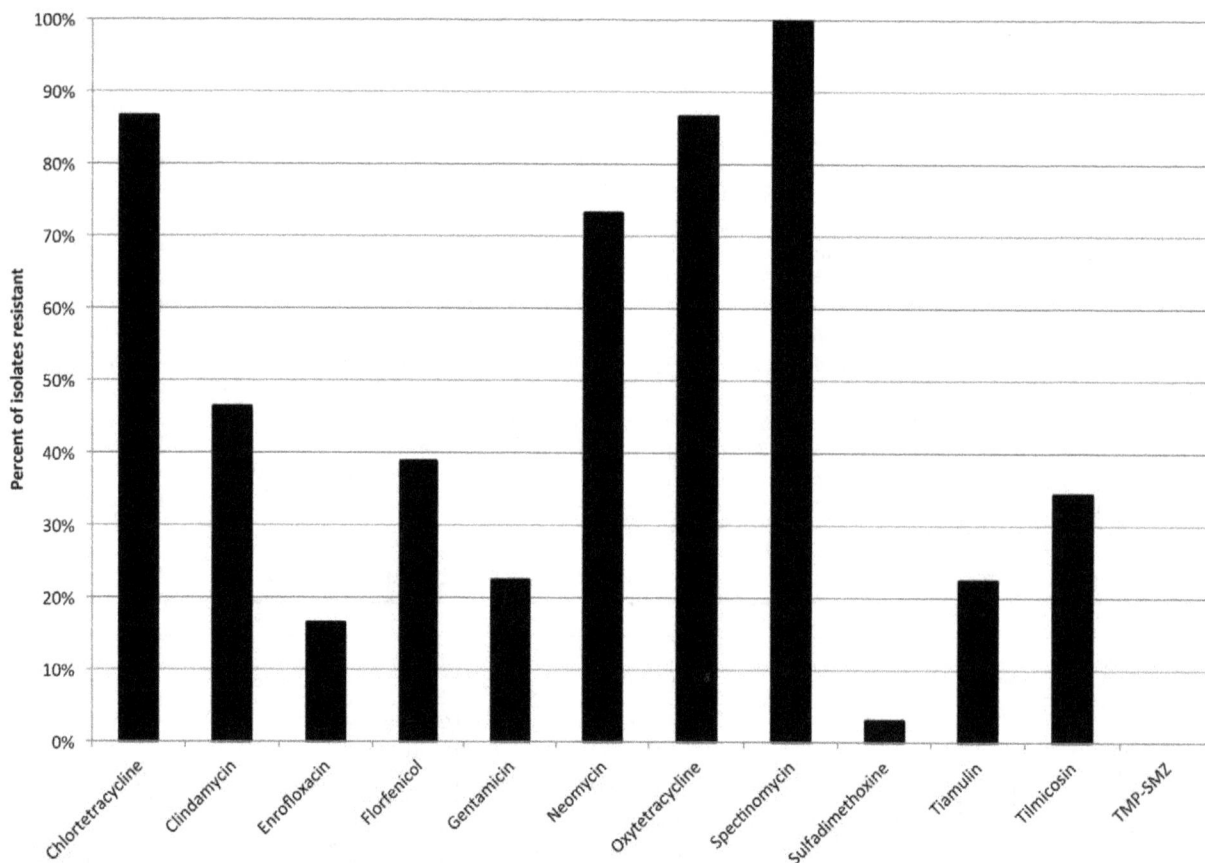

Figure 1. Antimicrobial resistance of MRSA isolates from pork farms and students. Results from 67 isolates tested.

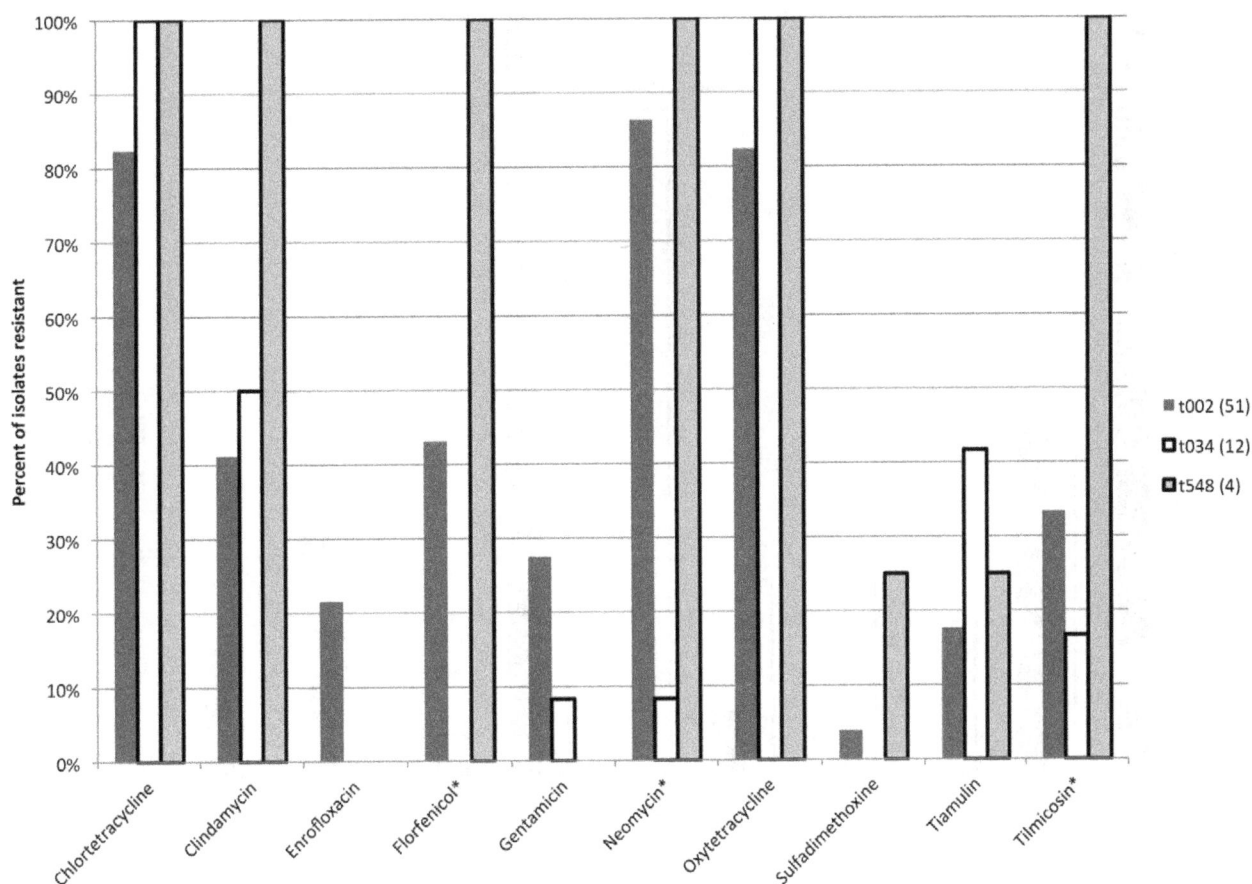

Figure 2. Antimicrobial resistance of MRSA isolates from pork farms and students. Number of isolates tested in parenthesis. Significantly different antimicrobial results across *spa* types indicated with asterisk (*).

studies indicating that this study may accurately represent the occupational exposure encountered by swine veterinarians. Additionally this study might provide insight into possible transmission risk to other sectors of the population with limited animal contact, such as agricultural fairgoers or petting zoo visitors. An advantage of this study over point-in-time prevalence studies is that participants were sampled frequently over time and therefore represents true incidence and temporal association to exposure. Although certain risk factors were investigated in this study (i.e. recent respiratory illness, SSTI, antibiotic use, hospitalization, pork farm visit), sample size limits the extent to which any conclusions can be drawn regarding these risk factors. Future studies targeting known MRSA-positive pork farms would increase the level of exposure and allow better assessment of human risk factors and MRSA colonization, but this would require a different approach than what could be achieved with the limitations associated with this study.

MRSA prevalence in pork farms

This study provides an estimate of the prevalence of MRSA on pork farms in the Midwestern U. S. While there have been a large number of studies examining prevalence of MRSA is pork farms in Europe [5,6,31–43], there have been rather few similar studies in the North America [7,8]. However, finding MRSA in 30% of the pork farms in this study is consistent with these studies (Smith 50%, Khanna 45%). If MRSA was detectable in a farm it was generally easily detectable by either pig or environmental samples.

MRSA was detected in approximately 60% of the samples collected at MRSA-positive farms. A higher level of detection was seen in pigs from MRSA-positive farms, but the results were not conclusive. In fact, in one farm all pigs were negative while MRSA was detectable in the environment. In all farms with both pig and environmental testing MRSA status matched 97.4% (37/38) of the time indicating either method is equally likely to detect MRSA from a positive farm. Environmental dust samples have been used for surveillance purposes in other studies [6,44] and in practice environmental samples are a more convenient method of collection versus live animals. Although this study was not designed to assess risk factors for MRSA on pork farms, there was a strong relationship between presence of young pigs (<10 weeks of age) and detection of MRSA (OR = 5.95). Other studies have reported an age-related association with MRSA status with highest prevalence reported in piglets between 6–12 weeks of age [8,45].

spa types

The findings of many studies investigating MRSA in pork farms have indicated that ST398 is the predominant MLST present. In fact, discovery of an untypeable strain of MRSA in the Netherlands and subsequent investigations linking this strain to ST398 and pork farms initiated the process leading to the term "livestock-associated" MRSA [4,5,9,31,46,47]. There were 6 *spa* types observed in this study (t002, t034, t126, t548, t1107, t10065) associated with 3 sequence types (ST5, ST398, ST72). However,

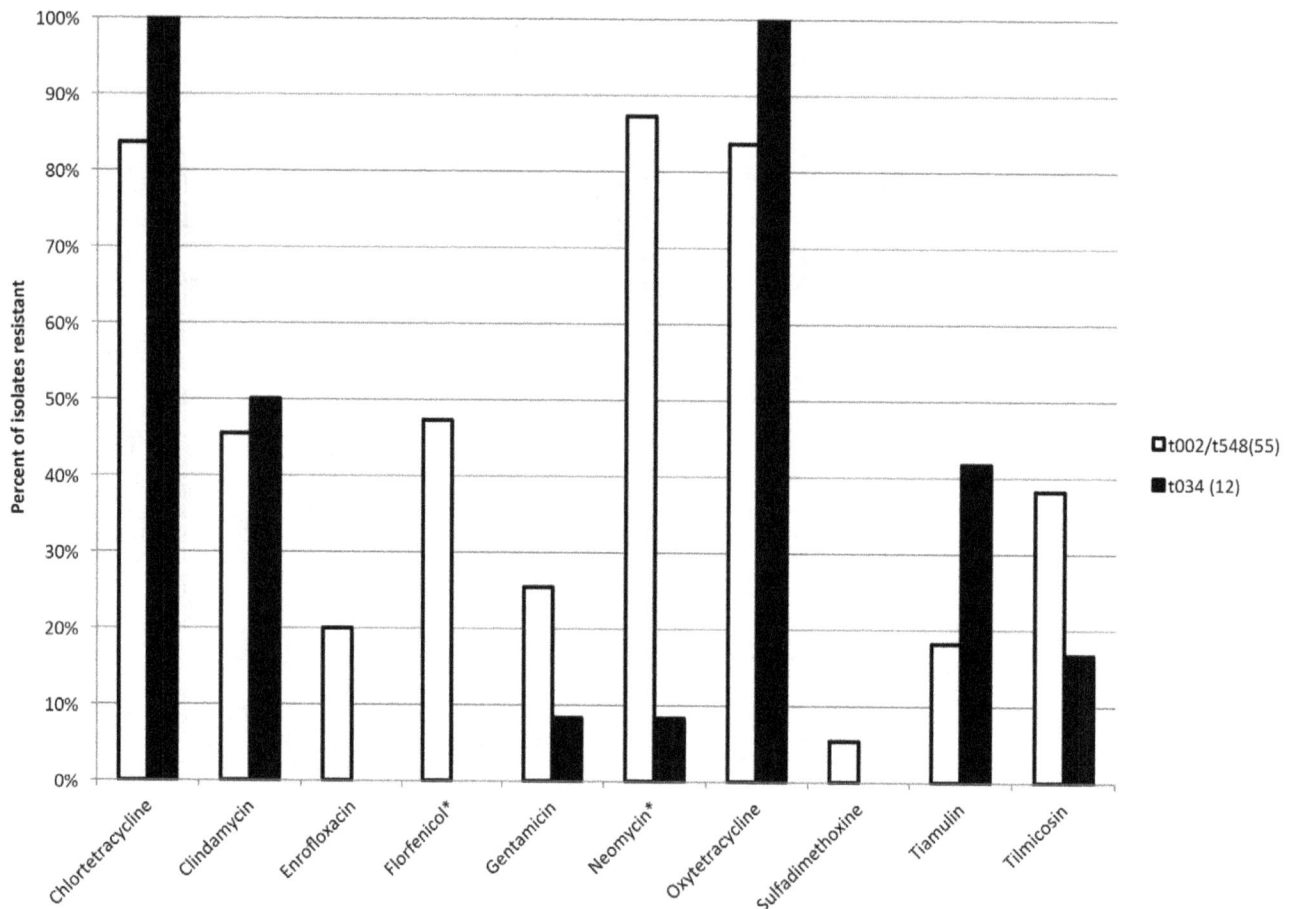

Figure 3. Antimicrobial resistance of MRSA isolates from pork farms and students by ST398 status. t034 considered ST398-associated and t002/t548 considered non-ST398-associated. Number of isolates tested in parenthesis. Significantly different antimicrobial results by *spa* types indicated with asterisk (*).

non-ST398 *spa* types (t002, t548, t1107) predominated and accounted for 84% of the *spa* types observed and were found on 75% MRSA-positive farms. On the other hand, ST398-associated *spa* types (t034, t10065) accounted for 15% of *spa* types observed and were found on only 3 of 12 MRSA-positive farms. MRSA ST5 has been isolated from backyard-raised pigs in Michigan [48] and MRSA t002 was found in Canadian pigs [7], pigs at agricultural fairs [49], U. S. pork products [50,51], and recently

from Ohio pork farms [52]. This study also documents MRSA ST5 subtypes (t002 or t548) directly from pork farms in the U.S. Other studies indicate that non-ST398 (ST9) MRSA strains can be found in pigs and pig carcasses in Asia [44,53–55]. Thus is appears that LA-MRSA is more diverse than ST398-associated strains and geographic differences exist.

Studies using whole-genome sequence typing have examined differences between livestock- origin and human- origin ST398

Table 4. Most prevalent antimicrobial resistant profiles found in MRSA isolates and associated *spa* types.

Resistance profile	No. isolates (%)	*spa* type(s) with pattern (#)
CHL-NEO-OXY-SPE	17/67 (25.4)	t002
CHL-CLI-FLO-NEO-OXY-SPE-TIL	10/67 (14.9)	t002 (7); t548 (3)
CHL-OXY-SPE	5/67 (7.5)	t034
CLI-ENR-FLO-GEN-NEO-SPE-TIL	3/67 (4.5)	t002
CHL-CLI-GEN-NEO-OXY-SPE-TIA	3/67 (4.5)	t002 (2); t034(1)
CHL-CLI-OXY-SPE-TIA	3/67 (4.5)	t034
CHL-FLO-NEO-OXY-SPE	3/67 (4.5)	t002

CHL = chlortetracycline, CLI = clindamycin, ENR = enrofloxacin, FLO = florfenicol, GEN = gentamicin, NEO = neomycin, OXY = oxytetracycline, SPE = spectinomycin, TIA = tiamulin, TIL = tilmicosin.

isolates [56,57]. The first study reported that human-associated isolates carried phages that were largely missing from livestock-associated isolates. These phages were associated with innate immunomodulatory genes and considered virulence factors in humans. The authors theorized that during the jump to livestock these genes were lost, antibiotic resistance genes gained, and the resulting strains became less capable of re-infecting humans. The Uhleman study similarly reported differences in mobile genetic elements between human- and livestock- associated ST398 strains, but also reported enhanced adhesion of human isolates to human skin keratinocytes and keratin. Both studies found that genes responsible for PVL toxin production were missing in all livestock-associated ST398 strains. Similarly, in our study all ST398 and non-ST398 isolates lack *lukS-lukF*. Taken together, a picture that appears to be emerging is one of initial transmission of human-associated *S. aureus* strains or subtypes to livestock facilitated by loss of human virulence factors. However once established in livestock, the ability to re-infect humans appears reduced, albeit not totally eliminated. MRSA ST398 is perhaps only one example of this process that may have occurred in other sequence types. A similar scenario was reported to be associated with the introduction of human *S. aureus* ST5 into chickens and broilers and subsequent global dissemination [58]. In that study, Lowder provided evidence that subtypes of ST5 found in poultry had undergone genetic diversification leading to acquisition of avian-specific accessory genes and inactivation of human virulence genes. This study suggests a similar process may have occurred with subtypes of ST5 leading to host-adaptation in swine with as yet only local distribution.

Antimicrobial resistance patterns

All isolates were resistant to spectinomycin, an aminocyclitol. Spectinomycin resistance in ST398 has been reported [59–61], however at lower levels than found here. Resistance to tetracycline derivatives (chlortetracycline, oxytetracycline) overall was quite high (87%). Tetracycline resistance is a common feature of ST398 [24,62], but was also found here with high frequency in non-ST398 isolates (84%). Aminoglycoside resistance (gentamicin, neomycin) averaged approximately 48% with neomycin resistance much higher than gentamicin. A striking difference in neomycin resistance between non-ST398 (87%) and ST398 (8%) isolates was observed. Macrolide resistance (tilmicosin) was 34% while lincosamide (clindamycin) resistance was just over 46%. As a class, the least resistance was seen with sulfonamides (sulfadimethoxine, trimethoprim/sulfamethoxazole). Fluoroquinolone (enrofloxacin) resistance was 16% and resistance to florfenicol, a phenicol derivative, was nearly 39%. A Belgian study [42] which tested 643 pig MRSA ST398 isolates reported similar resistant rates in comparable drug classes for tetracycline (100%), aminoglycosides (48%), macrolides (56%), and sulfonamides (2%). However, that study found higher resistance with lincosamides (73%), and fl17roquinolones (32%), and lower resistance to the phenicol derivative, chloramphenicol (5%). In this study pleuromutilin resistance (tiamulin) was 22%. Additionally, tiamulin resistance appeared to be associated with clindamycin resistance (12/15), which may indicate presence of *vga*(A) as recently reported in

ST398 [63]. There was a wide diversity of resistance phenotypes found in the isolates tested in this study with combined resistant to tetracyclines, neomycin, and spectinomycin seen most commonly particularly in ST5 subtypes. These subtypes were also more likely to be multidrug resistant.

Resistance patterns can be expected to vary based on location, drug approval, and farm level management. Due to study constraints, site-specific antimicrobial use was not recorded. Other limitations in this study include non-random selection of production sites and clustering of sites within production systems. Since the selection of pork production sites that were sampled was based on a request for assistance to the ISU Swine Production Group, presumably health-related problems existed at the farm. Management practices and farm conditions which contribute to health problems may also contribute to the presence of MRSA. Additionally, it is not uncommon for swine course diagnostic investigations to involve multiple pork farms within a common production system. Therefore, use of common practices, equipment, and breeding stock could lead to MRSA contamination of multiple farms and significantly affect the prevalence of particular MRSA strains. Detailed information on the pork farms was withheld in this study.

Conclusions

The findings from this study support some of the findings from other studies. We found that following short-term exposure to MRSA-positive pork farms MRSA could be detected in students 22% of the time, but this level of exposure did not lead to stable colonization in participants. The prevalence of MRSA in pork farms was 30%, which is lower than results from many prevalence studies in Europe, but similar to results from other studies in North America. One of the surprising findings was the predominance of ST5 subtypes on farms and in students. ST398 subtypes were not detected in any exposed student. It was interesting that some the characteristics of the these non-ST398 isolates resembled ST398 in that none contained the PVL toxin gene but were likely to be tetracycline resistant. However, non-ST398 isolates differed in their resistance profile particularly in regard to a high level of resistance to neomycin and association with multidrug phenotype. Further investigation of these isolates by molecular analysis is needed to determine if these isolates fit the pattern associated with LA-MRSA, but it seems likely that MRSA subtypes from multiple lineages have made the human-to-livestock leap. Whether the impediments to human re-adaptation remain in place is still unknown.

Acknowledgments

The authors would like to thank C. Wang and F. Liu at Iowa State University for their assistance with the data analysis.

Author Contributions

Conceived and designed the experiments: TSF ARB JMK LAK AR TCS. Performed the experiments: ARB BMH JMK LLL LAK AR. Analyzed the data: TSF ARB BMH. Contributed reagents/materials/analysis tools: TSF TCS. Wrote the paper: TSF ARB.

References

1. Gorwitz RJ, Kruszon-Moran D, McAllister SK, McQuillan G, McDougal LK, et al. (2008) Changes in the prevalence of nasal colonization with Staphylococcus aureus in the United States, 2001–2004. J Infect Dis 197: 1226–1234.
2. Klevens RM, Morrison MA, Nadle J, Petit S, Gershman K, et al. (2007) Invasive methicillin-resistant Staphylococcus aureus infections in the United States. JAMA 298: 1763–1771.
3. Armand-Lefevre L, Ruimy R, Andremont A (2005) Clonal comparison of Staphylococcus aureus isolates from healthy pig farmers, human controls, and pigs. Emerg Infect Dis 11: 711–714.
4. Voss A, Loeffen F, Bakker J, Klaassen C, Wulf M (2005) Methicillin-resistant Staphylococcus aureus in pig farming. Emerg Infect Dis 11: 1965–1966.

5. Huijsdens XW, van Dijke BJ, Spalburg E, van Santen-Verheuvel MG, Heck ME, et al. (2006) Community-acquired MRSA and pig-farming. Ann Clin Microbiol Antimicrob 5: 26.

6. EFSA (2009) Analysis of the Baseline Survey on the Prevalence of Methicillin-Resistant Staphylococcus aureus (MRSA) in Holdings with Breeding Pigs, in the EU, 2008 Part B: factors associated with MRSA contamination of holdings. Parma, Italy.

7. Khanna T, Friendship R, Dewey C, Weese JS (2008) Methicillin resistant Staphylococcus aureus colonization in pigs and pig farmers. Vet Microbiol 128: 298–303.

8. Smith TC, Male MJ, Harper AL, Kroeger JS, Tinkler GP, et al. (2009) Methicillin-resistant Staphylococcus aureus (MRSA) strain ST398 is present in midwestern U.S. swine and swine workers. PLoS One 4: e4258.

9. Wulf M, van Nes A, Eikelenboom-Boskamp A, de Vries J, Melchers W, et al. (2006) Methicillin-resistant Staphylococcus aureus in veterinary doctors and students, the Netherlands. Emerg Infect Dis 12: 1939–1941.

10. Wulf MW, Sorum M, van Nes A, Skov R, Melchers WJ, et al. (2008) Prevalence of methicillin-resistant Staphylococcus aureus among veterinarians: an international study. Clin Microbiol Infect 14: 29–34.

11. Moodley A, Nightingale EC, Stegger M, Nielsen SS, Skov RL, et al. (2008) High risk for nasal carriage of methicillin-resistant Staphylococcus aureus among Danish veterinary practitioners. Scand J Work Environ Health 34: 151–157.

12. Meemken D, Cuny C, Witte W, Eichler U, Staudt R, et al. (2008) [Occurrence of MRSA in pigs and in humans involved in pig production–preliminary results of a study in the northwest of Germany]. Dtsch Tierarztl Wochenschr 115: 132–139.

13. Cuny C, Nathaus R, Layer F, Strommenger B, Altmann D, et al. (2009) Nasal colonization of humans with methicillin-resistant Staphylococcus aureus (MRSA) CC398 with and without exposure to pigs. PLoS One 4: e6800.

14. van Cleef BA, Verkade EJ, Wulf MW, Buiting AG, Voss A, et al. (2010) Prevalence of livestock-associated MRSA in communities with high pig-densities in The Netherlands. PLoS One 5: e9385.

15. Wassenberg MW, Bootsma MC, Troelstra A, Kluytmans JA, Bonten MJ (2011) Transmissibility of livestock-associated methicillin-resistant Staphylococcus aureus (ST398) in Dutch hospitals. Clin Microbiol Infect 17(2): 316–9.

16. Bootsma MC, Wassenberg MW, Trapman P, Bonten MJ (2011) The nosocomial transmission rate of animal-associated ST398 meticillin-resistant Staphylococcus aureus. J R Soc Interface 8: 578–584.

17. Graveland H, Wagenaar JA, Bergs K, Heesterbeek H, Heederik D (2011) Persistence of livestock associated MRSA CC398 in humans is dependent on intensity of animal contact. PLoS One 6: e16830.

18. van Cleef BA, Graveland H, Haenen AP, van de Giessen AW, Heederik D, et al. (2011) Persistence of livestock-associated methicillin-resistant Staphylococcus aureus in field workers after short-term occupational exposure to pigs and veal calves. J Clin Microbiol 49: 1030–1033.

19. Louie L, Goodfellow J, Mathieu P, Glatt A, Louie M, et al. (2002) Rapid detection of methicillin-resistant staphylococci from blood culture bottles by using a multiplex PCR assay. J Clin Microbiol 40: 2786–2790.

20. Shopsin B, Gomez M, Montgomery SO, Smith DH, Waddington M, et al. (1999) Evaluation of protein A gene polymorphic region DNA sequencing for typing of Staphylococcus aureus strains. J Clin Microbiol 37: 3556–3563.

21. Ridom website. Available: http://www.ridom.de www.ridom.de. Accessed 2012 Aug 3.

22. Lina G, Piemont Y, Godail-Gamot F, Bes M, Peter MO, et al. (1999) Involvement of Panton-Valentine leukocidin-producing Staphylococcus aureus in primary skin infections and pneumonia. Clin Infect Dis 29: 1128–1132.

23. CLSI (2008) Performance Standards for Antimicrobial Disk and Dilution Susceptibility Tests for Bacteria Isolated From Animals. Approved Standard – Third Edition ed. Wayne, PA: Clinical and Laboratory Standards Institute.

24. Smith TC, Pearson N (2010) The Emergence of Staphylococcus aureus ST398. Vector Borne Zoonotic Dis: epub ahead of print.

25. Monecke S, Coombs G, Shore AC, Coleman DC, Akpaka P, et al. (2011) A field guide to pandemic, epidemic and sporadic clones of methicillin-resistant Staphylococcus aureus. PLoS One 6: e17936.

26. Strommenger B, Braulke C, Heuck D, Schmidt C, Pasemann B, et al. (2008) spa Typing of Staphylococcus aureus as a frontline tool in epidemiological typing. J Clin Microbiol 46: 574–581.

27. Van Den Broek IV, Van Cleef BA, Haenen A, Broens EM, Van Der Wolf PJ, et al. (2009) Methicillin-resistant Staphylococcus aureus in people living and working in pig farms. Epidemiol Infect 137: 700–708.

28. Huber H, Koller S, Giezendanner N, Stephan R, Zweifel C (2009) Prevalence and characteristics of meticillin-resistant Staphylococcus aureus in humans in contact with farm animals, in livestock, and in food of animal origin, Switzerland, 2009. Euro Surveill 15.

29. Wulf MW, Sørum M, van Nes A, Skov R, Melchers WJ, et al. (2008) Prevalence of methicillin-resistant Staphylococcus aureus among veterinarians: an international study. Clin Microbiol Infect 14: 29–34.

30. Garcia-Graells C, Antoine J, Larsen J, Catry B, Skov R, et al. (2012) Livestock veterinarians at high risk of acquiring methicillin-resistant Staphylococcus aureus ST398. Epidemiol Infect 140: 383–389.

31. de Neeling AJ, van den Broek MJ, Spalburg EC, van Santen-Verheuvel MG, Dam-Deisz WD, et al. (2007) High prevalence of methicillin resistant Staphylococcus aureus in pigs. Vet Microbiol 122: 366–372.

32. Guardabassi L, Stegger M, Skov R (2007) Retrospective detection of methicillin resistant and susceptible Staphylococcus aureus ST398 in Danish slaughter pigs. Vet Microbiol 122: 384–386.

33. Lewis HC, Molbak K, Reese C, Aarestrup FM, Selchau M, et al. (2008) Pigs as source of methicillin-resistant Staphylococcus aureus CC398 infections in humans, Denmark. Emerg Infect Dis 14: 1383–1389.

34. Denis O, Suetens C, Hallin M, Catry B, Ramboer I, et al. (2009) Methicillin-resistant Staphylococcus aureus ST398 in swine farm personnel, Belgium. Emerg Infect Dis 15: 1098–1101.

35. Van Hoecke H, Piette A, De Leenheer E, Lagasse N, Struelens M, et al. (2009) Destructive otomastoiditis by MRSA from porcine origin. Laryngoscope 119: 137–140.

36. Kehrenberg C, Cuny C, Strommenger B, Schwarz S, Witte W (2009) Methicillin-resistant and -susceptible Staphylococcus aureus strains of clonal lineages ST398 and ST9 from swine carry the multidrug resistance gene cfr. Antimicrob Agents Chemother 53: 779–781.

37. Kock R, Harlizius J, Bressan N, Laerberg R, Wieler LH, et al. (2009) Prevalence and molecular characteristics of methicillin-resistant Staphylococcus aureus (MRSA) among pigs on German farms and import of livestock-related MRSA into hospitals. Eur J Clin Microbiol Infect Dis 28: 1375–1382.

38. Pomba C, Hasman H, Cavaco LM, da Fonseca JD, Aarestrup FM (2009) First description of meticillin-resistant Staphylococcus aureus (MRSA) CC30 and CC398 from swine in Portugal. Int J Antimicrob Agents 34: 193–194.

39. Battisti A, Franco A, Merialdi G, Hasman H, Iurescia M, et al. (2010) Heterogeneity among methicillin-resistant Staphylococcus aureus from Italian pig finishing holdings. Vet Microbiol 142: 361–366.

40. Riesen A, Perreten V (2009) Antibiotic resistance and genetic diversity in Staphylococcus aureus from slaughter pigs in Switzerland. Schweiz Arch Tierheilkd 151: 425–431.

41. Morcillo A, Castro B, Rodríguez-Álvarez C, González JC, Sierra A, et al. (2012) Prevalence and characteristics of methicillin-resistant Staphylococcus aureus in pigs and pig workers in Tenerife, Spain. Foodborne Pathog Dis 9: 207–210.

42. Crombé F, Willems G, Dispas M, Hallin M, Denis O, et al. (2012) Prevalence and antimicrobial susceptibility of methicillin-resistant Staphylococcus aureus among pigs in Belgium. Microb Drug Resist 18: 125–131.

43. Horgan M, Abbott Y, Lawlor PG, Rossney A, Coffey A, et al. (2011) A study of the prevalence of methicillin-resistant Staphylococcus aureus in pigs and in personnel involved in the pig industry in Ireland. Vet J 190: 255–259.

44. Wagenaar JA, Yue H, Pritchard J, Broekhuizen-Stins M, Huijsdens X, et al. (2009) Unexpected sequence types in livestock associated methicillin-resistant Staphylococcus aureus (MRSA): MRSA ST9 and a single locus variant of ST9 in pig farming in China. Vet Microbiol 139: 405–409.

45. Weese JS, Zwambag A, Rosendal T, Reid-Smith R, Friendship R (2011) Longitudinal Investigation of Methicillin-Resistant Staphylococcus aureus in Piglets. Zoonoses Public Health 58: 238–243.

46. van Loo I, Huijsdens X, Tiemersma E, de Neeling A, van de Sande-Bruinsma N, et al. (2007) Emergence of methicillin-resistant Staphylococcus aureus of animal origin in humans. Emerg Infect Dis 13: 1834–1839.

47. van Duijkeren E, Ikawaty R, Broekhuizen-Stins MJ, Jansen MD, Spalburg EC, et al. (2008) Transmission of methicillin-resistant Staphylococcus aureus strains between different kinds of pig farms. Vet Microbiol 126: 383–389.

48. Gordoncillo MJ, Abdujamilova N, Perri M, Donabedian S, Zervos M, et al. (2012) Detection of methicillin-resistant Staphylococcus aureus (MRSA) in backyard pigs and their owners, Michigan, USA. Zoonoses Public Health 59: 212–216.

49. Dressler AE, Scheibel RP, Wardyn S, Harper AL, Hanson BM, et al. (2012) Prevalence, antibiotic resistance and molecular characterisation of Staphylococcus aureus in pigs at agricultural fairs in the USA. Vet Rec 170: 495.

50. O'Brien AM, Hanson BM, Farina SA, Wu JY, Simmering JE, et al. (2012) MRSA in conventional and alternative retail pork products. PLoS One 7: e30092.

51. Hanson BM, Dressler AE, Harper AL, Scheibel RP, Wardyn SE, et al. (2011) Prevalence of Staphylococcus aureus and methicillin-resistant Staphylococcus aureus (MRSA) on retail meat in Iowa. J Infect Public Health 4: 169–174.

52. Molla B, Byrne M, Abley M, Mathews J, Jackson CR, et al. (2012) Epidemiology and Genotypic Characteristics of Methicillin-Resistant Staphylococcus aureus Strains of Porcine Origin. J Clin Microbiol 50: 3687–3693.

53. Cui S, Li J, Hu C, Jin S, Li F, et al. (2009) Isolation and characterization of methicillin-resistant Staphylococcus aureus from swine and workers in China. J Antimicrob Chemother 64: 680–683.

54. Guardabassi L, O'Donoghue M, Moodley A, Ho J, Boost M (2009) Novel lineage of methicillin-resistant Staphylococcus aureus, Hong Kong. Emerg Infect Dis 15: 1998–2000.

55. Neela V, Mohd Zafrul A, Mariana NS, van Belkum A, Liew YK, et al. (2009) Prevalence of ST9 methicillin-resistant Staphylococcus aureus among pigs and pig handlers in Malaysia. J Clin Microbiol 47: 4138–4140.

56. Price LB, Stegger M, Hasman H, Aziz M, Larsen J, et al. (2012) Staphylococcus aureus CC398: host adaptation and emergence of methicillin resistance in livestock. MBio 3.

57. Uhlemann AC, Porcella SF, Trivedi S, Sullivan SB, Hafer C, et al. (2012) Identification of a highly transmissible animal-independent Staphylococcus aureus ST398 clone with distinct genomic and cell adhesion properties. MBio 3.

58. Lowder BV, Guinane CM, Ben Zakour NL, Weinert LA, Conway-Morris A, et al. (2009) Recent human-to-poultry host jump, adaptation, and pandemic spread of Staphylococcus aureus. Proc Natl Acad Sci U S A 106: 19545–19550.

59. Kadlec K, Ehricht R, Monecke S, Steinacker U, Kaspar H, et al. (2009) Diversity of antimicrobial resistance pheno- and genotypes of methicillin-resistant Staphylococcus aureus ST398 from diseased swine. J Antimicrob Chemother 64: 1156–1164.

60. Overesch G, Büttner S, Rossano A, Perreten V (2011) The increase of methicillin-resistant Staphylococcus aureus (MRSA) and the presence of an unusual sequence type ST49 in slaughter pigs in Switzerland. BMC Vet Res 7: 30.

61. Jamrozy DM, Fielder MD, Butaye P, Coldham NG (2012) Comparative Genotypic and Phenotypic Characterisation of Methicillin-Resistant Staphylococcus aureus ST398 Isolated from Animals and Humans. PLoS One 7: e40458.

62. Graveland H, Duim B, van Duijkeren E, Heederik D, Wagenaar JA (2011) Livestock-associated methicillin-resistant Staphylococcus aureus in animals and humans. Int J Med Microbiol 301: 630–634.

63. Mendes RE, Smith TC, Deshpande L, Diekema DJ, Sader HS, et al. (2011) Plasmid-borne vga(A)-encoding gene in methicillin-resistant Staphylococcus aureus ST398 recovered from swine and a swine farmer in the United States. Diagn Microbiol Infect Dis 71: 177–180.

24

Interleukin-13 Genetic Variants, Household Carpet Use and Childhood Asthma

Ching-Hui Tsai[1], Kuan-Yen Tung[1,2], Ming-Wei Su[1], Bor-Luen Chiang[3], Fook Tim Chew[4], Nai-Wei Kuo[1], Yungling Leo Lee[1,2]*

1 Institute of Epidemiology and Preventive Medicine, College of Public Health, National Taiwan University, Taipei, Taiwan, **2** Research Center for Genes, Environment and Human Health, College of Public Health, National Taiwan University, Taipei, Taiwan, **3** Department of Pediatrics, National Taiwan University Hospital, Taipei, Taiwan, **4** Department of Biological Sciences, National University of Singapore, Singapore

Abstract

Interleukin (IL)-13 genetic polymorphisms have shown adverse effects on respiratory health. However, few studies have explored the interactive effects between *IL-13* haplotypes and environmental exposures on childhood asthma. The aims of our study are to evaluate the effects of *IL-13* genetic variants on asthma phenotypes, and explore the potential interaction between *IL-13* and household environmental exposures among Taiwanese children. We investigated 3,577 children in the Taiwan Children Health Study from 14 Taiwanese communities. Data regarding children's exposure and disease status were obtained from parents using a structured questionnaire. Four SNPs were tagged accounting for 100% of the variations in *IL-13*. Multiple logistic regression models with false-discovery rate (FDR) adjustments were fitted to estimate the effects of *IL-13* variants on asthma phenotypes. SNP rs1800925, SNP rs20541 and SNP rs848 were significantly associated with increased risks on childhood wheeze with FDR of 0.03, 0.04 and 0.04, respectively. Children carrying two copies of h1011 haplotype showed increased susceptibility to wheeze. Compared to those without carpet use and h1011 haplotype, children carrying h1011 haplotype and using carpet at home had significantly synergistic risks of wheeze (OR, 2.5; 95% CI, 1.4–4.4; p for interaction, 0.01) and late-onset asthma (OR, 4.7; 95% CI, 2.0–10.9; p for interaction, 0.02). In conclusions, *IL-13* genetic variants showed significant adverse effects on asthma phenotypes among children. The results also suggested that asthma pathogenesis might be mediated by household carpet use.

Editor: Guoying Wang, John Hopkins Bloomberg School of Public Health, United States of America

Funding: This study was supported by the National Science Council (Grant #96-2314-B-006-053, #98-2314-B-002-138-MY3 and #101-2314-B-002-113-MY3). The funders had no role in study design, data collection and analysis, decision to publish, or preparation of the manuscript.

Competing Interests: The authors have declared that no competing interests exist.

* E-mail: leolee@ntu.edu.tw

Introduction

Asthma not only results in morbidity or school absence in school children [1,2] but also leads to raising medical costs and social burden [3]. The prevalence of childhood asthma/wheeze has been reported as increasing globally [4,5]. Diverse genetic and environmental components have been noted for this complex disease. Recent studies have suggested that many genetic variants were associated with childhood asthma-related diseases that occur when environmental factors trigger immune responses [6,7].

Interleukin (IL)-13 is an important T-helper type 2 (Th$_2$) cytokine involved in the inflammation of asthmatic airways [8]. In animal models, pulmonary expression of IL-13 was reported to include eosinophilic tissue inflammation, subepithelial fibrosis, mucus hypersecretion and airway hyperresponsiveness (AHR) to methacholine [9,10]. Many epidemiological studies also revealed that the variants in the *IL-13* gene were associated with total IgE level, increased eosinophil count, atopy and asthma among children [11,12,13,14].

The most important risk factor in the development of allergic diseases such as asthma is induction of IgE against indoor allergens, and imbalance between T-helper type 1 (Th$_1$) and Th$_2$ cytokine responses for skewing to Th$_2$ response [15]. Household carpet use is known to be a reservoir of major indoor allergens [16], which have been suggested to increase airway inflammation and asthma in children [17,18]. Previous studies have shown that household environmental tobacco smoke (ETS) and *IL-13* genetic variants may have interactive effects on asthma phenotypes [19,20]. However, there is no related literature concerning the association between childhood exposure to household carpet use and *IL-13* genetic polymorphisms that might be involved in asthma susceptibility. Haplotype analyses of *IL-13* were also unclear among the Chinese population.

Taiwan Children Health Study (TCHS) is a population-based study representing a wide range of environmental factors and genetic susceptibility. TCHS offers an opportunity to investigate the gene-environment interactive effects on respiratory health. In present study, we explored the associations between *IL-13* genotypes/haplotypes, household carpet use and asthma phenotypes among children.

Materials and Methods

Study population

We conducted a population-based survey for children's health in 2007 and the study protocol has been described in detail

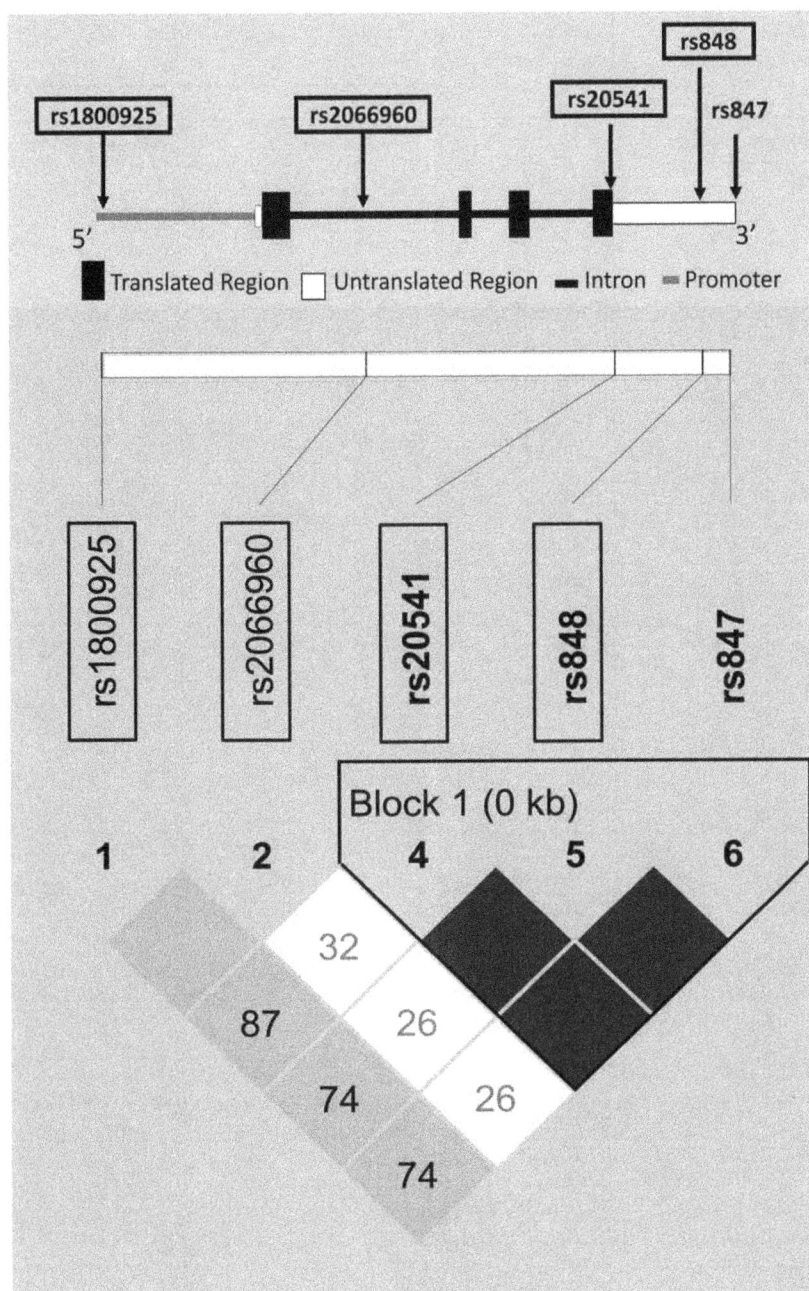

Figure 1. The location and LD of *IL-13* SNPs were plotted. D' is pairwise linkage disequilibrium using the Haploview program. The block structure of *IL-13* is defined by the confidence intervals of D'. D' values are displayed in the lozenge-shaped cells, and empty cells indicate D' = 1. Four SNPs (squared) are selected and they accounted for 100% of the variations in *IL-13*.

previously [21,22]. Briefly, TCHS recruited 5,082 middle-school children from 14 diverse communities in Taiwan. The parents or guardians of each participating student provided written informed consent at study entry. In this analysis, we randomly selected 3,577 seventh-grade children who provided their buccal cells as the DNA resource for genotyping, and there were no differences in the main characteristics between genotyped and non-genotyped subjects. The study protocol was approved by the Institutional Review Board.

Questionnaire of asthma phenotypes

The standard questionnaire for childhood exposures and health status was taken home by students and answered by parents or guardians. Children were considered to have asthma if there was a positive answer to the question "Has a doctor ever diagnosed this child as having asthma?" Wheeze was defined as any occurrence of the child's chest sounding wheezy or whistling. Early-onset asthma was defined as age of onset for asthma before 5 years of age. Late-onset asthma was onset after 5 years of age.

Table 1. Selected characteristics for participants in Taiwan Children Health Study.

	With genotyping (N = 3577)		All eligible participants (N = 5082)	
	N	%	N	%
Demographic information				
Sex				
Boy	1755	49.1	2464	48.5
Girl	1822	50.9	2618	51.5
Age, yr (Mean ± SD)	12.26±0.50		12.42±0.65	
Parental asthma†				
No	3335	96.9	4739	97.1
Yes	108	3.1	140	2.9
Parental atopy†				
No	2536	73.7	3617	74.1
Yes	907	26.3	1262	25.9
Home exposures†				
Carpet use	308	8.7	442	8.7
In utero exposures to maternal smoking	142	4.0	198	3.9
ETS at home	1544	43.4	2265	44.9
Respiratory Outcomes†				
Asthma	284	8.0	375	7.4
Wheeze	431	12.1	586	11.6
Early-onset asthma‡	184	5.3	239	4.9
Late-onset asthma§	92	2.7	123	2.6

†Number of subjects do not add up to total N because of missing data.
‡Early-onset: asthma diagnosed ≤5 yr of age.
§Late-onset: asthma diagnosed >5 yr of age.

Table 2. Genotype frequencies of *IL-13* in this study participants.

	N	%
IL-13 genotypes		
SNP rs1800925		
CC	2750	73.6
CT	877	23.5
TT	109	2.9
Minor allele frequency	0.15	
HWE	8×10^{-4}	
SNP rs2066960		
CC	1428	37.6
CA	1725	45.4
AA	645	17.0
Minor allele frequency	0.40	
HWE	0.01	
SNP rs20541		
CC	1774	46.5
CT	1653	43.3
TT	391	10.2
Minor allele frequency	0.33	
HWE	0.86	
SNP rs848		
GG	1718	45.9
GT	1599	42.7
TT	427	11.4
Minor allele frequency	0.33	
HWE	0.08	

HWE: Hardy-Weinberg equilibrium.

Exposure assessment and covariates

Household carpet use exposure was determined from the question "Have you ever used carpets in the living room, children's bedroom or other bedrooms in your house?" Basic demographic data and possible confounding variables were also collected, including sex, age, community, personal/family history of asthma or atopic diseases, *in utero* exposures to maternal smoking, ETS, dampness, incense burning, and pet ownership at home.

SNPs selection

A list of *IL-13* SNPs was provided by the Han Chinese in Beijing genome panel (CHB_GENO_PANEL) of Environmental Genome Project of National Institute of Environmental Health Sciences (NIEHS) (http://egp.gs.washington.edu/). We studied the genomic region of the *IL-13* and the region 2000 bp upstream of the gene. All SNPs were used as input files for the Haploview v4.1 (http://www.broadinstitute.org/mpg/haploview) to select tag SNPs and to investigate the linkage disequilibrium (LD) patterns for *IL-13*. One of the six SNPs was excluded due to minor allele frequency (MAF) less than 0.05 [23,24]. As shown in Fig. 1, one haplotype block in strong LD was defined by the confidence intervals of D' (where the upper CI limit was 0.98 and the lower CI limit was 0.70) [25]. Tagging SNPs were selected because of

pairwise tagging tests at the prescribed squared correlation (r^2) value ≥ 0.95 [24]. Pairwise tagging tests simply apply tag SNP represented to all the other SNPs, due to their highly correspondence [26]. The four tag SNPs of *IL-13* were SNP rs1800925, SNP rs2066960, SNP rs20541 and SNP rs848, and they captured 100% of allele's variations in *IL-13*.

DNA collection and genotyping

Genomic DNA was isolated from cotton swabs containing oral mucosa using phenol/chloroform extraction method [27]. The TaqMan assays were performed using a TaqMan PCR Core Reagent kit (Applied Biosystems, Foster City, CA) according to manufacturer's instructions. PCR amplification using 1.0~5.0 ng of genomic DNA was performed with an initial step of 95°C for 5 min followed by 40 cycles of 95°C for 30 s and 60°C for 30 s. The fluorescence profile of each well was measured in an ABI 7900HT Sequence Detection System (Applied Biosystems, Foster City, CA) and the results analyzed with Sequence Detection Software (Applied Biosystems, Foster City, CA). Experimental samples were compared with 36 controls to identify the three genotypes at each locus. Any samples that were outside the parameters defined by the controls were identified as non-informative and were retested. We also repeated 15% of randomly selected DNA samples to verify and confirm the results of genotyping for four *IL-13* SNPs. The details of primer and probe

Table 3. Association of IL-13 with asthma phenotypes, by additive genetic model.

SNP	Asthma				Wheeze				Early-onset asthma†				Late-onset asthma‡			
	OR	95% CI	P value	FDR	OR	95% CI	P value	FDR	OR	95% CI	P value	FDR	OR	95% CI	P value	FDR
rs1800925	1.2	(0.9,1.5)	0.21	0.41	1.3	(1.1,1.5)	0.01	0.03	1.2	(0.9,1.5)	0.23	0.60	1.2	(0.8,1.7)	0.41	0.76
rs2066960	0.9	(0.7,1.1)	0.12	0.41	0.9	(0.7,1.0)	0.02	0.04	1.0	(0.8,1.2)	0.60	0.60	0.7	(0.5,1.0)	0.03	0.13
rs20541	1.1	(0.9,1.3)	0.45	0.49	1.2	(1.0,1.4)	0.04	0.04	1.1	(0.9,1.4)	0.44	0.60	1.1	(0.8,1.5)	0.66	0.76
rs848	1.1	(0.9,1.3)	0.49	0.49	1.2	(1.0,1.4)	0.04	0.04	1.1	(0.9,1.3)	0.54	0.60	1.0	(0.8,1.4)	0.76	0.76

Models are adjusted for age, sex, parental history of asthma, parental history of atopy, *in utero* exposures to maternal smoking, ETS, dampness, incense burning, pet ownership at home and community.
†Early-onset: asthma diagnosed ≦5 yr of age.
‡Late-onset: asthma diagnosed >5 yr of age.

sequences were presented in table S1. The genotype completion rates were between 97% and 99% for all loci.

Statistical analysis

Unconditional multiple logistic regression models were fitted to estimate the individual effects of *IL-13* on asthma phenotypes. Models are adjusted for age, sex, parental history of asthma, parental history of atopy, *in utero* exposures to maternal smoking, ETS, dampness, incense burning, pet ownership at home and community. When considering the effects about *IL-13* additive genetic model was utilized. Selection of confounders that were included in the model was based on *a priori* consideration and the standard statistical procedure of 10% change in point estimates [28]. Subjects with missing covariate information were included in the model using missing indicators [29]. Estimates of measure-

Table 4. Haplotype frequencies of *IL-13* in this study participants.

Haplotype[a]	frequency
h0100	0.3314
h0000	0.3088
H0011	0.1356
H1011	0.1133
H0111[b]	0.0470
H0001[b]	0.0173
H1000[b]	0.0135
H1100[b]	0.0083
H0010[b]	0.0079
H1111[b]	0.0057
H1010[b]	0.0039
H0101[b]	0.0033
H0110[b]	0.0014
H1001[b]	0.0012
H1101[b]	0.0010
H1110[b]	0.0004

[a]0: common allele and 1: minor allele, by the order of SNP1 (rs1800925): C/T; SNP2 (rs2066960): C/A; SNP3 (rs20541): C/T; SNP4 (rs848): G/T.
[b]Haplotypes were collapsed into a category in the haplotype analyses.

ments of LD and r^2 in TCHS participants were obtained from Haploview.

Haplotype frequencies were estimated from the *IL-13* genotype data using the EM algorithm by TagSNPs [30]. The likelihood ratio test (LRT) was used to detect the global association of four variants of *IL-13* haplotypes with asthma phenotypes. We collapsed rare haplotypes (frequency <0.05) into a category in the log additive haplotype analyses. The numbers of copies of each haplotype a person carries and appropriate confidence intervals were estimated using a single imputation procedure [30]. Logistic regression models were based on the co-dominant (two copies of the haplotype vs. no copy and one copy of the haplotype vs. no copy) and dominant (at least one copy of the haplotype vs. no copy) inheritance model. We estimated the false-discovery rate (FDR) for multiple comparisons for main effect associations [31], and used FDR <0.05 as a criterion.

The interaction between genotype or haplotype and household carpet use was assessed by adding an interactive term in the logistic regression model and a likelihood ratio test was used to test its significance. All analyses were conducted using SAS software version 9.1 (SAS Institute, Cary, NC, USA).

Results

A total of 3,577 children with genotyping data were enrolled in current study. The mean age of participants was 12.3±0.5 years and all of them were of ethnic Han Chinese origin (Table 1). Among these children, 8.7% live in households with carpets, and 43.4% have ETS exposure at home. The prevalence of asthma was 8.0% and wheeze occurred in 12.1% of participants.

The genotype frequencies of *IL-13* were showed in Table 2 and distributions of the four selected SNPs were in Hardy-Weinberg equilibrium (p value cutoff >10^{-4}) [23]. The pairwise measures of LD for *IL-13* were presented in Table S2 and we could find SNP rs20541 and SNP rs848 in a strong LD.

After adjustment for age, sex, parental history of asthma, parental history of atopy, *in utero* exposures to maternal smoking, ETS, dampness, incense burning, pet ownership at home and community, *IL-13* SNPs showed statistical significance for the occurrence of wheeze (FDR<0.05) (Table 3 and Table S3). Children carrying T allele of SNP rs1800925 were associated with increased risks on wheeze (OR, 1.3; 95% CI, 1.1–1.5; FDR, 0.03). The variant allele of SNP rs2066960 was protective for wheeze (OR, 0.9; 95% CI, 0.7–1.0; FDR, 0.04). SNP rs20541 and SNP rs848 revealed a similar associated pattern with asthma phenotypes, the increased risks of wheeze were related to children with T allele in additive models.

Table 5. Association of *IL-13* haplotypes with asthma phenotypes among children.

	Asthma		Wheeze		Early-onset asthma[†]		Late-onset asthma[‡]	
	OR	95%CI	OR	95%CI	OR	95%CI	OR	95%CI
h0100[a]	1		1		1		1	
h0000[a]	1.1	(0.9,1.4)	1.1	(0.9,1.4)	1.0	(0.7,1.3)	**1.5**	**(1.0,2.2)**
h0011[a]	1.2	(0.9,1.6)	1.2	(0.9,1.5)	1.2	(0.8,1.6)	1.3	(0.8,2.1)
h1011[a]	1.2	(0.9,1.7)	**1.5**	**(1.2,1.8)**	1.2	(0.8,1.7)	1.5	(0.9,2.4)
Others	0.8	(0.6,1.2)	1.0	(0.8,1.4)	0.7	(0.5,1.2)	1.0	(0.5,1.9)
globe p value	0.22		**0.03**		0.34		0.21	

Models are adjusted for age, sex, parental history of asthma, parental history of atopy, *in utero* exposures to maternal smoking, ETS, dampness, incense burning, pet ownership at home and community.
[†]Early-onset: asthma diagnosed ≤5 yr of age.
[‡]Late-onset: asthma diagnosed >5 yr of age.
[a]0: common allele and 1: minor allele, by the order of SNP1 (rs1800925): C/T; SNP2 (rs2066960): C/A; SNP3 (rs20541): C/T; SNP4 (rs848): G/T.

Haplotype frequencies of the four SNPs were presented in Table 4, and the h0100 was the most common haplotype. The globe haplotype association using likelihood ratio test with 4 degrees of freedom was only significant for wheeze (Table 5). Compared with h0100 haplotype, children with h1011 haplotype had a significantly increased risk of wheeze (OR, 1.5; 95% CI, 1.2–1.8). The h0000 haplotype was correlated with late-onset asthma (OR, 1.5; 95% CI, 1.0–2.2).

The *IL-13* haplotype copy numbers analyses were presented in Table 6. Compared with children without h1011 haplotype, those with two copies of h1011 haplotype showed a significantly 2.4-fold increased risk of wheeze (95% CI, 1.3–4.5; FDR, 0.04). It also showed a dose-response relationship on the increased risks, with OR 1.3 (95% CI, 1.0–1.6; FDR, 0.23) for those with one copy of h1011 haplotype, and OR 2.4 (95% CI, 1.3–4.5; FDR, 0.04) for those with two copies.

Some household environmental factors were investigated in the TCHS (Table S4). We found no substantial differences on the effect of the *IL-13* genetic variants among children in relation to exposure to the other environmental factors, such as ETS, dampness, incense burning, and pet ownership at home. The association of household carpet use and ETS with asthma

phenotypes was shown in Table S5. Children in households with carpet use had an increased risk on late-onset asthma (OR, 1.8; 95% CI, 1.0–3.3; FDR, 0.07). To further investigate the interactions of household factors and *IL-13* variants on children's respiratory health, we examined the relationships of household carpet use with asthma phenotypes (Table 7). Joint exposure appeared to increase the individual effects of SNP rs1800925 and household carpet use on wheeze (OR, 2.0; 95% CI, 1.2–3.6; p for interaction, 0.03) and late-onset asthma (OR, 3.9; 95% CI, 1.7–9.1; p for interaction, 0.04). SNP rs20541 and SNP rs848 and household carpet use showed synergistic effects on late-onset asthma, with the OR 2.5 (95% CI, 1.2–5.2; p for interaction, 0.03) for those with T allele in SNP rs20541 and household carpet use, and with the OR 2.6 (95% CI, 1.2–5.3; p for interaction, 0.02) for those with T allele in SNP rs848 and household carpet use.

Because the effect of h1011 was greater than other haplotypes (Table 5), we investigated the association between h1011 haplotype, household carpet use and asthma phenotypes. Compared to those without household carpet use and h1011 haplotype, children carrying h1011 haplotype and living in homes with carpets had increased risks of wheeze (OR, 2.5; 95% CI, 1.4–4.4; p for interaction, 0.01) and late-onset asthma (OR, 4.7; 95% CI,

Table 6. Association of *IL-13* haplotype copy numbers with wheeze among children.

	OR	95%CI	P value	FDR		OR	95%CI	P value	FDR
h0100[a]					h0011[a]				
0 copies	1				0 copies	1			
1 copy	0.9	(0.7,1.1)	0.19	0.39	1 copy	1.1	(0.9,1.5)	0.41	0.65
2 copies	0.7	(0.5,1.0)	0.04	0.19	2 copies	1.1	(0.6,2.2)	0.75	0.89
≥1 copy	0.8	(0.7,1.0)	0.07	0.14	≥1 copy	1.1	(0.9,1.5)	0.39	0.52
h0000[a]					h1011[a]				
0 copies	1				0 copies	1			
1 copy	1.0	(0.8,1.3)	0.86	0.89	1 copy	1.3	(1.0,1.6)	0.08	0.23
2 copies	1.0	(0.7,1.4)	0.89	0.90	2 copies	2.4	(1.3,4.5)	0.01	0.04
≥1 copy	1.0	(0.8,1.3)	0.92	0.92	≥1 copy	1.4	(1.1,1.7)	0.02	0.07

Models are adjusted for age, sex, parental history of asthma, parental history of atopy, *in utero* exposures to maternal smoking, ETS, dampness, incense burning, pet ownership at home and community.
[a]0: common allele and 1: minor allele, by the order of SNP1 (rs1800925): C/T; SNP2 (rs2066960): C/A; SNP3 (rs20541): C/T; SNP4 (rs848): G/T.

Table 7. Joint effects of carpet use and *IL-13* genotypes on asthma phenotypes among children.

	Carpet use	Asthma OR	95%CI	Wheeze OR	95%CI	Early-onset asthma[†] OR	95%CI	Late-onset asthma[‡] OR	95%CI
SNP rs1800925									
CC	No	1		1		1		1	
CC	Yes	0.7	(0.4,1.2)	0.7	(0.5,1.2)	0.5	(0.2,1.2)	1.1	(0.5,2.6)
CT or TT	No	1.1	(0.8,1.5)	1.2	(0.9,1.5)	1.2	(0.8,1.7)	1.0	(0.6,1.7)
CT or TT	Yes	1.4	(0.7,3.0)	2.0	(1.2,3.6)	0.5	(0.1,1.9)	3.9	(1.7,9.1)
P for interaction		0.17		0.03		0.75		0.04	
SNP rs2066960									
CC	No	1		1		1		1	
CC	Yes	0.8	(0.3,1.9)	1.3	(0.7,2.3)	0.6	(0.2,2.1)	1.1	(0.3,3.7)
CA or AA	No	1.0	(0.7,1.2)	0.9	(0.7,1.1)	1.1	(0.8,1.6)	0.7	(0.4,1.0)
CA or AA	Yes	0.8	(0.5,1.5)	0.8	(0.5,1.3)	0.4	(0.2,1.1)	1.5	(0.7,3.1)
P for interaction		0.84		0.30		0.52		0.28	
SNP rs20541									
CC	No	1		1		1		1	
CC	Yes	0.6	(0.3,1.3)	0.7	(0.4,1.3)	0.6	(0.3,1.6)	0.7	(0.2,2.4)
CT or TT	No	1.0	(0.8,1.3)	1.1	(0.9,1.4)	1.2	(0.9,1.6)	0.8	(0.5,1.3)
CT or TT	Yes	1.1	(0.6,2.0)	1.4	(0.9,2.3)	0.4	(0.1,1.2)	2.5	(1.2,5.2)
P for interaction		0.30		0.15		0.36		0.03	
SNP rs848									
GG	No	1		1		1		1	
GG	Yes	0.6	(0.3,1.3)	0.7	(0.4,1.3)	0.6	(0.2,1.6)	0.7	(0.2,2.2)
GT or TT	No	1.0	(0.8,1.3)	1.2	(0.9,1.4)	1.2	(0.9,1.6)	0.8	(0.5,1.2)
GT or TT	Yes	1.1	(0.6,2.0)	1.5	(0.9,2.4)	0.4	(0.1,1.2)	2.6	(1.2,5.3)
P for interaction		0.26		0.13		0.39		0.02	

Models are adjusted for age, sex, parental history of asthma, parental history of atopy, *in utero* exposures to maternal smoking, ETS, dampness, incense burning, pet ownership at home and community.
[†]Early-onset: asthma diagnosed ≤5 yr of age.
[‡]Late-onset: asthma diagnosed >5 yr of age.

2.0–10.9; p for interaction, 0.02) (Table 8). However, we could not find the similar pattern for ETS at home on the effects of h1011 haplotype to asthma phenotypes in childhood (Table S6).

Discussion

To the best of our knowledge, this is the first study concerning the potential interactive associations between *IL-13*, household carpet use and childhood asthma. In our data, *IL-13* genetic variants showed significant adverse effects on asthma phenotypes. We found that children carrying h1011 haplotype have increased risks of the occurrence of wheeze. Household carpet use appears to modify the effects of *IL-13* gene on wheeze and late-onset asthma.

The *IL-13* gene is located on chromosome 5q, which has been suggested to be associated with the risk of elevated serum IgE levels, eosinophilia, airway hyper-sensitiveness and the occurrence of childhood asthma [13,14]. In our study, children with variant alleles of SNP rs1800925, SNP rs20541 and SNP rs848 have significantly higher risks for wheeze (Table 3). Previous studies have shown that promoter variant in *IL-13* (SNP rs1800925) could enhance *IL-13* transcription [32] and was associated with atopy, asthma and increased bronchial hyper-reactivity [13,33,34]. Another polymorphism in exon4 (SNP rs20541, Arg130Gln) also resulted in the occurrence of asthma, reduced lung function and

increased serum IgE [13,35,36]. Functional and association studies both showed that 130Gln was related to higher IL-13 levels and a stronger Th$_2$ immune response than 130Arg [37]. Few studies focused on rs848 polymorphism with asthma. Hunninghake *et al.* have indicated that SNP rs848 was in strong linkage disequilibrium with SNP rs20541 [13], which is consistent with our findings (Fig. 1 and Table S2). However, the effects of SNP rs2066960 variants in previous studies showed that minor allele (A allele) was associated with elevated serum IgE and early-transient wheeze [19,38]. In our data, we found that SNP rs2066960 A allele was associated with decreased risks of asthma phenotypes (Table 3). The different genetic association on asthma might be attributed to genotype frequencies in different ethnic populations. Based on the haplotype analyses in the present study, we found that three variants of 4 SNPs in *IL-13* gene might significantly affect risks of asthma phenotypes in children. Compared with the common haplotype, children carrying h1011 haplotype were more susceptible to development of wheeze (OR, 1.5; 95% CI, 1.2-1.8) (Table 5). Furthermore, the more copy numbers of the h1011 haplotype children carry, the higher risk of wheeze they would possess (Table 6).

IL-13, independent from IL-4, plays a central role for the development of asthma-related symptoms in animal models and

Table 8. Joint effects of carpet use and *IL-13* haplotype h1011 on asthma phenotypes among children.

| | | h1011[a] | | | | |
| | | No | | Yes | | |
	Carpet use	OR	95%CI	OR	95%CI	P for interaction
Asthma	No	1		1.1	(0.8,1.4)	0.06
	Yes	0.6	(0.3,1.1)	1.7	(0.8,3.6)	
Wheeze	No	1		1.2	(0.9,1.5)	0.01
	Yes	0.7	(0.4,1.1)	2.5	(1.4,4.4)	
Early-onset asthma†	No	1		1.1	(0.8,1.6)	0.98
	Yes	0.5	(0.2,1.1)	0.5	(0.1,2.2)	
Late-onset asthma‡	No	1		1.0	(0.6,1.7)	0.02
	Yes	1.0	(0.4,2.4)	4.7	(2.0,10.9)	

Models are adjusted for age, sex, parental history of asthma, parental history of atopy, *in utero* exposures to maternal smoking, ETS, dampness, incense burning, pet ownership at home and community.
†Early-onset: asthma diagnosed ≤5 yr of age.
‡Late-onset: asthma diagnosed >5 yr of age.
[a]0: common allele and 1: minor allele, by the order of SNP1 (rs1800925): C/T; SNP2 (rs2066960): C/A; SNP3 (rs20541): C/T; SNP4 (rs848): G/T.

human studies [10,39]. IL-13 was primarily produced by Th$_2$ CD4$^+$ T cells after allergen irritation, and it may induce the entire pathogenic pathway of asthma independently of traditional cells, such as mast cells and eosinophils [8]. Genetic variants in *IL-13* have been found to be associated with elevated serum levels of IL-13 [37]. Household carpet use is a significant reservoir of allergens, including house dust mite, dog and cat dander, and fungal concentrations [17,40]. House dust mites, *Dermatophagoides pteronyssinus* allergen 1 (*Der p* 1) and *Dermatophagoides farinae* (*Der f* 1), might play important roles in allergic sensitization, as well as in the development of asthma and asthma deterioration in children [41,42,43]. In our data, the interactive effects are consistent with *IL-13* genotypes and household carpet use on asthma phenotypes (Table 7). Especially in SNP rs1800925, joint exposure appeared to increase the individual effects of SNP rs1800925 T allele and household carpet use on wheeze (OR, 2.0; 95% CI, 1.2–3.6) and late-onset asthma (OR, 3.9; 95% CI, 1.7–9.1). It was suggested that the variant of promoter region, containing a binding site of the nuclear factor of activated T cells (NFAT) transcription factor, regulates *IL-13* and *IL-4* gene expression [33]. Additionally, our results indicated that children with h1011 haplotype and exposure to carpets may have increased risks for asthma phenotypes (Table 8). We believe that *IL-13* genetic variants and exposure to household carpet use may synergistically induce high IL-13 levels to inflammation, which would result in the occurrence of asthma phenotypes in children.

Up to the present, two studies concerning *IL-13*-environmental interaction on asthma phenotypes in children have been reported. Sadeghnejad and colleagues investigated SNP rs1800925, SNP rs2066960 and SNP rs20541 and demonstrated that the effect of ETS exposure at home was stronger on wheeze with the common *IL-13* haplotype compared to those without it [19]. Sorensen *et al.* reported that children exposed to maternal smoking during pregnancy and with SNP rs20541 C allele had increased risks on wheeze [20]. However, no significant interaction between *IL-13* polymorphisms (SNP rs20541 and SNP rs1800925) and ETS exposure at home were noted. In our data, we could not find

interactive effects between *IL-13* and ETS exposure at home in asthma phenotypes (Table S6). Several reasons, including differences in ethnicity or genotype frequencies, may explain this situation. For example, the genotype frequencies in SNP rs2066960 were 81.5, 17.6% and 0.9% for CC, CA and AA genotypes, respectively, in British population [19]. In SNP rs20541, the genotype frequencies were 61.8~64.4%, 32.1~33.1%, and 3.5~5.1% for CC, CT and TT genotypes, respectively, in European populations [19,20]. Our study showed distinctly different results: 37.6%, 45.4% and 17.0% for CC, CA and AA genotypes in SNP rs2066960, and 46.7%, 44.4% and 8.9% for CC, CT and TT genotypes in SNP rs20541 (Table 2). All of the results were similar to ethnic Han Chinese in the Beijing population from HapMap (data not shown). Our population did provide evidence for *IL-13* genetic variants on asthma phenotypes among Han children.

Age, sex, parental atopic history, maternal smoking during pregnancy, ETS, dampness, incense burning, and pet ownership at home were believed to contribute to asthma and wheeze in childhood [4,21,44,45,46]. We minimized interference from these confounders by recruiting lifelong non-smokers of similar age, and adjusting potential confounders by regression models. Difference in participation by children with respiratory outcomes who had different carpet exposure histories is unlikely to be significant enough to produce substantial bias, as participation rates in each classroom were high and the characteristics was similar between genotyping and all participants (Table 1). Because the differences in distribution are modest and are probably not associated with the genotypes, it is unlikely that selection of subjects biased the effect estimates in our results. As the study subjects were recruited in an unselected population, unbiased observations of the association between genetic effects and outcomes were expected.

Our definition of household carpet use might not indicate a good quantitative biomarker for measuring allergen levels in the houses. However, higher concentrations of indoor allergens have been reported to be associated with carpet use at home [16,47]. Exposure assessment from the questionnaire was likely to introduce some misclassification bias shifting the results toward the null. Moreover, the associations between household carpet use and childhood asthma were consistent in another case-control study from our group [18]. Another possible limitation is recall bias of respiratory outcomes. Asthma phenotypes in our study were ascertained by parental-reported questionnaire, so misclassification may have arisen from imperfect parental recall of events. Differential misclassification by *IL-13* genetic variants was probably not a major source of bias that accounts for our results, because disease status was defined without the knowledge of genotype. We found that large parts of significant effects were limited on wheeze and effect estimates of wheeze were also stronger than other asthma phenotypes. We believe that wheeze is the most common respiratory symptom in children when occurrence of airway inflammation induced by environmental stimuli. In Taiwan, parents of children with wheeze symptoms might be unlikely to seek medical care, and therefore physician-diagnosed asthma would be underreported. Consistent with previous well-known knowledge, we found the significant genetic association in *IL-13* gene, and wheeze is a good predictor for development of asthma in children.

In conclusions, our results showed that genetic variants in *IL-13*, especially h1011 haplotype, showed adverse effects on respiratory health in children. Household carpet use may influence the severity of diverse allergic inflammatory reactions induced by *IL-13* genetic variants. Additional long-term research is necessary to explore the roles played by other genes in determining genetic susceptibility on adverse respiratory outcomes. Identification of gene-environmental interactions in childhood asthma may lead to new and comprehensive insights into asthma pathogenesis and treatment.

Supporting Information

Table S1 Primer and probe sequences for *IL-13* genetic variants.

Table S2 Pairwise measures of linkage disequilibrium for *IL-13* in this study participants.

Table S3 Association of *IL-13* genotypes with asthma phenotypes, by co-dominant and dominant genetic model.

Table S4 Environmental questions of TCHS questionnaire.

Table S5 Association of household carpet use and ETS at home with asthma phenotypes among children.

Table S6 Joint effects of ETS exposure and *IL-13* haplotype h1011 on asthma phenotypes among children.

Acknowledgments

We thank all the field workers who supported data collection, the school administrators and teachers, and especially the parents and children who participated in this study.

Author Contributions

Conceived and designed the experiments: CHT KYT NWK MWS BLC FTC YLL. Performed the experiments: KYT NWK. Analyzed the data: CHT MWS. Contributed reagents/materials/analysis tools: BLC FTC. Wrote the paper: CHT YLL.

References

1. Spee-van der Wekke J, Meulmeester JF, Radder JJ, Verloove-Vanhorick SP (1998) School absence and treatment in school children with respiratory symptoms in The Netherlands: data from the Child Health Monitoring System. J Epidemiol Community Health 52: 359–363.

2. Silverstein MD, Mair JE, Katusic SK, Wollan PC, O'Connell E J, et al. (2001) School attendance and school performance: a population-based study of children with asthma. J Pediatr 139: 278–283.

3. Weiss KB, Sullivan SD (1994) Socio-economic burden of asthma, allergy, and other atopic illnesses. Pediatr Allergy Immunol 5: 7–12.

4. Lee YL, Lin YC, Hwang BF, Guo YL (2005) Changing prevalence of asthma in Taiwanese adolescents: two surveys 6 years apart. Pediatr Allergy Immunol 16: 157–164.

5. Maziak W, Behrens T, Brasky TM, Duhme H, Rzehak P, et al. (2003) Are asthma and allergies in children and adolescents increasing? Results from ISAAC phase I and phase III surveys in Munster, Germany. Allergy 58: 572–579.

6. Martinez FD (2007) Gene-environment interactions in asthma: with apologies to William of Ockham. Proc Am Thorac Soc 4: 26–31.

7. Hunninghake GM, Soto-Quiros ME, Lasky-Su J, Avila L, Ly NP, et al. (2008) Dust mite exposure modifies the effect of functional IL10 polymorphisms on allergy and asthma exacerbations. J Allergy Clin Immunol 122: 93–98, 98 e91–95.

8. Wills-Karp M, Chiaramonte M (2003) Interleukin-13 in asthma. Curr Opin Pulm Med 9: 21–27.

9. Zhu Z, Homer RJ, Wang Z, Chen Q, Geba GP, et al. (1999) Pulmonary expression of interleukin-13 causes inflammation, mucus hypersecretion, subepithelial fibrosis, physiologic abnormalities, and eotaxin production. J Clin Invest 103: 779–788.

10. Wills-Karp M, Luyimbazi J, Xu X, Schofield B, Neben TY, et al. (1998) Interleukin-13: central mediator of allergic asthma. Science 282: 2258–2261.

11. DeMeo DL, Lange C, Silverman EK, Senter JM, Drazen JM, et al. (2002) Univariate and multivariate family-based association analysis of the IL-13 ARG130GLN polymorphism in the Childhood Asthma Management Program. Genet Epidemiol 23: 335–348.

12. Graves PE, Kabesch M, Halonen M, Holberg CJ, Baldini M, et al. (2000) A cluster of seven tightly linked polymorphisms in the IL-13 gene is associated with total serum IgE levels in three populations of white children. J Allergy Clin Immunol 105: 506–513.

13. Hunninghake GM, Soto-Quiros ME, Avila L, Su J, Murphy A, et al. (2007) Polymorphisms in IL13, total IgE, eosinophilia, and asthma exacerbations in childhood. J Allergy Clin Immunol 120: 84–90.

14. Kim HB, Lee YC, Lee SY, Jung J, Jin HS, et al. (2006) Gene-gene interaction between IL-13 and IL-13Ralpha1 is associated with total IgE in Korean children with atopic asthma. J Hum Genet 51: 1055–1062.

15. Busse WW, Lemanske RF, Jr. (2001) Asthma. N Engl J Med 344: 350–362.

16. Spertini F, Berney M, Foradini F, Roulet CA (2010) Major mite allergen Der f 1 concentration is reduced in buildings with improved energy performance. Allergy 65: 623–629.

17. Tranter DC, Wobbema AT, Norlien K, Dorschner DF (2009) Indoor allergens in Minnesota schools and child care centers. J Occup Environ Hyg 6: 582–591.

18. Chen YC, Tsai CH, Lee YL (2011) Early-Life Indoor Environmental Exposures Increase the Risk of Childhood Asthma. Int J Hyg Environ Health (Accepted).

19. Sadeghnejad A, Karmaus W, Arshad SH, Kurukulaaratchy R, Huebner M, et al. (2008) IL13 gene polymorphisms modify the effect of exposure to tobacco smoke on persistent wheeze and asthma in childhood, a longitudinal study. Respir Res 9: 2.

20. Sorensen M, Allermann L, Vogel U, Andersen PS, Jespersgaard C, et al. (2009) Polymorphisms in inflammation genes, tobacco smoke and furred pets and wheeze in children. Pediatr Allergy Immunol 20: 614–623.

21. Tsai CH, Huang JH, Hwang BF, Lee YL (2010) Household environmental tobacco smoke and risks of asthma, wheeze and bronchitic symptoms among children in Taiwan. Respir Res 11: 11.

22. Hwang BF, Lee YL (2010) Air Pollution and Prevalence of Bronchitic Symptoms among Children in Taiwan. Chest 138: 956–964.

23. Balding DJ (2006) A tutorial on statistical methods for population association studies. Nat Rev Genet 7: 781–791.

24. de Bakker PI, Yelensky R, Pe'er I, Gabriel SB, Daly MJ, et al. (2005) Efficiency and power in genetic association studies. Nature Genetics 37: 1217–1223.

25. Gabriel SB, Schaffner SF, Nguyen H, Moore JM, Roy J, et al. (2002) The structure of haplotype blocks in the human genome. Science 296: 2225–2229.

26. Carlson CS, Eberle MA, Rieder MJ, Yi Q, Kruglyak L, et al. (2004) Selecting a maximally informative set of single-nucleotide polymorphisms for association analyses using linkage disequilibrium. Am J Hum Genet 74: 106–120.

27. Gill P, Jeffreys AJ, Werrett DJ (1985) Forensic application of DNA 'fingerprints'. Nature 318: 577–579.

28. Tong IS, Lu Y (2001) Identification of confounders in the assessment of the relationship between lead exposure and child development. Ann Epidemiol 11: 38–45.

29. Greenland S, Finkle WD (1995) A critical look at methods for handling missing covariates in epidemiologic regression analyses. Am J Epidemiol 142: 1255–1264.

30. Stram DO, Leigh Pearce C, Bretsky P, Freedman M, Hirschhorn JN, et al. (2003) Modeling and E-M estimation of haplotype-specific relative risks from genotype data for a case-control study of unrelated individuals. Hum Hered 55: 179–190.

31. Osborne JA (2006) Estimating the false discovery rate using SAS. SAS Users Group International Proceedings 190: 1–10.

32. Cameron L, Webster RB, Strempel JM, Kiesler P, Kabesch M, et al. (2006) Th2 cell-selective enhancement of human IL13 transcription by IL13-1112C>T, a polymorphism associated with allergic inflammation. J Immunol 177: 8633–8642.

33. van der Pouw Kraan TC, van Veen A, Boeije LC, van Tuyl SA, de Groot ER, et al. (1999) An IL-13 promoter polymorphism associated with increased risk of allergic asthma. Genes Immun 1: 61–65.

34. Hummelshoj T, Bodtger U, Datta P, Malling HJ, Oturai A, et al. (2003) Association between an interleukin-13 promoter polymorphism and atopy. Eur J Immunogenet 30: 355–359.

35. Heinzmann A, Jerkic SP, Ganter K, Kurz T, Blattmann S, et al. (2003) Association study of the IL13 variant Arg110Gln in atopic diseases and juvenile idiopathic arthritis. J Allergy Clin Immunol 112: 735–739.

36. Park HW, Lee JE, Kim SH, Kim YK, Min KU, et al. (2009) Genetic variation of IL13 as a risk factor of reduced lung function in children and adolescents: a cross-sectional population-based study in Korea. Respir Med 103: 284–288.

37. Arima K, Umeshita-Suyama R, Sakata Y, Akaiwa M, Mao XQ, et al. (2002) Upregulation of IL-13 concentration in vivo by the IL13 variant associated with bronchial asthma. J Allergy Clin Immunol 109: 980–987.

38. Ogbuanu IU, Karmaus WJ, Zhang H, Sabo-Attwood T, Ewart S, et al. (2010) Birth order modifies the effect of IL13 gene polymorphisms on serum IgE at age

10 and skin prick test at ages 4, 10 and 18: a prospective birth cohort study. Allergy Asthma Clin Immunol 6: 6.

39. Grunig G, Warnock M, Wakil AE, Venkayya R, Brombacher F, et al. (1998) Requirement for IL-13 independently of IL-4 in experimental asthma. Science 282: 2261–2263.

40. Vojta PJ, Randels SP, Stout J, Muilenberg M, Burge HA, et al. (2001) Effects of physical interventions on house dust mite allergen levels in carpet, bed, and upholstery dust in low-income, urban homes. Environ Health Perspect 109: 815–819.

41. Chan-Yeung M, Manfreda J, Dimich-Ward H, Lam J, Ferguson A, et al. (1995) Mite and cat allergen levels in homes and severity of asthma. Am J Respir Crit Care Med 152: 1805–1811.

42. Henderson FW, Henry MM, Ivins SS, Morris R, Neebe EC, et al. (1995) Correlates of recurrent wheezing in school-age children. The Physicians of Raleigh Pediatric Associates. Am J Respir Crit Care Med 151: 1786–1793.

43. Sporik R, Holgate ST, Platts-Mills TA, Cogswell JJ (1990) Exposure to house-dust mite allergen (Der p I) and the development of asthma in childhood. A prospective study. N Engl J Med 323: 502–507.

44. Tsai CH, Tung KY, Chen CH, Lee YL (2011) Tumour necrosis factor G-308A polymorphism modifies the effect of home dampness on childhood asthma. Occupational and Environmental Medicine.

45. Wang IJ, Tsai CH, Chen CH, Tung KY, Lee YL (2011) Glutathione S-transferase, incense burning and asthma in children. Eur Respir J 37: 1371–1377.

46. Takkouche B, Gonzalez-Barcala FJ, Etminan M, Fitzgerald M (2008) Exposure to furry pets and the risk of asthma and allergic rhinitis: a meta-analysis. Allergy 63: 857–864.

47. Mihrshahi S, Marks G, Vanlaar C, Tovey E, Peat J (2002) Predictors of high house dust mite allergen concentrations in residential homes in Sydney. Allergy 57: 137–142.

25

Autochthonous Leptospirosis in South-East Austria, 2004–2012

Martin Hoenigl[1,2*♋], **Carina Wallner**[1♋], **Franz Allerberger**[3], **Friedrich Schmoll**[3], **Katharina Seeber**[1], **Jasmin Wagner**[1], **Thomas Valentin**[1], **Ines Zollner-Schwetz**[1], **Holger Flick**[2], **Robert Krause**[1*]

1 Section of Infectious Diseases and Tropical Medicine, Department of Medicine, Medical University of Graz, Graz, Austria, **2** Division of Pulmonology, Department of Medicine, Medical University of Graz, Graz, Austria, **3** Austrian Agency for Health and Food Safety (AGES), Vienna, Austria

Abstract

Background: Leptospirosis is one of the world's mostly spread zoonoses causing acute fever. Over years, leptospirosis has been reported to occur rarely in Austria and Germany (annual incidence of 0.06/100,000 in Germany). Only imported cases have been on the increase. Objectives of this case-series study were to retrospectively assess epidemiologic and clinical characteristics of leptospirosis illnesses in South-East Austria, to describe risk exposures for autochthonous infections, and to compare patients with imported versus autochthonous infection.

Methodology/Principal Findings: During the 9-year period between 2004 and 2012, 127 adult patients (49 females, 78 males) who tested positive by rapid point-of-care test for *Leptospira*-specific IgM (Leptocheck®) were identified through electronic hospital databases. Follow-up telephone interviews were conducted with 82 patients. A total of 114 (89.8%) of the 127 patients enrolled had acquired leptospirosis within Austria and 13 (10.2%) had potentially imported infections. Most autochthonous cases were diagnosed during the months of June and July, whereas fewest were diagnosed during the winter months. Exposure to rodents, recreational activities in woods or wet areas, gardening, cleaning of basements or huts were the most common risk exposures found in autochthonous infection. Serogroups Australis (n = 23), Sejroe (n = 22), and Icterohaemorrhagiae (n = 11) were identified most frequently by MAT testing in autochthonous infections. Patients with imported leptospirosis were significantly younger, less likely to be icteric and had significantly lower liver transaminase levels (p = 0.004) than those with autochthonous infections.

Conclusions/Significance: Leptospirosis is endemic in South-East Austria. In contrast to reports from other countries we found a relatively high proportion of leptospirosis cases to be female (39% vs. ~10%), likely the result of differing risk exposures for South-East Austria.

Editor: Rudy A. Hartskeerl, Royal Tropical Institute, Netherlands

Funding: The authors have no support or funding to report.

Competing Interests: The authors have declared that no competing interests exist.

* E-mail: robert.krause@medunigraz.at (RK); martin.hoenigl@medunigraz.at (MH)

♋ These authors contributed equally to this work.

Introduction

In recent years, leptospirosis has gained increasing attention as an emerging infectious disease of global importance [1]. The clinical manifestations range from asymptomatic infection to severe and potentially fatal illness complicated by septic shock and organ failure [2–5]. The broad clinical spectrum is presumably one of the main reasons why diagnosis of this spirochaetal infection remains a challenge for clinicians. Over years, leptospirosis has been reported to occur rarely in Austria and Germany [6,7]. Diagnostic testing for the infection is therefore performed only in specialized reference hospitals. The low leptospirosis incidence rate reported for Germany and Austria appears discordant, however, with the high rate of *Leptospira* spp. seropositivity among healthy Austrian men identified by Poeppl and colleagues [8].

Hawaii has the highest reported annual incidence rate of leptospirosis in the United States, reaching 1.63 cases per 100,000 inhabitants [9]. Lower annual incidence rates have been reported from Central and Western Europe ranging from 0.06/100,000 per year in Germany over 0.1/100,000 in the United Kingdom and 0.25/100,000 in the Netherlands to 0.5/100,000 in France [6,7,10–12]. An increasing proportion of the leptospirosis infections diagnosed in many European countries is imported from abroad (25% to 60% of all infections) [10,12–14]. Most of the imported infections have been associated with sporting and adventurous vacation activities abroad [14–16].

The objectives of this study were to determine the epidemiology of leptospirosis in South-East Austria, to describe risk exposures for acquiring autochthonous infection, and to compare clinical characteristics of patients with imported to those with autochthonous infection.

Methods

Over a 9-year period (2004–2012), all patients with clinically compatible illness that have been tested positive by rapid point-of-care (POC) test for *Leptospira*-specific IgM (Leptocheck®, Zephyr Biomedicals, India) at the microbiology laboratory, University Hospital Graz, were included. The hospital has a capacity of more than 1500 beds and serves as reference hospital for about 1 million inhabitants in South-East Austria. If borderline positive test results were obtained with the routine microbiological evaluation, a repeat test was ordered within a few days to confirm the infection.

Microscopic agglutination testing (MAT) was performed on a subset of specimens at the Institute for Veterinary Disease Control in Moedling (AGES), for detection of the causative *Leptospira* serovar. A titre greater than 200 against any of the pathogenic antigens was considered positive. We defined all patients with positive POC test and clinically compatible illness as cases of leptospirosis, independent of MAT result, because the POC IgM test was recently shown to be more sensitive than MAT (85.6% versus 49.8%), with comparable specificity (96.2% versus 98.8%) in a study evaluating results in more than 1500 cases of leptospirosis [17]. In another recent study comparing prospectively three POC tests for *Leptospira*-specific IgM the Leptocheck® IgM POC test, which was also used in this study, showed the best results with an overall sensitivity of 78% and a specificity of 98% [18].

Data regarding course of disease as well as risk exposures (within three weeks before onset of infection) were collected via telephone questionnaires (n = 82; conducted between June 2012 and January 2013) and/or abstracted from electronic hospital databases (n = 127). Infections in patients that had travelled in foreign countries within three weeks before occurrence of symptoms were classified as potentially imported [17]. All other infections were classified as autochthonously acquired.

Questionnaire responses were entered into an electronic database. All statistical analyses were performed using the Statistical Package for Social Sciences version 20.0 (SPSS Inc., Chicago, IL, USA). Continuous data are presented as medians (inter-quartile ranges [IQR]) or means (95% confidence interval [CI]) and categorical data as proportions. Proportions were compared using the chi-squared or Fisher's exact test as appropriate. Analyses of continuous data were performed using the Mann-Whitney U test or Students T-test as appropriate. Bootstrapping was used to calculate the 95% CI for proportion by gender.

The study was conducted according to the principles expressed in the Declaration of Helsinki and was approved by the local ethics committee, Medical University of Graz. All data presented have been de-identified and are therefore not attributable to individual patients. At our center, information of all patients admitted is automatically stored in the electronic hospital database, and written informed consent of participating patients was waived by the local ethics committee.

Results

A total of 127 adult patients (range 18–89 years) with positive *Leptospira* specific IgM tests were identified while the test resulted negative in another 794 patients. 114/127 (89.8%) patients had acquired leptospirosis within Austria and 13 (10.2%) had potentially imported infections (Table 1). No outbreak was observed during the study period. In 80/127 (63%) patients single serum samples were received for MAT testing, which turned out positive in 61 (76%) and negative (i.e. titre <200) in 19/80 patients (24%). Cases per year (autochthonous and imported) are shown in

Table 1. Median duration of symptoms prior to presentation at the hospital was 5 days (IQR 3–9 days) and the median length of hospitalization was eight days (IQR 5–12 days); neither parameter differed between autochthonous and imported cases. Four autochthonous and two potentially imported cases had severe infections requiring ICU admission secondary to sepsis and organ failures; all six patients survived.

Characterisation of Autochthonous Cases

Overall 114 cases of autochthonous leptospirosis were diagnosed over a 9-year period, which is in average 12.6 cases a year. Considering that the Medical University Hospital Graz serves as a reference hospital for about 1 million inhabitants in South-East Austria this rate would correspond to an autochthonously acquired infection rate of 1.26 per 100,000 inhabitants per year in South-East Austria over the study period. After reaching a peak in 2007–2008 with more than 20 cases reported per year, the number of autochthonous cases declined in 2009 and remained stable at 5 to 6 cases per year through 2012 (Table 1). The male to female ratio was 1.6:1 for autochthonous cases. Most autochthonous cases were diagnosed during the months of June and July (n = 16 each), followed by October (n = 13), August (n = 12), April (n = 11) and March (n = 10), while fewer infections were diagnosed during the winter months (4 in December, 6 in January and 3 in February).

Commonly reported exposures for acquiring leptospirosis were activities in woods and wet areas, and exposure to rodents. Gardening or eating fruits/vegetables from the own garden/organic-farming markets was reported by 31/44 (70.5%) of female autochthonous cases. The proportion of patients reporting various risk exposures by subgroup are depicted in Table 1.

Serum samples were tested by MAT for 72/114 (63%) patients with autochthonous infection and 54 (75%) were positive. The following serogroups were identified: Australis (n = 23), Sejroe (n = 22), Icterohaemorrhagiae (n = 11), Ballum (n = 10), Grippotyphosa (n = 7), Canicola (n = 4), Bataviae (n = 2), Pyrogenes and Hebdomadis (n = 1).

The most frequently reported symptoms include fever (80/114; 70%), myalgia and/or arthralgia (41/114; 36%), abdominal pain and/or diarrhea (34/114; 30%), general weakness (31/114; 27%), jaundice (31/114; 27%), headache (24/114; 21%) and nausea and/or sickness (20/114; 18%). Laboratory results at admission revealed that 44/114 patients (39%) had thrombocytopenia (<140.000 cells/μL; 25/44 even <100.000 cells/μL). Elevated alanine aminotranferase levels (ALT >2 times normal value) were found in 55/114 (48%). There was no significant difference in the median ALT level for patients aged <50 years compared to older patients (median 75, IQR 29–456 vs median 80, IQR 42–149, respectively). Elevated serum creatinine levels (>1.2 mg/dL) were found in 45 (39%) patients with 25 patients having serum creatinine levels >2 mg/dL.

Comparison between Autochthonous and Imported Infections

Of the 13 cases with imported infections, five had been in South-East Asia within the incubation period, two in Africa, one in South America and five in Central Europe. Serogroups for the imported cases (samples received for MAT testing in 8/13 patients; positive result in 7/8) included Australis (n = 3), Ballum, Grippotyphosa, Icterohemorrhagiae (each n = 2), and Bataviae, Canicola, and Sejroe in one case each.

Patients with imported leptospirosis were significantly younger than those with autochthonous infections (p = 0.045; Students T Test). Jaundice at presentation was less common (p = 0.037; Fishers exact test) and ALT levels were significantly lower in

Table 1. Demographic data as well as recreational/occupational and residential risk exposures in autochthonous cases (overall, males, females) and imported cases.

Demographic data	Autochthonous cases N = 114	Autochthonous Males N = 70	Autochthonous Females N = 44	Imported cases N = 13
Male Sex (N; %; 95% CI)	70 (61%; 52–71%)			8
Female Sex (N; %; 95% CI)	44 (39%; 29–47%)			5
Age (years; mean, 95% CI)	33 (26–40)			43 (40–47)
Cases per year				
2004	10			4
2005	16			1
2006	18			3
2007	26			2
2008	23			2
2009	5			1
2010	5			0
2011	5			0
2012	6			0
Risk exposures				
Recreational/Occupational (N; %)				
Activities in woods/wet Areas	44 (39%)	31 (44%)	13 (30%)	7 (54%)
Gardening	36 (32%)	19 (27%)	17 (39%)	2 (15%)
Cleaning up/demolishing basement/hut/attic	28 (25%)	14 (20%)	14 (32%)	2 (15%)
Swimming/snorkelling/diving	9 (8%)	5 (7%)	4 (9%)	5 (38%)
Trekking	4 (4%)	3 (4%)	1 (2%)	5 (38%)
Excavation work	5 (4%)	4 (6%)	1 (2%)	2 (15%)
Camping	1 (1%)	1 (1%)	0	2 (15%)
Channel Digger	3 (3%)	3 (4%)	0	0
Surfing in a river	1 (1%)	1 (2%)	0	1 (8%)
Residential (N; %)				
Exposure to rats/mice	53 (46%)	32 (46%)	21 (48%)	8 (62%)
Contact to cats	29 (25%)	14 (20%)	15 (34%)	1 (8%)
Contact to dogs	20 (18%)	15 (21%)	5 (11%)	3 (23%)
Eating fruits/vegetables from the own garden	19 (17%)	10 (14%)	9 (20%)	0
Pond in surroundings	11 (10%)	9 (13%)	2 (5%)	4 (31%)
Farm Animals	11 (10%)	9 (13%)	2 (5%)	1 (8%)
Food from organic farming- markets or directly from farmer	8 (7%)	3 (4%)	5 (11%)	2 (15%)

Abbreviations: 95% CI, 95% confidence intervall; N, number.

patients with imported leptospirosis compared to autochthonous infections (median 24, IQR 14–40 U/L versus median 76, IQR 30–292; p = 0.004; Mann Whitney U test). No significant differences were found for other parameters.

Discussion

We found that leptospirosis is endemic in South-East Austria. Our findings would correspond to an autochthonously acquired infection rate of 1.26 per 100,000 inhabitants per year in South-East Austria over the study period. The estimated incidence probably reflects the more severe end of the clinical spectrum for leptospirosis, as mild forms of this disease are more likely to remain unrecognized and may have presented to smaller peripheral

hospitals or family doctors, i.e. settings where testing for leptospirosis is yet not performed.

Therefore we believe that the actual rate of leptospirosis in South-East Austria may be much higher than the rate reported here. Although it is required by law to report basic demographic data of all serologically confirmed leptospirosis cases to the Austrian Government the official numbers may suffer from underreporting for two reasons: (i) the fact that leptospirosis cases are rarely confirmed by serological tests in Austria as diagnostic testing for the infection is performed in a few specialized reference hospitals only, (ii) the suboptimal reporting behaviour of clinicians. It is interesting that a recent cross-sectional study demonstrated serological evidence of a high rate of exposure to *Leptospira* spp. among Austrian males [8].

In accordance with the literature exposure to rats or mice has been present in almost 50% of cases of our study cohort [10]. Other important risk exposures included recreational activities in woods or wet areas, gardening as well as cleaning basements or huts. Imported cases were less often icteric and presented with significantly lower transaminase levels when compared to autochthonous cases. This finding is consistent with a previous study of 60 cases of leptospirosis mostly from Germany [2]. In contrast to that study and other reports, we found, however, that in our hospital the number of both imported and autochthonous cases decreased over the study period [2,10]. While changes in temperature and rainfall may have been contributing factors, the reason for the decrease in autochthonous infections from 2008 to 2009 remains unknown [19].

Another surprising finding was that in our study 39% (95% CI 29–47%) of autochthonous leptospirosis cases occurred in females which stands in contrast to data from Hawaii, the Netherlands and UK where females accounted for less than 10% of leptospirosis cases [9,10,12]. In our setting the most frequently identified serogroups were Australis, Sejroe and Icterohaemorrhagiae. In accordance with a previous study from Austria and in contrast to the Netherlands, where the serogroup Canicola had disappeared after 1966, we found four patients autochthonously infected by this serogroup [10]. Two of these four patients had reported contact to dogs prior to occurrence of symptoms.

Limitations of the Study

A number of possible limitations have to be taken into account when interpreting the results of this study. First, we did not use the standard case definition that relies mainly on MAT testing but instead defined all patients with positive POC test and clinically compatible illness as cases of leptospirosis, independent of MAT result. We believe this approach is justifiable because the POC IgM test was recently shown to be more sensitive than MAT and has comparable specificity. Nevertheless, comparisons with other studies may be difficult due to the differences in the case definitions used. Second, the study design was retrospective and did not include a control group; therefore we cannot implicate specific risk exposures as the likely source of leptospirosis infection. Also, recall regarding exposures might have been adversely affected or biased by the fact that, in many cases, the phone interviews occurred years after the illness. Lastly, the overall sample size was relatively small and this limited our ability of making statistical comparisons between subsets of cases.

Conclusions

In summary, we report a high rate of leptospirosis occurring in South-East Austria between 2004 and 2012. The vast majority of cases were autochthonously acquired. The main risk exposures for acquiring leptospirosis reported were activities in woods and wet areas as well as exposure to rodents.

Acknowledgments

We thank Maria Mueller (AGES) for her help in collecting the MAT results and Christina Strempfl, Bernadette Neuhold and Verena Posch for their support in running Leptospira point-of-care (POC) tests.

Study results were presented in part at ICAAC 2012, San Francisco (poster number 1009), at IMED 2013, Vienna (poster number 21.051) and as oral presentation at ECCMID 2013, Berlin (oral presentation number 333).

Author Contributions

Conceived and designed the experiments: MH RK HF KS. Performed the experiments: MH CW FA FS. Analyzed the data: MH JW TV IZS. Contributed reagents/materials/analysis tools: RK FA FS. Wrote the paper: MH RK KS. Critically revised the intellectual content: FA FS CW JW TV IZS HF. Approved the final version to be published: MH CW FA FS KS JW TV IZS HF RK.

References

1. Vijayachari P, Sugunan AP, Shriram AN (2008) Leptospirosis: An emerging global public health problem. J Biosci 33: 557–569.
2. Hoffmeister B, Peyerl-Hoffmann G, Pischke S, Zollner-Schwetz I, Krause R, et al. (2010) Differences in clinical manifestations of imported versus autochthonous leptospirosis in austria and germany. Am J Trop Med Hyg 83: 326–335.
3. Levett PN (2001) Leptospirosis. Clin Microbiol Rev 14: 296–326.
4. Spichler A, Athanazio D, Buzzar M, Castro B, Chapolla E, et al. (2007) Using death certificate reports to find severe leptospirosis cases, brazil. Emerg Infect Dis 13: 1559–1561.
5. Tubiana S, Mikulski M, Becam J, Lacassin F, Lefevre P, et al. (2013) Risk factors and predictors of severe leptospirosis in new caledonia. PLoS Negl Trop Dis 7: e1991.
6. Jansen A, Schoneberg I, Frank C, Alpers K, Schneider T, et al. (2005) Leptospirosis in germany, 1962–2003. Emerg Infect Dis 11: 1048–1054.
7. Radl C, Muller M, Revilla-Fernandez S, Karner-Zuser S, de Martin A, et al. (2011) Outbreak of leptospirosis among triathlon participants in langau, austria, 2010. Wien Klin Wochenschr 123: 751–755.
8. Poeppl W, Orola M, Herkner H, Muller M, Tobudic S, et al. (2013) High prevalence of antibodies against leptospira spp. in male austrian adults: A cross-sectional survey, april to june 2009. Euro Surveill 18: 20509.
9. Katz AR, Buchholz AE, Hinson K, Park SY, Effler PV (2011) Leptospirosis in hawaii, USA, 1999–2008. Emerg Infect Dis 17: 221–226.
10. Goris MG, Boer KR, Duarte TA, Kliffen SJ, Hartskeerl RA (2013) Human leptospirosis trends, the netherlands, 1925–2008. Emerg Infect Dis 19: 371–378.
11. Baranton G, Postic D (2006) Trends in leptospirosis epidemiology in france. sixty-six years of passive serological surveillance from 1920 to 2003. Int J Infect Dis 10: 162–170.
12. Forbes AE, Zochowski WJ, Dubrey SW, Sivaprakasam V (2012) Leptospirosis and weil's disease in the UK. QJM 105: 1151–1162.
13. Perra A, Servas V, Terrier G, Postic D, Baranton G, et al. (2002) Clustered cases of leptospirosis in rochefort, france, june 2001. Euro Surveill 7: 131–136.
14. Picardeau M (2013) Diagnosis and epidemiology of leptospirosis. Med Mal Infect 43: 1–9.
15. Sejvar J, Bancroft E, Winthrop K, Bettinger J, Bajani M, et al. (2003) Leptospirosis in "eco-challenge" athletes, malaysian borneo, 2000. Emerg Infect Dis 9: 702–707.
16. Lagi F, Corti G, Meli M, Pinto A, Bartoloni A. (2013) Leptospirosis acquired by tourists in venice, italy. J Travel Med 20: 128–130.
17. Limmathurotsakul D, Turner EL, Wuthiekanun V, Thaipadungpanit J, Suputtamongkol Y, et al. (2012) Fool's gold: Why imperfect reference tests are undermining the evaluation of novel diagnostics: A reevaluation of 5 diagnostic tests for leptospirosis. Clin Infect Dis 55: 322–331.
18. Goris MG, Leeflang MM, Loden M, Wagenaar JF, Klatser PR, et al. (2013) Prospective evaluation of three rapid diagnostic tests for diagnosis of human leptospirosis. PLoS Negl Trop Dis 7: e2290.
19. [Anonymous]. Jahrbuch: Klimaübersicht österreich.

Permissions

All chapters in this book were first published in PLOS ONE, by The Public Library of Science; hereby published with permission under the Creative Commons Attribution License or equivalent. Every chapter published in this book has been scrutinized by our experts. Their significance has been extensively debated. The topics covered herein carry significant findings which will fuel the growth of the discipline. They may even be implemented as practical applications or may be referred to as a beginning point for another development.

The contributors of this book come from diverse backgrounds, making this book a truly international effort. This book will bring forth new frontiers with its revolutionizing research information and detailed analysis of the nascent developments around the world.

We would like to thank all the contributing authors for lending their expertise to make the book truly unique. They have played a crucial role in the development of this book. Without their invaluable contributions this book wouldn't have been possible. They have made vital efforts to compile up to date information on the varied aspects of this subject to make this book a valuable addition to the collection of many professionals and students.

This book was conceptualized with the vision of imparting up-to-date information and advanced data in this field. To ensure the same, a matchless editorial board was set up. Every individual on the board went through rigorous rounds of assessment to prove their worth. After which they invested a large part of their time researching and compiling the most relevant data for our readers.

The editorial board has been involved in producing this book since its inception. They have spent rigorous hours researching and exploring the diverse topics which have resulted in the successful publishing of this book. They have passed on their knowledge of decades through this book. To expedite this challenging task, the publisher supported the team at every step. A small team of assistant editors was also appointed to further simplify the editing procedure and attain best results for the readers.

Apart from the editorial board, the designing team has also invested a significant amount of their time in understanding the subject and creating the most relevant covers. They scrutinized every image to scout for the most suitable representation of the subject and create an appropriate cover for the book.

The publishing team has been an ardent support to the editorial, designing and production team. Their endless efforts to recruit the best for this project, has resulted in the accomplishment of this book. They are a veteran in the field of academics and their pool of knowledge is as vast as their experience in printing. Their expertise and guidance has proved useful at every step. Their uncompromising quality standards have made this book an exceptional effort. Their encouragement from time to time has been an inspiration for everyone.

The publisher and the editorial board hope that this book will prove to be a valuable piece of knowledge for researchers, students, practitioners and scholars across the globe.

List of Contributors

Zongzhuan Shen, Chao Xue, Jian Zhang, Rong Li and Qirong Shen
National Engineering Research Center for Organic-based Fertilizers, Key Laboratory of Plant Nutrition and Fertilization in Low-Middle Reaches of the Yangtze River, Ministry of Agriculture, Jiangsu Key Lab and Engineering Center for Solid Organic Waste Utilization, Jiangsu Collaborative Innovation Center for Solid Organic Waste Resource Utilization, Nanjing Agricultural University, Nanjing, China

Yunze Ruan
Hainan key Laboratory for Sustainable Utilization of Tropical Bio-resources, College of Agriculture, Hainan University, Haikou, China

Dongsheng Wang
Nanjing Institute of Vegetable Science, Nanjing, China

Miranda M. L. van Rijen
Laboratory for Microbiology and Infection Control, Amphia Hospital, Breda, the Netherlands

Thijs Bosch and Leo Schouls
Center for Infectious Disease Control Netherlands, National Institute for Public Health and the Environment, Bilthoven, the Netherlands

Erwin J. M. Verkade
Laboratory for Microbiology and Infection Control, Amphia Hospital, Breda, the Netherlands
Laboratory for Medical Microbiology and Immunology, St. Elisabeth Hospital, Tilburg, the Netherlands

Jan A. J. W. Kluytmans
Laboratory for Microbiology and Infection Control, Amphia Hospital, Breda, the Netherlands
Department of Medical Microbiology and Infection ControlJK, VUmc Medical University, Amsterdam, the Netherlands

Fabiana Fernandes Bressan, Felipe Perecin and Flávio Vieira Meirelles
Departamento de Medicina Veterinária, Faculdade de Zootecnia e Engenharia de Alimentos, Universidade de São Paulo, Pirassununga, Sco Paulo, Brazil

Juliano Rodrigues Sangalli and Rafael Vilar Sampaio
Departamento de Medicina Veterinária, Faculdade de Zootecnia e Engenharia de Alimentos, Universidade de São Paulo, Pirassununga, Sco Paulo, Brazil

Departamento de Cirurgia, Faculdade de Medicina Veterinária e Zootecnia, Universidade de São Paulo, São Paulo, São Paulo, Brazil
Department of Biomedical Science, Ontario Veterinary College, University of Guelph, Ontario, Canada

Reno Roldi de Araújo
Departamento de Medicina Veterinária, Faculdade de Zootecnia e Engenharia de Alimentos, Universidade de São Paulo, Pirassununga, Sco Paulo, Brazil
Departamento de Cirurgia, Faculdade de Medicina Veterinária e Zootecnia, Universidade de São Paulo, São Paulo, São Paulo, Brazil

Willian Allan King
Department of Biomedical Science, Ontario Veterinary College, University of Guelph, Ontario, Canada

Marcos Roberto Chiaratti
Departamento de Cirurgia, Faculdade de Medicina Veterinária e Zootecnia, Universidade de São Paulo, São Paulo, São Paulo, Brazil
Departamento de Genética e Evolução, Centro de Ciências Biológicas e da Saúde, Universidade Federal de São Carlos, São Carlos, Brazil

Tiago Henrique Camara De Bem
Departamento de Medicina Veterinária, Faculdade de Zootecnia e Engenharia de Alimentos, Universidade de São Paulo, Pirassununga, Sco Paulo, Brazil
Departamento de Genética, Faculdade de Medicina de Ribeirão Preto, Universidade de São Paulo, Ribeirão Preto, São Paulo, Brazil

Lawrence Charles Smith
Centre de recherche em reproduction animale, Faculté de médecine vétérinaire, Université de Montréal, St. Hyacinthe, Québec, Canada

David L. Williams
Department of Veterinary Medicine, Cambridge University, Cambridge, United Kingdom

Brenda K. Mann
SentrX Animal Care, Inc., Salt Lake City, Utah, United States of America,
Department of Bioengineering, University of Utah, Salt Lake City, Utah, United States of America

Benjamin L. Hart
Department of Anatomy, Physiology and Cell Biology, School of Veterinary Medicine, University of California Davis, Davis, California, United States of America

Lynette A. Hart and Abigail P. Thigpen
Department of Population Health and Reproduction, School of Veterinary Medicine, University of California Davis, Davis, California, United States of America

Neil H. Willits
Department of Statistics, University of California Davis, Davis, California, United States of America

Elena Rossi, Giovanna Camerino and Orsetta Zuffardi
Department of Molecular Medicine, Pavia University, Pavia, Italy

Orietta Radi, Lisa De Lorenzi and Pietro Parma
Department of Agricultural and Environmental Sciences, Milan University, Milan, Italy

Annalisa Vetro
Biotechnology Research Laboratories, Fondazione IRCCS Policlinico San Matteo, Pavia, Italy

Debora Groppetti
Department of Veterinary Science and Public Health, Milan University, Milan, Italy

Enrico Bigliardi
Department of Veterinary Science, Parma University, Parma, Italy

Gaia Cecilia Luvoni
Department of Health, Animal Science and Food Safety, Milan University, Milan, Italy

Ada Rota
Department of Veterinary Science, Torino University, Torino, Italy

Kathrin Deckardt and Qendrim Zebeli
Institute of Animal Nutrition and Functional Plant Compounds, Department for Farm Animals and Veterinary Public Health, Vetmeduni Vienna, Vienna, Austria

Barbara U. Metzler-Zebeli
Institute of Animal Nutrition and Functional Plant Compounds, Department for Farm Animals and Veterinary Public Health, Vetmeduni Vienna, Vienna, Austria
University Clinic for Swine, Department for Farm Animals and Veterinary Public Health, Vetmeduni Vienna, Vienna, Austria

Margit Schollenberger and Markus Rodehutscord
Institute of Animal Nutrition, University of Hohenheim, Stuttgart, Germany

Elihu Aranday-Cortes, Philip J. Hogarth, Daryan A. Kaveh, Adam O. Whelan, Bernardo Villarreal-Ramos and H. Martin Vordermeier
TB Research Group, Animal Health & Veterinary Laboratories Agency Weybridge, New Haw, Addlestone, Surrey, United Kingdom

Ajit Lalvani
Tuberculosis Immunology Group, National Heart and Lung Institute, Imperial College London, London, United Kingdom

Kevin L. Anderson, Maria T. Correa and Roberta Lyman
Department of Population Health and Pathobiology (PHP), North Carolina State University (NCSU) College of Veterinary Medicine, Raleigh, North Carolina, United States of America

Jorge Pinto Ferreira
Department of Population Health and Pathobiology (PHP), North Carolina State University (NCSU) College of Veterinary Medicine, Raleigh, North Carolina, United States of America
Department of Infectious Diseases, Duke University School of Medicine, Durham, North Carolina, United States of America

Felicia Ruffin, L. Barth Reller and Vance G. Fowler Jr.
Department of Infectious Diseases, Duke University School of Medicine, Durham, North Carolina, United States of America

Jie Zeng, Chuanbao Zhang, Haijian Zhao and Wenxiang Chen
Beijing Hospital and National Center for Clinical Laboratories, Ministry of Health, Beijing, China

Mo Wang, Shunli Zhang and Fei Cheng
Beijing Hospital and National Center for Clinical Laboratories, Ministry of Health, Beijing, China
Chinese Academy of Medical Sciences and Peking Union Medical College, Beijing, China

Yilong Li
Department of Laboratory Medicine, Beijing Hospital, Ministry of Health, Beijing, China

Songlin Yu
Department of Laboratory Medicine, Peking Union Medical College Hospital, Beijing, China

Gabriela Galateanu, Thomas Bernd Hildebrandt, Robert Hermes, Joseph Saragusty and Frank Göritz
Department of Reproduction Management, Leibniz Institute for Zoo and Wildlife Research, Berlin, Germany

Romain Potier and Baptiste Mulot
ZooParc de Beauval, Saint-Aignan, France

Alexis Maillot
Parc zoologique d'Amnéville, Amnéville-les-Thermes, France

Pascal Etienne
Parc zoologique de La Barben (Pélissane), La Barben, France

Rui Bernardino and Teresa Fernandes
Hospital Veterinário, Jardim Zoológico de Lisboa, Lisbon, Portugal

Jurgen Mews
Clinical Application Research Center, Toshiba Medical Systems Europe, Zoetermeer, The Netherlands

Marieke J. A. de Regt, Willem van Schaik, Miranda van Luit-Asbroek, Huberta A. T. Dekker, Marc J. M. Bonten and Rob J. L. Willems
Department of Medical Microbiology, University Medical Center Utrecht, Utrecht, the Netherlands

Engeline van Duijkeren
Department of Infectious Diseases and Immunology, Faculty of Veterinary Medicine, Utrecht University, Utrecht, the Netherlands

Catherina J. M. Koning
Department of Internal Medicine, University Hospital Maastricht, Maastricht, the Netherlands

Brian C. W. Kot, Michael T. C. Ying and Fiona M. Brook
Department of Health Technology and Informatics, The Hong Kong Polytechnic University, Hung Hom, Hong Kong SAR, China

Laura M. Laarhoven, Phebe de Heus, Jeanine van Luijn and Birgitta Duim
Department of Infectious Diseases and Immunology, Faculty of Veterinary Medicine, Utrecht University, Utrecht, The Netherlands

Jaap A. Wagenaar
Department of Infectious Diseases and Immunology, Faculty of Veterinary Medicine, Utrecht University, Utrecht, The Netherlands
Central Veterinary Institute of Wageningen UR, Lelystad, The Netherlands

Engeline van Duijkeren
Department of Infectious Diseases and Immunology, Faculty of Veterinary Medicine, Utrecht University, Utrecht, The Netherlands

Laboratory for Zoonoses and Environmental Microbiology, National Institute of Public Health and the Environment, Bilthoven, The Netherlands

Myrna M. T. de Rooij, Dick Heederik and Inge M. Wouters
Division of Environmental Epidemiology, Institute for Risk Assessment Sciences, Utrecht, the Netherlands

Wim van der Hoek and Barbara Schimmer
Centre for Infectious Disease Control, National Institute for Public Health and the Environment, Bilthoven, the Netherlands

Bart Versteeg
Centre for Infectious Disease Control, National Institute for Public Health and the Environment, Bilthoven, the Netherlands
Department of Medical Microbiology and Infection Control, Jeroen Bosch Hospital, 's-Hertogenbosch, the Netherlands

Peter Schneeberger
Department of Medical Microbiology and Infection Control, Jeroen Bosch Hospital, 's-Hertogenbosch, the Netherlands

Boyd R. Berends
Division of Veterinary Public Health, Institute for Risk Assessment Sciences, Utrecht, the Netherlands

Neeraj Suthar
Paul G. Allen School for Global Animal Health, College of Veterinary Medicine, Washington State University, Pullman, Washington, United States of America

Sandip Roy
Paul G. Allen School for Global Animal Health, College of Veterinary Medicine, Washington State University, Pullman, Washington, United States of America
School of Electrical Engineering and Computer Science, College of Veterinary Medicine, Washington State University, Pullman, Washington, United States of America

Douglas R. Call and Thomas E. Besser
Paul G. Allen School for Global Animal Health, College of Veterinary Medicine, Washington State University, Pullman, Washington, United States of America
Dept. of Veterinary Microbiology and Pathology, College of Veterinary Medicine, Washington State University, Pullman, Washington, United States of America

Margaret A. Davis
Paul G. Allen School for Global Animal Health, College of Veterinary Medicine, Washington State University, Pullman, Washington, United States of America

Dept. of Veterinary Clinical Sciences, College of Veterinary Medicine, Washington State University, Pullman, Washington, United States of America

Michelle R. Goulart and G. Elizabeth Pluhar
Department of Veterinary Clinical Sciences, University of Minnesota, Saint Paul, Minnesota, United States of America

John R. Ohlfest
Department of Pediatrics, University of Minnesota, Minneapolis, Minnesota, United States of America
Department of Neurosurgery, University of Minnesota, Minneapolis, Minnesota, United States of America

Victoriya V. Volkova, Zhao Lu and YrjöTapio Gröhn
Department of Population Medicine and Diagnostic Sciences, College of Veterinary Medicine, Cornell University, Ithaca, New York, United States of America,

Cristina Lanzas
Department of Biomedical and Diagnostic Sciences, College of Veterinary Medicine, The University of Tennessee, Knoxville, Tennessee, United States of America

Zakaria Bengaly and Augustin Z. Bancé
Centre International de Recherche-Développement sur l'Elevage en Zone subhumide (CIRDES), Bobo-Dioulasso, Burkina Faso

Issa Sidibé
Centre International de Recherche-Développement sur l'Elevage en Zone subhumide (CIRDES), Bobo-Dioulasso, Burkina Faso
Pan-African Tsetse and Trypanosomosis Eradication Campaign (PATTEC), Projet de Création de Zones Libérées Durablement de Tsé-tséet de Trypanosomoses (PCZLD), Bobo-Dioulasso, Burkina Faso

Adama Sow
Centre International de Recherche-Développement sur l'Elevage en Zone subhumide (CIRDES), Bobo-Dioulasso, Burkina Faso
Pan-African Tsetse and Trypanosomosis Eradication Campaign (PATTEC), Projet de Création de Zones Libérées Durablement de Tsé-tséet de Trypanosomoses (PCZLD), Bobo-Dioulasso, Burkina Faso
Ecole Inter-Etats des Sciences et Médecine Vétérinaires (EISMV), Dakar-Fann, Sénégal

Philippe Solano
Centre International de Recherche-Développement sur l'Elevage en Zone subhumide (CIRDES), Bobo-Dioulasso, Burkina Faso

Institut de Recherche pour le Développement (IRD), UMR 177 IRD-CIRAD INTERTRYP, Montpellier, France

Germain J. Sawadogo
Ecole Inter-Etats des Sciences et Médecine Vétérinaires (EISMV), Dakar-Fann, Sénégal

Marc J. B. Vreysen
Insect Pest Control Laboratory, Joint FAO/IAEA Programme of Nuclear Techniques in Food and Agriculture, Vienna, Austria

Renaud Lancelot
Institut Sénégalais de Recherches Agricoles, Laboratoire National d'Elevage et de Recherches Vétérinaires, Hann, Dakar, Sénégal

Jeremy Bouyer
Institut Sénégalais de Recherches Agricoles, Laboratoire National d'Elevage et de Recherches Vétérinaires, Hann, Dakar, Sénégal
UMR Contrôles des Maladies Animales et Emergentes, Centre de Coopération Internationale en Recherche Agronomique pour le Développement (CIRAD), Campus International de Baillarguet, Montpellier, France

Ute Philipp and Ottmar Distl
Institute for Animal Breeding and Genetics, University of Veterinary Medicine Hannover, Hannover, Germany

Andrea Vollmar
Veterinary Clinic for Small Animals, Wissen, Germany

Jens Häggström
Department of Clinical Sciences, Faculty of Veterinary Medicine and Animal Science, Swedish University of Agricultural Sciences, Uppsala, Sweden

Anne Thomas
ANTAGENE, Animal Genetics Laboratory, Limonest, France

Meghan F. Davis and Ellen K. Silbergeld
Department of Environmental Health Sciences, Johns Hopkins Bloomberg School of Public Health, Baltimore, Maryland, United States of America

Kenrad Nelson and Amy E. Peterson
Department of Epidemiology, Johns Hopkins Bloomberg School of Public Health, Baltimore, Maryland, United States of America

Cynthia J. Whitener, Kathleen G. Julian and Wallace H. Greene
Penn State Hershey Medical Center, Hershey, Pennsylvania, United States of America

222

Lance B. Price
Division of Pathogen Genomics, The Translational Genomics Research Institute (TGen North), Phoenix, Arizona, United States of America

René Van den Brom and Piet Vellema
Department of Small Ruminant Health, Animal Health Service, Deventer, The Netherlands,

Barbara Schimmer and Wim van der Hoek
Centre for Infectious Disease Control, National Institute for Public Health and the Environment, Bilthoven, The Netherlands

Peter M. Schneeberger
Department of Medical Microbiology and Infection Control, Jeroen Bosch Hospital, 's-Hertogenbosch, The Netherlands

Wim A. Swart
Department of Diagnostics, Research and Epidemiology, Animal Health Service, Deventer, The Netherlands

Timothy S. Frana, Aleigh R. Beahm, Joann M. Kinyon, Lori L. Layman, Locke A. Karriker and Alejandro Ramirez
Department of Veterinary Diagnostic and Production Animal Medicine, College of Veterinary Medicine, Iowa State University, Ames, Iowa, United States of America

Blake M. Hanson and Tara C. Smith
University of Iowa, Center for Emerging Infectious Diseases, Department of Epidemiology, College of Public Health, Iowa City, Iowa, United States of America

Ching-Hui Tsai, Ming-Wei Su and Nai-Wei Kuo
Institute of Epidemiology and Preventive Medicine, College of Public Health, National Taiwan University, Taipei, Taiwan

Yungling Leo Lee and Kuan-Yen Tung
Institute of Epidemiology and Preventive Medicine, College of Public Health, National Taiwan University, Taipei, Taiwan
Research Center for Genes, Environment and Human Health, College of Public Health, National Taiwan University, Taipei, Taiwan

Bor-Luen Chiang
Department of Pediatrics, National Taiwan University Hospital, Taipei, Taiwan

Fook Tim Chew
Department of Biological Sciences, National University of Singapore, Singapore

Carina Wallner, Katharina Seeber, Jasmin Wagner, Thomas Valentin, Ines Zollner-Schwetz and Robert Krause
Section of Infectious Diseases and Tropical Medicine, Department of Medicine, Medical University of Graz, Graz, Austria

Holger Flick
Division of Pulmonology, Department of Medicine, Medical University of Graz, Graz, Austria

Martin Hoenigl
Section of Infectious Diseases and Tropical Medicine, Department of Medicine, Medical University of Graz, Graz, Austria
Division of Pulmonology, Department of Medicine, Medical University of Graz, Graz, Austria

Franz Allerberger and Friedrich Schmoll
Austrian Agency for Health and Food Safety (AGES), Vienna, Austria

Index